Clinical Pain Management

Clinical Pain Management: A Practical Guide

Second Edition

EDITED BY

Mary E. Lynch, MD, FRCPC
Founder (Pain Medicine)
Professor
Department of Anesthesia, Pain Management and Perioperative Medicine
Department of Psychiatry
Department of Pharmacology
Dalhousie University
Halifax, Nova Scotia, Canada

Kenneth D. Craig, OC, PhD, FCAHS
Professor Emeritus
Department of Psychology
University of British Columbia
Vancouver, Canada

Philip W. Peng, MBBS, FRCPC
Founder (Pain Medicine)
Professor
Department of Anesthesiology and Pain Medicine
University Health Network and Sinai Health System
University of Toronto
Toronto, Canada

WILEY Blackwell

This second edition first published 2022

Edition History
John Wiley & Sons Ltd (1e, 2011)

Registered Offices
John Wiley & Sons, Inc., 111 River Street, Hoboken, NJ 07030, USA
John Wiley & Sons Ltd, The Atrium, Southern Gate, Chichester, West Sussex, PO19 8SQ, UK

Editorial Office
9600 Garsington Road, Oxford, OX4 2DQ, UK

For details of our global editorial offices, customer services, and more information about Wiley products visit us at www.wiley.com.

Wiley also publishes its books in a variety of electronic formats and by print-on-demand. Some content that appears in standard print versions of this book may not be available in other formats.

Library of Congress Cataloging-in-Publication Data

Names: Lynch, Mary E., editor. | Craig, Kenneth D., 1937– editor. | Peng, Philip W. H., editor.
Title: Clinical pain management : a practical guide / edited by Mary E. Lynch, Kenneth D. Craig, Philip W. Peng.
Other titles: Clinical pain management (Lynch)
Description: Second edition. | Hoboken, NJ : Wiley-Blackwell, 2022. | Includes bibliographical references and index.
Identifiers: LCCN 2021048524 (print) | LCCN 2021048525 (ebook) | ISBN 9781119701156 (paperback) | ISBN 9781119701187 (adobe pdf) | ISBN 9781119701163 (epub)
Subjects: MESH: Pain Management | Chronic Pain–therapy | Palliative Care–methods
Classification: LCC RB127.5.C48 (print) | LCC RB127.5.C48 (ebook) | NLM WL 704.6 | DDC 616/.0472–dc23/eng/20211015
LC record available at https://lccn.loc.gov/2021048524
LC ebook record available at https://lccn.loc.gov/2021048525

Cover Design: Wiley
Cover Image: © Dan Robitaille: Living with chronic pain has shaped my perception in many ways; positive, negative. Art is something that's allowed me to translate that perception, and use it to create perspective rather than distance.

Set in 8/12pt ITCStoneSerifStd by Straive, Pondicherry, India

SKY058859AA-E7E3-47F3-BD3F-19DCCADA430C_031122

This book is dedicated to our patients, their families and all people suffering with pain.

Contents

List of Contributors

Oli Abate Fulas MD PhD, Department of Anesthesia and Alan Edwards Centre for Research on Pain, McGill University, Montréal, Québec, Canada

Caroline Arbour PhD RN, Associate Professor, Center for Advanced Research in Sleep Medicine & Trauma Unit, Research Center, Centre Integre Sante et Services Sociaux du Nord Ile de Montreal (CIUSSS du NIM), Montréal, Québec, Canada; Faculty of Nursing, Université de Montréal, Québec, Canada

Lene Baad-Hansen DDS PhD, Professor, Section for Orofacial Pain and Jaw Function, Aarhus University, Aarhus, Denmark; Scandinavian Center for Orofacial Neurosciences (SCON), Aarhus University, Aarhus, Denmark

Misha Bačkonja MD, Department of Anaesthesiology and Pain Medicine, University of Washington Medical School, Seattle, Washington, USA

Louis de Beaumont PhD Center for Advanced Research in Sleep Medicine & Trauma Unit, Research Center, Centre Integre Sante et Services Sociaux du Nord Ile de Montreal (CIUSSS du NIM), Montréal, Québec, Canada; Faculty of Medicine, Université de Montréal, Québec, Canada

Inna Belfer MD, PhD, National Center for Complementary and Integrative Health (NCCIH), National Institutes of Health (NIH), Bethesda, Maryland, USA

Fabrizio Benedetti MD, Professor of Physiology and Neuroscience, University of Turin Medical School, Neuroscience Department, Turin, Italy; Medicine and Physiology of Hypoxia, Plateau Rosà, Switzerland

Klaus Bielefeldt MD PhD, George E. Wahlen Veterans Administration (VA) Medical Center, Salt Lake City, Utah, USA; Department of Medicine, University of Utah, Salt Lake City, Utah, USA

Kathryn A. Birnie PhD, Postdoctoral Fellow, Department of Anesthesiology, Perioperative, and Pain Medicine, University of Calgary, Calgary, Canada; Alberta Children's Hospital Research Institute, Calgary, Alberta, Canada

Laura Bockus-Thorne RD, BSN, Research Assistant, Department of Applied Human Nutrition, Mount Saint Vincent University, Halifax, Nova Scotia, Canada

Eduardo Bruera MD, Professor and Chair, Department of Palliative Care and Rehabilitation Medicine Unit 1414, University of Texas M.D. Anderson Cancer Center, Houston, Texas, USA

Kim J. Burchiel MD FACS, Professor and Chair, Department of Neurological Surgery, Oregon Health and Science University, Portland, USA

Chantel C. Burkitt PhD, Gillette Children's Specialty Healthcare, St. Paul, Minnesota, USA; Special Education Program, Department of Educational Psychology, University of Minnesota, Minneapolis, Minnesota, USA

Michael Butterfield MSc, MD, FRCPC (Psychiatry and Pain Medicine) Department of Psychiatry, Faculty of Medicine, University of British Columbia, Vancouver, British Columbia, Canada

Malin Carmland Danish Pain Research Center, Aarhus University, Aarhus, Denmark; Department of Neurology, Aarhus University Hospital, Aarhus, Denmark

Eugene J. Carragee MD, Professor and Vice Chairman, Department of Orthopedic Surgery, Stanford University School of Medicine, Redwood City, California, USA

James Chue MD, Fellow in Pain Medicine, Department of Anesthesiology, The Jacobs School of Medicine at the University of Buffalo, Buffalo, New York, USA

Terence J. Coderre PhD, Professor, Department of Anesthesia and Alan Edwards Centre for Research on Pain, McGill University, Montréal, Québec, Canada

Kenneth D. Craig OC, PhD, FCAHS, Department of Psychology, University of British Columbia, Vancouver, Canada

Melissa A. Day PhD, Associate Professor, School of Psychology, The University of Queensland, Brisbane, Australia; Affiliate Associate Professor, Department of Rehabilitation Medicine, University of Washington, Seattle, Washington, USA

Oscar A. de Leon-Casasola MD, Professor of Anesthesiology and Medicine, Senior Vice-Chair, Department of Anesthesiology, The Jacobs School of Medicine at the University at Buffalo, Buffalo, New York, USA; Chief, Division of Pain Medicine, Roswell Park Comprehensive Cancer Institute, Buffalo, New York, USA

Anthony H. Dickenson PhD FmedSci, Professor of Neuropharmacology, Department of Neuroscience, Physiology and Pharmacology, Division of Biosciences, University College, London, United Kingdom

Fernando Exposto DDS PhD, Assistant Professor, Section for Orofacial Pain and Jaw Function, Aarhus University, Aarhus, Denmark; Scandinavian Center for Orofacial Neurosciences (SCON), Aarhus University, Aarhus, Denmark

Cibele Dal Fabbro PhD, Center for Advanced Research in Sleep Medicine & Trauma Unit, Research Center, Centre Integre Sante et Services Sociaux du Nord Ile de Montreal (CIUSSS du NIM), Montréal, Québec, Canada

Timothy R. Deer MD, President and CEO, The Spine and Nerve Center of the Virginias, Charleston, West, Virginia, USA

Nanna Brix Finnerup MD PhD, Associate Professor, Danish Pain Research Center, Aarhus University, Aarhus, Denmark; Department of Neurology, Aarhus University Hospital, Aarhus, Denmark

Mary-Ann Fitzcharles MB ChB FRCP(C), Division of Rheumatology, McGill University Health Centre, Montréal, Québec, Canada; Alan Edwards Pain Management Unit, McGill University Health Center, Montréal, Québec, Canada

Elisa Frisaldi PhD, Postdoctoral Fellow, University of Turin Medical School, Neuroscience Department, Turin, Italy

Andrea D. Furlan MD PhD, Associate Professor, KITE, Toronto Rehabilitation Institute, University Health Network, Toronto, Ontario, Canada; Division of Physical Medicine & Rehabilitation, Department of Medicine, Faculty of Medicine, University of Toronto, Toronto, Ontario, Canada; Institute for Work & Health, Toronto, Ontario, Canada

Gerald F. Gebhart PhD, Professor Emeritus, Carver College of Medicine, University of Iowa, Iowa City, USA

Ian Gilron PMD MSc FRCPC, Professor, Departments of Anesthesiology & Perioperative Medicine and Biomedical & Molecular Sciences, Queen's University, Kingston, Ontario, Canada

Andrea Glenn PhD candidate, Department of Nutritional Sciences, University of Toronto, Toronto, Ontario, Canada

Douglas L. Gourlay MD, MSC, FRCPC, FASAM, Educational Consultant, Hamilton, Ontario, Canada

Shannan Grant PDt MSc PhD, Assistant Professor, Department of Applied Human Nutrition, Mount Saint Vincent Hospital, Halifax, Nova Scotia, Canada; Departments of Pediatrics and Obstetrics and Gynaecology, IWK Health Centre, Halifax, Nova Scotia, Canada

Katharine N. Gurba MD PhD, Assistant Professor Washington University Pain Center and Department of Anesthesiology, Washington University School of Medicine, St. Louis, Missouri, USA

Thomas Hadjistavropoulos PhD ABPP, Professor, Department of Psychology and Center on Aging and Health, University of Regina, Regina, Saskatchewan, Canada

Jonathan M. Hagedorn MD, Assistant Professor of Anesthesiology, Department of Anesthesiology and Perioperative Medicine, Division of Pain Medicine, Mayo Clinic, Rochester, Minnesota, USA

Simon Haroutounian PhD MSc Pharm, Chief of Division of Clinical and Translational Research, Chief of Clinical Pain Research, Associate Professor Washington University Pain Center and Department of Anesthesiology, Washington University School of Medicine, St. Louis, USA

Winfried Häuser MD, Associate Professor, Department Internal Medicine I and Interdisciplinary Center of Pain Medicine, Klinikum Saarbrücken, Germany; Department of Psychosomatic Medicine and Psychotherapy, Technische Universität München, Germany

Howard A. Heit MD, FACP, FASAM, Private Practice, Reston, Virginia, USA

Alberto Herrero Babiloni DDS, Center for Advanced Research in Sleep Medicine & Trauma Unit, Research Center, Centre Integre Sante et Services Sociaux du Nord Ile de Montreal (CIUSSS du NIM), Montréal, Québec, Canada; Division of Experimental Medicine, McGill University, Montréal, Québec, Canada

Marshall T. Holland MD, Assistant Professor, Department of Neurosurgery, Heersink School of Medicine, The University of Alabama at Birmingham, Birmingham, AL

Petra Hroch Tiessen MD, Department of Anesthesiology and Pain Medicine, University of Toronto, Toronto, Ontario, Canada

Robert N. Jamison PhD, Associate Professor, Departments of Anesthesia and Psychiatry, Brigham and Women's Hospital, Harvard Medical School, Chestnut Hill, Massachusetts, USA

David Jenkins MD PhD DSc, Professor, Associate Professor, Department of Nutritional Sciences, University of Toronto, Toronto, Ontario, Canada

Troels Staehelin Jensen MD PhD, Professor, Danish Pain Research Center, Aarhus University, Aarhus, Denmark; Department of Neurology, Aarhus University Hospital, Aarhus, Denmark

Joel Katz PhD, Department of Psychology, York University, Toronto, Canada; Department of Anesthesia and Pain Management, Toronto General Hospital, Toronto, Canada; Department of Anesthesia, University of Toronto, Toronto, Canada

Meaghan Kavanagh PhD candidate, Department of Nutritional Sciences, University of Toronto, Toronto, Ontario, Canada

Beatrice P. de Koninck Center for Advanced Research in Sleep Medicine & Trauma Unit, Research Center, Centre Integre Sante et Services Sociaux du Nord Ile de Montreal (CIUSSS du NIM), Montréal, Québec, Canada

Jacqueline Tu Anh Thu Lam, Consultant, Center for Advanced Research in Sleep Medicine & Trauma Unit, Research Center, Centre Integre Sante et Services Sociaux du Nord Ile de Montreal (CIUSSS du NIM), Montréal, Québec, Canada; Faculty of Medicine, Université de Montréal, Québec, Canada

Helene Langevin MD, National Center for Complementary and Integrative Health (NCCIH), National Institutes of Health (NIH), Bethesda, Maryland, USA

Gilles J. Lavigne DMD FRCD PhD, Professor and Dean, Faculty of Dental Medicine, Université de Montréal, Québec, Canada; Center for Advanced Research in Sleep Medicine & Trauma Unit, Research Center, Centre Integre Sante et Services Sociaux du Nord Ile de Montreal (CIUSSS du NIM), Montréal, Québec, Canada

Mary E. Lynch , MD, FRCPC, Founder (Pain Medicine) Department of Anesthesia, Pain Management and Perioperative Medicine, Department of Psychiatry, Department of Pharmacology, Dalhousie University, Halifax, Nova Scotia, Canada

Una E. Makris MD, Associate Professor, University of Texas Southwestern Medical Center, Dallas, Texas, USA

Marc O. Martel Assistant Professor, Division of Experimental Medicine, McGill University, Montréal, Québec, Canada; Faculty of Dentistry & Department of Anesthesia, McGill University, Montréal, Québec, Canada

Anjali Martinez MD, Assistant Professor, Obstetrics and Gynecology, George Washington University, Washington, DC, USA

Benjamin Matson MD, Assistant Professor , Department of Anesthesiology, The Jacobs School of Medicine at the University of Buffalo, Buffalo, New York, USA; Division of Pain Medicine, Roswell Park Comprehensive Cancer Institute, Buffalo, New York

Michael McGillion RN PhD, Assistant Professor, School of Nursing, McMaster University, Hamilton, Ontario, Canada

Lauren McNeill RD MPH, Tasting to Thrive, Toronto, Ontario, Canada

Vesanto Melina RD MS, Nutrispeak, Vancouver, British Columbia, Canada

Ronald Melzack Professor Emeritus, Department of Psychology, McGill University, Montréal, Québec, Canada

Alyssa Merbler MA, Department of Educational Psychology, University of Minnesota, Minneapolis, Minnesota, USA

Sarah E.E. Mills PhD, Academic Clinical Fellow, University of Dundee, Scotland, UK

Amir Minerbi MD PhD, Institute for Pain Medicine, Rambam Health Campus, Haifa, Israel

Laura Murphy PharmD, Assistant Professor, KITE, Toronto Rehabilitation Institute, University Health Network, Toronto, Ontario, Canada; Department of Pharmacy, University Health Network, Toronto, Ontario, Canada; Leslie Dan Faculty of Pharmacy, University of Toronto, Toronto, Ontario, Canada

Abagail Raiter BA, Gillette Children's Specialty Healthcare, Saint Paul, Minnesota, USA

Tim F. Oberlander MD FRCPC, Professor, Department of Pediatrics, School of Population and Public Health, Faculty of Medicine, University of British Columbia, University of British Columbia, Vancouver, British Columbia, Canada; Complex Pain Service, British Columbia Children's Hospital, Vancouver, British Columbia, Canada

M. Gabrielle Pagé PhD, Principal Scientist, Centre de recherche du Centre hospitalier de l'Université de Montréal (CRCHUM), Montréal, Canada; Département d'anesthésiologie et de medicine de la douleur, Faculté de médecine, et Département de Psychologie, Faculté des arts et des sciences, Université de Montréal, Montréal, Canada

Tonya M. Palermo PhD, Associate Professor, Department of Anesthesiology and Pain Medicine, Pediatrics and Psychiatry, University of Washington School of Medicine, Seattle Children's Hospital and Research Institute, Seattle, Washington, USA

Catherine Paré BA, Department of Psychology, McGill University, Montréal, Québec, Canada

Kushang V. Patel PhD, MPH, Research Associate Professor, Department of Anesthesiology and Pain Medicine, University of Washington, Seattle, USA

Philip W. Peng MBBS, FRCPC, Founder (Pain Medicine) Professor, Department of Anesthesiology and Pain Medicine, University Health Network and Sinai Health System, University of Toronto, Toronto, Canada

Tali Sahar Pain Relief Unit, Department of Anesthesia, Hadassah Medical Center, Jerusalem, Israel; Department of Family Medicine, Hebrew University of Jerusaleum, Jerusalem, Israel

Barry J. Sessle Professor, Faculties of Dentistry and Medicine, University of Toronto, Toronto, Ontario, Canada

Aziz Shaibani MD, Clinical Professor, Nerve and Muscle Center of Texas, Baylor College of Medicine, Houston, Texas, USA

Christine Short MD FRCPC, Associate Professor, Dalhousie University, Department of Medicine, Division of Physical Medicine and Rehabilitation; Department of Surgery, Division of Neurosurgery, Queen Elizabeth II Health Sciences Centre, Halifax, Nova Scotia, Canada

Stephen D. Silberstein MD, Jefferson Headache Center, Thomas Jefferson University, Philadelphia, Pennsylvania, United States

Andrew J. Smith MDCM, Interprofessional Pain and Addiction Recovery Clinic, Centre for Addiction and Mental Health, Toronto Academic Pain Medicine Institute, Toronto, Ontario, Canada

Blair H. Smith MD MEd FRCGP FRCP Edin, Clinical Professor, University of Dundee, Scotland, UK

Pam Squire MD CCFP CPE, Assistant Clinical Professor, University of British Columbia, Vancouver, British Columbia, Canada

Michael Stanton-Hicks MBBS DrMed FRCA ABPM FIPP, Pain Management Department, Centre for Neurological Restoration; Children's Hospital CCF Shaker Pediatric Pain Rehabilitation Program, Cleveland Clinic, Cleveland, Ohio, USA

Jennifer N. Stinson RN-EC PhD CPNP, Scientist, Child Health Evaluation Sciences, The Hospital for Sick Children, Toronto, Ontario, Canada; Department of Anesthesia and Pain Medicine, The Hospital for Sick Children, Toronto, Ontario, Canada; Lawrence S. Bloomberg, Faculty of Nursing, University of Toronto, Ontario, Canada

Agnes Stogicza MD FIPP CIPS, Department of Anesthesiology and Pain Medicine, Saint Magdolna Private Hospital, Budapest, Hungary

Michael J.L. Sullivan PhD, Professor, Department of Psychology, McGill University, Montréal, Québec, Canada

Peter Svensson Professor and Chairman, Section for Orofacial Pain and Jaw Function, Aarhus University, Aarhus, Denmark; Scandinavian Center for Orofacial Neurosciences (SCON), Aarhus University, Aarhus, Denmark; Faculty of Odontology, Malmø University, Malmø, Sweden

Frank J. Symons PhD, Distinguished McKnight University Professor, Special Education Program, Department of Educational Psychology, Center for Neurobehavioral Development, University of Minnesota, Minneapolis, Minnesota, USA

David M. Walton PhD, Assistant Professor, School of Physical Therapy, Western University, London, Ontario, Canada

Beverly E. Thorn PhD, Professor Emerita, Department of Psychology, The University of Alabama, Tuscaloosa, Alabama, USA

Rolf-Detlef Treede MD, Medical Faculty Mannheim, University of Heidelberg, Mannheim, Germany

Dennis C. Turk PhD, Department of Anesthesiology & Pain Medicine, University of Washington, Seattle, USA

Vishal P. Varshney MD FRCPC (Anesthesiology) FRCPC (Pain Medicine), Department of Anesthesia, Providence Healthcare, Vancouver, British Columbia, Canada; Department of Anesthesiology, Pharmacology and Therapeutics, Faculty of Medicine, University of British Columbia, Vancouver, British Columbia, Canada

Judith Versloot PhD, Institute for Health Policy, Management and Evaluation, University of Toronto, Toronto, Canada

Ashwin Viswanathan MD, Professor, Department of Neurosurgery, Baylor College of Medicine, Houston, Texas, USA

Aliza Weinrib PhD, Clinical Psychologist, Department of Anesthesia and Pain Management, Toronto General Hospital, Toronto, Canada

Timothy H. Wideman PhD, Associate Professor, School of Physical and Occupational Therapy, McGill University, Montréal, Canada

Sandra M. LeFort Faculty of Nursing, Memorial University of Newfoundland, St. John's, Newfoundland and Labrador, Canada

Karen Webber Faculty of Nursing, Memorial University of Newfoundland, St. John's, Newfoundland and Labrador, Canada

Chitra Lalloo Child Health Evaluation Sciences, The Hospital for Sick Children, Toronto, Ontario, Canada

Wen Chen National Center for Complementary and Integrative Health (NCCIH), National Institutes of Health (NIH), Bethesda, Maryland, USA

Emmeline Edwards National Center for Complementary and Integrative Health (NCCIH), National Institutes of Health (NIH), Bethesda, Maryland, USA

David Shurtleff National Center for Complementary and Integrative Health (NCCIH), National Institutes of Health (NIH), Bethesda, Maryland, USA

Maija Haanpää Department of Neurosurgery, Helsinki University Hospital, Helsinki, Finland

Amy Swan Department of Palliative Care and Rehabilitation Medicine Unit 1414, University of Texas M.D. Anderson Cancer Center, Houston, Texas, USA

See Wan Tham Department of Anesthesiology and Pain Medicine, University of Washington School of Medicine, Seattle Children's Hospital and Research Institute, Seattle, Washington, USA

Jeffery L. Koh Department of Anesthesiology and Peri-Operative Medicine, Oregon Health and Science University, Portland, Oregon, USA

Muhammad Saad Yousuf, Center for Advanced Pain Studies, School of Behavioral and Brain Sciences, University of Texas at Dallas, Dallas, Texas, USA

Allan I. Basbaum, Department of Anatomy, University of California at San Francisco. San Francisco, California, USA

Theodore J. Price, Center for Advanced Pain Studies, School of Behavioral and Brain Sciences, University of Texas at Dallas, Dallas, Texas, USA

Hance Clarke, Department of Anesthesia and Pain Management, Toronto General Hospital, Toronto, Canada; Department of Anesthesia and Pain Medicine, University of Toronto, Toronto, Canada

Foreword to First Edition

This excellent guide to clinical pain management covers every important facet of the field of pain. It describes recent advances in diagnosing and managing clinical pain states and presents procedures and strategies to combat a wide range of chronic pains. Unfortunately, many people suffer various forms of pain even though we have the knowledge to help them, but our educational systems have failed. This book is a valuable contribution to the field of pain by providing up - to - date knowledge that will stimulate a new generation of health professionals who are dedicated to abolishing pain.

Despite the impressive advances and optimistic outlook, many chronic pains remain intractable. Some people who suffer chronic headaches, backaches, fibromyalgia, pelvic pain and other forms of chronic pain are helped by several therapies that are now available, but most are not. For example, we have excellent new drugs for some kinds of neuropathic pains, but not for all. The continued suffering by millions of people indicates we still have a long way to go.

The field of pain has recently undergone a major revolution. Historically, pain has been simply a sensation produced by injury or disease. We now possess a much broader concept of pain that includes the emotional, cognitive and sensory dimensions of pain experience, as well as an impressive array of new approaches to pain management. Chronic pain is now a major challenge to medicine, psychology, and all the other health sciences and professions. Every aspect of life, from birth to dying, has characteristic pain problems. Genetics, until recently, was rarely considered relevant to understanding pain, yet sophisticated laboratory studies and clinical observations have established genetic predispositions related to pain as an essential component of the field. The study of pain therefore now incorporates research in epidemiology and medical genetics.

Clinical Pain Management: A Practical Guide highlights a mission for all of us: to provide relief of all pain, pain in children and the elderly, and for any kind of severe pain that can be helped by sensible administration of drugs and other pain therapies. We must also teach patients to communicate about their pain, and inform them that they have a right to freedom from pain. If we can pursue these goals together –as members of the full range of scientific and health professions –we can hope to meet the goal we all strive for: to help our fellow human beings who suffer pain.

Ronald Melzack
McGill University Montréal
Québec, Canada
2010

The editors would like to thank Ms. Sara Whynot for considerable assistance with every phase of the manuscript.

Foreword to Second Edition

In his Foreward to the first edition of this book, *Clinical Pain Management: A Practical Guide*, Ron Melzack emphasized that pain has many dimensions and that, despite advances in pain management and understanding, chronic pain in particular continues to be a major health concern. This, unfortunately, is still the case and many challenging problems still exist in managing and understanding chronic pain.

The Introductory chapter of this second edition of the book by its three editors, Drs. Lynch, Craig and Peng, draws attention to the challenges that exist for people living with chronic pain conditions, for the clinician trying to provide effective management of the patient's pain, for the scientist seeking to unravel the mechanisms underlying pain, and for society as a whole. These challenges stem from the complexity and multidimensional nature of chronic pain, the limited understanding of the processes underlying most chronic pain conditions, and the variety of diagnostic and therapeutic approaches advocated for pain management, some of which have little to no solid evidence base to support their use. Furthermore, chronic pain is in epidemic proportions in most countries, with a prevalence of around 20% or even higher, and the problem is compounded by problems with access to care and socioeconomic factors. Additionally, like many other chronic health disorders or diseases, the majority of chronic pain conditions are most common in the elderly. Therefore, unless effective steps are taken soon to address this crisis, their prevalence and associated problems will continue to grow over the coming decades because demographic predictions indicate that the elderly will comprise a growing proportion of the population in most countries.

Chronic pain can indeed be considered a "silent" epidemic because most people, including policymakers, have been unaware of this crisis and its ramifications. As a consequence, chronic pain has remained neglected to a large extent, despite clinical and scientific publications and pain-related societies and organizations pointing out its prevalence, the continuing difficulties and inequities with access to timely and appropriate care for many patients living with pain, and the enormous socioeconomic burden of chronic pain. The societal costs of chronic pain are reflected in patients' suffering and reduced quality of life, increased rates of depression and suicide, disrupted relationships with family and friends, and reduced employment or other responsibilities. The economic burden is also huge, amounting to many billions of dollars each year. Unfortunately, it has taken media attention in recent years to the misuse of drugs used for pain management, most notably opioids, to raise public awareness and to gain the attention of policymakers not only to the drug misuse, but also to the pain crisis itself and the socioeconomic toll of chronic pain in particular. It is hoped that this increased attention will translate into a comprehensive series of approaches targeting the many aspects of the pain crisis and result in a better understanding of pain and improved access and healthcare management for patients suffering from acute or chronic pain.

These approaches to address the pain crises have to include an increased emphasis on enhanced education of healthcare clinicians about pain because it has been well documented that most clinicians have only a limited knowledge base and understanding about pain and its management. This book offers the opportunity for clinicians to improve their knowledge about pain and apply that knowledge for the benefit of their patients. The three editors of this book have ensured that its second edition has built upon the first edition which was distinctive in its integration of the clinical, psychosocial and basic science topics related to the different types of pain and their management. As a result of the up-to-date information outlined in the 44 chapters of its second edition, this book provides a valuable resource about pain from a variety of perspectives. It will be particularly valuable not only for clinicians to help them assist their patients experiencing an acute pain or suffering from chronic pain, but also for scientists who wish to gain more insights into these pain conditions and their underlying processes.

Barry J. Sessle
Faculties of Dentistry and Medicine
University of Toronto
Toronto, Ontario, Canada
2021

Part 1

Basic Understanding of Pain Medicine

Chapter 1

The challenge of pain: a multidimensional phenomenon

Mary E. Lynch[1], Kenneth D. Craig[2], & Philip W. Peng[3]

[1]*Department of Anesthesia, Pain Management and Perioperative Medicine, Department of Psychiatry, Department of Pharmacology, Dalhousie University, Halifax, Nova Scotia, Canada*
[2]*Department of Psychology, University of British Columbia, Vancouver, Canada*
[3]*Professor, Department of Anesthesiology and Pain Medicine, University Health Network and Sinai Health System, University of Toronto, Toronto, Canada*

Pain is one of the most challenging problems in medicine and biology. It is a challenge to the sufferer who must often learn to live with pain for which no therapy has been found. It is a challenge to the physician or other health professional who seeks every possible means to help the suffering patient. It is a challenge to the scientist who tries to understand the biological mechanisms that can cause such terrible suffering. It is also a challenge to society, which must find the medical, scientific and financial resources to relieve or prevent pain and suffering as much as possible. (Melzack & Wall *The Challenge of Pain*, 1982)

Introduction

Last year, the International Association for the Study of Pain (IASP) introduced a revised definition of pain stating that pain is "an unpleasant sensory and emotional experience associated with, or resembling that associated with, actual or potential tissue damage [1]. Pain is divided into two broad categories: acute pain, which is associated with ongoing tissue damage, and chronic pain, which is generally taken to be pain that has persisted for longer periods of time. Many injuries and diseases are capable of instigating acute pain with sources including mechanical tissue damage, inflammation and tissue ischemia. Similarly, chronic pain can be associated with other chronic diseases, terminal illness, or may persist after illness or injury with uncertain biological mechanisms. The point at which chronic pain can be diagnosed may vary with the injury or condition that initiated it; however, for most conditions, pain persisting beyond 3 months is reasonably described as a chronic pain condition. In some cases, one can identify a persistent pain condition much earlier, for example, in the case of post-herpetic neuralgia subsequent to an attack of shingles, if pain persists beyond rash healing it indicates a persistent or chronic pain condition is present.

Exponential growth in pain research in the past five decades has increased our understanding regarding underlying mechanisms of the causes of chronic pain, now understood to involve a neural response to tissue injury. In other words, peripheral and central events related to disease or injury can trigger long-lasting changes in peripheral nerves, spinal cord and brain such that the system becomes sensitized and capable of spontaneous activity or of

Clinical Pain Management: A Practical Guide, Second Edition. Edited by Mary E. Lynch, Kenneth D. Craig, and Philip W. Peng.

responding to non-noxious stimuli as if painful. By such means, pain can persist beyond the point where normal healing takes place and is often associated with abnormal sensory findings. In consequence, the scientific advances are providing a biological basis for understanding the experience and disabling impact of persistent pain. Table 1.1 presents definitions of pain terms relevant to chronic pain.

Traditionally, clinicians have conceptualized chronic pain as a symptom of disease or injury. Treatment was focused on addressing the underlying cause with the expectation that the pain would then resolve. It was thought that the pain itself could not kill. We now know that the opposite is true. Pain persists beyond injury and there is mounting evidence that "pain can kill." In addition to contributing to ongoing suffering, disability and diminished life quality, it has been demonstrated that uncontrolled pain compromises immune function, promotes tumor growth and can compromise healing with an increase in morbidity and mortality following surgery [2, 3], as well as a decrease in the quality of recovery [4]. Clinical studies suggest that prolonged untreated pain suffered early in life may have long-lasting effects on the individual patterns of stress hormone responses. These effects may extend to persistent changes in nociceptive processing with implications for pain experienced later in life [5, 6]. Chronic pain is associated with the poorest health-related quality of life when compared with other chronic diseases such as emphysema, heart failure or depression [7] and has been found to double the risk of death by suicide compared to controls [8] and suicide rates remain higher even when controlling for mental illness [9]. Often chronic pain causes more suffering and disability than the injury or illness that caused it in the first place [10]. The condition has major implications not only for those directly suffering, but also family and loved ones become enmeshed in the suffering person's challenges, the work place suffers through loss of productive employees, the community is deprived of active citizens and the economic costs of caring for those suffering from chronic pain are dramatic.

Table 1.1 Definitions of pain terms.

Term	Definition
Allodynia	Pain due to a stimulus that does not normally provoke pain
Anesthesia dolorosa	Pain in a region that is completely numb to touch
Dysesthesia	An unpleasant abnormal sensation, whether spontaneous or evoked
Hyperalgesia	An increased response to a stimulus that is normally painful
Hyperpathia	A painful syndrome characterized by an abnormally painful reaction to a stimulus, especially a repetitive stimulus as well as an increased threshold
Neuropathic	Pain initiated or caused by a primary pain lesion or dysfunction in the nervous system
Nociceptor	A receptor preferentially sensitive to a noxious stimulus or to a stimulus that would become noxious if prolonged
Paresthesia	An abnormal sensation, whether spontaneous or evoked (use dysesthesia when the abnormal sensation is unpleasant)

Source: Based on Merskey H, Bogduk N, eds. (1994) *Classification of Chronic Pain, Descriptions of Chronic Pain Syndromes and Definitions of Pain Terms*, 2nd edn. Task Force on Taxonomy, IASP Press, Seattle.

Chronic pain is an escalating public health problem which remains neglected. Alarming figures demonstrate that more than 50% of patients still suffer severe intolerable pain after surgery and trauma [11–13]. Inadequately treated acute pain puts people at higher risk of developing chronic pain. For example, intensity of acute postoperative pain correlates with the development of persistent postoperative pain, which is now known to be a major and under-recognized health problem [13]. The prevalence of chronic pain subsequent to surgery has been found in 10–50% of patients following many commonly performed surgical procedures and in 2–10% this pain can be severe [12].

The epidemiology of chronic pain has been examined in high-quality surveys of general populations from several countries which have demonstrated that the prevalence of chronic pain is at least 18–20% [14-16]. These rates will increase with the aging of the population. In addition to the human suffering inflicted by pain there is also a large economic toll. Pain accounts for over 20% of doctor visits and 10% of drug sales and costs developed countries $1 trillion each year [17].

Chronic pain has many characteristics of a disease epidemic that is silent yet growing; hence addressing it is imperative. It must be recognized as a multidimensional phenomenon involving biopsychosocial aspects. Daniel Carr, in *IASP Clinical Updates*, expressed it most succinctly: "The remarkable restorative capacity of the body after common injury . . . is turned upside down (and) hyperalgesia, disuse atrophy, contractures, immobility, fear-avoidance, helplessness, depression, anxiety, catastrophizing, social isolation, and stigmatization are the norm" [18].

Such is the experience and challenge of chronic pain and it is up to current and future generations of clinicians to relieve or prevent pain and suffering as much as possible. The challenges must be confronted at biological, psychological and social levels. Not only is a better understanding needed, but reforms of caregiving systems that address medical, psychological and health service delivery must be undertaken.

References

1 Raja SN, Carr DB, Cohen M, *et al.* (2020) The revised International Association for the Study of Pain definition of pain: concepts, challenges, and compromises. *Pain* **161(9)**:1976–82.

2 Liebeskind, JC. 1991 Pain can kill. *Pain* **44**:3–4.

3 Page GG. Acute pain and immune impairment. *IASP Pain Clinical Updates* **XIII** (March 2005):1–4.

4 Wu CL, Rowlingson AJ, Partin AW, *et al.* (2005) Correlation of postoperative pain to quality of recovery in the immediate postoperative period. *Reg Anesth Pain Med*, 2005. **30**:516–22.

5 Finley, GA, Franck LS, Grunau RE *et al.* (2005) *Why children's pain matters. IASP Pain Clinical Updates* **XIII(4)**:1–6.

6 Beggs S. (2015) Long term consequences of neonatal injury. *Can J Psychiatry* **60**:176–80.

7 Choiniere M, Dion D, Peng P *et al.* (2010) The Canadian STOP-PAIN Project-Part 1: Who are the patients on the waitlists of multidisciplinary pain treatment facilities? *Can J Anesth* **57**:539–48.

8 Tang N and Crane C. (2006) Suicidality in chronic pain: review of the prevalence, risk factors and psychological links. *Psychol Med* **36**: 575–86.

9 Ratcliffe GE, Enns MW, Beluk S-L, Sareen J. (2008) Chronic pain conditions and suicidal ideation and suicide attempts: An epidemiologic perspective. *Clin J Pain* **24(3)**:204–10.

10 Melzack R and Wall, PD. (1988) *The Challenge of Pain*. Penguin Books, London.

11 Bond M, Breivik H, and Niv D. (2004). Global day against pain, new declaration. http://www.painreliefhumanright.com.

12 Kehlet H, Jensen TS, and Woolf CJ. (2006). Persistent postsurgical pain: risk factors and prevention. *Lancet* **367**:1618–25.

13 Haroutiunian S, Nikolajsen L, Finnerup NB, *et al.* (2013) The neuropathic component in persistent postsurgical pain: A systematic literature review. *Pain* **154**:95–102.

14 Lynch ME, Schopflocher D, Taenzer P, Sinclair C et al. (2009) Research funding for pain in Canada. *Pain Res Manage***14**:113–5.

15 Blyth FM, March LM, Brnabic AJM, *et al.* (2001) Chronic pain in Australia: a prevalence study. *Pain* **89**:127–34.

16 Eriksen JE, Jensen MK, Sjøgren P *et al.* (2003) Epidemiology of chronic non-malignant pain in Denmark. *Pain***106**:221–8.

17 Max MB and Stewart WF. (2008) The molecular epidemiology of pain: A new discipline for drug discovery. *Nat Rev Drug Discov* **7**:647–58.

18 Carr DB. (2009) What Does Pain Hurt? *IASP Pain Clinical Updates* **XVII(3)**:1–6.

Chapter 2

Epidemiology and economics of chronic and recurrent pain

Dennis C. Turk & Kushang V. Patel
Department of Anesthesiology and Pain Medicine, University of Washington, Seattle, Washington, USA

Introduction

Pain is prevalent worldwide and is among the most common symptoms leading patients to consult a physician in the United States (US) [1]. Recurrent and chronic non-cancer pain (CNCP) are not a set of single, cohesive disorders. Instead, recurrent and CNCP are generic classifications that include a wide range of disorders.

Individuals with recurrent pain and CNCP comprise disparate groups, with varying underlying pathophysiology, and widely diverse impacts on quality of life, function and demands on the healthcare provider and society. Thus, CNCP and recurrent pain have not only significant health consequences, but also personal, economic and societal implications. These conditions have both direct costs of health care and indirect costs (e.g., lost paid employment, disability compensation). In this chapter we provide a summary of the prevalence of some of the most common CNCP and recurrent pain disorders and describe their economic impact.

Epidemiology is, "The study of the occurrence and distribution of health-related states or events in specified populations, including the study of the determinants influencing such states, and the application of this knowledge to control the health problems" [2]. It is important to clarify the meaning of epidemiology and key concepts of incidence and prevalence.

Incidence is the number of new cases of a disease developing during a particular time period in a population at risk of developing the disease. Prevalence is the proportion of the at-risk population affected by a condition (i.e. total number of cases of disease present in the population at a specified time divided by the total number of persons in the population at that specified time). In this chapter, we will focus on prevalence of chronic pain in general as well as in specific diagnostic groups.

It is important to acknowledge at the outset that a number of factors will influence the prevalence rates of any chronic pain diagnosis as population estimates for the prevalence of chronic pain vary widely. Some of the variability in prevalence estimates reported in the literature result from the case definition used. In addition, ascertainment methods (telephone interview, in person interviews), wording of questions (e.g., any pain, pain that prevent respondent from daily activities, pain severe enough to induce healthcare seeking), timeframe (e.g. recall bias, differential time intervals such as pain over the last month versus last week, retrospective vs. current), sample (e.g., population-based) and time, place and population sampled (internet vs. in-person) will all influence the survey results.

One particularly important problem in establishing the prevalence of different chronic pain conditions is the inherent subjectivity of pain presents a fundamental impediment to increased

Clinical Pain Management: A Practical Guide, Second Edition. Edited by Mary E. Lynch, Kenneth D. Craig, and Philip W. Peng.

understanding of its mechanisms, control, and the epidemiology. The language used by any two individuals attempting to describe a similar injury and their pain experience often varies markedly. Similarly, clinicians and clinical investigators commonly use multiple terms that at times have idiosyncratic meanings. Needless to say, appropriate communication requires a common language and a classification system that is used in a consistent fashion.

In order to identify target groups, conduct research, prescribe treatment, evaluate treatment efficacy, to develop policy and for decision making, it is essential that some consensually validated criteria are used to distinguish groups of individuals who share a common set of relevant attributes. The primary purpose of such a classification is to describe the relationships of constituent members based on their equivalence along a set of basic dimensions that represent the structure of a particular domain. Infinite classification systems are possible, depending on the rationale about common factors and the variables believed to discriminate among individuals. The majority of the current taxonomies of pain are "expert-based" classifications.

Expert-Based Classification of Pain

Classifications of disease are usually based on a preconceived combination of characteristics (e.g., symptoms, signs, results of diagnostic tests), with no single characteristic being both necessary and sufficient for every member of the category, yet the group as a whole possesses a certain unity [3]. Most classification systems used in pain medicine (e.g., ICD [4], classification and diagnostic criteria for headache disorders, cranial neuralgias, and facial pain [5], IASP Classification of Chronic Pain [6], CRPS [7], whiplash-associated disorders [8], Research Diagnostic Criteria [RDC] for Temporomandibular Disorders in dentistry [9,10] and the Analgesic, Anesthetic, and Addiction Clinical Trial Translations, Innovations, Opportunities, and Networks [ACTTION]-American Pain Society Pain Taxonomy [AAPT] [11] and ACTTION-American Pain Society-American Academy of Pain Medicine [AAPM] Pain Taxonomy [AAAPT][12]) are based on the consensus reached by a group of "experts". In this sense, they reflect the inclusion or elimination of certain diagnostic features depending on agreement.

The original IASP Classification of Chronic Pain included 5 axes [i.e. (1) body region; (2) system whose abnormal functioning that might produce the pain; (3) temporal characteristics of pain and pattern of occurrence; (4) onset and intensity of pain; and (5) presumed etiology] and each diagnosis resulted in a unique code number. Thus, this approach moved beyond the location of symptoms and system involved.

Recently, IASP proposed a classification of chronic pain for inclusion in the ICD-11 [4]. The classification includes seven categories (i.e. "primary", cancer, postsurgical/posttraumatic, neuropathic, headache and orofacial, visceral and musculoskeletal). The primary category is somewhat of a mixed collection of pain disorders that cannot be explained by other chronic pain conditions and includes back pain that is neither identified as musculoskeletal nor neuropathic, chronic widespread pain, fibromyalgia (FM) or irritable bowel syndrome. The primary category is consistent with the lumping of this set of disorders in the category of The American Academy of Pain Medicine's (AAPM's) diagnosis of maldynia and central sensitivity disorders advocated by Clauw [13] and Yunus [14] among others. There may be some concern that this poorly defined category may imply the discredited psychogenic classification; that is, an artificial dichotomy where either the condition has a physical (i.e. somatogenic) basis or the absence is "primary" (i.e. psychogenic).

Recently, a consortium composed of Analgesic Clinical Trials Translations, Innovations, Opportunities, and Networks (ACTTION) (a public-private partnership support by the US Food and Drug Administration) partnered with the American Pain Society to create a chronic pain taxonomy – ACTTION American Pain Society Pain Taxonomy (AAPT) [11] and with the American Academy of Pain Medicine [12] to create an acute pain taxonomy – ACTTION, American Pain Society, and American Academy of Pain Medicine Pain taxonomy (AAAPT). AAPT and AAAPT are evidence-based pain taxonomies in which a multidimensional diagnostic framework has been applied to the most prevalent and important chronic and acute pain conditions. A major impetus for the AAPT/AAAPT initiative derived from observing the transformative impact of evidence-based diagnostic classifications that have been published by different medical specialties.

AAPT categorizes chronic pain conditions by organ system and anatomic structure, distinguishing (1) peripheral and central neuropathic pain, (2) musculoskeletal pain, (3) spine pain, (4) orofacial and head pain and (6) abdominal/pelvic/urogenital pain. Because certain types of chronic pain cannot be included in one of these groups, an additional category for disease-related pain not classified elsewhere includes pain associated with cancer and pain associated with sickle cell disease (pain associated with Lyme disease and with leprosy, among other conditions, would also be included in this group). It is important to emphasize that all types of headache were intentionally excluded from AAPT because the International Classification of Headache Disorders provides systematic, valid and widely used diagnostic criteria for these conditions [5].

The AAPT multidimensional framework comprises five dimensions that can be applied to *all* chronic pain conditions. This can be contrasted with the new IASP taxonomy in which psychosocial factors are "optional specifiers" for each diagnosis beyond the classification of "chronic primary pain"; psychosocial factors are given a prominent role as are interference with activities and participation in social roles (somewhat of a departure from the original IASP taxonomy where psychosocial factors are a significant consideration only for one diagnostic classification; namely, chronic primary pain) (see also [11]). Other than prioritizing core diagnostic criteria, which is the first AAPT dimension, the order of the dimensions does not reflect their importance. Indeed, as noted earlier, it is anticipated that AAPT diagnostic criteria will ultimately be based on the mechanisms of the specific chronic pain conditions, whereas in the current version of the taxonomy, these mechanisms constitute the final dimension.

Like the IASP classification, the AAPT also includes seven but somewhat different categories of chronic pain (i.e. peripheral nervous systems; central nervous system; spine; musculoskeletal; orofacial and head; visceral, pelvic, and urogenital; other [e.g., cancer, sickle cell]). The AAPT classification incorporates five dimensions for each condition within the seven categories (core diagnostic criteria [symptoms, signs, and diagnostic findings required for the diagnosis]; common features [including pain characteristics, non-pain features, lifespan], common medical and psychiatric comorbidities; neurobiological, psychosocial and functional consequences; and putative neurobiological and psychosocial mechanism, risk factors, and protective factors. Although the AAPT integrates important components of the classification of chronic pain conditions, there are no epidemiological data, thus far, that have been reported using this classification.

In this chapter, we will use a hybrid approach to classification, as the available epidemiological data tend to follow classification by body location (e.g., back pain, headache, pelvic pain, temporomandibular disorders (TMDs), irritable bowel syndrome (IBS), wide-spread) and etiology (i.e. osteoarthritis (OA), neuropathic whiplash-associated disorders). In the future, epidemiological research may advance our understanding of the prevalence of the diverse set of chronic pain disorders by using the more comprehensive IASP and AAPT classification.

Epidemiology of Chronic Noncancer Pain and Recurrent Pain

CNCP, typically assessed as pain that persists for longer than six months, remains a significant public health issue affecting millions of people worldwide [15]. Worldwide the prevalence is estimated to be over 20% of all adults, with 10% newly diagnosed each year [16, 17]. In 2015 the global point prevalence of activity-limiting low back pain (LBP) alone was 7.3% (540 million people) affected at any one point in time [18].

Based on data from the National Health Interview Survey (NHIS) conducted in 2012, a representative national population-based survey conducted annually by personal, home-based interviews by the National Center for Health Statistics, 25.3 million American adults report daily pain and 23.4 million reported having "a lot of pain" [19]. In a subsequent NHIS survey [20], 20.4% (50 million) of the adult US population reported chronic pain (defined as having pain on every day or most days over the past 6 months) and 8% (19.6 million) had "high-impact chronic pain" severe enough to interfere with their lives (i.e. limited life or work activities on most days or every day during the past 6 months).

The presence of high-impact chronic pain was strongly associated with an increased risk of disability after controlling for other chronic health conditions, where disability was more likely in those with chronic pain than in those with stroke or kidney failure, among other conditions [20]. In the US, pain (i.e. LBP, neck pain, other musculoskeletal pain, OA, migraine) accounts for 9.7 million years living with disability in comparison with 8.8 million years living with disability for the 12 leading medical conditions [21]. The high-impact chronic pain population reported more severe pain and more mental health and cognitive impairments than persons with CNCP or recurrent pain without disability and was also more likely to report worsening of health, more difficulty with self-care and greater health care use [22].

CNCP is estimated to account for 16.2% of all adult outpatient visits in 2015, having increased from 11.3% in 2000 [23]. CNCP is a highly common condition and accounts or 57% of health care encounters [24]. Interestingly, for some of the most prevalent pain conditions (e.g. LBP, FM, headache, pelvic pain) there is no clear objective evidence of any underlying physical pathology associated with reported pain in the majority of cases (e.g. [25-27]). One survey conducted in Australia, found that 65% of people had no clear medical diagnosis for their chronic pain and 33% identified no clear precipitant [28].

A secondary analysis of data from the 2016-2017 National Survey of Children's Health [29] indicated that CNCP and recurrent pain are not only problems for adults, but also for children. An estimated 8% of national sample (95% confidence interval [CI]: 7.5%-8.6%) of children (6-17) had chronic pain as rated by parents [30]. Chronic pain was defined by response to the question: "During the past 12 months, has this child had frequent or chronic difficulty with repeated or chronic physical pain, including headaches or other back or body pain?" The NSCH is an annual cross-sectional survey, conducted via in-person interviews of randomly sampled households, selected via a multistage process to represent the entire civilian, noninstitutionalized population of the US. Pediatric prevalence rates of chronic pain subtypes range across studies from 8% to 83% for headaches, 4% to 53% for abdominal pain, 14% to 24% for back pain, 4% to 40% for musculoskeletal pain, 4% to 49% for multiple pains and 5% to 88% for other pains. Several studies report that 5% of youth report experiencing severe pain that interferes with daily function [31,32].

Similar to adults, physical causes for reported pain are often difficult to identify. In only one-fifth of the patients are specific causes or medical diagnoses for their pain condition able to be identified, which further underscores chronic pain (and its related disability) as a medical syndrome unto itself [33].

Persistent pain in youth may continue to adulthood. A retrospective review of the onset of pain in adults seeking treatment in a pain clinic [34] found that 80% of adults with chronic pain reported that their current pain was a continuation of chronic pain they had experienced during childhood. It is important to note, however, that this estimate is based on patients from a tertiary pain clinic and therefore likely overestimates the proportion of adults with chronic pain who had also experienced chronic pain in childhood. Indeed, much of the burden of chronic pain occurs in later life [19, 35]. because of age-associated musculoskeletal conditions, such as OA.

Musculoskeletal pain

Musculoskeletal pain is perhaps the most commonly reported set of CNCP conditions. Based on the 2012 NHIS (n = 34,525) more than 50% of US adults (approximately 125 million) experience one or more musculoskeletal pain disorders [36]. In an earlier epidemiological study that differentiated among musculoskeletal conditions, the NHIS of 2007, reported 29,019,000 (12.8%) had neck pain, 57,070,000 (25.4%) had pain in the lower back and 9,062,000 (4%) had pain in the face or jaw in the 3 months preceding the interview [37].

Among musculoskeletal locations, the most commonly afflicted region is the lower back. Low LBP accounts for 34 million office visits annually by family physicians and primary care interests [38]. LBP is amongst the top six costliest health conditions, and one of the top three most disabling health conditions [39]. In fact, LBP is the highest ranked condition contributing to years lived with disability worldwide according to the most recent Global Burden of Disease Study and is associated with significant societal and individual cost [21,40, 41]. LBP is also the most common of chronic pain conditions reported by adolescents, however, the range of prevalence rates across studies is quite large, namely,

8–44% [42]. Some of the features of epidemiological surveys listed above many account for the variability observed.

Epidemiologic surveys in the US report a prevalence rate of 25% for LBP any time during a 3-month period [43]. Other industrialized nations, with prevalence rates for chronic LBP ranging 13–28% [42] with19% prevalence rate for CLBP during a 12-month period and a lifetime prevalence rate of 29.5% [44].

Rheumatological diagnoses

Osteoarthritis (OA) is a chronic debilitating condition typically observed within three specific areas in order of decreasing frequency; the hand, knee and hip. It is the most common rheumatological diagnosis [45]. As of 2020, there are an estimated 32.5 million adults in the US who have OA [46]. Using the 2013-15 data, Barbour et al. [47] concluded that 23.7 million (43.5%) had arthritis-attributable activity limitation (an age-adjusted increase of approximately 20% in the proportion of adults with arthritis activity limitations since 2002 [p-trend <0.001]) [47]. The prevalence of OA is projected to increase by about 40% in the next 25 years [48] with the number of affected individuals expected to rise to 78 million by 2040 [47].

The prevalence increases of OA steadily with age, affecting 29.9% in men aged 18–64 years, 31.2% in women aged 18–64 years, 55.8% in men aged 65 years and older and 68.7% in women aged 65 years and older [49]. Symptomatic knee OA alone affects approximately 12% of those aged 60 years and older. OA is more prevalent in women than in men, with a prevalence ratio varying between 1.5:1 and 4:1 [50]. In addition to age and sex, the prevalence of OA can vary due to several risk factors such as ethnicity, level of obesity, physical activity levels, bone density and trauma, as well as global factors such as geographical location [50, 52]. Barbour and his colleagues [47] tracked NHIS data from 2002-2014 and that by 2014 prevalence of OA was especially high among Blacks (42.3%) and Hispanics (35.8%).

Although OA is one of the most common diagnoses in general practice in the US [52], there are a number of other pain-related rheumatological disorders. Prevalence estimates for rheumatoid arthritis suggest that 1.3 million adults have this diagnosis. In addition, juvenile arthritis is estimated to affect 294,000 children; spondylarthritides affects 0.6-2.4 million adults; systemic lupus erythematosus affects from 161-322,000 adults, systemic sclerosis affects 49,000 adults; and primary Sjogren's syndrome affects from 0.4 million to 3.1 million adults [48].

Headache

Headache, an almost universal human experience, is one of the most common complaints encountered in medicine and, perhaps for this reason, the preponderance of data on the epidemiology of CNCP and recurrent pain disorders are found for headaches. According to the World Health Organization [53], half to three quarters of adults aged 18–65 years in the world have had headache in the last year and, among those individuals, 30% or more have reported migraine. When considering more chronic headache, the WHO estimated that the prevalence of headaches on 15 or more days every month affects 1.7–4% of the world's adult population. The life-long prevalence of headache is estimated to be 96% [54]. The 2011 NHIS [55] results reveal that 16.6% of US adults 18 or older reported having migraine or other severe headaches in the last 3 months.

Migraine and tension-type headaches are the most common primary headache disorders [56]. The main subtypes are migraine (vascular headache) with and without aura. An aura is a fully reversible set of nervous system symptoms, most often visual or sensory symptoms, that typically develops gradually, recedes, and is then followed by headache accompanied by nausea, vomiting, photophobia and phonophobia. Tension-type headache is a dull, bilateral, mild- to moderate-intensity pressure–pain without striking associated features that may be categorized as infrequent, frequent or chronic and is easily distinguished from migraine.

Migraine is more prevalent in females between the ages 18-44, with the overall age-adjusted 3-month prevalence of migraine in females was 19.1% and in males 9.0%, but varied substantially depending on age [56, 57, 58]. Data suggest that 70% to 80% of migraineurs have a family history. In the US, the impact of migraine appears to be greater in those who work part time or are unemployed, those with low socioeconomic status, and the uninsured [58]. The 2010 Global Burden of Disease Survey reported that migraine was the third most prevalent disorder and the seventh-highest cause of disability worldwide [56].

The National Headache Foundation estimated that more than 37 million American experience recurrent migraines [59]. However less than half of those who experience migraines have received a formal diagnosis from a health care provider [61]. Migraine alone affects 18% of women and 6% of men in the US and has an estimated worldwide prevalence of approximately 10% [60]. Pediatric prevalence rates range from 8% to 83%, depending on the sample, with the excessively high estimates based on clinical samples compared to the lower estimates from population samples [33].

After reviewing data from three national surveys (NAMCS, National Ambulatory Medical Care Survey (2010), the National Hospital Ambulatory Medical Care Survey (NHAMC [2010], and the NHIS (2005-2010), Burch et al. [58] concluded that migraine is a highly prevalent medical condition, affecting approximately 1 out of every 7 Americans annually and these estimates have been relatively stable over a period of eight years. The American Migraine Prevalence and Prevention study subdivided the migraine prevalence data into definite migraine and probably migraine. The authors concluded that the overall prevalence of migraine of 11.7% and probable migraine of 4.5%, for a total of 16.2% [61].

In the US, migraine accounted for 0.5% of all visits and other headache presentations for 0.4% of all ambulatory care visits. Overall, 52.8% of all visits for migraine occurred in primary care settings, 23.2% in specialty outpatient settings and 16.7% in emergency department (EDs) [55].

Although typically not as severe as migraine, tension-type headache is far more common, with a lifetime prevalence in the general population of up to 80%. The global active prevalence of tension-type headache is approximately 40% and migraine 10% [56].

Headache or pain in the head was the fourth leading cause of visits to the ED in 2009-2010, accounting for 3.1% of all ED visits. The 3-month prevalence of migraine or severe headache was 26.1% [58].

Neuropathic Pain

Neuropathic pain arises as a direct consequence of a lesion or disease affecting the somatosensory system. It can be peripheral in origin as a result of nerve injury or disease (e.g. lumbar radiculopathy, postherpetic neuralgia, diabetic or HIV-related neuropathy, or postsurgical pain), or central (e.g. poststroke or spinal cord injury). Other diseases known to cause neuropathic pain that are diagnosed during childhood include erythromelalgia, toxic and metabolic neuropathies, mitochondrial disorders, paroxysmal extreme pain disorder and Fabry disease. Moreover, there has been increasing recognition that some classically "nonneuropathic" painful conditions (e.g. OA, FM) can give rise to symptoms more commonly associated with neuropathic pain.

Neuropathic pain is characterized by unpleasant symptoms, such as shooting or burning pain, numbness, allodynia and other sensations that are very difficult to describe. "Definite" neuropathic pain can relatively rarely be confirmed, particularly in nonspecialist settings [63, 64]. Neuropathic pain conditions have proven to be particularly recalcitrant to treatment [63].

Much less is known about the prevalence of neuropathic pain disorders compared with other chronic and recurrent pain disorders (e.g. headache, back pain, arthritis). General population studies have reported prevalences of 8% and 6.9% in the United Kingdom and France, respectively [65, 66]. It is important to note that cases identified in these studies were described as having "pain of predominantly neuropathic origin" or "pain with neuropathic characteristics," rather than "neuropathic pain" [64]. A systematic review of population-based prevalence studies considered the true prevalence of pain with neuropathic characteristics to be 7% to 10% [67]. Furthermore, neuropathic pain is estimated to be present in 17% of adult patients with other CNCP disorders, with as many as 30% of adults seen in pain clinics are estimated to experience neuropathic pain [66, 68].

Pelvic Pain

Pelvic pain is characterized by intermittent or constant pain in the lower abdomen or pelvis for at least 6 months that may or may not be associated with menstruation. However, the pain should not be exclusively associate with menstruation, sexual intercourse or pregnancy. The most common diagnoses for pelvic pain are endometriosis, pelvic inflammatory disease and interstitial cystitis [bladder pain syndrome]. Pelvic pain is estimated to account for 20% of general practitioners' referrals to gynecologists [69].

CPP has a considerable impact on the well-being of women and is a cause of significant distress and disability. It has been reported to be associated with poor quality of life, fatigue, depression, anxiety and marital and sexual dysfunction [70]. Patients with CPP tend to spend days in bed due to illness and report poorer physical and mental health compared with the general population [71]. A study showed that 58.4% of women with CPP reported that they use analgesics and/or nonsteroidal anti-inflammatory drugs on a weekly or daily basis without medical prescription [72].

The heterogeneity of the definitions used for chronic pelvic pain (CPP) introduced challenges for comparing results across different studies. The American Congress of Obstetricians and Gynecologists defines CPP as noncyclical pain in the pelvis, severe enough to require medical attention, located below the umbilicus in the region of the anterior abdominal wall, lumbosacral back or buttocks lasting for at least 6 months [73].

A number of studies have reported the prevalence of CPP in women, but most of them have used sampling frames such as hospital patients which are unable to provide accurate estimates of the prevalence of CPP in the general population. The relatively few population-based studies have reported prevalence ranging from 6.4% [74] to 25.4% [75]. The studies were conducted using randomly selected women from representative sampling frames.

In a US population-based study conducted by the Gallup Organization, 14.7% of eligible women (773/5263, 1 in 7) reported pelvic pain in the last 3 months, 61% of women with pelvic pain symptoms did not have a clear diagnosis, 15% of employed women with chronic pelvic pain reported that they lost time from pain work and 45% overall reported reduced work productivity due to their pain [70]. Worldwide estimates suggest that 24% of women experience CPP [76]. All the studies on the epidemiology of pelvic pain have been conducted among women of reproductive age. Older women who are believed to be less susceptible to CPP have been traditionally excluded from prevalence studies. More recent population studies have also confirmed significant reporting of CPP among older women. For example, the highest rate reported in one of study was in women aged 18–25 years (17%), whereas women older than 75 years had a rate of 13% [77].

Temporomandibular Disorders

Temporomandibular disorders (TMD) are disorders of the jaw muscles (i.e. muscle of mastication), temporomandibular joints and the nerves associated with chronic facial pain. Any problem that prevents the complex system of muscles, bones and joints from working together in harmony may result in a TMD. The exact cause of a person's TMD is often difficult to determine. Pain may be due to a combination of factors, such as genetics, muscle hyperfunction, arthritis, jaw injury or hormonal influences. Some people who have jaw pain also tend to clench or grind their teeth (bruxism), although many people habitually clench or grind their teeth and never develop TMD.

TMDs are common, in some studies affecting approximately 25% of adults [78]. Further, TMD is associated with substantial morbidity, affecting quality of life and work productivity. As an example, it is estimated that for every 100 million working adults in the United States, TMD contributes to 17.8 million lost work days annually [79].

Over 2 decades of NHIS surveys (1989 to 2009), the prevalence of self-reported TMD symptoms remained stable, affecting 5% of US adults [80]. Based on a national population-based survey, it is estimated that 11.2-12.4 million Americans have symptoms related to TMDs [81].

IASP Primary classification (also referred to as chronic widespread pain and Central Sensitivity Syndromes (CSS))

Clinical practitioners commonly see patients with pain and other somatic symptoms that they cannot adequately explain based on the degree of damage or inflammation noted in peripheral tissue. If no cause is found, these individuals are often given a diagnostic label that merely connotes that the patient has pain in a region of the body [82] or chronic widespread pain Central Sensitivity Syndromes (CSS) or "primary pain" in the IASP taxonomy [83].

Depending on the practitioner a patient sees, there are a number of related and overlapping conditions, which have recently been referred to as chronic overlapping pain conditions or functional pain disorders. Some examples of the many conditions that have been included within the CSS classification are FM, chronic fatigue syndrome, IBS, chronic pelvic pain and TMD [84, 85]. FM is the current term used for chronic widespread musculoskeletal pain for which no alternative cause can be identified. In conjunction with having a diagnosis of chronic widespread pain, the development of the American College of Rheumatology (ACR) criteria for FM also saw an increase in cases observed in clinical settings [42]. Prevalence rates of FM reported in other high-income countries range 0.7–4% [42].

There are consistent prevalence estimates reported for chronic widespread pain, ranging 10–14%, in both adults and adolescents [42]. Population estimates from the prevalence of chronic pain in the United Kingdom suggest that up to 16.5% of the general population reporting chronic widespread pain [86].

These chronic overlapping pain conditions are thought to have similar underlying pathology with alterations in central nervous system function leading to augmented nociceptive processing and the development of central nervous system (CNS)-mediated somatic symptoms of fatigue, sleep, memory and mood difficulties. The widespread nature of the pain is a key clinical feature in these individuals and a number of other CNS-mediated symptoms (e.g., fatigue, memory difficulties, sleep and mood disorders) are frequent comorbidities. Together, this supports that the CNS is amplifying pain, and there is a fundamental problem with augmented pain or sensory processing in the CNS.

Central sensitization (CS) is defined as an amplified response and/or increased responsivity of nociceptive (pain) neurons in the CNS to sensory stimuli, hence, labelled CSS [84, 87]. Within the past decade, a number of common chronic pain conditions, historically viewed as independent, have been included under the rubric of CSS due to their overlapping features.

The underlying etiology and pathophysiology of CSSs are incompletely understood at this time [87]; however, as the name suggests, CS is viewed as primarily occurring in the CNS. Clinically, this can manifest as a patient who reports pain being widespread and present in multiple body regions or pain occurring after activities that are generally viewed as mundane and painless (e.g. taking a short walk or cooking a meal).

Factors associated with chronic and recurrent pain

There is a growing consensus that all pain conditions reflect an amalgam of biologic, psychologic and social factors that is best assessed with a multidimensional perspective to determine further evaluation and treatment options [88]. The IASP has recently updated the original 1979 definition to reflect advancements in the understanding of pain and to acknowledge that pain may exist even in the absence of objective physical pathology [89]. The revised definition states that pain is "an unpleasant sensory and emotional experience associated with, or resembling that associated with, actual or potential tissue damage," and is expanded upon by the addition of six key notes and the etymology of the word "pain" for further valuable context:

1 Pain is always a <u>personal experience</u> that is influenced to varying degrees by biological, psychological, and social factors.

2 <u>Pain and nociception are different</u> phenomena. Pain cannot be inferred solely from activity in sensory neurons.

3 <u>Through their life experiences, individuals learn the concept of pain</u>.

4 A <u>person's report of an experience as pain should be respected</u>.

5 Although pain usually serves an adaptive role, it <u>may have adverse effects on function and social and psychological well-being</u>. [emphasis added]

Thus, as noted, recurrent and CNCP are not medical conditions that can be solely pinpointed to specific tissue pathology. For the vast majority of patients with back pain, headache and FM, no objective pathology is detectable (e.g. [25-27]). The biopsychosocial model of pain elaborates on the complex interplay of physical, psychological, social and environmental factors that exacerbate and perpetuate the pain condition [90]. For painful conditions that persist beyond the usual period of healing, the development of a pain–stress cycle may result in anger and distress at the situation. A prolonged state of the pain–stress cycle often results in the development of comorbid psychopathology. Individuals with chronic pain are at risk for adopting the sick-role and engaging in maladaptive behaviors that perpetuate the pain–stress cycle, resulting in both physical and psychological deconditioning. Thus, in considering the epidemiology and costs of various chronic pain diagnoses, it is important to consider some of the factors that may impact on the prevalence of these conditions.

Demographic factors

The most commonly identified demographic factors that have significant associations with CNCP are age, sex and socioeconomic status [42]. Older age is significantly associated with increased prevalence of CNCP. This increasing trend for prevalence with age was noted among patients with shoulder pain, LBP, arthritis and other joint disorders and chronic widespread pain. Several factors [42] may account for the observed increase in prevalence among older adults, including degenerative processes, reduced physical activity and recurrent episodes of pain.

There are also pronounced differences in the prevalence rate of various CNCP disorders between males and females. Marked increases in prevalence rates have been observed among females for CNCP disorders such as shoulder pain, LBP, arthritis and chronic widespread pain, as well as migraine. This sex difference persists even when other factors such as age are accounted for. Several hypotheses have been advanced to explain these sex differences, and include a difference between the sexes in hormones, body focus, evaluation and appraisal of symptoms, increased sensitivity or lower thresholds among females, differences in symptom reporting and healthcare seeking behaviors and differential exposure to risk factors (e.g. childbearing) [42,91].

Increased prevalence of CNCP has also been observed among individuals with lower socioeconomic status, which includes dimensions such as household income, employment status, occupational class and level of education. Specifically, the strongest associations with CNCP were observed for lower level of education, lower household income and unemployment [42]. However, socioeconomic status may not be a direct risk factor for CNCP, but significantly associated with underlying psychosocial factors consequent to the onset of pain [42].

Occupational factors

Several population-based prospective studies have confirmed occupational-related stressors as a risk factor for CNCP. These factors included high job demands, low requirement for learning new skills and repetitive work. Furthermore, they were associated with later onset of persistent pain, independent of occupational class, shift work, working hours and job satisfaction levels. The association between these stressors and onset of pain was more pronounced among individuals with relatively lower levels of education. In addition, a study conducted by the World Health Organization included a cohort from 14 nations with a 12-month follow-up [92]. The strongest predictor for development of chronic pain was occupational role disability at baseline due to an injury. Risk of CNCP was 3.6 times greater among those with occupational role disability and it was a stronger predictor than the presence of initial anxiety or major depressive disorders.

Role of disability compensation

The complex and often adversarial nature of the medicolegal system associated with disability compensation may result in the development of "secondary gain" factors that have a role as barriers to recovery. Indeed, in a review investigating the effect of disability compensation for whiplash injuries following motor vehicle collisions, there was some evidence indicating that increased legal complexity under tort laws was associated with longer periods until disability claims are closed. Additionally, in a prospective cohort study on people involved in rear-end collisions in a country with no compensation for whiplash injuries, neck pain and headaches resolved within days of the collision. Such an effect due to the medicolegal barriers to recovery may contribute towards the prevalence rate of CNCP.

However, it should be noted that there is some contradictory evidence. For example, the prevalence rate of FM has been reported to be equivalent in a non-litigious population with no disability compensation relative to populations that had a disability compensation system in place and associated litigation [93]. Therefore, it is possible that the increased incidences of "secondary gain" related to litigation observed in some studies were mediated by the stress of being involved in potentially protracted legal battles. Furthermore, as reviewed in an earlier section on the prevalence of CNCP, similarities in the range of prevalence estimates have been observed across nations with differing systems of disability compensation and healthcare structures. As noted in a review of "secondary gain" concepts in the literature, there is inconsistent evidence for the isolation of the effect of disability compensation and litigation as a secondary factor that perpetuates the chronic pain condition [94].

Economic impact of chronic pain

The economic impact of healthcare in general has been serious enough to have spurred debates about healthcare reforms aimed at managing costs. In addition, there have been calls for legislative reforms to contain the costs of healthcare and to make these costs manageable for all stakeholders. The effect of CNCP is certainly one of the drivers of healthcare costs. For example, in a review of costs documented by a US State Workers' Compensation system, a small minority of patients with chronic LBP (7%) were responsible for approximately 75% of the annual costs incurred [95].

The economic costs of chronic pain are comprised of two general categories: direct costs (i.e. health care provider services, medical devices, medications, hospital services and diagnostic tests) and the even greater indirect costs related to employment (e.g. absenteeism, lost productivity), household activities and disability compensation, among others related to the impact of chronic pain.

Nationally, chronic pain conditions have an immense economic impact. Prior appraisals of annual costs emerging from these conditions range from $560 to $635 billion in the US, and include direct costs of medical care, along with indirect costs such as lost wages and productivity and disability payments [96]. Notably, according to the Institute of Medicine (US) Committee on Advancing Pain Research, Care, and Education, these costs surpass those of other high-impact diseases such as cancer, heart disease and diabetes [97]. The total direct cost of moderate–severe pediatric chronic pain in the US is estimated to cost another $19.5 billion/year [98]. According to the US Center for Disease Control and Prevention, painful rheumatological conditions and spinal problems are the most common causes of disability, two to three times more prevalent than the next most common cause of disability – heart problems [99].

Direct costs

CNCP is associated with a high utilization rate of healthcare services. In the US, approximately 17% of patients in primary care settings report persistent pain [100]. This subset of patients is also among the highest utilizers of healthcare services. For example, the presence of CNCP was shown to be associated with a twofold increase in the number of primary care visits and hospitalizations and also a five-fold increase in the number of visits to emergency rooms. In a review of cost data obtained from a large US Workers' Compensation database, the overall direct costs associated with healthcare utilization increased exponentially as a function of disability duration [101]. Specifically, the cost-per-claim for patients disabled for more than 18 months due to musculoskeletal injuries was $67,612. In contrast, patients disabled for 4–8 months and 11–18 months in duration incurred total medical costs-per-claim of $21,356 and $33,750, respectively. Among the biggest cost drivers for the direct costs associated with healthcare utilization are the costs associated with pharmaceuticals and surgeries.

The cost of pharmaceuticals for pain management amounts to $18.3 billion annually for prescription analgesics and an additional $2.6 billion for non-prescription analgesics [102, 103], and these costs are increasing annually. Overall pharmaceutical costs per claim in a Workers' Compensation setting reveal exponential increases as a function of disability duration due to CNCP.

Similar variations in costs are noted for surgical procedures often used to treat CNCP. The most current estimates of surgical costs are available from the US Centers for Medicare and Medicaid Services (CMS) [101]. These surgical costs range $5,708–23,555 per surgery, with lumbar fusions being the costliest of these surgical procedures for common musculoskeletal disorders. The costs reported by CMS are a conservative estimate and may not necessarily reflect the true costs billed which vary by geographic region. Taking lumbar fusion as an example, the most recent estimate for the annual frequency of lumbar fusion surgery for degenerative conditions is 122,316 cases during year 2001 [104]. Therefore, costs of lumbar fusions alone amounted to approximately $2.9 billion annually [104].

Pharmaceutical and surgical costs, while substantial, are only two aspects of the variety of costs incurred by CNCP patients. Other direct costs that substantially add to the total cost of illness over the lifetime of CNCP include costs associated with health care provider visits, diagnostic and imaging, injection therapeutics, hospital admissions, physical therapy, complementary and alternative medicine (e.g. chiropractic, acupuncture), psychological services, comprehensive pain management programs and medical and case management services.

The costs to treat CNCP in adults in the US exceeds costs to treat coronary artery disease, cancer, and AIDS combined [105]. Again, the total direct cost of moderate-severe pediatric chronic pain in the United States is extrapolated to $19.5 billion per year [98].

Indirect costs

In addition to these direct costs associated with healthcare utilization, there are substantial indirect costs associated with CNCP. Indirect costs incurred due to CNCP include disability compensation, lost productivity, legal fees associated with litigation for injuries, lost tax revenue, and any additional healthcare costs associated with comorbid medical and psychological disorders consequent to CNCP. Projected annual estimates for some of these indirect costs due to back pain alone, range $18.9–71 billion in disability compensation, $6.9 billion in lost productivity due to disability and $7 billion in legal fees [106].

Back pain cases have been estimated to result in approximately 149 million lost work days at an estimated cost of $14 billion [107]. The estimated annual lost productive work time cost from arthritis in the US workforce was $7.11 billion, with 65.7% of the cost attributed to the 38% of workers with pain exacerbations [108]. Lost productive time from common pain conditions among workers cost an estimated $61.2 billion per year. The majority (76.6%) of the lost productive time was explained by reduced performance while at work and not work absence [109]. The total cost of lost productive time in the US workforce due to arthritis, back pain and other musculoskeletal pain from August 2001 to July 2002 was estimated at approximately $40 billion, including $10 billion for absenteeism and $30 billion for employees who were at work but impaired by pain ("presenteeism") [109].

On a per-patient basis, using estimates from a Workers' Compensation setting for chronic musculoskeletal disorders (≥ 4 months' duration), the average cost of disability compensation ranges $7,328–$36,790 [101]. Similarly, the estimated productivity losses, based on pre-injury earnings, ranges $12,547–$73,075 [101]. Both estimates have a range that depends on the duration of disability, from 4–8 months at the lower limit to > 18 months for the upper limit.

Estimates for the total cost (both direct and indirect) of CNCP and recurrent pain for adults in the US may exceed $600 billion annually [96]. Such estimates can be broken down by trying to identify costs associated with some of the most prevalent pain conditions. As noted, the societal costs of pediatric chronic pain are estimated to be $19.5 billion USD/year, exceeding costs of childhood asthma and obesity [98].

Back Pain

LBP is the third costliest medical condition in the United States, behind only diabetes and heart disease, and costs have been increasing at the second fastest rate over the past 10 years [110]. In 2010, chronic LBP was ranked as the condition with the highest number of years lived with disability (YLDs) and sixth in terms of disability-adjusted life years (DALYs) [111]. Chronic pain accounted for more than 2.3 million hospital inpatient stays were related to back problems in 2008. The overall costs for inpatient stays primarily for back problems was more than $9.5 billion accounting for nearly 3% of the total national hospital bill and making it the 9th most expensive condition treated in US hospitals [112].

Overall, LBP is estimated to be responsible for between $100 and $200 billion dollars a year in direct costs in the US [52]. Compared to a cohort of non-LBP patients, health care costs were significantly higher among chronic LBP patients with total direct medical costs estimated at $8,386 - $17,507, compared to $3,607 - $10,845 in the control group [113]. Health expenditures were estimated to have a total cost of $102 billion in the US [114]. Costs for spinal surgeries are substantial, some of which exceed $400,000 USD for the surgery alone [115].

Indirect costs for LBP add to the overall costs. In a study conducted over 20 years ago, back pain cases were estimated to result in a total of approximately 149 million lost work days [107]. These numbers have likely increased substantially during the ensuing years. Indirect costs related to employment and household activities were estimated to be between $7 billion and $20 billion [39, 108, 109]. LBP causes more years lived with disability than any other health condition [41].

Osteoarthritis

OA is one of the leading causes of disability in the US, impacting patient's activities of daily living [116]. The economic burden associated with OA is substantial. According to the US Bone and Joint Commission, the direct costs (i.e. medical expenditures) and indirect costs (i.e. lost earnings) of OA are $65 billion and $71 billion, respectively, totaling to $136 billion annually in the US alone [117]. In 2009, OA was the fourth most common cause of hospitalization, and the leading indication for joint replacement surgery, resulting in a cost of $42.3 billion driven by knee and hip replacement [118].

The estimated annual lost productive work time cost from arthritis in the US workforce was $10.3 billion, with 65.7% of the cost attributed to the 38% of workers with pain exacerbations [108]. Evidence from US National Survey data in 2010 found that aggregate annual absenteeism costs due to OA were $10.3 billion, which is substantial compared with other major chronic diseases)[119].

In a study of workers with OA, Xie et al. [120] estimated that the direct costs exceeded US $10,000 (e.g. medication) and Indirect costs (e.g. absenteeism) to vary from US$7,227 for mild OA pain, to US$29,935 for severe OA pain. Recently, the annual total healthcare costs and lost wages among adults with OA relative to those without OA were $17781 and $189 per person, respectively, resulting in estimated national excess costs of $45 billion and $1.7 billion, respectively [121].

Headache

According to the National Headache Foundation [122], chronic headaches account for losses of $50 billion a year to absenteeism and medical expenses and an excess of $4 billion spent on over-the-counter medications alone.

Absenteeism and presenteeism most commonly occur in migraineurs between 25 and 55 years old and contribute to the loss of $13 billion each year for employers in the US [57]; Migraine fact sheet [122].

Pelvic Pain

In the UK, care for women with pelvic pain was estimated to cost the National Health Service is estimated approximately £326 million based on indices from the hospital and community services index [123]. In the US, the total annual direct cost for physician visits and out-of-pocket cost was estimated to be US$2.8 billion in 1996 [71]. This is equivalent to US $5.68 billion currently according to the figures in the medical care component of the Consumer Price Index [124]. A study found that loss of work productivity in endometriosis was majorly driven by pelvic pain and disease severity [125]. This work productivity loss translated into substantial cost per woman per week of $4 in the US.

Mental Health

A number of studies have reported on the high comorbidity rate of pain and mental health problems (e.g. [126-128]). Epidemiological research has shown that the presence of chronic pain at baseline is significantly associated with higher rates of depressive symptoms and suicidal ideation and attempts at baseline and at 1-year follow-up [129,130]. For example, Kroenke et al. [131] reported that pain and depression co-occur with rates of 30% to 50% and Elman et al. [132] note that chronic pain is second only to bipolar disorder as a medical cause of suicide.

Perhaps the most commonly prescribed treatment of CNCP historically has been opioids. More recently, there have been concerns about the high prevalence of opioid misuse and addiction associated with prescriptions of opioids [133]. Individuals with concurrent chronic pain and opioid misuse are considered to be at high risk for opioid-related morbidity and mortality [134]. However, the current body of literature on concurrent chronic pain and opioid misuse presents a range of conflicting research on the prevalence, risk factors, and clinical management approaches specific to this growing sub-population.

Minozzi et al. [135] found a 0.5% incidence (range: 0%–24%) and 4.5% prevalence (range: 0%–31%) of opioid dependence syndrome (defined by DSM-IV or ICD-10 criteria) across 17 studies of patients receiving opioids for pain, whereas Chou et al. [136] found a prevalence of 3%–26% for opioid dependence among chronic pain patients prescribed long-term opioid therapy in primary care settings. Vowles et al. [137] sought to measure more precise estimates of problematic opioid use among adult CNCP patients by using more explicitly defined terms. The overall rate of problematic use across 38 studies ranged from <1% to 81%, with rates of misuse, abuse, and addiction ranging from 21%–29%, 8% (based on one study), and 8%–12%, respectively. In comparison, other reviews found ranges from 8%–16% for opioid misuse [136], 0.43%–8% for opioid abuse [136, 138] and 0.05%–14% for opioid addiction [136,138].

The cost estimates detailed above do not take into account the expenditures for medical and psychological treatments that are incurred by those with chronic pain and their significant others for mental health problems.

Conclusions

The estimated population prevalence of CNCP varies substantially, depending on the study. The wide range is a result of several factors (e.g. the population sampled, definition of CNCP by duration, body parts targeted, sampling methodology, phrasing of survey items and the survey response rate). Overall, the perpetuation of chronic painful disorders may exceed a total annual cost of $650 billion in the US, which includes direct costs associated with healthcare utilization as well as indirect costs associated with disability compensation losses in productivity, lost tax revenue and out-of- pocket expenses. Therefore, CNCP and recurrent pain have a significant impact on society, resulting in poorer quality of life for those afflicted, imposing substantially on the costs of healthcare and exacting societal costs in terms of disability compensation and productivity losses.

Chronic pain has multiple associated physical, psychological and social factors. The development of chronic pain has been related to a set of factors: namely, genetics, demographics (e.g. age, sex, ethnicity and cultural background, socioeconomic background, occupation and employment status), lifestyle and behavior (e.g. smoking, alcohol use, physical activity, nutrition, BMI, sleep), clinical factors (e.g. number of pain sites and location, comordibidites, mental health, surgical and medical history and interventions) and other factors (e.g. attitudes, beliefs, and expectations, history of abuse and trauma) [139]. Thus, epidemiological studies in the future might be more informative by using the more comprehensive, multidimensional IASP and AAPT classification.

References

1 Hing E, Cherry DK, Woodwell DA. (2006). *Advance Data from Vital Health Statistics: no. 374.* National Center for Health Statistics, Hyattsville, MD.

2 Porta M. (2014) *A Dictionary of Epidemiology*, 6th edition. Oxford University Press, Oxford.

3 Turk DC, Okifuji A. (2019) Pain terms and taxonomies of pain. In: Ballantyne J, Rathmell J, Fishman S, eds. *Bonica's Management of Pain, 5th edition*. Philadelphia: Lippincott, Williams & Wilkins, pp 11–23.

4 Treede RD, Rief W, Barke A *et al.* (2019) Chronic pain as a symptom or a disease: the IASP Classification of Chronic Pain for the International

Classification of Diseases (ICD-11). *Pain* **160(1)**: 19–27.

5 Headache Classification Subcommittee of the International Headache Society. (2004) The International Classification of Headache Disorders: 2nd edition. *Cephalalgia* **24(suppl 1)**:1–160.

6 Merskey H, Bogduk N. (1994) *Classification of Chronic Pain: Descriptions of Chronic Pain Syndromes and Definitions of Pain Terms.* 2nd ed. Seattle, WA: IASP Press.

7 Harden RN, Bruehl S, Stanton-Hicks M *et al.* (2007). Proposed new diagnostic criteria for complex regional pain syndrome. *Pain Med* **8**:326–31.

8 Spitzer WO, Skovron ML, Salmi LR *et al.* (1995) Scientific monograph of the Quebec Task Force on Whiplash-Associated Disorders: redefining "whiplash" and its management. *Spine (Phila Pa 1976)* **20(8)**(suppl):1S–73S.

9 Dworkin SF, LeResche L. (1992) Research diagnostic criteria for temporomandibular disorders: review, criteria, examinations and specifications, critique. *J Craniomandib Disord* **6**:301–55.

10 Schiffman E, Ohrbach R, Truelove E *et al.* (2014) Diagnostic criteria for temporomandibular disorders (DC/TMD) for clinical and dental research applications: recommendations of the International RDC/TMD Consortium Network and Orofacial Pain Special Interest Group. *J Oral Facial Pain Headache* **28**:6–27.

11 Fillingim RB, Bruehl S, Dworkin RH *et al.* (2014) The ACTTION-American Pain Society Pain Taxonomy (AAPT): an evidence-based and multidimensional approach to classifying chronic pain conditions. *J Pain* **15**:241–9.

12 Kent ML, Tighe PJ, Belfer I *et al.* (2017) The ACTTION-APS-AAPM Pain Taxonomy (AAAPT) multidimensional approach to classifying acute pain conditions. *J Pain* **18**:479–89.

13 Clauw DJ. (2015) Fibromyalgia and related conditions. *Mayo Clinic Proc* **90**:680–92.

14 Yunus MB. (2008) Central sensitivity syndromes: a new paradigm and group nosology for fibromyalgia and overlapping conditions, and the related issue of disease versus illness. *Semin Arthritis Rheum* **37**:339–52.

15 Goldberg DS, McGee SJ. (2011) Pain as a global public health priority. *BMC Public Health* **11**,770. https://doi.org/10.1186/1471-2458-11-770.

16 Langley PC. (2011) The prevalence, correlates and treatment of pain in the European Union. *Curr Med Res Opin* **272**:463–80.

17 Elzahaf RA, Tashani OA, Unsworth BA *et al.* (2012) The prevalence of chronic pain with an analysis of countries with a Human Development Index less than 0.9: a systematic review without meta-analysis. *Curr Med Res Opin* **28**:1221–9.

18 Hartvigsen J, Hancock MJ, Kongsted A *et al.*, on behalf of the Lancet Low Back Pain Series Working Group. (2018) What low back pain is and why we need to pay attention. *Lancet* **391(18)**:2356–67.

19 Nahin RL. Estimates of pain prevalence and severity in adults, United States, 2012. (2015) *J Pain* **16**:769–80.

20 Dahlhamer J, Lucas J, Zelaya C *et al.* (2018) Prevalence of chronic pain and high-impact chronic pain among adults—United States, 2016. *MMWR Morb Mortal Wkly Rep* **67**:1001–6.

21 Murray CJ, Vos T, Lozano R *et al.* (2012) Disability-adjusted life years (DALYs) for 291 diseases and injuries in 21 regions, 1990-2010: a systematic analysis for the Global Burden of Disease Study 2010. *Lancet* **380**:2197–223.

22 Pitcher MH, Von Korff M, Bushnell MC *et al.* (2019) Prevalence and profile of high–impact chronic pain in the United States. *J Pain* **20 (2)**:146–60.

23 Rusu RS, Vouthy K, Crowl AN *et al.* (2014) Cost of pain medication to treat adult patients with nonmalignant pain in the United States. *J Managed Care & Specialty Pharmacy* **20**:921–8.

24 Sauver JLS, Warner DO, Yawn BP *et al.* (2014) Why patients visit their doctors: assessing the most prevalent conditions in a defined American population. *Mayo Clinic Proceedings* **88(1)**:56–67.

25 Brinjikji W, Luetmer PH, Comstock B *et al.* (2014) Systematic literature review of imaging features of spinal degeneration in asymptomatic populations. *Spine (Phila Pa 1976)* **36**:811–16.

26 Maher C, Underwood M, Buchbinder R. (2017) Non-specific low back pain. *Lancet* **389**:736–47.

27 Farrell SF, Smith AD, Hancock MJ *et al.* (2019) Cervical spine findings on MRI in people with neck pain compared with pain-free controls: a systematic review and meta-analysis. *J Magn Reson Imaging* **49(6)**:1638–54.

28 Blythe FM, March LM, Cousins MJ. (2003) Chronic pain-related disability and use of analgesia and health services in a Sydney community. *Med J Austral* **179(2)**:84–7.

29 Child and Adolescent Health Measurement Initiative. 2016-2017. (2018) Data Resource Center on Child and Adolescent Health. *National Survey of Children's Health*. **2018**. Available at: www.childhealthdata.org/learn-about-the-nsch/NSCH. Accessed July 1, 2019.

30 Groenewald CB, Tham SW, Palermo TM. (2020) Impaired school functioning in children with chronic pain. National Perspective. *Clin J Pain* **36(9)**:693–9.

31 Huguet A, Miró J. (2006) The severity of chronic pediatric pain: an epidemiological study. *J Pain* **9**:226–36.

32 King S, Chambers CT, Huguet A *et al*. (2011) The epidemiology of chronic pain in children and adolescents revisited: a systematic review. *Pain* **152**:2729–38.

33 Roth-Isigkeit A, Thyen U, Stoven H *et al*. (2005) Pain among children and adolescents: restrictions in daily living and triggering factors. *Pediatrics* **115**:e152–e62

34 Hassett AL, Hilliard PE, Goesling J *et al*. (2013) Reports of chronic pain in childhood and adolescence among patients at a tertiary care pain clinic. *J Pain* **14**:1390–7.

35 Patel KV, Guralnik JM, Dansie EJ *et al*. (2013) Prevalence and impact of pain among older adults in the United States: findings from the 2011 National Health and Aging Trends Study. *Pain* **154(12)**:2649–57.

36 Clarke TC, Nahin RL, Barnes PM et al. (2016) Use of complementary health approaches for musculoskeletal pain disorders among adults: United States, 2012. *National Health Statistics Reports; no 98*. Hyattsville, MD: National Center for health Statistics.

37 Pleis JR, Lucas JW. (2009) Summary health statistics for U.S. Adults: National Health Interview Survey, 2007. National Center for Health Statistics. *Vital Health Stat* **10**:242.

38 Licciardone JC. (2008) The epidemiology and medical management of low back pain during ambulatory medical care visits in the United States. *Osteopath Med Primary Care* **2**:11.

39 Dagenais S, Caro J, Haldeman S. (2008) A systematic review of low back pain costs of illness studies in the United States and internationally. *Spine J* **8**:2–80.

40 Henschke N, Maher CG, Refshauge KM *et al*. (2008) Prognosis in patients with recent onset low back pain in Australian primary care: inception cohort study. *BMJ* **337**:1–7.

41 Vos T, Flaxman AD, Maghavi M *et al*. (2012) Years lived with disability (YLDs) for 1160 sequelae of 289 diseases and injuries1990-2010: a systematic analysis for the Global Burden of Disease Study 2010. *Lancet* **380**:2163–96.

42 McBeth J, Jones K. (2007) Epidemiology of chronic musculoskeletal pain. *Best Pract Res Clin Rheumatol* **21(3)**:403–25.

43 National Center for Health Statistics. (2006) *Health, United States, 2006 with Chartbook on Trends in the Health of Americans. National Center for Health Statistics*, Hyattsville, MD.

44 Von Korff M, Crane P, Lane M *et al*. (2005) Chronic spinal pain and physical-mental comorbidity in the United States: results from the national comorbidity survey replication. *Pain* **113(3)**:331–9.

45 Lawrence RC, Felson DT, Helmick CG *et al*. (2008) Estimates of the prevalence of arthritis and other rheumatic conditions in the United States, Part II. *Arthritis Rheumat* **58(1)**: 26–35.

46 Centers for Disease Control and Prevention. (2020) Osteoarthnritis. Retrieved from: https://www.cdc.gov/arthritis/basics/osteoarthritis.htm, September 24, 2020

47 Barbour KE, Helmick C, Boring M *et al*. (2017) Prevalence of doctor-diagnosed arthritis and arthritis-attributable activity limitation – United States, 2013-2015. *MMWR Morb Mortal Wkly Rep* **66**:246–53.

48 Helmick CG, Felson DT, Lawrence RC *et al*. for the National Arthritis Data Workgroup. (2008) Estimates of the prevalence of arthritis and other rheumatic conditions in the United States. Part I. *Arthritis Rheum* **58**:15–25.

49 Jafarzadeh SR, Felson DT. (2018) Updated estimates suggest a much higher prevalence of arthritis in United States adults than previous ones. *Arthritis Rheumatol* **70(2)**:185–92.

50 Litwic A, Edwards M, Dennison E *et al*. (2013) Epidemiology and burden of osteoarthritis. *Br Med Bull* **105**:185–99.

51 Maiese K, (2016) Picking a bone with WISP1 (CCN4): new atrategies gainst degenerative joint disease. *J Transl Sci* **1(3)**:83–5.

52 Ma VY, Chan L, Carruthers KJ. (2014) Incidence, prevalence, costs, and impact on disability of common conditions requiring rehabilitation in the United States: stroke, spinal cord injury, traumatic brain injury, multiple sclerosis, osteoarthritis, rheumatoid arthritis, limb loss, and back pain. *Arch Phys Med Rehabil* **95(5)**:986–95.e1.

53 World Health Organization. (2016) Headache Disorders. *Fact Sheet*. Geneva, Switzerland: WHO.

54 Rissoli P, Mullaly WJ. (2018) Headache. *Am J Med* **131(1)**:17–24.

55 Landy SH, Runken MC, Bell CF *et al*. (2011) Assessing the impact of migraine onset on work productivity. *J Occup Environ Med* **53**:74–81.

56 Stovner LJ, Hagen K, Jensen R *et al*. (2007) The global burden of headache: a documentation of headache prevalence and disability worldwide. *Cephalalgia* **27**:193–210.

57 Robbins MS, Lipton RB. (2010) The epidemiology of primary headache disorders. *Semin Neurol* **30**:107–19.

58 Burch RC, Loder S, Loder E *et al*. (2015) The prevalence and burden of migraine and severe headache in the United States: updated statistics from government health surveillance studies. *Headache* **55(1)**:21–34.

59 National Headache Foundation. (2004) Chicago, Ill.

60 Sheffield RE. (1998) Migraine prevalence: a literature review. *Headache* **38(8)**:595–601.

61 Buse DC, Manack AN, Fanning K *et al*. (2012) Chronic migraine prevalence, disability, and sociodemographic factors: results from the American Migraine Prevalence and Prevention Study. *Headache* **52(10)**:1456–70.

62 Minen MT, Tanev K, Friedman BW. (2014) Evaluation and treatment of migraine in the emergency department: a review. *Headache* **54**:1131–45.

63 Treede RD, Jensen TS, Campbell JN *et al*. (2008) Neuropathic pain: redefinition and a grading system for clinical and research purposes. *Neurology* **70**:1630–5.

64 Smith BH, Hebert HL, Veluchamy A. (2020) Neuropathic pain in the community: prevalence, impact, and risk factors. *Pain* **161 (Suppl 1)**:S127–S37.

65 Torrance N, Smith BH, Bennett MI *et al*. (2006) The epidemiology of chronic pain of predominantly neuropathic origin. Results from a general population survey. *J Pain* **7**:281–9.

66 Bouhassira D, Lanteri-Minet M, Attal N *et al*. (2008) Prevalence of chronic pain with neuropathic characteristics in the general population. *PAIN* **136**:380–7.

67 Van Hecke O, Austin SK, Khan RA *et al*. (2014) Neuropathic pain in the general population: a systematic review of epidemiological studies. *PAIN* **155**:654–62.

68 Rayment C, Hjermstad MJ, Aass N *et al*. (2013) Neuropathic cancer pain: prevalence, severity, analgesics and impact from the European Palliative Care Research Collaborative-Computerised Symptom Assessment study. *Palliat Med* **27**:714–21.

69 Howard FM. (2003) The role of laparoscopy in the chronic pelvic pain patient. *Clinical Obstet Gynecol* **46**:749–66.

70 Mathias SD, Kuppermann M, Liberman RF *et al*. (1996) Chronic pelvic pain: prevalence, health-related quality of life, and economic correlates. *Obstet Gynecol* **87**:321–27.

71 Leserman J, Zolnoun D, Meltzer-Brody S *et al*. (2006) Identification of diagnostic subtypes of chronic pelvic pain and how subtypes differ in health status and trauma history. *Am J Obstet Gynecol* **195(2)**:554–60.

72 Coelho L, Brito L, Chein M *et al*. (2014) Prevalence and conditions associated with chronic pelvic pain in women from São Luís, Brazil. *Braz J Med Bio Res* **47(9)**:818–25.

73 ACOG Committee on Practice B. ACOG Practice Bulletin No. 51. (2003) Chronic pelvic pain. *Obstet. Gynecol.* **103(3)**:589–605.

74 Garcia-Perez H, Harlow SD, Erdmann CA *et al*. (2010) Pelvic pain and associated characteristics among women in northern Mexico. *Int Perspect Sex Reprod Health* **36(2)**,90–8.

75 Grace VM, Zondervan KR. (2004) Chronic pelvic pain in New Zealand: prevalence, pain severity, diagnoses and use of the health services. *Aust NZ J Public Health* **28(4)**:369–75.

76 Latthe P, Mignini L, Gray R *et al*. (2006) Factors predisposing women to chronic pelvic pain: systematic review. *BMJ* **332(7544)**:749–55.

77 Loving S, Thomsen T, Jaszczak P *et al*. (2014) Female chronic pelvic pain is highly prevalent in

Denmark. A cross-sectional population-based study with randomly selected participants. *Scand J Pain* **5(2)**: 93–101.

78 Liu F, Steinkeler A. (2013) Epidemiology, diagnosis, and treatment of temporomandibular disorders. *Dent Clin North Am* **57(3)**:465.

79 Maixner W, Diatchenko L, Dubner R *et al.* (2011) Orofacial pain prospective evaluation and risk assessment study--the OPPERA study. *J Pain* **12**:T4–11.e1-e2.

80 Slade GD. (2014) Epidemiology of temporomandibular joint disorders and related painful conditions. *Mol Pain* **10 (Suppl 1)**. doi: 10.1186/1744-8069-10-S1-O16

81 Isong U, Gansky SA, Plesh O. (2008) Temporomandibular joint and muscle disorder-type pain in US adults: The National Health Interview Survey. *J Orofac Pain* **22(3)**:317–22.

82 Adams LM, Turk DC. (2018) Central sensitization and the biopsychosocial approach to understanding pain. *J Appl Biobehavioral Res* **11(3)**:218–32.

83 Treede RD, Rief W, Barke A *et al.* (2015) A classification of chronic pain for the *ICD-11*. *Pain* **156**:1003–7.

84 Yunus MB. (2007). Role of central sensitization in symptoms beyond muscle pain, and the evaluation of a patient with widespread pain. *Best Pract. Res. Clin. Rheumatol.* **21(3)**:481–97.

85 Yunus MB. (2015). An update on central sensitivity syndromes and the issues of nosology and psychobiology. *Curr Rheumatol Rev* **11(2)**: 70–85.

86 Beasley M, Macfarlane GJ. (2014). Chronic widespread pain versus multi-site pain: does the distribution matter? *Arthritis Rheumatol* **66**:S908–09.

87 Woolf CJ. (2011) Central sensitization: implications for the diagnosis and treatment of pain. *Pain* **152(3 Suppl)**:S2–S15.

88 Turk DC, Fillingim RB, Ohrbach R et al. (2016) Assessment of psychosocial and functional impact of chronic pain. *J Pain* **17(9 Suppl)**:T21–49.

89 Raja SN, Carr DB, Cohen M *et al.* (2020) The revised International Association for the Study of Pain definition of pain: concepts, challenges, and compromises. *Pain.* **161**:1976–82.

90 Turk DC, Monarch ES. (2018) Biopsychosocial perspective on chronic pain. In: Turk DC, Gatchel RJ, eds. *Psychological Approaches to Pain Management: A Practitioner's Handbook*, 3rd edn. Guilford, New York. pp. 3–24.

91 Bartley EJ, Fillingim RB. (2013) Sex differences in pain: a brief review of clinical and experimental findings. *Br J Anaesth* **111(1)**:52–8.

92 Gureje O, Simon GE, Von Korff M. (2001) A cross-national study of the course of persistent pain in primary care. *Pain* **92(1–2)**:195–200.

93 White LA, Robinson RL, Yu AP *et al.* (2009) Comparison of health care use and costs in newly diagnosed and established patients with fibromyalgia. *J Pain* **10(9)**:976–83.

94 Fishbain DA, Rosomoff HL, Cutler RB *et al.* (1995) Secondary gain concept: a review of the scientific evidence. *Clin J Pain* **11(1)**:6–21.

95 Hashemi L, Webster BS, Clancy EA *et al.* (1997) Length of disability and cost of workers' compensation low back pain claims. *J Occup Environ Med* **39(10)**:937–45.

96 Gaskin DJ, Richard P. (2012) The economic costs of pain in the United States. *J Pain* **13(8)**:715–74.

97 Institute of Medicine (US) Committee on Advancing Pain Research, Care, and Education. (2011). *Relieving pain in America: A Blueprint for Transforming Prevention, Care, Education, and Research.* National Academies Press, Washington, D.C.

98 Groenewald CB, Essner BS, Wright D, et al. (2014) The economic costs of chronic pain among a cohort of treatment-seeking adolescents in the United States. *J Pain* **15(9)**:925–33.

99 Center for Diseasse Control and Prevention. (2009) Prevalence and most common causes of disability among adults – United States, 2005. *MMWR Mor Mortal Wkly Rep* **58**:421–6

100 Gureje O, Von Korff M, Simon GE *et al.* (1998) Persistent pain and well-being: a World Health Organization Study in Primary Care. *JAMA* **280(2)**:147–51.

101 Theodore BR. (2009) Cost-effectiveness of early versus delayed functional restoration for chronic disabling occupational musculoskeletal disorders. *Dissertation Abstracts International* **B 70/05** (Publication Number: AAT 3356104).

102 Stagnitti MN. (2006) The top five therapeutic classes of outpatient prescription drugs ranked by total expense for adults age 18 and older in

the US civilian non-institutionalized population, 2004. Statistical Brief 154. Agency for Healthcare Research and Quality.

103 Rasu RS, Vouthy K, Crowl AN *et al.* (2014) Cost of pain medication to treat adult patients with nonmalignant chronic pain in the United States. *J Manag Care Spec Pharm* **20**:921–8.

104 Deyo RA, Gray DT, Kreuter W, *et al.* (2005) United States trends in lumbar fusion surgery for degenerative conditions. *Spine (Phila Pa 1976)* **30(12)**:1441–5; discussion 1446–7.

105 Gupta A, Mehdi A, Duwell MA *et al.* (2010) Evidence-based review of the pharmacoeconomics related to the management of chronic nonmalignant pain. *J Pain Palliat Care Pharmacother* **24**:152–6.

106 Katz JN. (2006) Lumbar disc disorders and low back pain: socioeconomic factors and consequences. *JBJS* **88-A** (**Suppl 2**): 21–4

107 Guo HR, Tanaka S, Halperin WE *et al.* (1999) Back pain prevalence in US industry and estimates of lost workdays. *Am J Public Health* **89(7)**:1029–35.

108 Ricci JA, Stewart WF, Chee E *et al.* (2005) Pain exacerbation as a major source of lost productive time in US workers with arthritis. *Arthritis Rheum* **53(5)**:673–81.

109 Stewart WF, Ricci JA, Chee E *et al.* (2003) Lost productive time and cost due to common pain conditions in the US workforce. *JAMA* **290(18)**:2443–54.

110 Dieleman JL, Baral R, Birger M *et al.* (2016) US spending on personal health care and public health 1996-2013. *JAMA* **316**:2627–46.

111 Hoy D, March L, Brooks P et al. (2014) The global burden of low back pain: estimates from AHRQ Healthcare Cost and utilization Project. http://www.hcup-us.ahrq.gov/reports/statbriefs/sb105.jsp 2011. (accessed May 24, 2011).

112 Gore M, Sadosky A, Stacey BR *et al.* (2012). The burden of chronic low back pain: clinical comorbidities, treatment patterns, and health care costs in usual care settings. *Spine* **37(11)**:E668–77.

113 Shmagel A, Foley R, Ibrahim H. (2016) Epidemiology of chronic low back pain in US adults: National Health and Nutrition Examination Survey 2009–2010. *Arthritis Care Res* **68(11)**:1688–94.

114 Jain NB, Ayers GD, Fan R *et al.* (2018) Predictors of pain and functional outcomes after operative treatment for rotator cuff tears. *J Shoulder Elbow Surg* **27**:1393–400.

115 Neogi T. (2013) The epidemiology and impact of pain in osteoarthritis. *Osteoarthritis Cartilage* **21(9)**:1145–53.

116 *United States Bone and Joint Initiative. The Burden of Musculoskeletal Diseases in the United States (BMUS). In: In. Fourth ed. Rosemont, IL. 2018: Available at* https://www.boneandjointburden.org/fourth-edition. Accessed on November 8, 2020

117 Murphy L, Helmick CG. (2012) The impact of osteoarthritis in the United States: a population-health perspective. *Am J Nursing* **112(3 Suppl 1)**:S13–9.

118 Kotlarz H, Gunnarsson CL, Fang H *et al.* (2009) Insurer and out-of-pocket costs of osteoarthritis in the US: evidence from national survey data. *Arthritis Rheum* **60**:3546–53.

119 Xie F, Kovic B, Jin X *et al.* (2016) Economic and humanistic burden of osteoarthritis: a systematic review of large sample studies. *PharmacoEconomics* **34**:1087–100.

120 Zhao X, Shah S, Ghandi K *et al.* (2019) Clinical, humanistic, and economic burden of osteoarthritis among noninstitutionalized adults in the United States. *Osteoarthr. Cartilage* **27(11)**:1618–26.

121 Migraine fact sheet [Migraine Research Foundation web site].2012. Available at: http://www.migraineresearchfoundation.org/fact-sheet.html. Accessed May 1, 2014.

122 Curtis L. (2014) *Unit Costs of Health and Social Care 2014. Personal Social Services Research Unit,* University of Kent, Kent, UK. www.pssru.ac.uk/project-pages/unit-costs/2014/index.php

123 Ayorinde AA, Macfarlane GJ, Saraswat L *et al.* (2012). Chronic pelvic pain in women: an epidemiological perspective. *Womens Health* **11(6)**:851–64.

124 Nnoaham KE, Hummelshoj L, Webster P *et al.* (2011) Impact of endometriosis on quality of life and work productivity: a multicenter study across ten countries. *Fertil Steril* **96(2)**:366–73.

125 Bair MJ, Robinson RL, Katon W, et al. (2003) Depression and pain comorbidity: a literature review. *Arch Intern Med* **163**:2433–45.
126 Asmundson GJG, Katz, J. (2009) Understanding the co-ocurrence of anxiety disorders and chronic pain: state-of –the-art. *Depression & Anxiety* **26(10)**:888–901.
127 Racine M. (2017) Chronic pain and suicide risk: a comprehensive review. *Prog Neuropsychopharmacol Biol Psychiatry* **87(B)**:169–280.
128 van Tilburg MAL, Spence NJ, Whitehead WE *et al.* (2011) Chronic pain in adolescents is associated with suicidal thoughts and behaviors. *J Pain* **12**:1032–9.
129 Koenig J, Oelkers-Ax R, Parzer P *et al.* (2015) The association of self-injurious behaviour and suicide attempts with recurrent idiopathic pain in adolescents: evidence from a population based study. *Child Adolesc Psychiatry Ment Health* **9**:1–9.
130 Kroenke K, Wu J, Bair MJ *et al.* (2011) Reciprocal relationship between pain and depression: a 12-month longitudinal analysis in primary care. *J Pain* **12**:964–73.
131 Elman I, Borsook D, Volkow ND. (2013) Pain and suicidality: insights from reward and addiction neuroscience. *Progress in Neurobiology* **109**:1–27.
132 Voon P, Karamouzian M, Kerr T. (2017) Chronic pain and opioid misuse: a review of reviews. *Subst Abuse Treat Prev Policy* **12(1)**:36
133 Dowell D, Haegerich TM, Chou R. (2016) CDC guideline for prescribing opioids for chronic pain United States, 2016. *MMWR Recomm Rep* **65**:1–49.
134 Minozzi S, Amato L, Davoli M. (2013) Development of dependence following treatment with opioid analgesics for pain relief: a systematic review. *Addiction* **108**:688–98.
135 Chou R, Turner JA, Devine EB *et al.* (2015). The effectiveness and risks of long-term opioid therapy for chronic pain: a systematic review for a National Institutes of Health pathways to prevention workshop. *Ann Intern Med* **162**:276–86.
136 Vowles KE, McEntee ML, Julnes PS *et al.* (2015) Rates of opioid and data synthesis. *Pain* **156**:569–76.
137 Noble M, Tregear SJ, Treadwell JR *et al.* (2008) Long-term opioid therapy for chronic noncancer pain: a systematic review and meta-analysis of efficacy and safety. *J Pain Symptom Manag* **35**:214–28.
138 Mills SEE, Nicholson KP, Smith BH. (2019) Chronic pain: a review of its epidemiology and associated factors in population-based studies. *BJA* **123**:e273–e83.

Chapter 3

Basic mechanisms and pathophysiology

Muhammad Saad Yousuf[1], Allan I. Basbaum[2], & Theodore J. Price[1]

[1] *Center for Advanced Pain Studies, School of Behavioral and Brain Sciences, University of Texas at Dallas, Dallas, Texas, USA*
[2] *Department of Anatomy, University of California at San Francisco. San Francisco, California, USA*

Introduction

The ability to experience pain is essential for survival and wellbeing and the pathological consequences of the inability to experience pain are particularly well-illustrated by the extensive injuries experienced by children with congenital insensitivity to pain [1]. On the other hand, the need for better pain relief therapeutics is urgent and, in particular for chronic pain, has been a contributing factor to the international opioid crisis [2]. The neural basis of pain processing, including afferent fibers (nociceptors) that respond to injury, and the circuits engaged by these afferents, not only generate reflex withdrawal to injury, but also provide a protective function following tissue or nerve injury. These pain sensitizing mechanisms following an injury promote tissue repair and enhance evolutionary fitness of an organism [3, 4]. In these situations, neurons in the pain processing circuitry become sensitized such that normally innocuous stimuli are perceived as painful (allodynia), and normally noxious stimuli are perceived as even more painful (hyperalgesia). The sensitization process is presumably an adaptive response, in that it promotes protective guarding of an injured area. In some cases, however, sensitization can be long-lasting, leading to the establishment of chronic pain syndromes. In this situation, the sensitization outlives its usefulness, persisting well after the acute injury has resolved. In these pathological, often debilitating conditions, aberrant plasticity in pain circuitry establishes a maladaptive condition in which pain no longer serves as an acute warning system.

The ability to prevent or treat such conditions is critically dependent upon a comprehensive understanding of the basic mechanisms through which pain signals are generated by nociceptors, how this information is transmitted to the central nervous system (CNS) as well as how the CNS modulates incoming nociceptive information. In this chapter, we focus on the molecules and cell types that underlie normal pain sensation, with specific emphasis on the nociceptor and on second order neurons in the spinal cord. We also discuss how these circuits are altered following tissue or nerve injury and in persistent pain states.

Primary afferent neurons

The detection of somatosensory stimuli is initiated by primary sensory neurons that have their cell bodies in the trigeminal (TG) and dorsal root ganglia (DRG). These pseudo-unipolar neurons extend an efferent branch that innervates peripheral target tissues, and a central afferent branch that targets the spinal cord dorsal horn or medullary nucleus caudalis (for trigeminal afferents). Primary afferents that innervate somatic tissue are traditionally classified

Clinical Pain Management: A Practical Guide, Second Edition. Edited by Mary E. Lynch, Kenneth D. Craig, and Philip W. Peng.

into three categories: Aβ, Aδ and C fibers, based on axon diameter, degree of myelination, and conduction velocity. These physiological differences are associated with distinct functional contributions to somatosensation. The largest diameter cell bodies give rise to myelinated Aβ fibers that rapidly conduct nerve impulses and detect innocuous mechanical stimulation. In contrast, noxious thermal, mechanical, and chemical stimuli are detected by medium diameter, thinly myelinated Aδ fibers, and by small diameter, unmyelinated C fibers. These latter two groups constitute the nociceptors and represent a dedicated system for the detection of stimuli capable of causing tissue damage, as they are only excited when stimulus intensities reach the noxious range [5]. The Aδ nociceptors mediate the fast, pricking sensation of "first pain," and the C fibers convey information leading to the sustained, often burning quality of "second pain". Another lesser-known class of C fibers are C-low threshold mechanoreceptors (C-LTMRs) that innervate hairy skin and are typically associated with affective aspects of touch. The contribution of C-LTMRs to pain modulation has only recently come to light [6, 7].

Nociceptor subtypes

Electrophysiology studies have identified two main classes of Aδ nociceptor. The first class is readily activated by intense mechanical stimulation. These neurons are relatively unresponsive to short duration, noxious heat stimulation, but respond more robustly to extended periods of heat stimulation [8]. The second class is insensitive to mechanical stimulation but is robustly activated by heat [8]. The majority of C-fiber nociceptors show polymodal response properties. They are activated by multiple modalities of painful stimuli, including thermal, chemical and mechanical. Although rarer, modality-specific (e.g. exclusively heat-responsive) C fibers also exist. These molecularly defined C-fiber subtypes make functionally distinct contributions to the detection of noxious stimuli of different modalities [9].

Recent advances in RNA sequencing-based transcriptomics, largely in mice, have further delineated sensory neurons into at least 11 different subtypes based on their unique RNA expression profiles [10] (Figure 3.1). These neurons are further grouped into 4 main categories consisting of large diameter

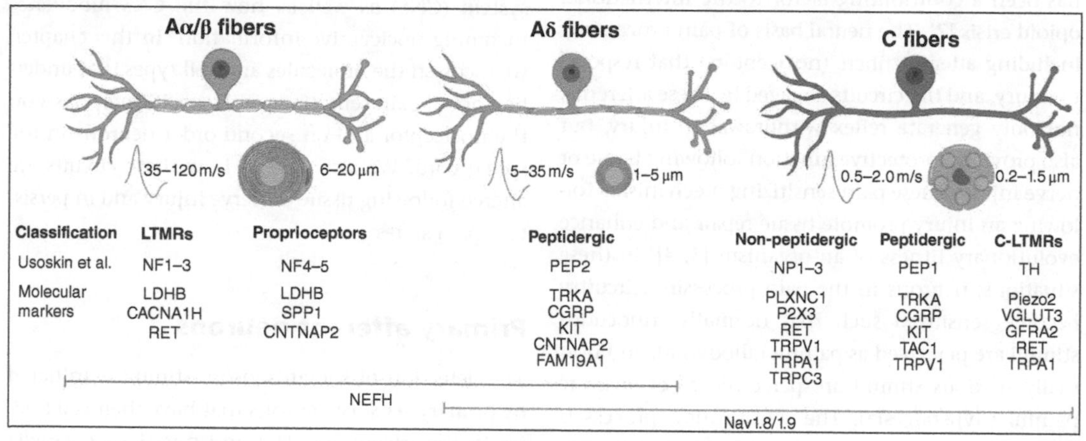

Figure 3.1 Primary sensory neuron characteristics. Primary sensory neurons are categorized based on their conduction velocity, degree of myelination and thickness of their axons and cell bodies. While the axons of Aα/β large-diameter and Aδ medium-diameter neurons are thickly and thinly myelinated, respectively, C fibres are unmyelinated and supported by Schwann cells organized in Remak bundles. Recent single cell RNA sequencing by Usoskin, Furlan [10] has revealed 11 sensory neuronal subtypes based on their molecular composition. Aα/β fibres are classified as low-threshold mechanoreceptors (LTMRs) and proprioceptors. Nociceptors (Aδ and C fibres) are further grouped by whether they produce neuropeptides (peptidergic), like calcitonin-gene related peptide (CGRP), or not (non-peptidergic). C-low threshold mechanoreceptors (C-LTMRs), a special class of C fibres, are involved in non-noxious, affective touch and are characterized by their expression of tyrosine hydroxylase. Myelinated fibres (Aα/β and Aδ) express the heavy neurofilament polypeptide (NEFH). Nociceptors (Aδ and C) are characterized by the presence of voltage-gated sodium channels 1.8 and 1.9 (Nav1.8/1.9). Other molecular markers are summarized (Color Plate 1).

myelinated afferents that express the 200kD neurofilament protein (NEFH), peptidergic afferents that express neuropeptides [including calcitonin gene-related peptide (CGRP)], non-peptidergic afferents that lack neuropeptides and bind the isolectin B4 (IB4) and tyrosine hydroxylase-expressing C-LTMRs. Additional characteristics of these sensory neurons are presented in Figure 3.1. Single cell sequencing and other cellular characterization methods are now being used in non-human primate [11] and human DRG studies [12]. Importantly, molecular identification of sensory neuron subtypes in mice has enabled identification of genetic tools to elucidate cell-type specific functions in the behaving animal. These experimental tools should provide powerful insights into conserved, and divergent, functions of genes in nociceptors, across species and should also improve target identification and validation for clinical translation.

Nociceptors and noxious stimulus detection

The peripheral terminal of the nociceptor is specialized to detect and transduce noxious stimuli. This process depends on the presence of specific ion channels and receptors at the peripheral terminal (Figure 3.2). Among these are the acid-sensing ion channels (ASICs), purinergic P2X receptors, voltage-gated sodium, calcium and potassium channels and the transient receptor potential (TRP) family of ion channels [8, 13]. Notably, many of these molecules are uniquely or preferentially expressed in nociceptors, compared to other parts of the nervous system.

The activation thresholds of several peripheral receptors closely match the psychophysical demarcation between the perception of innocuous and noxious thermal stimuli. For example, the heat pain threshold in humans, which rests around 43°C, matches the activation threshold for the sensory ion channel, TRPV1, and mice lacking TRPV1 exhibit deficits in cellular and behavioral responses to noxious heat [13]. In addition, several other receptors contribute to the detection of noxious thermal stimuli, including TRPV2, TRPV3, TRPV4 and TRPM2 ion channels [13].

Cold sensitive neurons are a mix of low-threshold and high-threshold thermoreceptors, each of which respond to a gradient of cool temperatures from mild to extreme. Low-threshold cold-sensitive neurons are tonically active and respond to cooler temperatures by increasing their firing frequency. On the contrary, high threshold cold-sensitive neurons are only active in the noxious temperature range, below about 20°C. At subzero temperatures all nociceptors, even cold-insensitive ones, fire action potentials, possibly due to tissue damage. TRPM8, an ion channel sensitive to menthol, is activated by temperatures below 20°C, and mice lacking this receptor show a drastic reduction in their responses to a range of cool and cold temperatures [14]. More importantly, TRPM8 knockout animals still have preserved sensitivity to noxious cold stimuli suggesting that another cold-sensitive channel may also contribute to discriminating painful cold stimuli. As such, TRPA1 is activated at temperatures below 10°C in recombinant assays and may further encode noxious cold sensation [14]. However, there remains a debate as to whether TRPA1, which responds to a host of irritants, is a genuine cold receptor.

Several candidate receptors have been proposed to underlie the transduction of mechanical stimuli. Rapidly adapting neurons have a low threshold to mechanical stimulation and are involved in innocuous touch and proprioception. Mechano-sensitive nociceptors, however, include rapidly, moderately and slowly adapting currents with high activation thresholds, allowing them to encode noxious stimuli. Various members of the degenerin/ epithelial Na^+ channel (DEG/ENaC) families, the TRP family (e.g. TRPV2, TRPV4 and TRPA1), and the Piezo family (Piezo1 and Piezo2) have been implicated in mechanonociception. Piezos are the most important family of mechanically-gated channels in the mammalian genome. Piezo2 is predominantly expressed in the sensory nervous system and is gated by mechanical stimulation following gentle touch [15]. Its contribution to mechanical allodynia has only recently been described. Notably, individuals with loss-of-function mutations in the Piezo2 channel fail to develop mechanical allodynia following skin inflammation; however, their sensitivity to noxious mechanical stimulation is preserved [16, 17]. TACAN was recently identified as a mechanically-activated ion channel that is encoded by the *Tmem120A* gene [18]. This mechanically-activated channel is expressed in nociceptors and may be involved in mechanical hyperalgesia [18, 19].

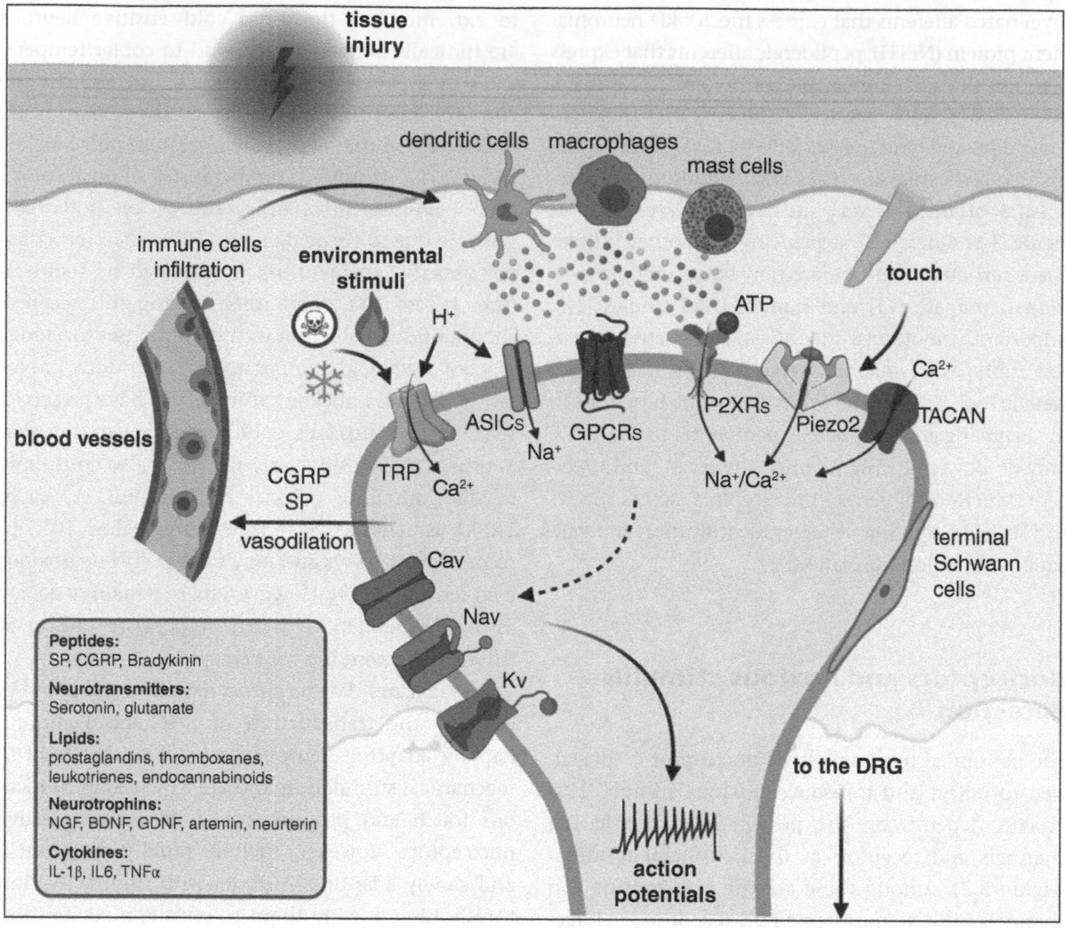

Figure 3.2 Primary afferent terminals. The sensory afferent terminal preferentially responds to a plethora of stimuli using a panoply of receptors and ion channels. Heat, cold and chemical toxins are encoded by Ca^{2+}-permeable transient receptor potential (TRP) channels such as TRPV1, TRPM8, and TRPA1. Low pH (pH<6) is also known to activate acid-sensing ion channels (ASICs). Purinergic receptors, particularly P2X receptors, respond to extracellular ATP usually released in response to an inflammatory insult. Recent characterization of pressure-sensitive receptors has identified Piezo2 and TACAN channels as selective mechanosensors important for the development of mechanical allodynia and hyperalgesia. More recently, a class of Schwann cells that transduce tactile nociception were discovered to ensheathe free nerve endings [86]. Tissue injury and inflammation causes the release of various factors that enhance the activity of nerve fibres and promote sensitization. These factors are summarized in the figure (Color Plate 2).

Noxious chemical stimuli activate a range of receptors found in nociceptor terminals. Among these are the ASICs and ATP-responsive purinergic receptors, which may be especially relevant in the setting of tissue injury (where pH changes and ATP release are common). Some TRP channels (e.g. TRPV1) are also regulated by pH and many are targets of plant-derived irritants, including capsaicin (TRPV1), menthol (TRPM8) and the pungent ingredients in mustard and garlic plants (TRPA1). TRPA1 also responds to a host of environmental irritants [20]. Undoubtedly there are endogenous chemical mediators that activate the different TRP channel subtypes. These mediators may be especially critical in the setting of injury to visceral tissue, the afferent innervation of which is not accessible to exogenous chemical or intense thermal stimuli.

Finally, nociceptors have recently been implicated in host defense. These neurons respond directly to bacterial infection through mechanisms that can be mediated directly by bacterial factors that form pores in nociceptor membranes or through direct actions of bacterial mediators on host receptors [21, 22]. An excellent example of the latter is sulfolipid-1 a product of the tuberculosis pathogen that evokes cough through a direct action on nociceptors [23]. Nociceptors also respond to type I interferons, which are rapidly produced in response to viral infection [24]. Moreover, the activation of nociceptor nerve endings leads to the release of CGRP and substance P (SP) that then promote neurogenic inflammation. CGRP functions as a vasodilator and SP causes vascular leakiness both of which ultimately promote immune infiltration. Therefore, nociceptors are clearly important contributors in the response to infection.

Conduction of nociceptive signals

Nociceptors express a panoply of voltage-gated ion channel subtypes. Among these are the sensory neuron-specific sodium channels Nav1.8 and 1.9, which, along with the more broadly expressed sodium channel Nav1.7, contribute to the generation and transduction of action potentials in nociceptors [1, 25]. A pivotal role for Nav1.7 in nociception has been demonstrated by the report that loss-of-function mutations of this channel in humans lead to the inability to detect painful stimuli, while gain-of-function mutations lead to disorders characterized by intense burning pain [1, 25]. Mice lacking Nav1.7 fail to develop pain hypersensitivity to noxious heat, mechanical and chemical (e.g. formalin) stimuli [1]. Furthermore, these animals are unaffected by complete Freund's adjuvant treatment, suggesting that inflammatory pain relies on Nav1.7-mediated spike generation. Interestingly, deleting Nav1.7 in Nav1.8-positive sensory neurons prevents the development of mechanical allodynia but not heat hypersensitivity [1]. Particularly provocative is the recent report that the loss of function after NaV1.7 deletion occurs concomitantly with a naloxone-reversible increase in enkephalin-mediated inhibitory controls in the dorsal horn [26, 27].

With over 20 different K^+ channels coupled with a plethora of auxiliary subunits, K^+ channels have versatile electrophysiology properties that are integral to the falling phase of the action potential [28]. Following nerve injury, K^+ currents are typically attenuated, which accommodate persistent action potential generation. The KCNQ type of potassium channel produces M-currents that determine the repolarization time of nociceptors [28]. Importantly, many inflammatory mediators, including interleukin 1β, can modulate these K^+ currents in nociceptors resulting in an increase overall excitability and neurotransmitter release [28].

Once an action potential invades the central terminal of a nociceptor, neurotransmitter release is evoked via the activation of N-, P/Q- and T-type voltage-gated calcium channels. Although glutamate is the predominant, if not the obligatory, excitatory neurotransmitter in all nociceptors, many nociceptors co-release release substance P (SP) and CGRP [8]. Receptors for these neurotransmitters, including N-methyl-D-aspartic acid (NMDA) and α-amino-3-hydroxy-5-methyl-4-isoxazolepropionic acid (AMPA) receptors for glutamate, neurokinin 1 receptors for SP and CGRP receptors, are located in appropriate regions of the spinal cord dorsal horn, and mediate the postsynaptic response to primary afferent activation [29].

Organization of the "pain system"

The afferent terminal

Nociceptors not only transmit pain messages, centrally to the spinal cord, but also release a variety of molecules from their peripheral terminals. These molecules (e.g. the neuropeptides SP and CGRP) influence the local tissue environment by acting on blood vessels and other cells to cause vasodilatation and plasma extravasation, key features of neurogenic inflammation (Figure 3.2). Neurogenic inflammation alters the extracellular milieu of the peripheral terminals of nociceptors, which can sensitize the nociceptor to subsequent stimulation. It is now understood that these sensory neuropeptides are also involved in immune responses to infection [30, 31] and in immunological tissue homeostasis [32] (Figure 3.2). In addition to detecting noxious insults, nociceptors likely play a key homeostatic role that contributes to overall fitness.

The biochemical complexity of nociceptor subtypes is paralleled by their distinct peripheral innervation patterns. For example, some markers delineate populations of nociceptors whose peripheral innervation is restricted to particular tissues. Thus, nociceptors that express the Mrgprd subtype of G-protein coupled receptor innervate skin, but not visceral organs [33, 34]. Interestingly, these Mrgprd+ neurons in the trigeminal ganglion innervate the meninges of the brain, a specialized tissue that protects the brain and forms the blood brain barrier [35].

Central projections of nociceptors

The central branches of primary afferents terminate in the dorsal horn of the spinal cord, which is classically divided into six parallel laminae, based on cytoarchitectural grounds [29]. Neurons in lamina III and IV are innervated by myelinated fibers that respond to innocuous touch (Figure 3.3). In contrast, neurons in laminae I, II and V receive inputs from nociceptive afferents and are therefore important relays in the transmission of pain-related information, both locally and via projection neurons of laminae I and V that target the brain [29]. Lamina VI neurons receive input from muscle. Recent single-cell RNA sequencing experiments have identified 15 inhibitory and 15 excitatory neuronal subtypes in the dorsal horn, revealing a diverse, heterogeneous population of spinal neurons [36].

The remarkable stratification of spinal cord inputs is further demonstrated by the distinct projection patterns of Aδ and C-fiber nociceptors (Figure 3.3). Lamina I spinal cord neurons are innervated by both Aδ and C fibers. Consistent with this input, the majority of neurons in lamina I are selectively activated by noxious stimuli and are thus referred to as nociceptive-specific neurons. Lamina I also contains so-called wide dynamic range (WDR) neurons, which receive convergent monosynaptic input from nociceptors and polysynaptic input from non-nociceptive fibers. Neurons that appear to encode selectively innocuous sensations such as cooling, itch and sensual touch are also found in lamina I [37, 38]. Although most lamina I neurons are interneurons that are engaged in local dorsal horn circuits, a small but critical number (~10%) are projection neurons that directly access pain processing centers in the brain [29].

Lamina II predominantly contains nociresponsive interneurons and can be further subdivided into outer (IIo) and inner (IIi) regions, which respectively receive inputs from peptidergic and non-peptidergic afferents, at least in rodents (Figure 3.3). In the human spinal cord, the distinction between peptidergic and non-peptidergic afferent terminals is less clear, likely because peptidergic markers are more broadly expressed in the human DRG [39]. The most ventral part of lamina II is characterized by a group of excitatory interneurons that express the gamma isoform of protein kinase C (PKCγ). In contrast to the predominant nociceptor input to the dorsal most part of lamina II, the PKCγ neurons are targeted by myelinated non-nociceptive afferents and by low threshold C mechanoreceptors and participate in the process of nerve-injury induced persistent pain [29, 40].

Although some lamina V neurons are nociceptive-specific, most are WDR neurons that receive convergent innocuous and noxious monosynaptic inputs from Aβ and δ fibers, respectively, and indirect polysynaptic input from C fibers. As for lamina I, a portion of neurons of lamina V are projection neurons that carry information to the brain [29].

Ascending nociceptive pathways

Projection neurons in laminae I and V are at the origin of multiple ascending pathways. Among these are the spinothalamic and spinoreticular tracts, which project to various brain regions implicated in pain processing, including the thalamus, periaqueductal gray (PAG), parabrachial region, reticular formation of the medulla, hypothalamus and amygdala [41]. From these areas, nociceptive information is transferred to brain regions involved in sensory-discriminatory (somatosensory cortex) and affective-motivational (insula and anterior cingulate cortex) aspects of the pain experience, as well as to areas that are involved in descending modulation of spinal cord neurons that transmit pain messages to the brain (rostral ventromedial medulla; RVM) [42-44].

Descending pain modulation

The perception of pain is a phenomenon that integrates the noxious sensory input with higher cognitive processes: state of awareness, mood and consciousness. Neurons in the brainstem receive inputs from higher order regions of the brain. These neurons, in turn, project to spinal cord circuits

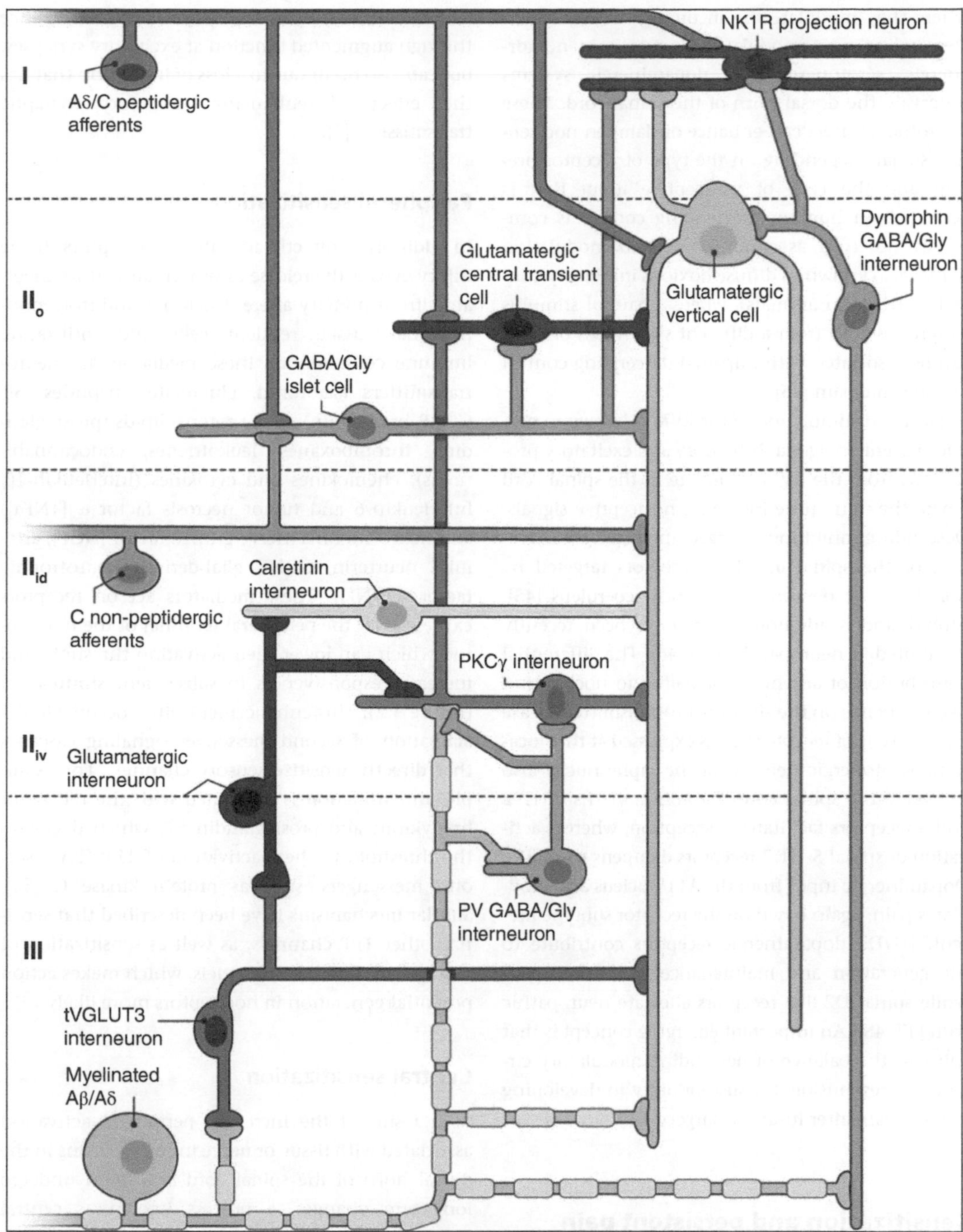

Figure 3.3 Spinal dorsal horn circuitry. The complex circuitry of the spinal cord allows for the integration of incoming noxious and non-noxious stimuli prior to relaying them forward to the brain. Nociceptive afferents terminate in lamina I and II while low-threshold mechanoreceptors (Aβ) terminate in deeper laminae. Local excitatory and inhibitory interneurons act as "gates", suppressing certain information while allowing other information to pass through. Spinal inhibitory circuits are impaired following neuropathy and inflammation, giving rise to hyperalgesia and allodynia. Peirs, Williams [59] recently described engagements of different microcircuits in the development of pain hypersensitivity following nerve injury and inflammation. Peirs, Williams [59] recently demonstrated that a loss of inhibitory tone following spared nerve injury allows Aβ fibres to activate PKCγ interneurons which ultimately lead to the activation of projection neurons. Inflammatory stimuli, such as carrageenan, instead engages calretinin interneurons that further transmit information to projection neurons. This figure is from Peirs and Seal [29] and was reproduced with permission from the American Association for the Advancement of Science (Color Plate 3).

where they modulate the incoming sensory input. Descending neuromodulatory inputs from noradrenergic, serotonergic and dopaminergic systems innervate the dorsal horn of the spinal cord. These neurotransmitters can enhance or dampen nociceptive signals depending on the type of receptor present and the type of nociceptive input that is activated. In humans, descending control is commonly observed as conditioned pain modulation (CPM; also known as diffuse noxious inhibitory control or DNIC in animals), where a painful stimulus suppresses pain from a different site. A loss of CPM can be associated with impaired descending control and chronic pain [45].

Electrical stimulation of the RVM is known to produce potent analgesia. Inhibitory and excitatory projections from the RVM terminate in the spinal cord where they fine tune incoming nociceptive signals. Descending inhibition is largely mediated by activation of the spinal α2-adrenoreceptors targeted by noradrenergic neurons of the locus coeruleus [45]. Alpha1 and ß adrenoreceptors have been recently implicated in neuropathic pain [46]. The differential contribution of adrenergic signaling to nociception likely depends on the site of neurotransmitter release and the type of receptor that is expressed at that location. Serotonergic neurons of the raphe nuclei also innervate the spinal cord. Serotonin, via its 5-HT 2 and 3 receptors facilitates nociception, whereas activation of spinal 5-HT 7 receptors dampens pain [47]. Dopaminergic input from the A11 nucleus also modulates pain, again based on the receptor subtype present. D1/D5 dopaminergic receptors contribute to the generation and maintenance of chronic pain while spinal D2-like receptors alleviate neuropathic pain [47, 48]. An important emerging concept is that shifts in the balance of descending modulatory circuits are responsible for susceptibility to developing chronic pain after injury or surgery [49].

Sensitization and persistent pain

In the setting of injury, complementary and sometimes contemporaneous mechanisms underlie the process of sensitization that leads to allodynia and hyperalgesia. One involves peripheral sensitization usually of the nociceptor itself. Another, central sensitization, can result from increased excitability of CNS circuits in the nociceptive pathway, for instance through augmented function at excitatory synapses, but can also occur due to a loss of inhibition that has the effect of enhancing excitatory synaptic transmission [5].

Peripheral sensitization

In addition to directly activating nociceptors, tissue injury evokes the release of pro-inflammatory mediators from primary afferent neurons and from non-neuronal, tissue resident cells and infiltrating immune cells. Among these mediators are neurotransmitters (serotonin, glutamate), peptides (SP, CGRP, bradykinin), ATP, protons, lipids (prostaglandins, thromboxanes, leukotrienes, endocannabinoids), chemokines and cytokines (interleukin-1β, interleukin-6 and tumor necrosis factor α [TNFα]) and neurotrophins (nerve growth factor [NGF], artemin, neurterin, GDNF, glial-derived neurotrophic factor [GDNF]). These mediators act on receptors expressed by the peripheral terminal of the nociceptor, which can lower their activation threshold and increase responsiveness to subsequent stimulation (Figure 3.2). This enhancement often occurs via the activation of second messenger signaling cascades that directly sensitize sensory channels. For example, inflammation is associated with the release of bradykinin and prostaglandin E2, which decreases the threshold for heat activation of TRPV1 via second messengers, such as protein kinase C [50]. Similar mechanisms have been described that sensitize other TRP channels, as well as sensitization of voltage-gated sodium channels, which makes action potential generation in nociceptors more likely.

Central sensitization

As a result of the increased peripheral activation associated with tissue or nerve injury, neurons in the dorsal horn of the spinal cord and brain undergo long-term changes, a process known as central sensitization. Central sensitization shares many properties with other forms of long-term plasticity observed in the CNS [51]. In the spinal cord, this form of plasticity is characterized by significant changes in the firing properties of neurons: decreased activation thresholds, increased receptive field size and increased spontaneous activity.

A variety of mechanisms have been proposed to underlie the development of central sensitization. The most well-studied involves activation of the NMDA subtype of glutamate receptor, a process that is functionally similar to the neuronal plasticity implicated in memory formation. Acute stimulation of nociceptors evokes the release of glutamate from primary afferent terminals. The glutamate activates calcium-impermeable AMPA and kainate receptors, but fails to activate NMDA receptors. However, following sustained release of glutamate, such as in the setting of persistent tissue or nerve injury, the postsynaptic spinal cord neurons are sufficiently depolarized to engage calcium-permeable NMDA receptors. Calcium influx through these channels leads to long-term molecular changes in spinal cord neurons, thereby strengthening synaptic connections between these neurons and nociceptors, and enhancing the central effects of subsequent nociceptive (and even non-noxious) inputs [52].

Loss of inhibitory control is also a major contributor to central sensitization. Inhibitory interneurons are densely distributed throughout the spinal cord dorsal horn, and these neurons regulate the transmission of noxious information by dampening excitatory inputs and preventing overactivation of nociceptive circuits. Following injury, however, there is a decrease in the efficacy of inhibitory inputs to superficial spinal cord neurons, which enhances spinal cord output in response to painful stimuli and can additionally unmask inputs from non-nociceptive primary afferents [53, 54]. This process is often referred to as disinhibition. There is evidence that disinhibition can result from a shift in the effect of normally inhibitory transmitters (e.g. gamma-aminobutyric acid (GABA) and glycine) such that they may even depolarize, rather than hyperpolarize, postsynaptic neurons. There is also evidence for alterations of inhibitory receptors on spinal cord neurons, making them less responsive to inhibitory transmitters [54, 55]. Frank loss of inhibitory interneurons secondary to nerve injury has also been reported [56, 57], although this has been an area of much debate. Nevertheless, transplanting embryonic GABAergic neurons back into the spinal cord to restore inhibitory balance has proven to be efficacious in reducing pain across several rodent pain models [58]. Importantly, mechanical allodynia brought about by inflammation or nerve injury appear to engage separate classes of inhibitory interneurons (Figure 3.3). This suggests that different spinal pathways are likely involved in promoting mechanical allodynia depending on the type of insult [59]. Therefore, the microcircuitry involved in the loss of inhibition in the dorsal horn is likely a disease-dependent phenomenon.

Central sensitization also involves interactions among microglia, astrocytes and spinal cord neurons. In response to soluble factors released from the terminals of injured primary afferent fibers, microglia are activated and accumulate in the superficial dorsal horn. In turn, the microglia release a host of pathophysiologic signaling molecules, including interleukin-1β, interleukin-6, TNFα, fractalkine and brain-derived neurotrophic factor (BDNF), which promote central sensitization and therefore contribute to persistent pain states [60]. Recent studies suggest that these microglial effects are at least partially male-specific [61], although a sufficiency for microglial activation promoting chronic pain in female rodents has been demonstrated [62]. Microglia are monocytes present in the CNS. They are similar to macrophages that are found in the periphery. Some macrophages are resident to the DRG. These cells also play an important role in neuropathic pain where they influence neuropathic pain development in male and female mice but a specific signaling factor called colony stimulating factor 1 (CSF1) is exclusively required for this mechanism in male mice [63]. Astrocytes are also activated in the spinal cord following many types of injury that promote pain. Although their contribution to central sensitization is less clear and potential sex-differences have not been clearly elucidated, astrocytes are critical for both the induction and the maintenance of persistent pain [64].

Finally, sensitization of the pain pathway can result from changes in the brainstem. In addition to their more commonly recognized role in descending inhibition of pain processing, neurons of the midbrain PAG and RVM can facilitate the processing of pain signals at the level of the spinal cord. Under certain persistent pain conditions, this facilitatory effect is enhanced. In fact, the persistence of the pain may require sustained facilitatory inputs from brainstem neurons to the spinal cord. For example, in a model of nerve injury-induced (neuropathic) pain, the resulting mechanical allodynia can be blocked by injections of lidocaine into the RVM [65]. Sensitization of the supraspinal facilitatory circuits likely occurs via mechanisms similar to those involved in sensitization of spinal cord neurons. Thus, activation of NMDA receptors has been implicated in the sensitization of RVM neurons and, a BDNF and microglial contribution to the process has also been suggested [66, 67].

Analgesic targets

Our increased knowledge of the mechanisms that produce pain, in particular the process of sensitization, has identified a number of novel targets for its management. In addition, we have come to better understand the mechanisms of action of traditional analgesics, including opioids, non-steroidal anti-inflammatory drugs (NSAIDs) and local nerve blockers like lidocaine. As with any pharmacotherapy, the goal is to treat pain while limiting adverse side effects, which arise from drug binding at sites unrelated to those generating the pain.

For this reason, targets enriched or exclusively expressed in elements of the pain pathway are of great interest, notably subtypes of voltage-gated sodium channels which predominate in nociceptors. Although it has proven difficult to design drugs selective for these channels (e.g. Nav 1.7 and 1.8), it is significant that tricyclic antidepressants, which are beneficial in the treatment of neuropathic pain (notably diabetic neuropathy and post-herpetic neuralgia), are not only monoamine uptake inhibitors, but also excellent use-dependent sodium channel blockers. It is thus possible that their utility involves blockade of action potential generation and transmission in nociceptors. Some reports claimed development of selective Nav1.7 channel inhibitors, but to date these have not successfully completed clinical trials for drug approval. An interesting recent study suggests that these Nav1.7 inhibitors may need to penetrate the spinal dorsal horn because Nav1.7 may play a more important role in regulating neurotransmitter release at nociceptor spinal terminals than has previously been recognized [26].

The importance of targeting nociceptors is further demonstrated by the approval of high dose topical capsaicin for neuropathic pain [68], an approach that likely produces a transient degeneration of nociceptor terminals. As many of the elements of the inflammatory milieu exert their effects via TRPV1 (e.g. in preclinical models of metastatic bone cancer), the development of TRPV1 antagonists for the treatment of pain is also being pursued extensively [69]. Finally, there is very encouraging evidence that targeting pro-inflammatory mediators, like TNFα, and neuropeptides, namely CGRP, with neutralizing antibodies is effective in the treatment of chronic pain conditions such as arthritis and migraines, respectively [70, 71]. There is also considerable evidence that antibodies directed against NGF have significant utility in the management of osteoarthritis [72], but these drugs have also not yet been approved.

Other classes of analgesic do not specifically target the nociceptor but act at different levels of the neural circuits that transmit pain-provoking injury messages. These agents include the opioids (e.g. morphine), but also a variety of calcium channel blockers that notably include ziconotide, a cone snail derived toxin that targets N-type calcium channels [73]. Also included in these more general agents are anticonvulsants (e.g. gabapentin and pregabalin), which constitute the first line therapy for neuropathic pain. Although the target of gabapentin and pregabalin is likely the α2δ subunit of calcium channels, there is evidence that binding of gabapentinoids regulates transport of Ca^{2+} channels. Thus, the mechanism of action of these compounds is still unclear [74]. Given the prominent role of NMDA receptors in the development of central sensitization, this channel remains a very attractive target. To date ketamine remains the most common approach to pain management via interaction with the NMDA receptor. However, as NMDA receptors are ubiquitously expressed throughout the nervous system, the potential for adverse side effects of targeting this receptor is high.

Sensitization is associated with changes in gene expression leading to the production of new proteins that are required to maintain chronic pain states. Regulating mRNA translation presents a novel therapeutic target for chronic pain [75]. In response to nerve injury, phosphorylation of eukaryotic initiation factor 4E (eIF4E) by MAP-kinase interacting serine/threonine kinases (MNK) can shift the preference of mRNA translation towards the synthesis of pro-nociceptive proteins. In addition, phosphorylation of eIF2α, part of a process known as the integrated stress response (ISR) suppresses overall protein synthesis while promoting the translation of select mRNA transcripts. Inhibitors of MNK (e.g. eFT508) and the ISR have shown promise in various preclinical models of pain and are now undergoing clinical trials [76-79]. Of course, gene therapy provides another promising approach. Of particular interest is the report of Weir, Middleton [80] who intrathecally injected an adeno-associated virus that expresses a chimeric inhibitory effect that can be targeted by an oral drug. The receptor is expressed in sensory neurons and binding of the drug (ivermectin) resulted in strong inhibition of firing [80]. The approach proved effective in a preclinical model of neuropathic pain.

Finally, new approaches are being developed to prevent the contribution of glial cells to chronic pain. Thus, glial modulators, which directly affect glial cell function, and purinergic drugs, which prevent the glial activation by ATP, are candidate drugs for the treatment of neuropathic pain [81]. Despite the challenges, the future of pharmacologic management of pain is encouraging, as evidence by the approval since 2019 of many new drugs for migraine. As more details of nociceptive processing and sensitization mechanisms are uncovered, there is no question that the opportunities for drug development will continue to grow.

Clinical considerations

One of the greatest challenges in developing effective analgesics is the translation of preclinical studies performed in animal models, typically rodents, to clinical trials performed on human subjects. Unfortunately, the majority of clinical trials in the pain space have failed either due to safety concerns or to lack of efficacy. There have been many proposed reasons for this lack of translation, including the need for new preclinical models that do not rely on reflex endpoints. Another recently highlighted issue is the divergence in the neurochemistry of neurons in the pain pathway, in particular nociceptors, between humans, non-human primates and rodents. There are now many examples of markers associated with a variety of nociceptor subtypes in mice that are differentially expressed or not well represented in human nociceptors and in non-human primates [11, 82]. A particularly striking example, as mentioned above, is that human sensory neurons have significant overlap between peptidergic (CGRP+) and non-peptidergic (P2X3R+) nociceptor markers. This difference is also represented in the spinal dorsal horn where human peptidergic and non-peptidergic neurons terminate uniformly throughout lamina I and II [39]. It is unclear how these differences in gene expression might affect neuronal physiology but recent advances in a variety of techniques that enable the study of human nociceptors will likely fill this gap in knowledge in the near future [83-85]. A hope is that this rapidly expanding understanding of gene expression and physiology of human nociceptors will dramatically improve clinical translation for emerging therapeutic targets for pain. This area of work can also serve as a foundation to better utilize preclinical models for therapeutic validation and proof of concept.

References

1 Bennett DL, Clark AJ, Huang J, Waxman SG, Dib-Hajj SD. (2019) The role of voltage-gated sodium channels in pain signaling. *Physiol Rev* **99(2)**:1079–151.

2 Sheikh S, Booth-Norse A, Holden D, Henson M, Dodd C, Edgerton E, *et al.* (2021) Opioid overdose risk in patients returning to the emergency department for pain. *Pain Med.* **22(9)**:2100–5.

3 Crook RJ, Dickson K, Hanlon RT, Walters ET. (2014). Nociceptive sensitization reduces predation risk. *Curr Biol* **24(10)**:1121–5.

4 Price TJ, Dussor G. (2014) Evolution: the advantage of 'maladaptive' pain plasticity. *Curr Biol* **24(10)**:R384–6.

5 Basbaum AI, Bautista DM, Scherrer G, Julius D. (2009) Cellular and molecular mechanisms of pain. *Cell* **139(2)**:267–84.

6 Habig K, Schanzer A, Schirner W, *et al.* (2017) Low threshold unmyelinated mechanoafferents can modulate pain. *BMC Neurol* **17(1)**:184.

7 Kambrun C, Roca-Lapirot O, Salio C, Landry M, Moqrich A, Le Feuvre Y. (2018) TAFA4 reverses mechanical allodynia through activation of GABAergic transmission and microglial process retraction. *Cell Rep* **22(11)**:2886–97.

8 Lolignier S, Eijkelkamp N, Wood JN. (2015) Mechanical allodynia. *Pflugers Arch* **467(1)**:133–9.

9 Cavanaugh DJ, Lee H, Lo L, *et al.* (2009) Distinct subsets of unmyelinated primary sensory fibers mediate behavioral responses to noxious thermal and mechanical stimuli. *Proc Natl Acad Sci USA* **106(22)**:9075–80.

10 Usoskin D, Furlan A, Islam S, *et al.* (2015). Unbiased classification of sensory neuron types by large-scale single-cell RNA sequencing. *Nat Neurosci* **18(1)**:145–53.

11 Kupari J, Usoskin D, Parisien M, *et al* (2021) Single cell transcriptomics of primate sensory neurons identifies cell types associated with chronic pain. *Nat Commun* **12(1)**:1510.

12 Tavares-Ferreira D, Shiers S, Ray PR, *et al.* (2021) Spatial transcriptomics reveals unique molecular fingerprints of human nociceptors. *bioRxiv* 2021.02.06.430065.

13 Naziroglu M, Braidy N. (2017) Thermo-sensitive TRP channels: novel targets for treating chemotherapy-induced peripheral pain. *Front Physiol* **8**:1040.

14 MacDonald DI, Wood JN, Emery EC. (2020) Molecular mechanisms of cold pain. *Neurobiol Pain* **7**:100044.

15 Fang XZ, Zhou T, Xu JQ, *et al.* (2021) Structure, kinetic properties and biological function of mechanosensitive Piezo channels. *Cell Biosci* **11(1)**:13.

16 Szczot M, Liljencrantz J, Ghitani N, *et al.* (2018) PIEZO2 mediates injury-induced tactile pain in mice and humans. *Sci Transl Med* **10(462)**:eaat9892.

17 Murthy SE, Loud MC, Daou I, *et al.* (2018) The mechanosensitive ion channel Piezo2 mediates sensitivity to mechanical pain in mice. *Sci Transl Med* **10(462)**:eaat9897.

18 Beaulieu-Laroche L, Christin M, Donoghue A, *et al.* (2020) TACAN Is an ion channel involved in sensing mechanical pain. *Cell* **180(5)**:956–67 e17.

19 Bonet IJM, Araldi D, Bogen O, Levine JD. (2021) Involvement of TACAN, a mechanotransducing ion channel, in inflammatory but not neuropathic hyperalgesia in the rat. *J. Pain* **22(5)**:498–508.

20 Silverman HA, Chen A, Kravatz NL, Chavan SS, Chang EH. (2020) Involvement of neural transient receptor potential channels in peripheral inflammation. *Front Immunol* **11**:590261.

21 Chiu IM, Heesters BA, Ghasemlou N, *et al.* (2013) Bacteria activate sensory neurons that modulate pain and inflammation. *Nature* **501(7465)**:52–7.

22 Blake KJ, Baral P, Voisin T, *et al.* (2018) *Staphylococcus aureus* produces pain through pore-forming toxins and neuronal TRPV1 that is silenced by QX-314. *Nat Commun.* **9(1)**:37.

23 Ruhl CR, Pasko BL, Khan HS, *et al.* (2020) *Mycobacterium tuberculosis* sulfolipid-1 activates nociceptive neurons and induces cough. *Cell* **181(2)**:293–305 e11.

24 Barragan-Iglesias P, Franco-Enzastiga U, Jeevakumar V, *et al.* (2020) Type I interferons act directly on nociceptors to produce pain sensitization: implications for viral infection-induced pain. *J Neurosci* **40(18)**:3517–32.

25 Goodwin G, McMahon SB. (2021) The physiological function of different voltage-gated sodium channels in pain. *Nat Rev Neurosci* **22(5)**:263–74.

26 MacDonald DI, Sikandar S, Weiss J, *et al.* (2021) A central mechanism of analgesia in mice and humans lacking the sodium channel NaV1.7. *Neuron* **109(9)**:1497–512.e6.

27 Pereira V, Millet Q, Aramburu J, Lopez-Rodriguez C, Gaveriaux-Ruff C, Wood JN. (2018) Analgesia linked to Nav1.7 loss of function requires micro- and delta-opioid receptors. *Wellcome Open Res* **3**:101.

28 Smith PA. (2020) K^+ channels in primary afferents and their role in nerve injury-induced pain. *Front Cell Neurosci* **14**:566418.

29 Peirs C, Seal RP. (2016) Neural circuits for pain: Recent advances and current views. *Science* **354(6312)**:578–84.

30 Baral P, Umans BD, Li L, *et al.* (2018) Nociceptor sensory neurons suppress neutrophil and gammadelta T cell responses in bacterial lung infections and lethal pneumonia. *Nat Med* **24(4)**:417–26.

31 Lai NY, Musser MA, Pinho-Ribeiro FA *et al.* (2020) Gut-innervating nociceptor neurons regulate Peyer's patch microfold cells and SFB levels to mediate *Salmonella* host defense. *Cell* **180(1)**:33–49 e22.

32 Huang S, Ziegler CGK, Austin J *et al.* (2021) Lymph nodes are innervated by a unique population of sensory neurons with immunomodulatory potential. *Cell* **184(2)**:441–59 e25.

33 Wang H, Zylka MJ. (2009) Mrgprd-expressing polymodal nociceptive neurons innervate most known classes of substantia gelatinosa neurons. *J Neurosci* **29(42)**:13202–9.

34 Rau KK, McIlwrath SL, Wang H, *et al.* (2009) Mrgprd enhances excitability in specific populations of cutaneous murine polymodal nociceptors. *J Neurosci* **29(26)**:8612–9.

35 von Buchholtz LJ, Lam RM, Emrick JJ, Chesler AT, Ryba NJP. (2020) Assigning transcriptomic class in the trigeminal ganglion using multiplex in situ hybridization and machine learning. *Pain* **161(9)**:2212–24.

36 Haring M, Zeisel A, Hochgerner H, *et al.* (2018) Neuronal atlas of the dorsal horn defines its architecture and links sensory input to transcriptional cell types. *Nat Neurosci* **21(6)**:869–80.

37 Koch SC, Acton D, Goulding M. (2018) Spinal circuits for touch, pain, and itch. *Annu Rev Physiol* **80**:189–217.

38 Duan B, Cheng L, Ma Q. (2018) Spinal circuits transmitting mechanical pain and itch. *Neurosci Bull* **34(1)**:186–93.

39 Shiers SI, Sankaranarayanan I, Jeevakumar V, Cervantes A, Reese JC, Price TJ. (2021) Convergence of peptidergic and non-peptidergic protein markers in the human dorsal root ganglion and spinal dorsal horn. *J Comp Neurol* **529(10)**:2771–88.

40 Seal RP, Wang X, Guan Y, *et al.* (2009) Injury-induced mechanical hypersensitivity requires C-low threshold mechanoreceptors. *Nature* **462(7273)**:651–5.

41 Wercberger R, Basbaum AI. (2019) Spinal cord projection neurons: a superficial, and also deep, analysis. *Curr Opin Physiol* **11**:109–15.

42 Vierck CJ, Whitsel BL, Favorov OV, Brown AW, Tommerdahl M. (2013) Role of primary somatosensory cortex in the coding of pain. *Pain* **154(3)**:334–44.

43 Lu C, Yang T, Zhao H, *et al.* (2016) Insular cortex is critical for the perception, modulation, and chronification ofpPain. *Neurosci Bull* **32(2)**:191–201.

44 Chen Q, Heinricher MM. (2019) Descending Control Mechanisms and Chronic Pain. *Curr Rheumatol Rep* **21(5)**:13.

45 Bannister K, Dickenson AH. (2017) The plasticity of descending controls in pain: translational probing. *J Physiol* **595(13)**:4159–66.

46 Llorca-Torralba M, Borges G, Neto F, Mico JA, Berrocoso E. (2016) Noradrenergic Locus Coeruleus pathways in pain modulation. *Neuroscience* **338**:93–113.

47 Li C, Liu S, Lu X, Tao F. (2019) Role of descending dopaminergic pathways in pain modulation. *Curr Neuropharmacol* **17(12)**:1176–82.

48 Megat S, Shiers S, Moy JK, *et al.* (2018) A critical role for dopamine D5 receptors in pain chronicity in male mice. *J Neurosci* **38(2)**:379–97.

49 Denk F, McMahon SB, Tracey I. (2014) Pain vulnerability: a neurobiological perspective. *Nat Neurosci* **17(2)**:192–200.

50 Kawabata A. (2011) Prostaglandin E2 and pain--an update. *Biol Pharm Bull* **34(8)**:1170–3.

51 Price TJ, Inyang KE. (2015) Commonalities between pain and memory mechanisms and their meaning for understanding chronic pain. *Progress in molecular biology and translational science* **131**:409–34.

52 Latremoliere A, Woolf CJ. (2009) Central sensitization: a generator of pain hypersensitivity by central neural plasticity. *J Pain* **10(9)**:895–926.

53 Price TJ, Cervero F, Gold MS, Hammond DL, Prescott SA. (2009) Chloride regulation in the pain pathway. *Brain Res Rev* **60(1)**:149–70.

54 Price TJ, Prescott SA. (2015) Inhibitory regulation of the pain gate and how its failure causes pathological pain. *Pain* **156(5)**:789–92.

55 Zeilhofer HU, Wildner H, Yevenes GE. (2012) Fast synaptic inhibition in spinal sensory processing and pain control. *Physiol Rev* **92(1)**: 193–235.

56 Inquimbert P, Moll M, Latremoliere A, *et al.* (2018) NMDA receptor activation underlies the loss of spinal dorsal horn neurons and the transition to persistent pain after peripheral nerve injury. *Cell Rep* **23(9)**:2678–89.

57 Meisner JG, Marsh AD, Marsh DR. (2010) Loss of GABAergic interneurons in laminae I-III of the spinal cord dorsal horn contributes to reduced GABAergic tone and neuropathic pain after spinal cord injury. *J Neurotrauma* **27(4)**:729–37.

58 Braz JM, Sharif-Naeini R, Vogt D, *et al.* (2012) Forebrain GABAergic neuron precursors integrate into adult spinal cord and reduce injury-induced neuropathic pain. *Neuron* **74(4)**:663–75.

59 Peirs C, Williams SP, Zhao X, *et al.* (2015) Dorsal horn circuits for persistent mechanical pain. *Neuron* **87(4)**:797–812.

60 Buchheit T, Huh Y, Maixner W, Cheng J, Ji RR. (2020) Neuroimmune modulation of pain and

regenerative pain medicine. *J Clin Invest* **130(5)**:2164–76.

61 Sorge RE, Mapplebeck JC, Rosen S, *et al.* (2015) Different immune cells mediate mechanical pain hypersensitivity in male and female mice. *Nat Neurosci* **18(8)**:1081–3.

62 Yi MH, Liu YU, Umpierre AD, *et al.* (2021) Optogenetic activation of spinal microglia triggers chronic pain in mice. *PLoS Biol* **19(3)**:e3001154.

63 Yu X, Liu H, Hamel KA, *et al.* (2020) Dorsal root ganglion macrophages contribute to both the initiation and persistence of neuropathic pain. *Nat Commun* **11(1)**:264.

64 Ji RR, Donnelly CR, Nedergaard M. (2019) Astrocytes in chronic pain and itch. *Nat Rev Neurosci* **20(11)**:667–85.

65 Saade NE, Al Amin HA, Barchini J, *et al.* (2012) Brainstem injection of lidocaine releases the descending pain-inhibitory mechanisms in a rat model of mononeuropathy. *Exp Neurol* **237(1)**:180–90.

66 Dai S, Ma Z. (2014) BDNF-trkB-KCC2-GABA pathway may be related to chronic stress-induced hyperalgesia at both the spinal and supraspinal level. *Med Hypotheses* **83(6)**:772–4.

67 Guo W, Robbins MT, Wei F, Zou S, Dubner R, Ren K. (2006) Supraspinal brain-derived neurotrophic factor signaling: a novel mechanism for descending pain facilitation. *J Neurosci* **26(1)**:126–37.

68 Maloney J, Pew S, Wie C, Gupta R, Freeman J, Strand N. (2021) Comprehensive review of topical analgesics for chronic pain. *Curr Pain Headache Rep* **25(2)**:7.

69 Honore P, Chandran P, Hernandez G, *et al.* (2009) Repeated dosing of ABT-102, a potent and selective TRPV1 antagonist, enhances TRPV1-mediated analgesic activity in rodents, but attenuates antagonist-induced hyperthermia. *Pain* **142(1-2)**:27–35.

70 Cohen JM, Ning X, Kessler Y, *et al.* (2021) Immunogenicity of biologic therapies for migraine: a review of current evidence. *J Headache Pain* **22(1)**:3.

71 Caso F, Lubrano E, Del Puente A, *et al.* (2016) Progress in understanding and utilizing TNF-alpha inhibition for the treatment of psoriatic arthritis. *Expert Rev Clin Immunol* **12(3)**:315–31.

72 Lane NE, Schnitzer TJ, Birbara CA, *et al.* (2010) Tanezumab for the treatment of pain from osteoarthritis of the knee. *N Engl J Med* **363(16)**: 1521–31.

73 Viswanath O, Urits I, Burns J, *et al.* (2020) Central neuropathic mechanisms in pain signaling pathways: current evidence and recommendations. *Adv Ther* **37(5)**:1946–59.

74 Alles SRA, Smith PA. (2018) Etiology and pharmacology of neuropathic pain. *Pharmacol Rev* **70(2)**:315–47.

75 Yousuf MS, Shiers SI, Sahn JJ, Price TJ. (2021) Pharmacological manipulation of translation as a therapeutic target for chronic pain. *Pharmacol Rev* **73(1)**:59–88.

76 Costa-Mattioli M, Walter P. (2020) The integrated stress response: from mechanism to disease. *Science* **368(6489)**:eaat5314.

77 Shiers S, Mwirigi J, Pradhan G, *et al.* (2020) Reversal of peripheral nerve injury-induced neuropathic pain and cognitive dysfunction via genetic and tomivosertib targeting of MNK. *Neuropsychopharmacology* **45(3)**:524–33.

78 Moy JK, Kuhn JL, Szabo-Pardi TA, Pradhan G, Price TJ. (2018) eIF4E phosphorylation regulates ongoing pain, independently of inflammation, and hyperalgesic priming in the mouse CFA model. *Neurobiol Pain* **4**:45–50.

79 Yousuf MS, Samtleben S, Lamothe SM, *et al.* (2020) Endoplasmic reticulum stress in the dorsal root ganglia regulates large-conductance potassium channels and contributes to pain in a model of multiple sclerosis. *FASEB J* **34(9)**:12577–98.

80 Weir GA, Middleton SJ, Clark AJ, *et al.* (2017) Using an engineered glutamate-gated chloride channel to silence sensory neurons and treat neuropathic pain at the source. *Brain* **140(10)**:2570–85.

81 Ji RR, Berta T, Nedergaard M. (2031) Glia and pain: is chronic pain a gliopathy? *Pain* **154 Suppl 1(Supplement 1)**:S10–S28.

82 Shiers S, Klein RM, Price TJ. (2020) Quantitative differences in neuronal subpopulations between mouse and human dorsal root ganglia demonstrated with RNAscope in situ hybridization. *Pain* **161(10)**:2410–24.

83 Valtcheva MV, Copits BA, Davidson S, *et al.* (2016) Surgical extraction of human dorsal root ganglia from organ donors and preparation of primary sensory neuron cultures. *Nat Protoc* **11(10)**:1877–88.

84 Wangzhou A, McIlvried LA, Paige C, *et al.* (2020) Pharmacological target-focused transcriptomic analysis of native vs cultured human and mouse dorsal root ganglia. *Pain* **161(7)**:1497–517.

85 Schrenk-Siemens K, Rosseler C, Lampert A. (2018) Translational model systems for complex sodium channel pathophysiology in pain. *Handb Exp Pharmacol* **246**:355–69.

86 Abdo H, Calvo-Enrique L, Lopez JM, et al. (2019) Specialized cutaneous Schwann cells initiate pain sensation. *Science* **365(6454)**:695–9.

Chapter 4

Psychosocial perspectives on chronic pain

Kenneth D. Craig[1] & Judith Versloot[2]

[1] *Department of Psychology, University of British Columbia, Vancouver, Canada*
[2] *Institute for Health Policy, Management and Evaluation, University of Toronto, Toronto, Canada*

Introduction

Understanding the psychosocial determinants of pain is crucial to optimal delivery of care. Pain is widely recognized to be a complex subjective experience with multiple features requiring consideration in the course of deciding upon appropriate interventions. The International Association for the Study of Pain defines pain as "An unpleasant sensory and emotional experience associated with, or resembling that associated with, actual or potential tissue damage" [1]. The definition carefully explains that an association with tissue damage is a feature of the experience, but it also establishes that it is not necessarily the exclusive or sufficient cause, thereby pointing to important roles for psychosocial determinants. Psychological and social challenges may be of great importance to patients irrespective of whether a pathophysiological basis for pain can be identified. This characterization of attributes of the experience appropriately acknowledges sensory and emotional attributes, but it appears too narrow as cognitive and social attributes are not made explicit [2, 3]. These aspects are important particularly in applications of psychosocial interventions, for example, cognitive behavioral therapy or self-management approaches. What the individual is thinking about and the social challenges they confront may be central to providing appropriate care. They become increasingly important as chronic pain persists [4, 5].

The psychological and social factors deserving attention in understanding an individual's unique pattern of pain experience and expression are complex, but increasingly well-defined. Perceptual processes, emotions and mood, thought patterns, personality characteristics and pain-related behavior have been implicated. Further, exploring how the individual's current life situation and history of personal and social experiences influence pain and pain-related disability may be crucial in delivery of care. The capacity to pursue typical roles at work or with family and friends is likely to be important and should be considered in the broader contexts of socioeconomic status, ethnocultural and familial backgrounds. Appraisal of psychosocial determinants of pain typically leads to important targets and specific interventions for working with patients. This chapter describes fundamental psychosocial processes and their clinical relevance, with the chapters on psychological assessment (Chapter 11) and psychological interventions (Chapters 25 to 27) applying the perspective, among other chapters in this volume.

Clinical Pain Management: A Practical Guide, Second Edition. Edited by Mary E. Lynch, Kenneth D. Craig, and Philip W. Peng.

Modeling the network of biological, psychological and social determinants of pain

Biopsychosocial perspective

This volume endorses the biopsychosocial model of health and illness that posits biological, psychological and social factors must be considered in understanding human health or illness, whether one is interested in being well-informed about the nature of pain or caring for an individual [6]. Figure 4.1 illustrates dimensions of the model, signifying the importance of each component to the wellbeing of the person. It has been embraced by those arguing the necessity of multidisciplinary care for people suffering from chronic pain and calls for the integration of contributions from various healthcare practitioners, including medicine, nursing, physical therapy, psychology, social work and rehabilitation. Multidisciplinary care is demonstrably more effective and cost-efficient than single practice care [7, 8]. Nevertheless, attention to biological phenomena overwhelms the field; psychologically based approaches are often ignored by those with strong biomedical orientations, and social determinants of pain have received relatively minimal attention. Healthcare professionals who do not have competencies in all domains must engage in consultation to insure comprehensive care. Integrative care models ensure interdisciplinary collaboration in the use of multimodal therapies for persistent pain [9, 10, 11].

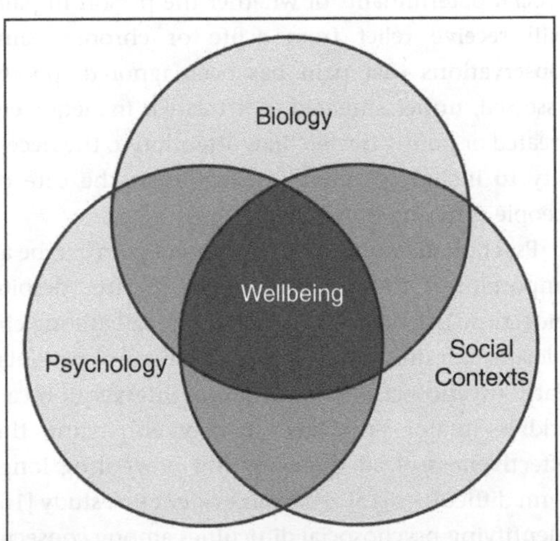

Figure 4.1 The biopsychosocial approach to human disease and injury. Optimal wellbeing arises through consideration of the whole person – biological, psychological and social factors are important when addressing an individual's pain and related disability.

Social Communication Model of Pain

This systemic model begins to provide a detailed framework for describing the complex interactions among psychological and social factors of pain (see Figure 4.2) [12, 13]. The model is structured around the typical temporal sequence of events during a painful episode: (a) there is exposure to events in a person variably disposed to experience pain; (b) pain is perceived; (c) the distress becomes manifest in pain expression; (d) pain may be inferred by an observer; and (e) observer decisions are made concerning delivery of care. Note inclusion of persons other than the suffering person in the model as their role is typically important to the continuing process. Benevolent care is not the only possibility – indifference and malevolent exploitation are not unusual in human relationships, but less common in clinical settings. The model directs attention to both intrapersonal (biological and psychological) and interpersonal (social) determinants of the experience and its overt expression, as well as to the caregiver's perception of the person's distress and the process whereby decisions are made concerning delivery of care. Both intrapersonal and interpersonal determinants of each stage are important to an understanding of this dynamic temporal sequence.

Intrapersonal determinants concern the personal dispositions to experience or express pain, in the case of the patient. Similar dispositions govern the reactions of caregivers. For the person in pain, the dispositions are embodied in the biological substrates that support pain. These are plastic and dynamic. While inherited dispositions to respond to noxious events with pain are important [14], the biological substrates of pain also reflect personal life experiences, including the individual's medical and social history. Personal life histories include a myriad of personal, familial and ethnocultural events that are formative of the individual's experiences and modes of painful expression. A parallel analysis is needed for caregiver dispositions during assessment and treatment. Their reactions, both in terms of

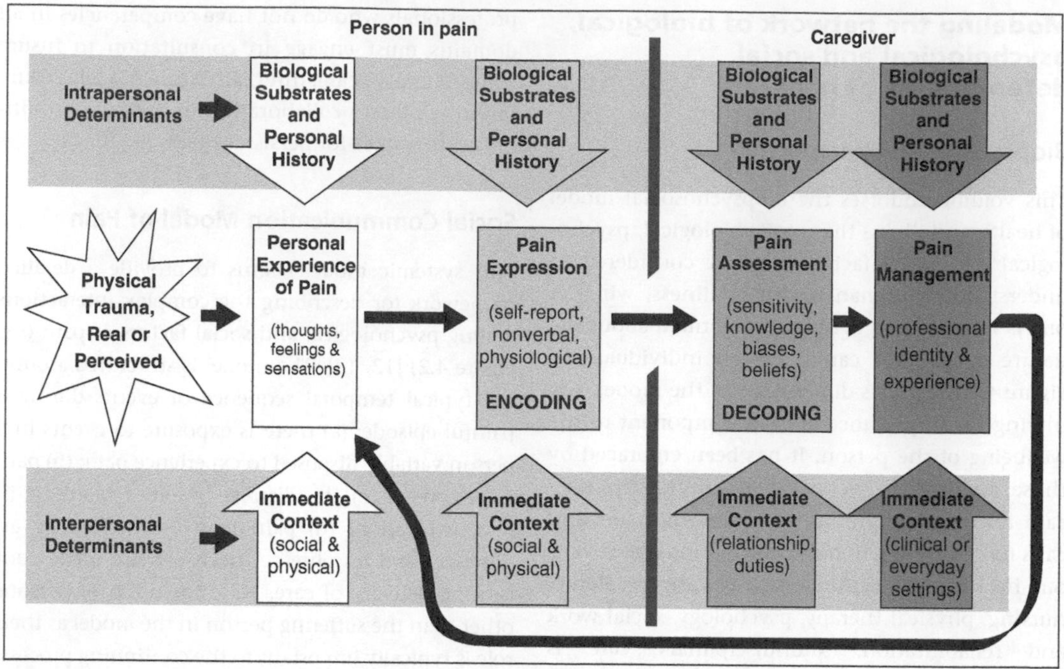

Figure 4.2 The Social Communication Model of Pain. This framework identifies biological, psychological and social features of pain through the sequence of events during typical injury and exacerbation of chronic pain, including reactions of caregivers, and identifies both intrapersonal and interpersonal determinants of the stages of the sequence.

what they perceive and how they respond, are similarly constrained by biological systems and reflect informal and formal education and life experience.

The interpersonal context interacts with the intrapersonal dispositions to determine the individual's unique response at the time pain is experienced and expressed. Patients often confront difficult work, family and other interpersonal challenges which influence pain, personal coping, pain-related disability and demands for healthcare. These, and the immediate context, are related to the substantial variability in how people experience pain and express their distress as well as how observing people interpret and respond to those reactions. The social context and the manner in which those present treat the person in pain have a potent impact on the individual's current and future status. Access to a clinician able to deliver effective interventions is a key feature of the patient's interpersonal context.

Clinicians serve as pivotal social agents who control services provided to individuals, with public health and institutional policies dictating availability of resources, including determining whether and which caregivers will be available. Their training and competence in delivering effective interventions are crucial determinants of whether the person in pain will receive relief from acute or chronic pain. Observations that pain has been ignored, poorly assessed, underestimated, not treated, inadequately treated or poorly treated draw attention to the necessity to include psychosocial factors in the care of people suffering from pain.

Psychological and social features of pain can be as important as their biological counterparts, despite biocentric orientations that often prevail among clinicians, administrators, policy makers and patients. Early psychosocial assessment and intervention can address major problems, thereby enhancing the effectiveness of all therapies and preventing long-term difficulties [15]. This was evident in a study [16] identifying psychosocial difficulties among consecutive new patients (a total of 1242 patients were enrolled) referred to a tertiary care, hospital-based pain clinic. Both psychosocial and biomedical issues were important in 51% of the patients. For an additional 20.9% of the patients, no medical factors could be established and painful experience and disability were attributed to psychological factors. Importantly, the pain of only 25.5% of the patients could be attributed directly to general medical conditions. About 75% of the patients had detectable biomedical pathology and close to 72% had diagnosable psychological issues. Similarly, mental health problems, including depression (61%) and anxiety (45%) were common in patients with chronic pain presenting as unable to cope with chronic pain to an emergency department [17]. Life challenges were also evident among 935 patients presenting to a community-based multidisciplinary chronic pain clinic, as 50% lived below the poverty line, 30% were not working due to disability and 63% reported severe functional disability [18]. Evidence of high levels of psychosocial difficulties indicate the importance of treating the whole person rather than focusing exclusively on physical pathology.

Psychosocial factors in best practice

The Social Communication Model of Pain (Figure 4.2) encourages consideration of best clinical practice with respect to its numerous dimensions. The following examines components of the model.

The person in pain

Pain experience

Clinical care begins with careful attention to the subjective experience of the patient. Pain is typically initially assessed as a unidimensional construct, using self-report of numerical and verbal descriptor scales focusing upon pain severity; however, these reports obscure the complexity of the experience [19] and should be conceptualized as integrating sensory/discriminative, emotional/motivational, cognitive/appraisal and social dimensions, thereby offering focused targets for different forms of intervention [20].

Intrapersonal determinants

Patients bring to any painful episode, acute or chronic, dispositions to respond that often vary substantially, both in sensitivity to pain and qualitatively [21]. These variable dispositions are determined by genetic inheritance [22] and personal life histories of environmental interactions with both physical and social worlds. Each person represents a relatively unique embodiment of the interaction between these "nature" and "nurture" determinants of pain reactivity. Tissue damage, or the perception of tissue damage, would account for modest to moderate proportions of variations in pain experience, expression, functional capacity and risk of persistence of pain-related disability, in addition to these dispositions [21, 22].

Assessment of personal, medical, family and social history often discloses the formative role of life history events. Several chapters in this book discuss excessive stress reactivity and emotional reactions (e.g. debilitating fear of pain or depression), destructive thinking (e.g. catastrophizing, passive coping), behavioral maladjustment (excessive avoidant behavior and inactivity) and deteriorating social relationships as risk factors for excessive pain and disability, including failure to respond to treatment.

Intrapersonal factors also have been identified that protect against the debilitating impact of painful injury or disease and the development of disability. Key protective factors include:

1 A strong sense of self-efficacy, or confidence in one's ability to follow a course of action that will accomplish desired outcomes (e.g. control of pain) [24, 25].

2 Effective use of cognitive, affective and behavioral coping skills, such as muscle relaxation, distraction, commitment to activity and an ability to redefine situations in less catastrophic ways [26].

3 A readiness or willingness to engage in active roles that are contradictory to lapsing into maladaptive patterns of thinking, feeling and behaving [24, 27].

4 A capacity for accepting certain limitations or handicaps, thereby avoiding one's life being consumed by unsuccessful efforts to eliminate pain [28, 29].

These processes not only describe resilience to pain and pain-related disability, but they represent reasonable objectives for therapeutic intervention.

Firmly entrenched beliefs concerning the importance of the pathophysiological factors in pain among healthcare practitioners, patients and the public ensure efforts to provide specific and accurate biomedical diagnoses. There also is general agreement that clear feedback to patients should be provided, whether a firm medical diagnosis is available or not. A careful and complete diagnosis reduces the likelihood that dissatisfied patients will seek further opinions and/or additional testing, which is often expensive, unnecessary and sometimes harmful [30, 31]. Perseverating on medical diagnosis can trap patients in self-perpetuating roles as invalids as they seek medical care exclusively. Knowing a pathophysiological source of discomfort, with the potential for medical treatment to eliminate it can be very comforting, whereas discomfort from unknown sources with unknown futures can be very disturbing. To the disappointment of many patients and their physicians, tissue damage arising from injury and disease very often does not account for patient complaints [32]. Efforts to identify peripheral and central neurophysiological mechanisms responsible for dysfunctional central regulation and long-term persistence of chronic pain offer promising alternative explanations [33].

Interpersonal determinants

Recognizing the impact of the immediate setting on pain experience is important in understanding variability in patient behavior. Demands for intense engagement in activities can diminish the experience of pain, as in the case of injured athletes or others in life-threatening situations.

Perhaps more important would be the social environment as a source of stress reactivity, with vocational, familial and other sources of social stress able to exacerbate pain. Dubin & King-Van Vack [34] observed dramatic increases in medical visits, use of analgesics and hospital admissions to coincide with major life events, including conflicts with employers, insurers and lawyers and financial distress. Being compelled to abandon usual roles, such as a worker, family member or friend, also leads to deteriorating social relationships. Stress and strain in interactions with others, lapsing into the role of the sick person or invalid and social isolation are common problems for people with chronic pain.

Interpersonal determinants are also evident when gender, familial and ethnocultural variation is observed. Family life provides considerable exposure to others who instruct in appropriate patterns of emotional reactivity, patterns of appraisal (beliefs and attitudes) and interpretation of the meaning of painful events and coping strategies [35]. Conformity to the role standards of others typically has favorable consequences, thereby promoting stable and persistent patterns of emotion and thinking that relate to persistence or recovery from persistent pain [36]. While our understanding of these factors is improving [37], in general, we need to know more about the social modulation of pain [38, 39].

Pain expression

Pain and other features of subjective experience must be inferred through overt manifestations. Various actions, including self-report, qualities of speech and other vocalizations, facial expression, body activity and escape or avoidance behavior and evidence of physiological activity may signal pain and associated psychological states to others. While some of these patterns represent physiological and behavioral coping with the noxious event, others, such as self-report and facial grimaces, appear to function to enhance coping through communication with others [40].

Intrapersonal determinants

The biological basis for painful expression is governed by both automatic (reflexive, unintentional) and controlled (intentional, purposive) neuroregulatory processes [40, 41]. Automatic expressions of pain (e.g. reflexive escape, facial grimaces, guarded posture) represent the immediate biological reaction to sudden tissue insult or exacerbation of chronic pain. In contrast, controlled expression reflects the complex features of painful experience as processed through higher levels of executive control, including memory, problem solving and planning as modulating influences. Non-verbal expression and self-report typically are recognized as different categories of pain response with different sources. Self-report can provide a valid estimate of pain in the competent well-motivated person, but the clinician must recognize that self-report can be biased by the individual's perception of their best interests and requires a high level of linguistic and social competency. Non-verbal expression typically adds context and meaning to self-report and usually is perceived as less amenable to conscious control than verbal report. It is noteworthy to add that non-verbal expression is not invariably reflexive but is subject to misrepresentation and can confound spontaneous with socially predicated expression [42].

Interpersonal determinants

Self-report and non-verbal expressions typically are only modestly correlated, with contextual factors determining the magnitude of the relationship [43, 44]. Pain expression is modulated contingent upon the audience. If the audience is comprised of those who are close and sympathetic, more expressive behavior can be expected; if the audience is comprised of strangers or enemies, expression of painful distress is likely to be diminished or very carefully controlled. This influence is not always straightforward. A study in patients with rheumatoid arthritis found that when the support of a spouse is perceived as satisfying, a reduction in pain expression and an increase in the use of adaptive coping strategies results. When patients became disappointed in their support, efforts to engage in adaptive ways of coping became derailed [45]. Thus, the expression of pain is best recognized as an integrated product of somatosensory events, life history and sensitivity to the immediate context.

Particularly problematic is the potential for exaggerated or suppressed pain expression under purposive control in the interests of intentionally manipulating audiences. Both self-report and non-verbal expression can be deliberately controlled, as evident in both children [46] and adults [47], and clinicians may be challenged to identify circumstances in which pain is deliberately misrepresented [48, 49].

Caregivers

Pain assessment

Clinicians confront a considerable challenge in understanding expressions of painful distress. While manifestations can be highly objective (e.g., what the person says, what they write on paper, reproducible video recordings of non-verbal activity], their relationship to subjective experience may not be so clear. Added to the complex mix of data would be information concerning events leading to injury or disease, evidence of tissue damage and biomedical status and general understanding of the individual's history and life status. From all this, clinicians infer subjective states and are disposed to attributing causes to the actions [50-52].

Intrapersonal determinants

Clinicians are variable in their sensitivity, knowledge and biases. Some features of the response to pain in other people appear biologically prepared or hard-wired, whereas others represent cognitive interpretation. Witnessing another's immediate reaction to painful events is capable of instigating a "visceral" or "gut level" emotional experience. In parallel, the observer will be challenged to attach meaning and understand the event. In this manner, the "bottom-up" external sources of information come to be subjected to "top-down" influences, as the observer appraises the situation and applies knowledge, beliefs, expectancies, attitudes and biases to achieve understanding [48]. It is not surprising that estimates of pain in others frequently underestimate self-report [53-55]. The challenge for the observer is heightened when only self-report or other controlled expressions of pain are available. Given the potential for suppressing or enhancing pain expression, concerns regarding credibility often develop [56]. Systematic use of assessment strategies, including structured interviews and objective psychometric scales (Chapter 12), tend to minimize personal bias.

Interpersonal determinants

Professional education and socialization, training experiences, clinical setting, peer influences and many other social and contextual factors can be expected to have an impact on judgments of pain in others. The evidence indicates clinicians and others tend to be "good enough" rather than "perfectly accurate" in estimating the pain of others [57]. Perfect empathy for another's pain is improbable, given the pain will have distinct sensory components related to injury or disease, although the emotional impact of witnessing others in pain can lead to "vicarious traumatization." Work on burn units, emergency and intensive care units can be difficult and clinicians come to use cognitive and social strategies to minimize personal distress, thereby increasing the likelihood of delivering objective professional care to people experiencing high levels of distress. Similarly, clinicians tend to be cognizant that patients realize they must provide a convincing case for delivery of care services to them. The challenge is particularly demanding for patients with chronic pain. Werner & Malerud [58] provided accounts of women with medically unexplained pain encountering skepticism and lack of comprehension, rejection in addition to being blamed for their condition and experiencing feelings of being ignored or belittled. Socially marginalized people appear particularly vulnerable to neglect [59]. The current opioid overdose epidemic further demonstrates the complexities of clinician judgments as chronic pain patients perceive their clinicians as "They think you're trying to get the drug [60]." Clearly, these are situations to be avoided.

Pain management

Decisions to treat pain and how this should be accomplished again represent the consequences of complex factors, many already described in the foregoing and other papers [61]. Conceptualizing pain as having sensory, emotional, cognitive and social parameters supports utilizing the broad range of interventions described in this volume. The overall assessment of the patient should identify salient challenges permitting treatment tailored to the needs of the patient. Medically focused assessment is likely to identify a pathophysiological basis, if present, whereas psychosocial assessment will be oriented towards emotional, cognitive and social challenges. This broad assessment should be followed by a comprehensive treatment plan that considers all potential targets of intervention if treatment is to reduce pain and to improve quality of life.

Intrapersonal determinants

Decisions concerning whether to deliver care and the type of care provided follow from an assessment of patient needs and inevitably reflect practitioner training and individual differences in personal background and experience in clinical settings. The demands on clinicians are considerable and pain education should be substantial and formal [62]. Given the diversity of causes potentially implicated in any given person's painful condition and disability, the full range of biomedical, psychological and social interventions must be considered. This book provides a compendium of treatment options available to practitioners with different backgrounds and competencies for understanding specific clinical states and special populations.

Interpersonal determinants

Given the importance of public and institutional policy to the delivery of care, availability and accessibility of care for any given individual will reflect the nature of the healthcare system in particular jurisdictions and policies and practices concerning assessment and delivery of pain management in a given setting. The importance of facilitative policies cannot be underestimated and it is conceivable that more can be done to enhance quality of care for people suffering from pain through efforts to change policies than efforts to improve service delivery on the part of any given practitioner [63-65].

Conclusions

The biopsychosocial perspective and the Social Communication Model of Pain provide a useful framework for consideration of best practice in delivery of care to patients. Integrated and interdisciplinary care providing for multimodal treatment has proven superior to unidimensional care in ensuring emotional, cognitive and social challenges are addressed.

References

1 International Association for the Study of Pain. (2018) *IASP Terminology*. International Association for the Study of Pain. https://www.iasp-pain.org/Education/Content.aspx?ItemNumber=1698 Accessed November 25, 2020.

2 Williams AC de C, Craig KD. (2016 Updating the definition of pain. *Pain* **157(11)**:2420–3.

3 Craig KD, MacKenzie NE. (2021). What is pain: are cognitive and social features core components? *Paediatr Pain*00:1–13.

4 Gatchel RJ, Peng YB, Peters ML, Fuchs PN, Turk DC. (2007) The biopsychosocial approach to chronic pain: scientific advances and future directions. *Psychol Bull* **133(4)**:581–624.

5 Turk DC, Monarch ES. Biopsychosocial perspective on chronic pain. (2018) In: Turk DC, Gatchel RJ, eds. *Psychological approaches to pain management: a practitioner's handbook*, 3rd edn. Cambridge University Press, Cambridge. pp. 3–25.

6 Engel GL. (1977) The need for a new medical model: a challenge for biomedicine. *Science* **196(4286)**:129–36.

7 Gatchel RJ, Howard KJ. (2021) The biopsychosocial approach. *Pract Pain Manag* https://www.practicalpainmanagement.com/treatments/psychological/biopsychosocial-approach?page=0,3.

8 Guzman J, Esmail R, Karjalainen K, Malmivaara A, Irvin E, Bombardier C. (2021) Multidisciplinary rehabilitation for chronic low back pain: systematic review. *Br Med J* **322**:1511–6.

9 Gibson CA. (2012) Review of posttraumatic stress disorder and chronic pain: the path to integrated care. *JRRD* **49**:753–76.

10 Lambeek LC, van Mechelen W, Knol DL, Loisel P, Anema JR. (2010) Randomised controlled trial of integrated care to reduce disability from chronic low back pain in working and private life. *BMJ* **340**:c1035.

11 Leasure WB, Leasure EL. (2017) The role of integrated care in managing chronic pain. *Focus (Am Psychiatr Publ)* **15(3)**:284–91.

12 Craig KD. (2009) The social communication model of pain. *Can Psychol* **50(1)**:22–32.

13 Hadjistavropoulos T, Craig KD, Duck S, *et al.* (2011) A biopsychosocial formulation of pain communication. *Psychol Bull* **137(6)**:910–39.

14 Mogil JS. (2009) Are we getting anywhere in human pain genetics? *Pain* **146(3)**:231–2.

15 Melzack R, Katz J. (2005) Pain assessment in adult patients. In: McMahon SB, Koltzenburg M, eds, *Melzack and Wall's Textbook of Pain*, 5th edn. Churchill-Livingstone, London. pp. 291–304.

16 Mailis-Gagnon A, Yegneswaran B, Lakha SF, *et al.* (200) Pain characteristics and demographics of patients attending a university-affiliated pain clinic in Toronto, Ontario. *Pain Res Manag* **12(2)**:93–9.

17 Poulin PA, Nelli J, Tremblay S, *et al.* (2016) Chronic pain in the emergency department: a pilot mixed-methods cross-sectional study examining patient characteristics and reasons for presentations. *Pain Res Manag* **2016**:3092391.

18 May C, Brcic V, Lau B. (2018) Characteristics and complexity of chronic pain patients referred to a community-based multidisciplinary chronic pain clinic. *Can J Pain* **2(1)**:125–34.

19 Williams AC de C, Davies HT, Chadury Y. (2000) Simple pain rating scales hide complex idiosyncratic meanings. *Pain* **85**:457–63.

20 Melzack R. (1975) The McGill Pain Questionnaire: major properties and scoring methods. *Pain* **1(3)**:277–99.

21 Fillingim RB. (2017) Individual differences in pain: understanding the mosaic that makes pain personal. *Pain* **158(Suppl 1)**:S11–S18.

22 Carragee EJ, Don AS, Hurwitz EL, *et al.* (2009). Does discography cause accelerated progression of degeneration changes in the lumbar disc: a ten-year matched cohort study. *Spine* 34(**21**):2338–45.

23 Belfer I, Diatchenko L. (2013) *Pain Genetics: Basic to Translational Science*. Hoboken, John Wiley & Sons.

24 Peters Ml, Vlaeyen JW, Weber WE. (2005) The joint contribution of physical pathology, pain-related fear and catastrophizing to chronic back pain disability. *Pain* **113**:45–50.

25 Turk DC, Okifuji A. (2002) Psychological factors in chronic pain: evolution and revolution. *J Consult Clin Psychol* **70(3)**:678–90.

26 Jackson T, Wang Y, Wang Y, Fan H. (2014) Self-efficacy and chronic pain outcomes: A meta-analytic review. *Pain* **15**:800–14.

27 Morley S, Eccleston C, Williams A. (1999) Systematic review and meta-analysis of randomized controlled trials of cognitive behaviour therapy and behaviour therapy for chronic pain in adults, excluding headache. *Pain* 1999;80(**1–2**):1–13.

28 Higgins N, Bailey SJ, LaChapelle DL, Harman K, Hadjistavropoulos T. (2014) Coping styles, pain expressiveness, and implicit theories of chronic pain. *J Psychol.* **149**:737–750.

29 McCracken LM, Eccleston C. (2005) A prospective study of acceptance of pain and patient functioning with chronic pain. *Pain* **118(1–2)**: 164–9.

30 Wetherell JL, Afari N, Rutledge T, *et al.* (2011) A randomized, controlled trial of acceptance and

commitment therapy and cognitive-behavioral therapy for chronic pain. *Pain* **152(9)**: 2098–107.

31 Carragee EJ, Don AS, Hurwitz EL, *et al.* (2009) Does discography cause accelerated progression of degeneration changes in the lumbar disc: a ten-year matched cohort study. *Spine* **34(21)**:2338–45.

31 Hadler NM. (2003) MRI for regional back pain: need for less imaging, better understanding. *JAMA* **289(21)**:2863–5.

32 Mayer EA, Bushnell MC, eds. (2009) *Functional Pain Syndromes: Presentation and Pathophysiology*. Seattle, IASP Press.

33 Tracey I, Bushnell MC. (2009) How neuroimaging studies have challenged us to rethink: is chronic pain a disease? *J Pain* **10(11)**:1113–20.

34 Dubin R, King-Van Vlack C. (2010) The trajectory of chronic pain: can a community-based exercise/education program soften the ride? *Pain Res Manag* **15(6)**:361–8.

35 Goubert L, Vlaeyen JW, Crombez G, Craig KD. (2011) Learning about pain from others: an observational learning account. *J Pain* 12:167–74.

36 Main CJ, Foster N, Buchbinder R. (2010) How important are back pain beliefs and expectations for satisfactory recovery from back pain? *Best Pract Res Clin Rheumatol* **24**:205–17.

37 Vervoort T, Karos K, Trost Z, Prkachin KM.(2010) *Social and Interpersonal Dynamics in Pain: We Don't Suffer Alone*. Springer Nature, Cham.

38 Karos K, Williams AC de C, Meulders A, Vlaeyen JW. (2018) Pain as a threat to the social self: a motivational account. *Pain* **159**:1690–5.

39 Krahe C, Springer A, Weinman JA, Fotopoulou A. (2013) The social modulation of pain: Others as predictive signals of salience—a systematic review. *Front Hum Neurosci* **7**:386.

40 Craig KD, Versloot J, Goubert L *et al.* (2010) Perceiving others in pain: automatic and controlled mechanisms. *J Pain* **11(2)**:101–8.

41 Hadjistavropoulos T, Craig KD. (2002) A theoretical framework for understanding self-report and observational measures of pain: a communications model. *Behav Res Ther* **40(5)**:551–70.

42 Hill ML, Craig KD. (2002) Detecting deception in pain expressions: the structure of genuine and deceptive facial displays. *Pain* **98(1)**: 135–44.

43 Peeters PA, Vlaeyen JW. (2011) Feeling more pain, yet showing less: The influence of social threat on pain. *J Pain* **12**:1255–61.

44 Versloot J, von Baeyer CL, Craig, KD. (2013) Children give different self-reports of pain intensity to different people: The influence of social display rules. *Pediatric Pain Letter* **15**:19–22.

45 Holtzman S, Newth S, Delongis A. (2004) The role of social support in coping with daily pain among patients with rheumatoid arthritis. *J Health Psychol* **9(5)**:677–95.

46 Larochette AC, Chambers CT, Craig KD. (2006) Genuine, suppressed and faked facial expressions of pain in children. *Pain* **126(1–3)**:64–71.

47 Craig KD, Badali MA. (2004) Introduction to the special series on pain deception and malingering. *Clin J Pain* **20(6)**:377–82.

48 Goubert L, Craig KD, Vervoort T, *et al.* (2005) Facing others in pain: the effects of empathy. *Pain* **118(3)**:286–8.

49 Steinkopf L. (2016) An evolutionary perspective on pain communication. *Evol Psychol*

50 Schiavenato M, Craig KD. (2010) Pain assessment as a social transaction: beyond the "Gold Standard". *Clin J Pain* **26**: 667–76.

51 Wideman TH, Edwards RR, Walton DM, Martel MO, Hudon A, Seminowicz DA. (2019) The multimodal assessment of pain. *Clin J Pain* **35**:212–21.

52 Ruben MA, Hall JA. (2013) "I know your pain": proximal and distal predictors of pain detection accuracy. *Pers Soc Psychol Bull* **39**:1346–1358.

53 Chambers CT, Reid GJ, Craig KD, *et al.* (1998) Agreement between child and parent reports of pain. *Clin J Pain* **14(4)**:336–42.

54 Prkachin KM, Solomon PA, Ross AJ. (2007) The underestimation of pain among health-care providers. *Can J Nurs Res* **39(2)**:88–106.

55 Kappesser J, Williams AC, Prkachin KM. (2006) Testing two accounts of pain underestimation. *Pain* **124(1–2)**:109–16.

56 Craig KD. Hill ML. (2003) Detecting voluntary misrepresentation of pain in facial expression. In: Halligan P, Bass C, Oakley D. editors. *Malingering and Illness Deception*. Oxford University Press, Oxford. po. 336–47.

57 Goubert L, Craig KD, Buysse A. (2009) Perceiving others in pain: experimental and clinical evidence on the role of empathy. In: Decety J, Ickes

WJ, eds. *The Social Neuroscience of Empathy*. MIT Press, Cambridge. pp. 153–66.

58 Werner A, Malterud K. (2003) It is hard work behaving as a credible patient: encounters between women with chronic pain and their doctors. *Soc Sci Med* **57(8)**:1409–19.

59 Wallace B, Varcoe C, Holmes C, *et al*. (2021) Towards health equity for people experiencing chronic pain and social marginalization. *Int J Equity Health* **20**:53.

60 Dassieu L, Heino A, Develay E, *et al*. (2021) "They think you're trying to get the drug": qualitative investigation of chronic pain patients' health care experiences during the opioid overdose epidemic in Canada. *Can J Pain*. **5(1)**:66–80.

61 Rababa, M. (2018) The role of nurses' uncertainty in decision-making process of pain management in people with dementia. *Pain Res Treat* **2018**:7281657.

62 Fishman SM, Young HM, Lucas Arwood E, *et al*. Core competencies for pain management: results of an interprofessional consensus summit. *Pain Med* **14(7)**:971–81.

63 Blyth FM, Macfarlane GJ, Nicholas MK. (2007) The contribution of psychosocial factors to the development of chronic pain: the key to better outcomes for patients. *Pain* **129(1-2)**:8–11.

64 McGrath PJ, Finley GA, eds. *Pediatric Pain: Biological and Social Context*. Seattle IASP Press.

65 Rashiq S, Schopflocher D, Taenzer P *et al*. eds. *Chronic Pain: A Health Policy Perspective*. Weinheim: Wiley-VCH.

Chapter 5

Identification of risk and protective factors in the transition from acute to chronic post surgical pain

Joel Katz[1,2,3], M. Gabrielle Pagé[4,5], Aliza Weinrib[2], & Hance Clarke[2,3]

[1] *Department of Psychology, York University, Toronto, Canada*
[2] *Department of Anesthesia and Pain Management, Toronto General Hospital, Toronto, Canada*
[3] *Department of Anesthesia and Pain Medicine, University of Toronto, Toronto, Canada*
[4] *Centre de recherche du Centre hospitalier de l'Université de Montréal (CRCHUM), Montréal, Canada*
[5] *Département d'anesthésiologie et de medicine de la douleur, Faculté de médecine, et Département de Psychologie, Faculté des arts et des sciences, Université de Montréal, Montréal, Canada*

Introduction

Every chronic pain was once acute. Yet not all acute pain becomes chronic. Some pains develop spontaneously. Others arise as the result of surgery, accident, or illness. Regardless of the cause, most people recover and do not develop persistent pain. Nevertheless, there is obvious interest in determining the factors responsible for the transition of acute, time-limited pain to chronic, intractable, pathological pain [1]. Identification of causal risk factors is the first step in developing effective treatments to prevent and manage pain. In this chapter we focus on the transition of acute to chronic pain after surgery. For several reasons, the study of pain after surgery can serve as a model for the transition to chronicity for other types of pain: (1) Chronic postsurgical pain (CPSP) develops in an alarming proportion of patients; (2) Research into the transition from acute to chronic pain has already revealed specific risk factors that predict who develops CPSP (3); Elective surgery is unique in that the timing and nature of the physical injury are known in advance. This facilitates identification of risk and protective factors that predict the course of recovery; (4) There is a growing body of literature examining preventive efforts to minimize the development of CPSP.

The aim of this chapter is to provide a selective overview of CPSP. We review the basic epidemiology of CPSP according to surgery type; define the concept of a risk factor and the requirements for determining causality; describe the surgical, psychosocial, social-environmental, and patient-related factors that confer a greater risk of developing CPSP; review the rationale and evidence for a preventive analgesic approach to surgery designed to reduce the incidence and intensity of CPSP; and describe preliminary outcomes from a multi-professional Transitional Pain Service specifically designed to prevent the transition from acute to chronic pain after surgery.

Clinical Pain Management: A Practical Guide, Second Edition. Edited by Mary E. Lynch, Kenneth D. Craig, and Philip W. Peng.

Definition and Epidemiology of CPSP

The most recent revision of the International Classification of Diseases (ICD-11) defines chronic postsurgical pain (CPSP) as pain that [1] develops or increases in intensity after a surgical procedure, [2] has been present for at least 3 months (i.e., persists beyond the typical healing time), [3] is localized to the surgical field or projected/referred to a dermatome or deeper structures subserved by involved nerves, and [4] is not caused by other factors (e.g., pre-existing pain, infection, cancer recurrence) [2]. Some authors have suggested the additional criterion, not currently part of the ICD-11 definition, that CPSP must interfere substantially with everyday activities [3]. ICD-11 sub diagnoses include CPSP after amputation, arthroplasty, breast surgery, herniotomy, hysterectomy, spinal surgery and thoracotomy, although other surgical procedures also result in CPSP.

Although most patients who undergo major surgery do not develop CPSP, the incidence of CPSP following certain surgical procedures is unacceptably high [2, 4–6] (Table 5.1). The one-year incidence of CPSP is variable and surgery-specific, ranging from upwards of approximately 30% after modified radical mastectomy and hysterectomy to more than 50% after joint arthroplasty, hernia repair, spinal surgery and thoracotomy and almost 80% for limb amputation. Across surgery types, the one-year CPSP incidence of moderate-to-severe pain has been estimated to be between 8% and 39% [6]. We know next to nothing about CPSP beyond the one-year mark: Pain persists in 8.1% - 19% of patients up to 6 years after hernia repair with severe or very severe pain occurring in 1.8%. Two years after amputation, approximately 60% and between 21%-57% of amputees report phantom limb pain and stump pain, respectively. These statistics are alarming considering the total number of patients worldwide who undergo surgery each year. That almost 25% of patients referred to chronic pain treatment centers have CPSP reflects the intractability of the problem.

Table 5.1 Incidence of chronic postsurgical pain (CPSP) after various surgical procedures

Surgical Procedure	Incidence of CPSP	Follow-up Time after Surgery
Amputation	59-79%	1-2 years
Arthroplasty	13-65%	12 months
Breast surgery	13-33%	12 months
Herniotomy	19-57%	1-5 years
Hysterectomy	21-28%	12 months
Spinal surgery	56%	12 months
Thoracic surgery	41-51%	1-1.5 years

Data from the following sources: Schug et al. [2]; Katz & Seltzer [4] Fletcher et al. [6]

Understanding Risk and Attributing Causality to Outcomes

An important goal of epidemiological and clinical research is to identify the necessary and sufficient conditions under which specific health-related outcomes arise. This typically is achieved over the course of many years involving progressively more sophisticated research designs from observation and description through to experimental manipulation. Initially, an understanding is developed through careful observation of the conditions under which the phenomenon occurs. The next stage involves prediction; specifying in advance the situations under which the phenomenon occurs and the factors that reliably predict its occurrence. The final stage involves prevention and control, which requires detailed knowledge of the causal mechanisms that give rise to the phenomenon and specialized tools to facilitate or inhibit its occurrence. In the field of CPSP, the process of moving from understanding through prediction to control is linked to the concept of risk and to accurately identifying the (risk and protective) factors that place an individual at greater or lesser likelihood of developing CPSP.

A risk factor is defined as a "measurable characterization of each subject in a specified population that precedes the outcome of interest and can be used to divide the population into . . . high-risk and . . . low-risk groups . . ." [7]. Merely identifying a risk factor however does not provide information about risk estimation, and this is particularly relevant for studies with large sample sizes. Risk estimation should always be based on the relative potency of a risk factor. Tools to evaluate the potency of a risk factor include odds ratio, risk ratio, and Cramer's V [8].

A relevant and often overlooked issue pertinent to the concept of risk is that of correlation versus causality, necessitating a distinction between the terms causal risk factor and correlated risk factor [7]. As described above, to meet the requirements for a risk factor, the observed variable must precede the outcome of interest. If the factor is measured at the same time as, or after, the outcome, then it may be a symptom or consequence of the outcome. When the temporal criterion of precedence is not met, as for example in a cross-sectional study, the observed variable is simply a correlate of the measured outcome. Moreover, the temporal criterion of precedence is necessary, but not sufficient, to infer causality. Thus, even if a risk factor is shown to precede the development of the outcome, it does not imply causality and may be a correlate. A risk/protective factor is determined to be causal if its manipulation increases/decreases the risk associated with the measured outcome [7]. Determining the status of a given risk factor as causal or non-causal is essential to progress in understanding the development of CPSP and in prevention and treatment efforts; attempts to manipulate a non-causal risk factor (i.e., a correlate) will have no effect on the outcome (see Figure 5.1E). A major objective of epidemiological research is to identify causal, modifiable risk factors. Demonstrating the causal role of specific risk factors for CPSP is time-consuming, expensive, and requires an evidence base of many randomized, controlled trials. Figure 5.2 shows a schematic illustration of the risk and protective factors involved in the transition to CPSP and disability and how they interact across the pre-operative, intra-operative, and post-operative phases of the peri-operative period.

The increased availability of large datasets and continuously evolving computational approaches, such as machine learning, has also introduced new methodologies to build prediction models [9]. While often such models make it difficult to pinpoint specific risk factors that could become the target of preventive measures, they are becoming increasingly precise in predicting presence or absence of CPSP [10].

Factors Associated with CPSP

Surgical Factors

The following surgical factors are associated with a greater risk of developing CPSP: increased duration of surgery, low (vs high) volume surgical unit, open (vs laparoscopic) approach, peri-costal (vs intracostal) stitches for thoracotomy, conventional hernia repair and intraoperative nerve damage [4]. Whether the above factors are causally related to the development of CPSP is not yet known. However, these factors appear to be associated with greater surgical trauma, and, in particular, they point to intraoperative nerve injury as a likely causal mechanism and the main culprit in producing both acute and chronic neuropathic pain. Thus, one useful preventive measure that can be taken is to avoid intraoperative nerve damage. This is not possible for certain surgeries such as limb amputation that involve ligation and section of major nerve trunks. However, the practice of intentionally transecting nerves for surgical convenience can be avoided and doing so will reduce the incidence of CPSP.

Psychosocial Factors

Several psychosocial risk factors for CPSP or CPSP disability have been identified, including heightened negative affective states such as preoperative state anxiety; preoperative trait anxiety; preoperative pain catastrophizing; fear of surgery; an introverted personality; and "psychic vulnerability", a construct linked to somatization [4, 11, 12]. It remains to be established whether these factors are causally linked to the development of CPSP.

Social Support and Social Environmental Factors

The operant conditioning model proposes that in offering pain contingent help (e.g., taking over household jobs) in response to pain behaviors (e.g., guarding, limping) and verbal expressions of pain, well-intentioned spouses may unwittingly negatively reinforce the patient's pain behaviors leading to an increase in their frequency of occurrence. Greater social support and less spousal solicitousness one month after lower limb amputation has been reported to be associated with improvement in pain interference scores two years later [13].

Patient-Related Factors

Concurrent or past pain is the most consistent patient-related risk factor for the development of CPSP [4]. The presence, intensity, or duration of

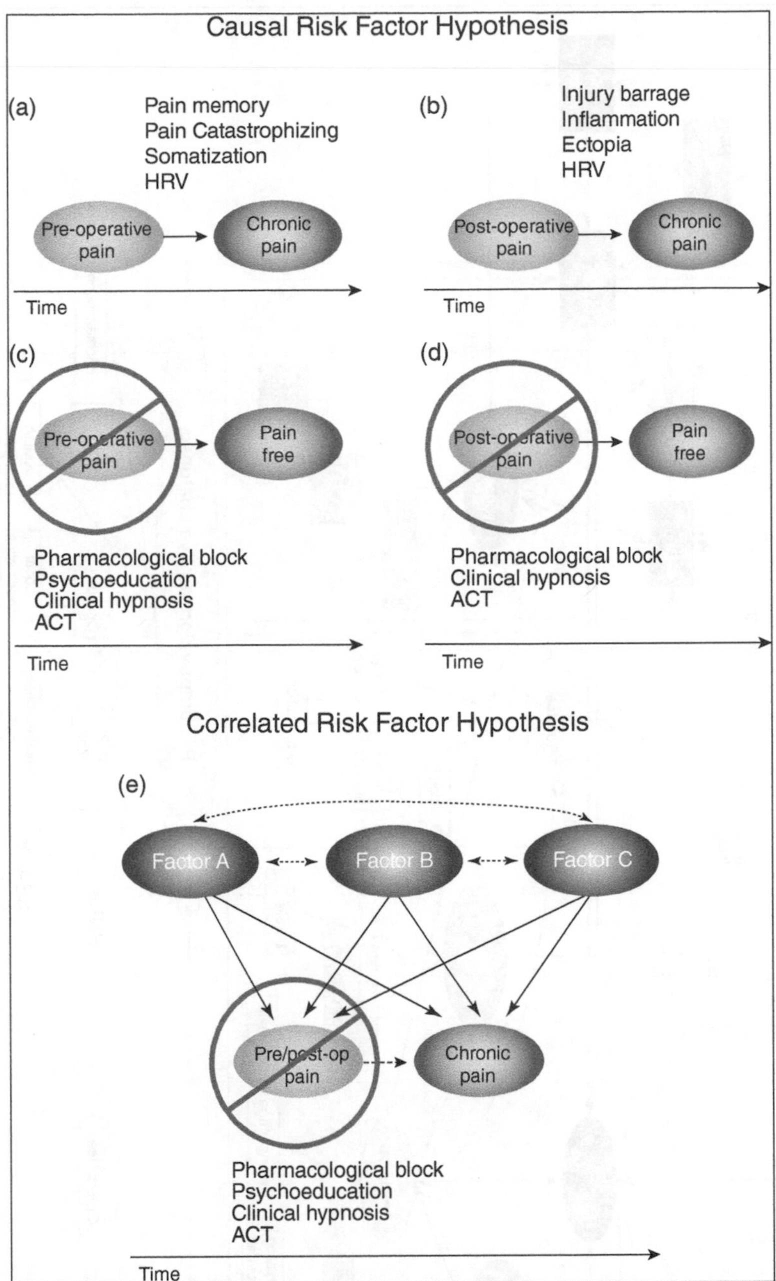

Figure 5.1 Figure depicting causal (top) and associative (bottom) hypotheses predicting the prevention and non-prevention of CPSP by pharmacologic blockade and/or psychological management at various times throughout the perioperative period. Top. Transition to chronicity (A, B) may be prevented by pharmacological blockade or psychological management of preoperative pain (C) and/or acute postoperative pain (D) assuming the former causes the latter. Bottom. Transition to chronicity will not be prevented if pains are merely correlated and caused by one or more higher-order, inter-related factors (E). HRV = heart rate variability; ACT = Acceptance and Commitment Therapy (Color Plate 4).

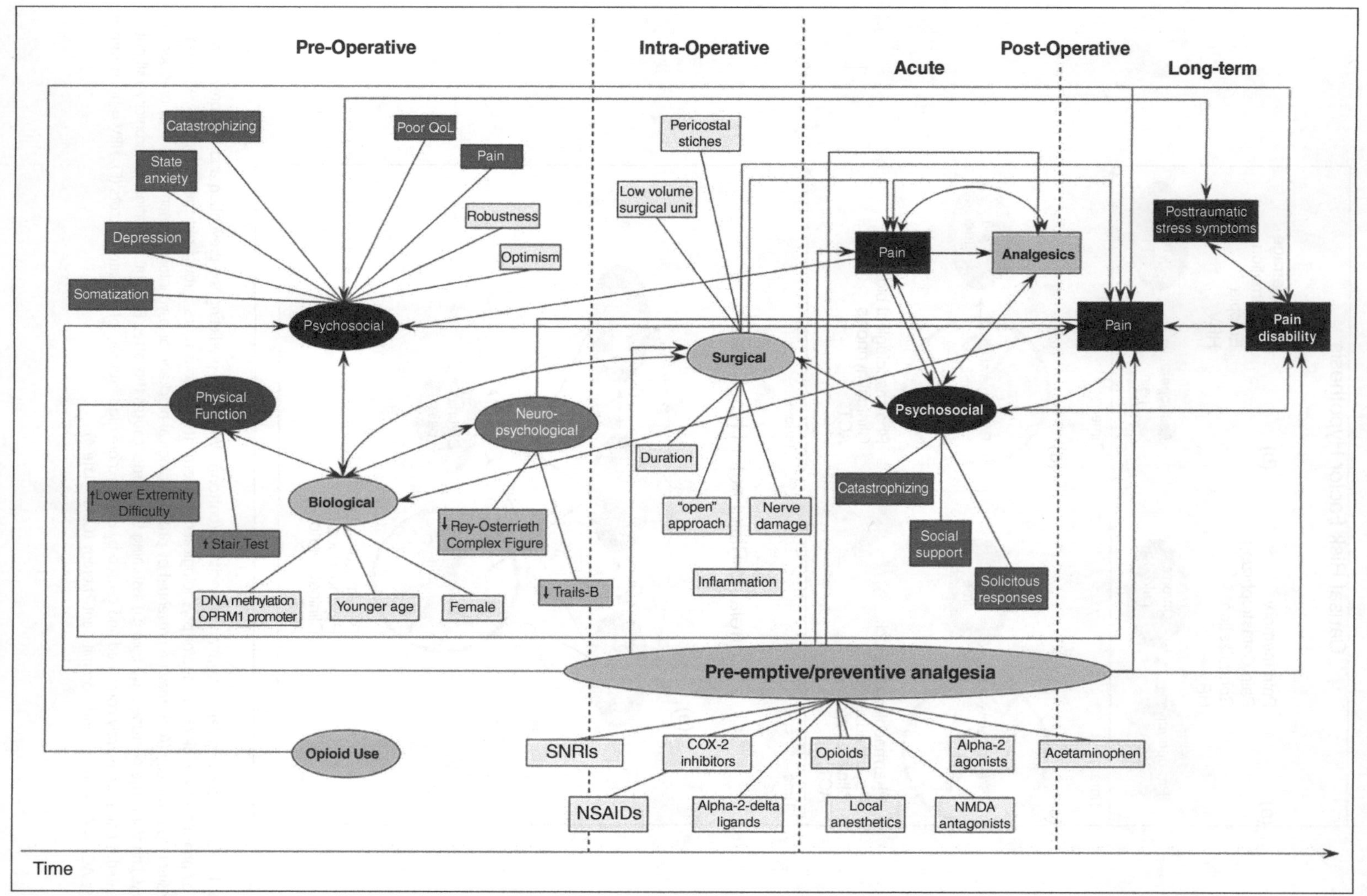

Figure 5.2 Schematic illustration of the processes involved in the development of CPSP and CPSP disability showing relationships (arrows) among pre-operative, intra-operative and post-operative factors. Lines with double arrows between variables show associative relationships reported in the literature. Lines with a single arrow show causal relationships based on randomized controlled trials of preventive analgesia (Color Plate 5).

preoperative pain is a risk factor for the development of CPSP as is the severity of acute postoperative pain in the days and weeks after surgery. Pre-operative and acute post-operative opioid use, a proxy for intense pain, is also a risk factor for CPSP. No other individual difference factor is as consistently related to the development of future pain problems as is pain itself. Younger age and female gender are markers of CPSP but neither predicts CPSP as consistently or strongly as does pain itself. What is essential to determine, however, is the precise feature(s) of pain that is (are) predictive. There are many possibilities for why pain predicts pain, including those that propose a causal or correlative role; however, the evidence to date has not advanced to the point where we can identify pain as a causal risk factor. We propose the following non-mutually-exclusive possibilities [4]:

1 intraoperative nerve damage and the injury barrage that it produces;

2 sensitization of nociceptors in the surgical field;

3 early postoperative ectopic activity of injured afferent fibers and of somata of intact neurons in dorsal root ganglia neighboring those associated with damaged nerves;

4 collateral sprouting from intact nociceptive A-delta afferents that are proximal to the field innervated by injured afferents;

5 central sensitization induced by the surgery and maintained by peripheral input;

6 structural changes in the CNS induced by perioperative nociceptive activity (e.g., loss of anti-nociceptive inhibitory interneurons in the spinal dorsal horn, centralization of pain and somatosensory pain 'memories');

7 as yet unidentified pain genes that confer increased risk of developing intense acute pain and CPSP;

8 consistent response bias over time. Some people report more intense pain than others and they would therefore do so immediately after surgery as well as in the long term;

9 psychosocial factors including greater pain catastrophizing, somatization and less social support;

10 social environmental factors, such as greater solicitous responding from significant others;

11 publication bias in which studies that do not show a significant relationship between pain before and after surgery are not published.

Multi-modal Preventive Approaches

The current practice of treating pain only after it has become well entrenched is slowly being supplanted by a preventive approach that aims to proactively identify and manage patients at high risk of developing CPSP. From an anesthesiology perspective, this entails blocking the primary afferent injury discharge, the inflammatory response and ensuing ectopic activity associated with surgery. The idea is that acute postoperative pain is amplified by a state of central neural hyperexcitability induced by incision. This concept has been expanded to include the sensitizing effects of preoperative noxious inputs and pain, other noxious intraoperative stimuli as well as perioperative peripheral and central inflammatory mediators and ectopic neural activity. From a psychological perspective, research and more recently, clinical practice, have advanced to the point of identifying and modifying the deleterious effects of pre-operative psychosocial factors on CPSP through preoperative psychoeducation [14] and perioperative clinical interventions [15–19].

As shown in Figure 5.1, it is critical to determine the precise causal mechanisms that underlie the relationship between pain at time one (e.g., preoperative pain or acute post-operative pain) and pain at time two (e.g., CPSP 1 year after surgery). The idea that pain is in some way etched into the CNS (e.g., via a pain 'memory' or other memory-like processes) has been at the heart of efforts to halt the transition to chronicity by blocking noxious perioperative impulses from reaching the CNS using a preventive pharmacological approach or by intervening in a psychotherapeutic manner to reduce the deleterious effects preoperative emotional and psychological factors have on the development of CPSP [16, 20]. The assumption has been that pain or some aspect of it (e.g., the peripheral nociceptive barrage associated with surgery, central sensitization, psychological functioning) is a causal risk factor for CPSP (Figure 5.1A-D). However, if the relationship between preoperative or acute postoperative pain and CPSP is merely correlative, and both are caused by one or more higher-order factors that themselves are interrelated, then interventions targeting these correlated risk factors will not prevent the development of CPSP (Figure 5.1E). Our task is to determine the causal modifiable risk factors for CPSP and intervene to prevent its development through multi-professional, multi-modal management.

Preventive Analgesia. The focus of preventive multi-modal analgesia is on attenuating the impact of the peripheral nociceptive barrage associated with noxious preoperative, intraoperative, and/or postoperative events/stimuli. The rationale is to capitalize on the combined effects of several analgesic agents, administered across the preoperative, intraoperative, and postoperative periods, in reducing peripheral and central sensitization. Reviews of the preventive analgesia literature indicate that, across a variety of classes of agents, preventive analgesia reduces acute postoperative pain, analgesic consumption, or both [21–23]. Although the evidence favors a preventive approach for acute postoperative pain, fewer studies have examined the possibility that CPSP can be prevented or attenuated.

Randomized, controlled trials have been conducted to evaluate the long-term efficacy of preventive analgesia. The studies vary in several fundamental ways including sample size, patient population, nature and extent of surgery, pharmacologic agent, route and timing of administration relative to incision and follow-up time after surgery. Space limitations preclude a detailed discussion of the results; however, taken together, the results are equivocal. There is some evidence that CPSP can be minimized by an analgesic approach involving aggressive perioperative multi-modal treatment, but other studies fail to show this benefit [21–23].

Transitional Pain Service. A multi-professional, multi-modal preventive approach to CPSP recently has been instituted at the Toronto General Hospital [11, 15, 18–20]. The Transitional Pain Service (TPS) involves intensive, perioperative psychological, physical and pharmacological monitoring and management designed to prevent and treat the known risk factors for CPSP, pain-related disability and prolonged opioid use. The aim of the TPS is to offer timely and effective treatment for high-risk patients scheduled for surgical procedures for cancer, cardiac disease and organ transplants. Patients are assessed and offered treatment as early as the preoperative visit. Treatment is extended in-hospital after surgery and is maintained for up to 6 months after surgery, as necessary. The treatment team comprises anesthesiologists, psychologists, nurse practitioners, physical therapists and other professionals as needed. The main psychological approaches involve Acceptance and Commitment Therapy (ACT), mindfulness and clinical hypnosis. Opioid tapering and weaning are critical components of the TPS, achieved through compassionate and realistic patient-centered methods that respect the individuality of the patient.

In the first of 2 clinical practice-based studies, we compared patients receiving TPS psychological services (ACT group) to those not receiving psychological services (no ACT group) in a non-randomized trial [20]. Compared with the no ACT group, the ACT group had a significantly higher prevalence of mental health conditions before surgery and, at the first post-surgical visit, were consuming a significantly larger daily dose of opioids. These pre-treatment differences are not surprising because patients who are referred for TPS psychology services are typically emotionally distressed and having difficulty coping. By the last TPS visit, although both groups reported significant reductions in pain, pain-related interference, catastrophizing, anxiety, and opioid use, the ACT group showed even greater reductions in opioid use and pain interference than the no ACT group. In addition, only the ACT group reported a significant reduction in symptoms of depression by the last TPS visit. Group differences in treatment duration raise the possibility that the no ACT group might have achieved the same level of improvement given an equivalent follow-up time. Moreover, the lack of randomization introduces a selection bias that may explain the observed differences in outcomes. Nevertheless, these results provide preliminary support for the TPS in targeting and successfully managing patients at risk of CPSP and persistent opioid use.

In a second clinical practice-based study [18], we compared opioid consumption and opioid weaning rates at the last TPS visit an average of 6 months after surgery between TPS patients who were opioid-naïve or opioid-experienced before surgery. Figure 5.3 shows the relationship between opioid dose at hospital discharge and at the last TPS visit ~6 months after surgery for the opioid-naïve and opioid experienced patients depicting treatment success and failures based on the recommended guideline that patients take no more than 90 mg/day in morphine equivalent dosing.

At the last TPS visit ~6 months after surgery, opioid-experienced patients had reduced their

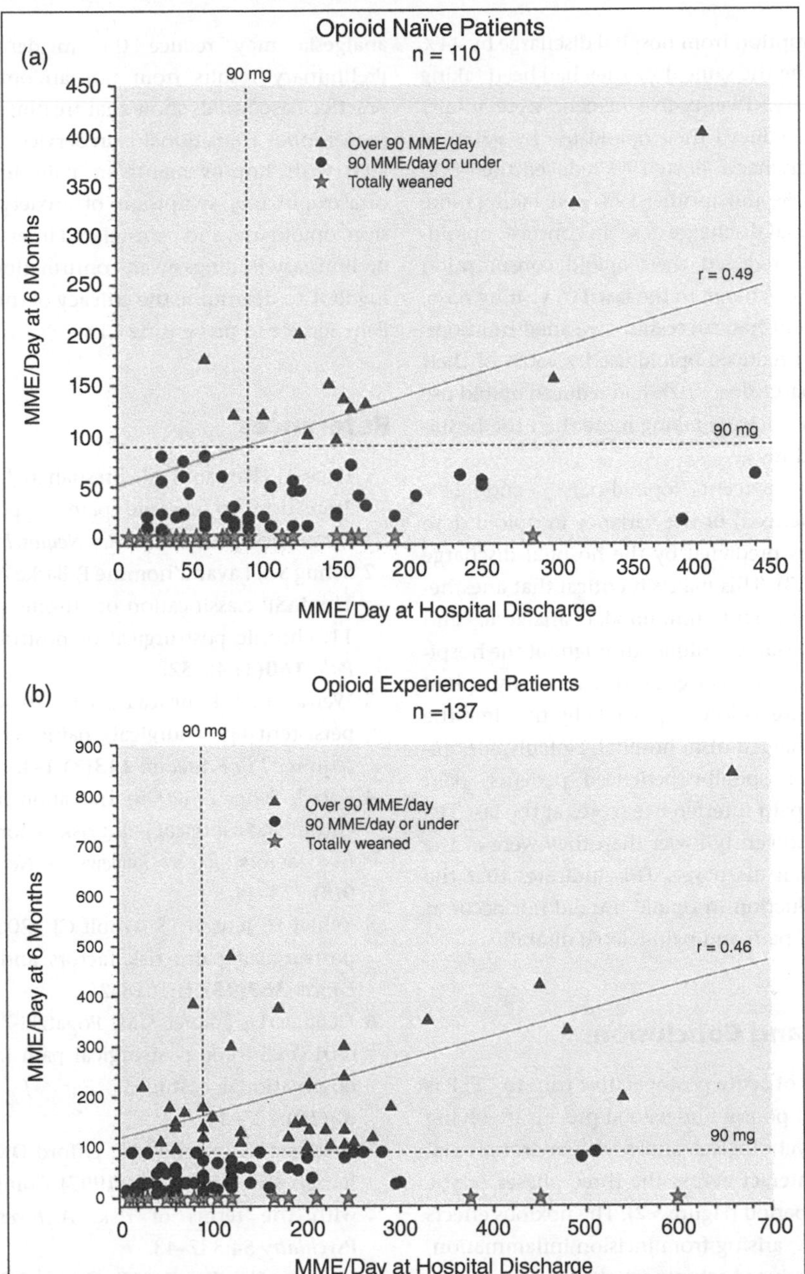

Figure 5.3 Mean daily opioid use in mg morphine equivalents (MME/day) at the end of Transitional Pain Service (TPS) treatment 6 months after surgery shown as a function of MME/day at hospital discharge prior to the first outpatient TPS visit among 110 patients (A) who were not taking opioids before surgery (opioid-naïve) and 137 patients (B) who were (opioid experienced). Also shown is the best-fitting straight line and correlation between MME/day at hospital discharge and at 6 months indicating that 21% and 24% of the latter dose can be predicted by the former for opioid-naïve and opioid experienced patients, respectively. The maximum dose of 90 MME/day recommended by the USA and Canadian opioid guideline is depicted by the dashed lines. Based on the maximum recommended dose, patients in the two lower quadrants (green shading) represent TPS treatment successes and those in the two upper quadrants (red shading) represent TPS treatment failures. Green circles represent patients who were under 90 MME/day at the end of TPS treatment 6 months after hospital discharge; cyan stars represent patients who were totally weaned (MME/day = 0) by 6 months; red triangles represent patients who were over 90 MME/day at 6 months (Color Plate 6). Adapted from Clarke et al. [18].

opioid consumption from hospital discharge by 44% and were taking the same dose they had been taking prior to surgery. Twenty-five percent were totally weaned, 36% reduced their opioid use by >50% of the hospital discharge dose, 19% reduced their opioid use by <50%, and another 19% were taking more than the hospital discharge dose. In contrast, opioid-naïve patients reduced their opioid consumption from hospital discharge to the last TPS visit by 65%. Forty-six percent had successfully weaned from opioids, 35% had reduced opioid use by >50% of their hospital discharge dose, 10% had reduced opioid use by <50%, and 8% were taking more than the hospital discharge dose.

Twenty-one percent (opioid-naïve) and 24% (opioid-experienced) of the variance in opioid dose at 6 months is predicted by the hospital discharge dose (Figure 5.3). This makes it critical that anesthesiologists implement multimodal analgesic and regional/neuraxial techniques throughout the hospital stay to ensure postsurgical pain and daily opioid requirements are as low as possible by the time the patient is discharged from hospital. Notably, for opioid naïve and opioid-experienced patients, pain intensity and pain interference scores at the last TPS visit were significantly lower than they were at the time of hospital discharge. This indicates that the significant reduction in opioid use did not occur at the expense of pain and pain-related disability.

Summary and Conclusion

The transition of acute postoperative pain to CPSP is a complex and poorly understood process involving biological, psychological and social-environmental factors that interact across the three phases of the perioperative period (Figure 5.2). The noxious effects of surgery (e.g., arising from incision inflammation, nerve-injury induced ectopic activity, central sensitization), in conjunction with the competing, protective effects of preventive analgesia, interact with pre-existing and concurrent pain, psychological and emotional factors as well as the social environment to determine the nature, severity, frequency and duration of CPSP. There is good evidence to support that avoiding nerve damage in the surgical field and maximizing pain control in the peri and postoperative periods improves pain outcomes. In certain cases, perioperative, multi-modal preventive analgesia may reduce the incidence of CPSP. Preliminary results from nonrandomized, clinical practice-based trials show that treatment by a multiprofessional Transitional Pain Service team is associated with improvements in pain intensity, pain catastrophizing, symptoms of anxiety and depression, opioid use, and pain-related interference. These preliminary findings await confirmation of an ongoing RCT to determine the efficacy of the Transitional Pain Service in preventing CPSP.

References

1 Price TJ, Basbaum AI, Bresnahan J, *et al.* (2018) Transition to chronic pain: opportunities for novel therapeutics. *Nat Rev Neurosci* **19(7)**:383–4.

2 Schug SA, Lavand'homme P, Barke A, *et al.* (2019) The IASP classification of chronic pain for ICD-11: chronic postsurgical or posttraumatic pain. *Pain* **160(1)**:45–52.

3 Werner MU, Kongsgaard UE. (2014) I. Defining persistent post-surgical pain: is an update required? *Br J Anaesth* **113(1)**:1–4.

4 Katz J, Selter Z. (2009) Transition from acute to chronic postsurgical pain: risk factors and protective factors. *Expert Reviews of Neurotherapeutics* **9(5)**:723–44.

5 Kehlet H, Jensen TS, Woolf CJ. (2006) Persistent postsurgical pain: risk factors and prevention. *Lancet* **367(9522)**:1618–25.

6 Fletcher D, Stamer UM, Pogatzki-Zahn E, *et al.* (2015) Chronic postsurgical pain in Europe: an observational study. *Eur J Anaesthesiol* **32(10)**:725–34.

7 Kraemer HC, Kazdin AE, Offord DR, Kessler RC, Jensen PS, Kupfer DJ. (1997) Coming to terms with the terms of risk. *Archives of General Psychiatry* 54:337–43.

8 Kraemer HC, Kazdin AE, Offord DR, Kessler RC, Jensen PS, Kupfer DJ. (1999) Measuring the potency of risk factors for clinical or policy significance. *Psychological Methods* **4(3)**:257–71.

9 Lotsch J, Ultsch A. (2018) Machine learning in pain research. *Pain* **159(4)**:623–30.

10 Lotsch J, Sipila R, Tasmuth T, *et al.* (2018) Machine-learning-derived classifier predicts absence of persistent pain after breast cancer surgery with high accuracy. *Breast Cancer Res Treat* 171(**2**):399–411.

11 Katz J, Weinrib AZ, Clarke H. (2019) Chronic postsurgical pain: From risk factor identification to multidisciplinary management at the Toronto General Hospital Transitional Pain Service. *Canadian Journal of Pain* **3(2)**:49–58.

12 Giusti EM, Lacerenza M, Manzoni GM, (2021) Psychological and psychosocial predictors of chronic postsurgical pain: a systematic review and meta-analysis. *Pain* **162(1)**:10–30.

13 Hanley MA, Jensen MP, Ehde DM, Hoffman AJ, Patterson DR, Robinson LR. (2004) Psychosocial predictors of long-term adjustment to lower-limb amputation and phantom limb pain. *Disabil Rehabil* **26(14-15)**:882–93.

14 Horn A, Kaneshiro K, Tsui BCH. (2020) Preemptive and preventive pain psychoeducation and its potential application as a multimodal perioperative pain pontrol option: a systematic review. *Anesth Analg* **130(3)**: 559–73.

15 Katz J, Weinrib A, Fashler SR, *et al*. (2015) The Toronto General Hospital Transitional Pain Service: development and implementation of a multidisciplinary program to prevent chronic postsurgical pain. *J Pain Res* **8**:695–702.

16 Nicholls JL, Azam MA, Burns LC, *et al*. (2018) Psychological treatments for the management of postsurgical pain: a systematic review of randomized controlled trials. *Patient Relat Outcome Meas* **9**:49–64.

17 Weinrib AZ, Azam MA, Birnie KA, Burns LC, Clarke H, Katz J. (2017) The psychology of chronic post-surgical pain: new frontiers in risk factor identification, prevention and management. *Br J Pain* **11(4)**:169–77.

18 Clarke H, Azargive S, Montbriand J, *et al*. (2018) Opioid weaning and pain management in postsurgical patients at the Toronto General Hospital Transitional Pain Service. *Canadian Journal of Pain* **2(1)**:236–47.

19 Weinrib AZ, Burns LC, Mu A, *et al*. (2017) A case report on the treatment of complex chronic pain and opioid dependence by a multidisciplinary transitional pain service using the ACT Matrix and buprenorphine/naloxone. *J Pain Res* **10**:747–55.

20 Azam MA, Weinrib AZ, Montbriand J, *et al*. (2017) Acceptance and Commitment Therapy to manage pain and opioid use after major surgery: preliminary outcomes from the Toronto General Hospital Transitional Pain Service. *Canadian Journal of Pain* **1(1)**.

21 Clarke H, Bonin RP, Orser BA, Englesakis M, Wijeysundera DN, Katz J. (2012) The prevention of chronic postsurgical pain using gabapentin and pregabalin: a combined systematic review and meta-analysis. *Anesth Analg* **115(2)**:428–42.

22 Clarke H, Poon M, Weinrib A, Katznelson R, Wentlandt K, Katz J. (2015) Preventive analgesia and novel strategies for the prevention of chronic post-surgical pain. *Drugs* **75(4)**:339–51.

23 Katz J, Clarke H, Seltzer Z. (2011) Review article: preventive analgesia: quo vadimus? *Anesth Analg* **113(5)**:1242–53.

Chapter 6

Placebo/nocebo: a two-sided coin in the clinician's hand

Elisa Frisaldi[1], Aziz Shaibani[2], & Fabrizio Benedetti[1,3]

[1] *University of Turin Medical School, Neuroscience Department, Turin, Italy*
[2] *Nerve and Muscle Center of Texas, Baylor College of Medicine, Houston, Texas, USA*
[3] *Medicine and Physiology of Hypoxia, Plateau Rosà, Switzerland*

Introduction

The use of placebos dates back to the origins of medicine itself. Much of the ongoing confusion about the term, still pervading both the society and the scientific community, probably derives from the shifting focus on its different aspects across the centuries, such as: an inert medication given more to please than to benefit, a deceiving expedient to trick the naive layman, a means to detect the mystifying patient, a tool to isolate specific drugs effects in the course of clinical trials and, finally, an additional therapeutic aid. Current neurobiological and pharmacological evidence has placed placebo effects at the intersection between expectation, hope, desire, anxiety and previous experience (conditioning), involving both patient and attending staff, and has provided scientific ground for their exploitation. Interest in the placebo's evil twin, the nocebo, is more recent. If a placebo is a sham treatment inducing a positive outcome, a nocebo is a sham treatment inducing a negative one. It could actually be the same inert substance (e.g. coupled to opposite verbal instructions to reverse the patient's expectations). As for placebos, the whole context surrounding the therapeutic act impacts on different psychological aspects to produce the end result. In modern clinical practice, ethical concerns have been raised about the legitimacy of placebo administration. Informed consent and patient deceit seem irreconcilable; still a more widespread awareness of the importance of the patient–provider interaction and the introduction of specific therapeutic protocols can represent a way to exploit placebo effects to the patient's advantage while at the same time avoiding nocebo effects.

In this chapter a brief overview on current knowledge of the biology of placebo and nocebo effects is outlined, followed by some suggestions for clinical application. Emphasis is on pain studies and pain treatment, but it should be remembered that placebo and nocebo effects have been described in many other clinical conditions, such as Parkinson's disease and depression; in different systems, like the endocrine and immune systems; and even outside the medical domain, as in sport performance. Indeed, they pervade our everyday life, at the conscious and unconscious level, affecting our evaluations and decisions.

The interested reader is referred to a number of reviews and books that address these topics in greater detail [1–7].

Clinical Pain Management: A Practical Guide, Second Edition. Edited by Mary E. Lynch, Kenneth D. Craig, and Philip W. Peng.

Before we begin: a few facts on placebo/nocebo

Q1: *Is the placebo effect the same as the placebo response?*

A. The two terms are often used synonymously. However, a recent consensus paper stated that the placebo response is that observed in the placebo arm of a clinical trial, which is produced by the placebo biological phenomenon in addition to other potential factors contributing to symptom amelioration, such as natural history, regression to the mean, biases and judgment errors. The placebo effect, on the other hand, designates the biological phenomenon in isolation, as can best be studied in specifically designed experimental protocols [8].

Q2: *Is the placebo an inert treatment?*

A. Yes and no. The adjective "inert" correctly suggests that the substance or treatment is devoid of specific effects for the condition being treated. However, it cannot by definition be inert if it produces an effect. The solution to the conundrum can be found by shifting the attention from the treatment to the patient who receives it: it is in fact the symbolic meaning of the treatment, rather than the treatment itself, which by different mechanisms triggers active processes in the patient's brain, ultimately producing the placebo effect. The placebo need not be a "treatment" either. Its archetype is, of course, the sugar pill, but more subtle or more general factors work equally well. For example, the symbolic meaning can be ascribed to one or all aspects of the context surrounding the therapeutic act, and the simulation of a therapeutic situation can thus adequately replace the sugar pill.

Q3: *Is a nocebo effect the opposite of a placebo effect?*

A. Yes, the nocebo has been defined as negative placebo. As expectations of amelioration can lead to clinical improvement, expectations of worsening can result in negative outcome. The term nocebo (Latin "I shall harm") was originally introduced to designate noxious effects produced by a placebo (e.g. side effects of the drug the placebo is substituting for). In that case, however, the negative outcome is produced in spite of an expectation of benefit. True nocebo effects, on the other hand, are always the result of negative expectations, specific or generic (like a pessimistic attitude).

Proposed mechanisms of placebo/ nocebo effects

Different explanatory mechanisms have been proposed for both placebo and nocebo effects, each supported by experimental evidence. They need not be mutually exclusive and can actually be at work simultaneously.

Classical conditioning

This theory posits the placebo/nocebo effect as the result of Pavlovian conditioning. In this process, the repeated co-occurrence of an unconditioned response to an unconditioned stimulus (e.g. salivation after the sight of food) with a conditioned stimulus (e.g. a bell ringing) induces a conditioned response (i.e. salivation that is induced by bell ringing alone). Likewise, aspects of the clinical setting (e.g. taste, color, shape of a tablet, as well as white coats or the peculiar hospital smell) can also act as conditioned stimuli, eliciting a therapeutic response in the absence of an active principle, just because they have been paired with it in the past. In the same way, the conditioned response can be a negative outcome, as in the case of nausea elicited by the sight of the environment where chemotherapy has been administered in the past. Classical conditioning seems to work best where unconscious processes are at play, as in placebo/nocebo effects involving endocrine or immune systems, but it has also been documented in clinical and experimental placebo analgesia and nocebo hyperalgesia.

Expectations

This theory conceives the placebo effect as the product of cognitive engagement, with the patient consciously foreseeing a positive or negative outcome, based on factors as diverse as verbal instructions, environmental clues, previous experience, emotional arousal and the interaction with care-providers. This anticipation of the future outcome in turn triggers internal changes resulting in specific experiences (e.g. analgesia or hyperalgesia). Desire, self-efficacy and self-reinforcing feedback all interact with expectation, potentiating its effects. Desire is the experiential dimension of wanting something to happen or wanting to avoid something happening [7], while self-efficacy is the belief to be able to manage the disease, performing the right actions to induce positive changes (e.g. to withstand and lessen pain). Self-reinforcing feedback is a positive loop whereby the subject attends selectively to signs of improvement, taking them as evidence that the placebo treatment has worked. This is also called the somatic focus (i.e. the degree to which individuals focus on their symptoms) [7]. A related proposed mechanism posits that anxiety reduction also has a role in placebo responses, because the subject interpretation of ambiguous sensations is changed from noxious and menacing to benign and unworthy of attention.

Embodiment

Central to the constructionist view of the placebo experience held by medical anthropologists is the concept of embodiment, which states that the human mind is strongly influenced and shaped by aspects of the body, such as the sensory systems and our interaction with the environment and the society. Thus, our experiences can not only be consciously stored as memories, but also imprinted straight onto our body, without involvement of any cognitive process. An example of how sociocultural experiences can impact on the individual's physiology is offered by trauma or stress, as in post-traumatic stress disorder (PTSD), where symptoms such as sleep disorders or frightening thoughts are the result of an implicit perception, the literal "incorporation" of a terrifying event in the external world, which bypassed conscious awareness. According to this view, the placebo effect is a positive effect of embodiment and the nocebo effect a negative one. Lived positive experiences can be channeled into objects or places, which then acquire potential to trigger healing responses. Importantly, this process needs not involve conscious expectation or conscious attribution of symbolic meaning to the object or place [7].

Performative efficacy

Therapeutic performances may have *per se* a convincing persuading effect; just by the ritual of the therapeutic act, a change in the body can be achieved. The performance inducing a placebo effect may be social, as in sham surgery in clinical trials with positive outcomes in the placebo arm, or in the case of a mother's kiss on a child's wound; or it may be internal, as for athletes mentally rehearsing before a competition. In this framework, a placebo effect could result from the internal act of imagining a specific change of state of the body. It is tempting to speculate that as mirror motor neurons fire when observing somebody perform a motor task (in the same way as they would when the individual performs the task himself), so could neural pathways be activated by the internal performance of healing change, in turn facilitating healing itself. Central in the performative efficacy of the ritual is the patient–provider relationship, with factors such as empathy, prestige of the healer, gesture and recitation all contributing to the treatment success.

All these mechanisms may contribute to the final placebo/nocebo effect in varying proportion, or combine differently in specific cases. To some extent, some of them can influence one another, as for conditioning and expectation, which both represent a form of learning; thus, conditioning can bring about conscious expectations. Many forms of learning may take place, including social observational learning: observing beneficial effects in a demonstrator induced stronger analgesic placebo responses than those induced by verbal suggestions alone, and as potent as those induced by a conditioning procedure.

The importance of each mechanism can be different in placebo vs. nocebo effects. For example, it has been shown in healthy volunteers in a pain conditioning/expectation protocol that conditioning was more important than verbal instructions (inducing expectation) for placebo effects, while the opposite was true for nocebo effects.

Neurobiology of placebo analgesia

The last decade has witnessed the beginning of clarification of neurochemical and pharmacological details of placebo analgesia. In 1978, a pioneering study by Levine *et al.* [7] showed that the opiate antagonist naloxone was able to reduce the placebo response in dental postoperative pain. That was the first indication that endogenous opioids were involved in placebo analgesia. Subsequent experiments provided ever more compelling evidence that the secretion of endogenous opioids in the brain was the key event in placebo pain modulation. Placebo responders had levels of β-endorphin in the cerebrospinal fluid that were more than double those of non-responders; opioids released by a placebo procedure displayed the same side effects as exogenous opiates; naloxone-sensitive cardiac effects could be observed during placebo-induced expectation of analgesia. Indirect support also came from the placebo-potentiating role of the cholecystokinin (CCK) antagonist proglumide. In fact, the CCK system effects counteracted those of opioids, delineating a picture where the placebo effect seems to be under the opposing influence of facilitating opioids and inhibiting CCK. In some situations, however, a placebo effect can still occur after blockade of opioid mechanisms by naloxone, indicating that systems other than opioids are also implicated. For example, with a morphine conditioning and/or expectation-inducing protocol, naloxone was able to completely reverse placebo analgesia induced in experimental ischemic arm pain. Conversely, with the use of ketorolac (a non-opioid analgesic) in the same protocol, only a partial blockade could be observed. Almost nothing is currently known on these non-opioid systems, and further research is needed to clarify them (Fig. 6.1).

The advent of neuroimaging techniques and of their use for experimental purposes added anatomic and temporal details to the neurochemical information. The first positron emission tomography (PET) study to investigate placebo analgesia was conducted in 2002. It showed overlapping in the brain activation pattern generated by opioid-induced analgesia (by the μ-agonist remifentanil) and by placebo-induced analgesia. Common activated areas included the rostral anterior cingulate cortex (rACC) and the orbitofrontal cortex. In the following years, in spite of some discrepancies likely explained by methodological and procedural differences, PET, functional magnetic resonance imaging (fMRI) and magneto-electroencephalography (MEG) studies all suggested placebo activation of the descending pain control system, with modulation of activity in areas such as periaqueductal gray (PAG), the ventromedial medulla, the parabrachial nuclei, the ACC, the orbitofrontal cortex, the hypothalamus and the central nucleus of the amygdala. Notably, direct demonstration of endogenous opioid release was obtained through [^{11}C] carfentanil displacement by the activation of opioid neurotransmission, with the decrease

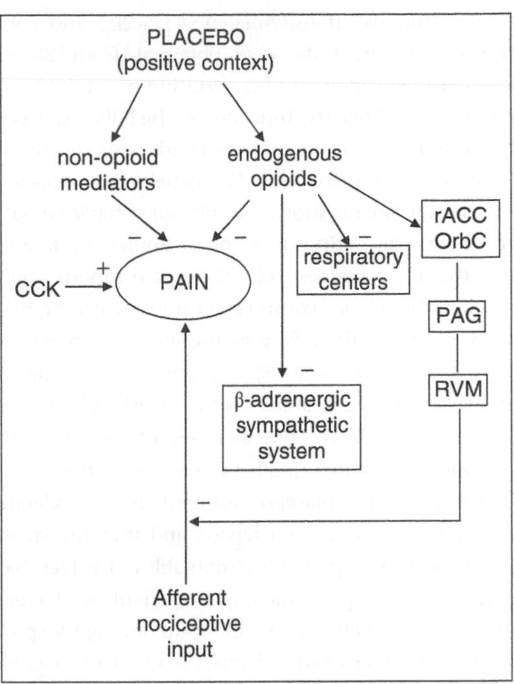

Figure 6.1 Cascade of events that may take place during a placebo procedure. Pain is inhibited by the activation of a descending inhibitory network involving the rostral anterior cingulate cortex (rACC), the orbitofrontal cortex (OrbC), the periacqueductal gray (PAG) and the rostral ventromedial medulla (RVM). Endogenous opioids inhibit pain through this descending network and/or other mechanisms. The respiratory centers may be inhibited by opioid mechanisms as well. The β-adrenergic sympathetic system is also inhibited during placebo analgesia. Non-opioid mechanisms are also involved. Cholecystokinin (CCK) counteracts the effects of the endogenous opioids, thus antagonizing placebo analgesia.

in binding correlating with placebo reduction of pain intensity reports. Recently, naloxone was observed to block placebo-induced responses in pain modulatory cortical structures and in key structures of the descending pain control system (for a review on neuroimaging studies see 9).

Further clarification to the functional neuroanatomy of placebo analgesia comes from a more recent meta-analysis aimed at assessing whether the neurological pain signature (NPS), which represent the set of brain regions involved in pain processing, is specifically affected by placebos [10]. In this analysis, Medline (PubMed) was searched from inception to May 2015 and involved studies of functional neuroimaging of the human brain with evoked pain delivered under stimulus intensity-matched placebo and control conditions. Data were obtained from 20 of 28 identified eligible studies, resulting in a total sample size of 603 healthy individuals. The NPS responses to painful stimulation compared with baseline conditions were positive in 575 participants (95.4%). Placebo treatments showed significant behavioral outcomes on pain ratings in 17 of 20 studies (85%) and also moderate analgesic effects on pain reports compared with matched control conditions. However, placebo effects on the NPS response were significant in only 3 of 20 studies (15%) and were small. Similarly, analyses restricted to studies with low risk of bias indicated small effects, and analyses of just placebo responders indicated small effects as well. These findings indicate that placebo treatments have moderate analgesic effects on pain reports and that the small effects on NPS are probably attributable to the fact that placebos affect pain via brain mechanisms largely independent of effects on bottom-up nociceptive processing. In other words, placebos may act on regions other than the neurological pain signature.

Also of interest is the fact that knowledge of placebo analgesia can be gained by focusing on changes in brain activity that take place with modulation of expectation alone. In fact, expectation of benefit can induce a placebo effect even without the physical administration of a placebo. Because no placebo is actually given, these effects may be more appropriately called "placebo-like" effects. Thus, activity in pain areas following a constant painful stimulus can be modulated, at least in part, just by varying the subject's expectation of the level of stimulation: the higher the *expected* level of the stimulus, the stronger the activity in ACC and other areas implicated in the activation of the descending inhibitory pathway. Taken together, these studies show how the same result (i.e. the activation of the same receptors in the brain) can be obtained by a pharmacologic (drug) or a psychologic (placebo) means. A more comprehensive description of the studies mentioned here can be found in [7].

Neurobiology of nocebo hyperalgesia

Compared to placebo effect research, the investigation of the nocebo effect raises more ethical difficulties, especially in the clinical setting. However, in recent times a few experimental studies have begun to shed light on this phenomenon, focusing mainly on the model of nocebo hyperalgesia. In the protocols used, an inert treatment is given along with verbal suggestions of pain worsening, resulting in exacerbation of pain. It has been suggested that the anticipatory anxiety about the impending pain, brought about by negative expectations, triggers the activation of CCK, which in turn facilitates pain transmission and results in hyperalgesia. Accordingly, this hyperalgesia can be blocked by proglumide, a non-specific CCK-1 and CCK-2 antagonist, in a dose-dependent manner. The proglumide block is related specifically to nocebo/anxiety-induced hyperalgesia rather than to the more general process of nocebo-induced anxiety, as it is selectively exerted on nocebo hyperalgesia but not on the concurrent stress-induced hypothalamic-pituitary-adrenal axis hyperactivity (Fig. 6.2).

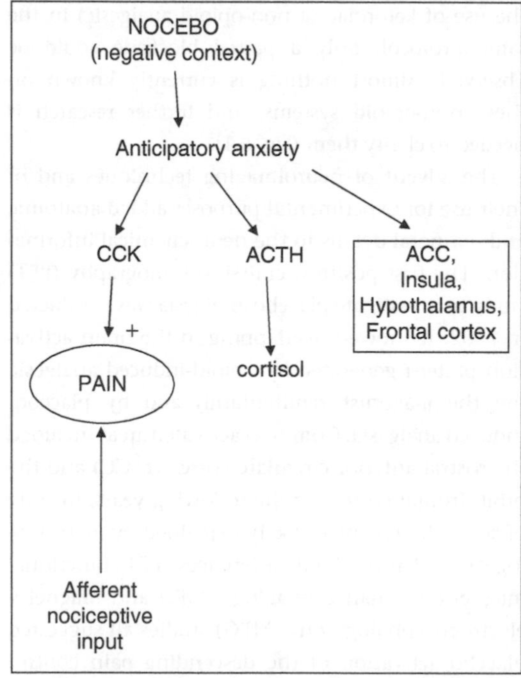

Figure 6.2 Events that may occur during a nocebo procedure. Nocebo induces anticipatory anxiety which, in turn, affects both the hypothalamus-pituitary-adrenal axis (adrenocorticotropic hormone [ACTH] and cortisol) and pain mechanisms. The link between anxiety and pain is represented by cholecystokinin (CCK), which has a facilitating effect on pain. Anticipatory anxiety about the impending pain also activates different brain regions that are involved in pain processing.

Proglumide also exhibits placebo-potentiating effects, raising the question of how the two endogenous systems, CCK and opioids, may interact in producing negative or positive outcomes. It can be speculated that the placebo/nocebo phenomenon is a continuum, with opioid and CCK-ergic systems acting as the mediators of opposing effects. Recent experimental evidence also suggests that nocebo effects involve the cyclooxygenase pathway as well [11].

As for placebo analgesia, neuroimaging techniques have also brought important contributions to the knowledge of nocebo hyperalgesia. Here again, expectations without the physical administration of a nocebo treatment have been exploited ("nocebo-like" effects). Inducing negative expectations resulted in both amplified unpleasantness of innocuous stimuli as assessed by psychophysical pain measures (subject report) and increased fMRI responses in ACC, insula, hypothalamus, secondary somatosensory areas and prefrontal cortex. From these studies it appears that the circuitry underlying nocebo hyperalgesia largely involves, with opposite modulation, the same areas engaged by placebo analgesia (see [7] for a review).

The effects of nocebo on the spinal cord have also been found for complex psychological factors, such as value information about a drug, e.g. the price tag. Tinnermann et al. [12] discovered that labelling an inert treatment as expensive medication led to stronger nocebo hyperalgesia than labelling it as cheap medication. This effect was mediated by the activity in the prefrontal cortex and coupling between prefrontal areas, brainstem and spinal cord. This might represent a mechanism through which higher cognitive representations, such as value, can modulate early pain processing.

The coin in the clinician's hand

What is the relevance of placebo/nocebo studies to clinical practice and how can patients benefit from the application of these research findings? It could be argued that today's ethical restrictions prevent the widespread use of placebos that was commonplace in ancient times. Still, its practice is common, and physicians surveyed in many countries reported using placebos to calm patients, avert requests for unnecessary medications or as a supplement treatment. But from what we know today, deception is not necessarily involved in the use of placebo. We have learned that anything inducing expectation of benefit (e.g. analgesia) can act as a placebo, positively impacting on the patient's (pain) brain circuitry. In fact, every real treatment administered in routine health care has two distinct components: the active constituent and the placebo (psychosocial) factor. Every effort should be made to enhance the latter to maximize the benefit of the therapeutic act. This behavior is perfectly acceptable and does not challenge ethical imperatives. Central in the psychosocial context is the patient–provider relationship, with empathy, perceived skill, correct attitudes and words, ceremony and encouragement all contributing to a positive outcome.

The reverse actions represent nocebos, and they may lessen the effectiveness of therapeutic agents. Although the harmful effect of natural situations such as the impact of negative diagnoses or the patient's disbelief in a therapy are sometimes difficult to circumvent, care should be given to at least eliminate negligence and minimize distrust. Of note, nocebo suggestions can be more powerful than placebo ones, as reversing the verbal instructions can turn a placebo analgesic response into a hyperalgesic nocebo one, in spite of previous placebo conditioning. Even a seemingly innocuous act such as communicating to the patient that a therapy is going to be interrupted can have a negative impact, as showed by the faster and larger intensity relapse of pain after open versus hidden interruption of morphine analgesic therapy.

Conclusions

Thus, the clinician has in his hand a coin with two sides: when the coin is tossed on the "plus" side the clinician has an extra tool to minimize the patient's distress. When tossed on the "minus" side, the clinician unintentionally minimizes drug efficacy. Although a positive doctor–patient relationship and good medical practice have long been known to affect the therapeutic outcome and the patient's quality of life, what is new today is that we are beginning to understand the underlying biological mechanisms. It is to be hoped that awareness and good knowledge of placebo/nocebo mechanisms will govern the physician's conduct, rather than the random toss of a coin.

References

1 Benedetti F (2013) Placebo and the new physiology of the doctor-patient relationship. *Physiol Rev* **93**:1207–46.

2 Benedetti F (2014) Placebo effects: from the neurobiological paradigm to translational implications. *Neuron* **84**: 623–37.

3 Benedetti F, Carlino E, Piedimonte A (2016) Increasing uncertainty in CNS clinical trials: the role of placebo, nocebo, and Hawthorne effects. *Lancet Neurol* **15**:736–47.

4 Shaibani A, Frisaldi E, Benedetti F (2017) Placebo response in pain, fatigue, and performance: possible implications for neuromuscular disorders. *Muscle & Nerve* **56**: 358–67.

5 Colloca L, Barsky AJ (2020) Placebo and nocebo effects. *N Engl J Med* **382**:554–61.

6 Finniss DG, Miller F, Kaptchuk T, Benedetti F (2010) Biological, clinical, and ethical advances of placebo effects. *Lancet* **375**:686–95.

7 Benedetti F (2020) *Placebo effects*. 3rd Edition, Oxford University Press, Oxford.

8 Evers AWM, Colloca L, Blease C, Annoni M, Atlas LY et al (2018) Implications of placebo and nocebo effects for clinical practice: Expert consensus. *Psychotherapy & Psychosomatics* **87**:204–10.

9 Wager TD, Atlas LY (2015) The neuroscience of placebo effects: connecting context, learning and health. *Nat Rev Neurosci* **16**:403–18.

10 Zunhammer M, Bingel U, Wager TD, Atlas L, Benedetti F et al (2018) Placebo effects on the neurologic pain signature: A meta-analysis of individual participant functional magnetic resonance imaging data. *JAMA Neurology* **75**:1321–30.

11 Benedetti F, Durando J, Vighetti S (2014) Nocebo and placebo modulation of hypobaric hypoxia headache involves the cyclooxygenase-prostaglandins pathway. *Pain* **155**:921–8.

12 Tinnermann A, Geuter S, Sprenger C, Finsterbusch J, Büchel C (2017). Interactions between brain and spinal cord mediate value effects in nocebo hyperalgesia. *Science*, **358**:105–8.

Chapter 7

Knowledge transfer to patients experiencing pain and poor sleep and sleep disorder

Gilles J. Lavigne[1,2], Alberto Herrero Babiloni[1,3], Beatrice P. De Koninck[1], Marc O. Martel[3,6], Jacqueline Tu Anh Thu Lam[1,4], Cibele Dal Fabbro[1], Louis de Beaumont[1,4], & Caroline Arbour[1,5]

[1] Center for Advanced Research in Sleep Medicine & Trauma Unit, Research Center, Centre Integre Sante et Services Sociaux du Nord Ile de Montreal (CIUSSS du NIM), Montréal, Québec, Canada
[2] Faculty of Dental Medicine, Université de Montréal, Québec, Canada
[3] Division of Experimental Medicine, McGill University, Montréal, Québec, Canada
[4] Faculty of Medicine, Université de Montréal, Québec, Canada
[5] Faculty of Nursing, Université de Montréal, Québec, Canada
[6] Faculty of Dentistry & Department of Anesthesia, McGill University, Montréal, Québec, Canada

Sleep is a state with partial isolation from vigilance, the dominant state during wake. Despite being apparently obvious, it must be remembered that sleep is not coma nor anesthesia. During sleep, sound, temperature changes, touch and pain can be perceived, thus maintaining the capacity to react to external stimuli (such as a baby's cry) or to maintain comfort [1].

Approximately 10% of the general population and 50% of individuals with chronic pain complain of poor sleep quality, reporting their sleep to be non-restorative or unrefreshing. These numbers go as high as 70% in individuals with widespread pain syndrome/fibromyalgia. Many sleep disorders, described in more detail below, may contribute to exacerbate pain and complicate its relief. It has been reported that nearly 44% of people living with chronic pain present sleep disorders with insomnia (72%), sleep apnea and periodic limb movement (32% each) being the most frequent [2]

This narrative practical review will describe the interactions between pain and sleep and how pain is processed during sleep. Furthermore, it will overview the most frequent sleep disorders in chronic pain and it will provide advice for clinicians to guide patients in the management of sleep in the absence or in the presence of sleep disorders. For patients suffering from poor sleep and pain the *one size fits all* treatment approach has never been a choice as multimodal avenues are the most likely route to be successful as described in this chapter. Thus, it is important for clinicians to gain the expertise and knowledge in providing advice and guide patients toward optimal treatment and, when needed, refer to other health professionals.

Clinical Pain Management: A Practical Guide, Second Edition. Edited by Mary E. Lynch, Kenneth D. Craig, and Philip W. Peng.

Assessment of pain and sleep interactions

Sleep quality can be easily estimated in pain and sleep clinics through patients' self-reports, via semi-structures interviews, which include use of visual analogue scales and screening questionnaires when sleep disorders are suspected. Several sleep disorder screening tools are widely used, but not specifically validated for the sleep and pain interaction. These include the Epworth Sleepiness Scale (ESS), the Pittsburgh Sleep Quality Index (PSQI), the Insomnia Severity Index (ISI) and the STOP-Bang for sleep apnea, which all are currently available online. The classical self-reports related to poor sleep, which are not exclusive to people living with chronic pain, are depicted in Figure 7.1.

Polysomnography (PSG) at home or in a sleep laboratory supervised by a physician are both important tools to assess sleep quality and the presence of sleep disorders. Objective testing such as PSG improves diagnosis accuracy from possible (self-reports on sleep and interview) to probable (screening tools and examination) and definitive, as confirmed for the majority of sleep disorders [3]. Sleep recording is recommended in chronic pain cases: 1) when excessive sleepiness and/or fatigue (a dominant complaint in women) are noted; 2) when sleep comorbidities are suspected; 3) or when there is no clear response to usual treatments. Sleep disorders can be concomitant to chronic pain and have synergic influence on sleep quality and on pain intensity and ability to coping with its burdens. From PSG recordings specifically, several pieces of information can be extracted from people living with chronic pain can be extracted, including: lack of sleep continuity (i.e. frequent sleep stage shifts, periodic limb movement and breathing disruption such as apneas), trouble to initiate or maintaining sleep or long sleep latency, which are frequent characteristics of insomnia. These features can also be monitored at home by using a sleep agenda and/or actigraphy watch (a movement sensor as a proxy to assess quiet period and delay of sleep onset) or home limited number of channel devices recording system. Smart phone applications may increase patient collaboration and motivation according to emerging research.

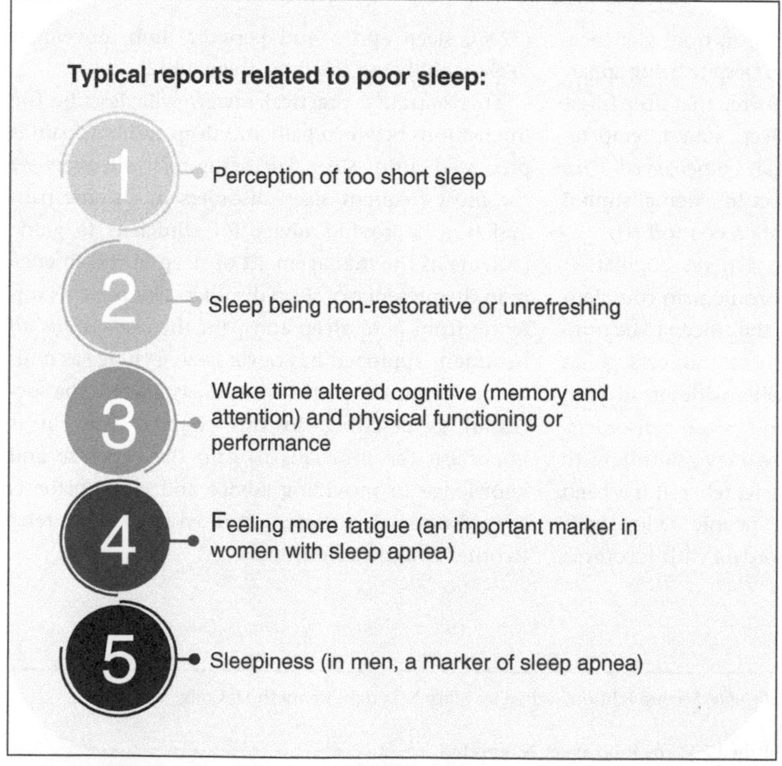

Typical reports related to poor sleep:
1
Perception of too short sleep
2
Sleep being non-restorative or unrefreshing
3
Wake time altered cognitive (memory and attention) and physical functioning or performance
4
Feeling more fatigue (an important marker in women with sleep apnea)
5
Sleepiness (in men, a marker of sleep apnea)

Figure 7.1 Classical self-reports related to poor sleep.

In chronic pain (i.e. pain lasting more than 3 months) [4], it is frequent for patients to complain of poor home- or work-related performance due to fatigue. Cognitive impairments such as attention, memory or executive function alterations are either noticed or reported. Furthermore, clinicians have to take into consideration the fact that both pain and sleep have interlaced socio-psychological impacts [1].

Even in acute pain situations (e.g. after a surgery or a trauma, or in an emergency room), sleep can be disrupted for a few nights [5,6]. In these cases, all of the above socio-psychological impacts are usually transients. In order to prevent risk of chronicity, it may be wise for clinicians to provide patient guidance as explained in the last section of this chapter.

The circular pain and sleep interactions

In the pain and sleep literature, a simple circular model has been commonly used to investigate and depict the reciprocal impact of sleep and pain disturbances [1]. In the later model, it was proposed that a bad day with pain (regardless of intensity) could be followed by a night with poor sleep, whereas a bad night of sleep could be followed by pain exacerbations on the next day. Nowadays, experiential evidence has made it clearer that a bad day with pain is not the dominant trigger of poor sleep quality; individual vulnerability or comorbidities have to be taken into consideration [1]. However, the impact of a poor sleep night has been shown to exacerbate pain during the first half of the following day [7]. Additionally, women with chronic pain and menopause seem to get longer sleep duration when higher pain is reported, potentially as a means to numb the pain [8]. This recent finding challenges the strength and uniqueness of a circular effect of a day with pain driving a poor sleep quality night or shorter sleep. Furthermore, little evidence is available on the exact contribution of deleterious influences of fatigue and exhaustion, life pressure or task overload. Similarly, although it is clinically reported as a way to cope with fatigue and pain, the benefit of rest and nap on pain symptomatology needs further investigation. Circadian rhythms also shape the pain and sleep interaction, a topic of specific interest for investigators in the field [9]. Therefore, the impact of many independent or synergic risk or protective or palliative factors (e.g., older age, gender/female, life style, sleep hygiene, napping, exercise, substance, or medication misuse or abuse and mood and sleep disorders) need to be identified individually.

Sleep disruption in people living with chronic pain may have different effects between individuals depending on risk factors that have not yet been clearly identified. The search of socio-psychobiological vulnerability (e.g. gender, age, healthy life behavior, inflammatory response) or specific phenotype (circadian rhythm and/or breathing physiology) are paths for future research [9, 10].

Pain processing during sleep and its consequences

The sleeping brain remains reactive to any type of inputs, including potentially painful ones. Experimental pain and sleep studies, using cutaneous heat pain or sub-cutaneous infusion of hypertonic saline or laser stimulation, have challenged brain reactivity and persistence of placebo analgesia in sleep as described below [11-13].

During sleep, the pre-alerting reaction (i.e. brief arousal lasting 3–15 seconds without return of consciousness) and the ready to react awakening (i.e. not fully conscious but towards awake state) remain dominant in light sleep (stages 1 and 2: 40–50% response), whereas it is less dominant in deep sleep (stage 3; less than 30%). In REM or paradoxical sleep (i.e. a stage with low responsiveness, muscle paralysis and intense metabolic activity), this reaction is more variable [12, 13].

A piece of the puzzle came from studies on placebo analgesia paradigm applied to sleep studies. The brain can still process pain related information during sleep following induction of conditioned analgesia. In placebo studies, there are non-responders and responders. Indeed, placebo responders are individuals who typically had a prior positive experience with a therapeutic modality [14]. The latter is among variables that seem to moderate hypoalgesia or pain relief expectation. In experimental protocols, 50–60% of healthy individuals can be identified as placebo responders. For several reasons, some individuals can be responders in a specific context, in a given time, but not in others. In relation to sleep, experimental investigations from Dr. Lavigne's laboratory have shown that the placebo effect remains active during sleep as individuals who had a higher pain relief expectation while awake before sleep experienced more placebo analgesia following a night of sleep. Indeed, individuals with high analgesia expectation prior to sleep had shorter REM sleep, experienced less pain, reported better sleep and were less anxious [11]. The role of REM sleep in potentiating the placebo analgesia via expectation was further documented with use of clonidine, a medication that suppresses REM sleep [11].

Retention of placebo analgesia during sleep may also be associated to learning processes; considerable evidence supports the conclusion that learning is consolidated during sleep [11]. The *'sleep on it'* idiom illustrates that sleep is an active process also involved in memory consolidation and learning [15]. The neuropsychological process associated with these functions may contribute to explain some of the discrepancies between experimental studies performed on healthy subjects vs. chronic pain subjects [16, 17]. Indeed, in individuals with chronic pain, working memory and episodic memory performance are altered, which seems to be independent of age but related to the more specific 'pain attention deficit state' [17]. Moreover, sleep and sensory/pain processing are sleep stage dependent and inter-related [12, 13]. Noxious and sensory inputs activate mid and prefrontal cortex, the insula and the opercular cortex up to sensory motor cortex in order to prepare for movements; this is a normal gradation in preparing a response to a threatening event such as pain [18].

Ideally, sleep duration should be between 7 to 9 hours per day for most individuals. Duration of sleep of less than 6 or more than 9 hours influences pain perception and report the next day [19]. In fact, mood, social reactivity and pain are exacerbated by short sleep duration (4 instead of 7-8 hours) as tested experimentally by inducing a few days up to 3 weeks of sleep deprivation [20]. Experimental short-term sleep deprivation alters endogenous 'relief' mechanisms and exacerbates pain in heathy individuals [21]. Recent brain imaging studies have shown that cortical pain sensory motor processing, including periaqueductal gray matter and accumbens adenosinergic activities, are enhanced, whereas thalamic, insula and striatum plus accumbens dopaminergic activities are blunted following acute sleep deprivation [22, 23]. Likewise, activities in structures associated to pain modulation and to deficient pain-reward reactivity are exacerbated by lack of sleep [1].

Sleep Disorders in Patients With Pain

Insomnia and its management related to pain

Insomnia can be acute, transient or chronic and can be comorbid [24]. It is characterized by complaint or dissatisfaction about sleep quantity or quality, related to a series of criteria. As examples:

1 Difficulty to initiate sleep, usually taking more than 20 minutes in a child and or young adult and up to 30 minutes in adult (but it can be longer if the individual nap during late afternoon);

2 Difficulty to resume sleep if the individual awakes at night to go to the bathroom or other reasons, or;

3 The *'petit matin'* or early morning insomnia that is described by complains of awaking too early with expectations to get longer sleep to prevent fatigue and improve performance.

Insomnia is classified as *Chronic Insomnia Disorder* if complaints occur at least 3 times per week for at least 3 months and as *Short-term Insomnia Disorder* if insomnia symptoms are present for less than 3 months in an irregular pattern. Both need to be reported as a problem by the individual[24]. Some individuals have atypical sleep patterns and cope well with it. Insomnia is frequently associated with mood alterations, hypervigilance, fatigue, chronic pain, brain trauma and sometimes addiction[25].

According to the DSM-IV and ICSD-3 criteria, the prevalence of insomnia in the general population is 6-10% and is age related [26]. However, in a Canadian survey, 29.9% of the general population self-reported insomnia symptoms, with 9.5% of complaints consistent with insomnia syndrome [27]. In the EPISONO general population sample (Brazil), the estimated self-reported insomnia prevalence was 32%, for symptoms and only about 15% meet the DSM-IV criteria for insomnia syndrome [28]. Interestingly, the prevalence of insomnia seems to have increased over recent decades. A Finish survey reported a 4.5% rise from 2008 to 2013 in occasional insomnia symptoms, with no change for chronic insomnia [29]/ Similarly, a comparative 10-year study (1999/2000–2009/2010) in Norway found that insomnia cases increased from 11.9% to 15.5% using the DSM-IV criteria [30].

Changes in sleep quality and risk of emerging insomnia, may concur to predict chronic pain, and chronic insomnia is a dominant comorbidity in people living with chronic pain of various origins [2, 31]. Many studies suggest that insomnia, lack of sleep quantity or quality and mood disorders are important risk factors or mediators for chronic pain [25, 32]. This is illustrated by one study, carried out over 6 years in a large sample of the Netherlands population, that revealed that both insomnia and short sleep had hazard ratios of 1.6 and 1.5, respectively, for onset of new chronic multisite musculoskeletal pain [32]. Importantly, suicidal risk needs to be considered when chronic pain and insomnia overlap [33].

Sleep disorders breathing

Sleep disorders breathing (SDB) includes snoring to respiratory effort related arousal (RERA), obstructive sleep apnea (OSA) and central sleep apnea (CSA) [24].

Snoring is a frequent precursor sign of a sleep breathing problem, whereas OSA is the dominant sleep breathing disorder in the population. RERA is a respiratory event in which there is a sequence of breath lasting > 10 seconds, characterized by increasing respiratory effort or by fattening of the inspiration waveform leading to arousal [24 34]. OSA is observed on sleep recoding by a combination of partial reductions (hypopneas) and complete pauses (apneas) in breathing that last at least 10 seconds or more with oxygen desaturation (3% or 4%). CSA occurs due to a lack of input form the brain respiratory network to motor centers of breathing.

Opioids, benzodiazepines and gabapentin (an anticonvulsant frequently used to manage chronic pain) may contribute to CSA in a subgroup of vulnerable individuals not yet well characterized [35, 36]. Thereby, phenotyping or disease characterization based on individual traits is an active domain of research in sleep breathing disorders [37[.

In this context, many anatomical risk factors are associated to OSA, including narrow upper airway due to small oral development (retrognathia) or large tissue (macroglossia, large tonsil and pharyngeal pillar, which is fat accumulation at the base of the tongue). Obesity also concurs to exacerbate that risk and being a male or a post-menopausal woman is also part of the equation. Identified non-anatomical risk factors are: 1) low muscle tone or responsiveness that prevent airway patency to be optimal; 2) low arousal threshold that contribute to interrupt sleep continuity; and 3) high loop-gain, that is an excessive breathing activity or "overshoot", when the oxygen level is too low causing irregular breathing and poor sleep maintenance [37].

OSA prevalence with a mild apnea-hypopnea index (AHI ≥ 5 and <15) ranges from 9% to 38% and moderate (IAH ≥15 and <30) to severe (IAH ≥ 30) range from 6% to 17%; OSA prevalence is higher in male and increase with age [38]. OSA is associated with headache (a marker of therapy success is when it disappears), cognitive alterations (memory, executive function), sexual dysfunction and sleepiness in men, fatigue (dominant in woman), increased risk of transportation or work accidents and increased risk of cardiovascular disease, diabetes and depression in both sexes [39]. Overall mortality and cancer is higher in OSA [40].

SDB, mainly OSA, is present in 30 to 90% of people living with chronic pain with a higher incidence in opioid users seen in sleep clinics [2, 41, 42]. Based on a recent meta-analysis of 9 studies (n=3791 individuals), CSA in people living with chronic pain represent 33% of sleep clinic and 20% of pain clinic patients [42]. Prescription medications such opioids and gabapentin can aggravate OSA and CSA [35, 43]. Caution is recommended before treating pain patients under suspicion of having a sleep breathing disorder. PSG monitoring is recommended to assess treatment safety in opioid users [44].

Other sleep disorders with a putative link to pain

Periodic limb movement (PLM) or its awake feature, restless leg syndrome (RLS), is a condition reported by about 8% of the population. When occurring during wakefulness, RLS/PLM is associated with discomfort and pain in limbs in addition to irresistible desire to move. During sleep, PLM is observed by the presence of repetitive leg or arms twitches. PLM contributes to sleep disruption and fragmentation, is associated to dopamine and ferritin deficiency, and can be diagnosed by sleep or neurology physicians with PSG. Moreover, it is present in about 1/3 of patients with chronic pain at a lower frequency of PLM index per hour of sleep than in typical individuals with RLS/PLM [2]. This sleep disorder is managed with medications addressing its pathophysiology (dopamine agonists and α2δ calcium channel ligands up to ferritin injection or use of codeine) [45, 46].

Sleep bruxism (SB) is associated with repretitive jaw movements with tooth grinding and jaw clenching. It is present in 8–12% of the adult general population. For most individuals, it is a transient behavior expressed during intense or stressful life periods. In some cases, it is a concomitant condition to insomnia, OSA and more rarely to sleep epilepsy and REM behavior disorders. SB is a potential additive factor that can alter sleep and exacerbate pain, namely the temporomandibular/orofacial pains, and may be concomitant to OSA, although level of evidence is low and strength of the associations debated [47–49]. [47-49]

Finally, as it can be associated with heightened clinical pain intensity [50], narcolepsy (associated with genetic predisposition and clinically observed with/without cataplexy and excessive sleepiness) is another sleep disorder to consider.

Advice Helping Pain and Sleep Patients: Behavioral to Medical (see Figures 7.2 and 7.3).

Develop healthy sleep and life habits/ behaviors:

Sleep hygiene: Sleep time requirements differ from individual to individual. Some need longer than others. Normal values are between 7-9 hours; as described above, less than 6 and more than 9 hours can be deleterious for pain and mood. Ideally, patients should not be attentive with their sleep duration; it is normal to have great night of sleep with shorter or longer duration. Quality of sleep perception is 'subjective'. Still, individuals should try to get regular sleep schedule, time to go to bed and to waking time; a "yoyo" sleep pattern is not ideal.

Siesta/naps: Napping can help some subjects to recover from fatigue and sleep deprivation. Some individuals have a monotonic chronotype (e.g. regular 8 hr of sleep/16 hrs of activity) whereas others have a polyphasic one (one or more shorter periods of sleep or nap over 24 hrs). The level of evidence supporting the benefits of short naps (ideally less than 20 min) is low, but it may be useful for patients with chronic pain. Importantly, naps should not be taken in late afternoon to avoid delaying sleep onset/ insomnia.

Diet: Heavy diet or late meals do not contribute to good sleep and fatty food and red meat may exacerbate sleep breathing problems [51]. Few recent meta-analyses and Cochrane reviews provide some insight on benefit, although modest, for exercise (ideally not too late in evening) as a beneficial contributor to improve sleep quality. Diet control combined with regular exercising also contribute to slightly reduce the AHI (reduced by a mean of about 8 events/hour sleep) and improve sleep as well as reducing pain [52–54].

Along with these approaches, meditation and yoga seem to have an additive and modest effect possibly related to length of practice and regular adherence to the activity [55]./

Privileged sleep environment

Although there is not much science on the following recommendations for the specific pain and sleep interaction, many individuals report better sleep with they are implemented (Figure 7.2).

If the sleep partner is noisy (e.g. snoring, tooth grinding or excessive movements), patients have to realize that the partner has no major control except if the noise is due to an untreated sleep disorder (e.g. OSA, PLM). The use of earplugs is a convenient possibility. In some cases, however, it is wise to use a separate bedroom to reduce the impact of a 'noisy' (e.g. breathing sounds) or 'active' (e.g. movements, wake) sleep partner. This is a simple way to cope and recover from fatigue and pain. The other 'back-up' bedroom should be as comfortable as the regular one and can be use in alternated sequence by sleep partners.

Psychotherapy

Psychotherapy can help to modify sleep habits, pain and/or sleep expectations and catastrophizing behaviors. Moreover, it has been shown that hybrid

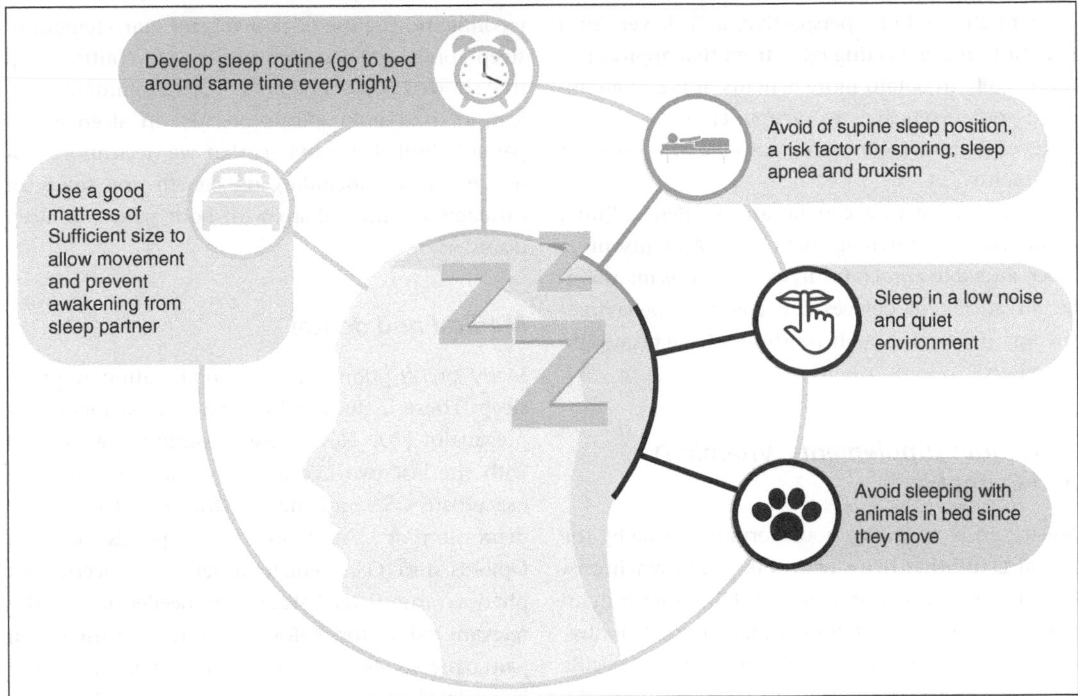

Figure 7.2 Advice and recommendations for a better sleep.

approaches targeting sleep and pain can be even more helpful [56]. Cognitive and behavioral therapy can be done in presence of patient or through an electronic medium. For insomnia, psychotherapy is a beneficial approach with fewer side effects and with more durable benefits than sleep medications [25]. Sleep medications can be prescribed for the transition period from the medical appointment to beginning of psychotherapy.

Physical Therapy

Recent Cochrane reviews and trials revealed modest benefits for physical therapy alone, and in some cases the addition of cognitive and behavioral advice seem to be advantageous [53, 57]. Despite the low level of evidence, many patients report a better sleep and decrease pain with physical therapy.

Acupuncture

Acupuncture seems to help some individuals with insomnia, sleep apnea and pain. However, acupuncture effects cannot be generalized and they are subject to inconsistencies in the literature as assessing their benefits appears to be a methodological challenge [58].

Two recent systematic reviews were recently published showing acupuncture as an effective option of management of insomnia, as well in OSA patients, but the methodological quality of most of the studies and the quality of evidence were low, especially in the Insomnia paper. The OSA systematic review and meta-analysis recently published, including nine RCTs with 584 participants, showed that acupuncture therapy is effective for these patients in reducing AHI and sleepiness (ESS) and in improving the oxygen saturation (SaO_2) of various severities, especially in moderate and severe OSA patients [59].

Another recent review showed that the effectiveness of acupuncture is explained by a variety mechanisms, as follows: inhibiting the oxidative stress response, modulating the local inflammation, reducing TNF-α, IL-1β, and IL-6 (in the inflamed area) and improving the anti-inflammatory response (cholinergic pathway). Additionally, it has been shown that acupuncture improves the nociceptive inflammatory mediators (IL-1β, and IL-6) and improves the ANS (autonomic nervous system) by neuroregulation, contributing to the functional recuperation [60].

From the authors' perspective, a "believer" or a patient that is expecting relief from that approach is more likely to obtain more benefits. It is a phenomenon not exclusive to acupuncture, as "non-believers" are known to not respond well to most treatments.

Also, acupuncture can be an excellent adjunct approach to the management of OSA or insomnia when added to regular forms of control, as mandibular advancement devices and cognitive behavioral therapy (CBT), although no studies have been published yet.

Melatonin supplements, Vitamin D and Cannabis

Melatonin is an endogenous hormone made by the pineal gland that helps with wake/sleep synchrony. Melatonin pills are not sleep pills, but rather contain a substance that facilitates circadian and sleep ultradian rhythms. Briefly, melatonin binds to specific receptors in the brain thus helping to adjust the wake and sleep rhythm [61]. Although little evidence is yet available for the efficacy and safety of melatonin in the management of the complex disruption associated to chronic pain and sleep problems, it is a well-accepted adjunct therapy by many patients [62]. Again, an individual can be a melatonin responder or non-responder; it is not expected that every patient gets beneficial effects.

Supplementation with vitamin D was suggested to help with the challenging interaction between pain and sleep, but more evidence is needed to confirm this path and its putative mechanism of action on hyperalgesia and inflammation [63].

Cannabis and prescribed cannabinoids are reported to improve pain and sleep [65, 65]. The two main components are THC and CBD and each has different mechanism of action and psycho-biological effects [66]. Nonetheless, their efficiency (efficacy and safety / low risk of addiction or craving or mixture with other medications or drug inducing respiratory depression) is not yet fully demonstrated. More knowledge is available for pain than for sleep and little is known when these conditions are comorbid [67]. CBD dominant derivatives seem to have beneficial effect on insomnia but the lack of solid randomized trial invites caution [68]. Indeed, the American Academy of Sleep Medicine does not recommend the use of cannabis for management of sleep apnea and a recent randomized control sleep trial showed that dronabinol, a THC dominant medication, had mild effects on AHI in sleep apnea patients [69]. It is obvious that we need more evidence before concluding on benefit and safety of cannabis for individuals with both pain and sleep disorders.

Medical and dental

Many prescription drugs in combination improve sleep. These include duloxetine and gabapentin or pregabalin [70]. Nevertheless, caution is warranted with the last two because they may contribute to exacerbate OSA and increase the risk of breathing depression or CSA if used with opioids [43, 71]. Opioids and OSA remain a serious concern, but phenotyping-derived studies are needed to identify relevant risk factors before rejecting their use for all pain patients [44].Other medications with modest to lower level of evidence include non-steroidal anti-inflammatories, antidepressants such as milnacipran or amitriptyline and cyclobenzaprine, a muscle relaxant, for the sleep and pain overlap notably in fibromyalgia patients [72].

The most common sleep medications for insomnia include benzodiazepines, Z-drugs or hypnotics such as zolpidem and zopiclone and "off-label" medications such as the atypical antidepressant trazodone, the latter being popular due to its reduced costs and reduced risk of dependence [73]. Moreover, it seems that trazodone can also decrease AHI in OSA patients by increasing arousal thresholds [74]. Even though so far no definitive pharmacological tool has demonstrated constant and clear benefits in OSA, a combination of atomoxetine and oxybutynin, the latter preventing drop in upper airway muscle tone, is considered as promising [75].

Sleep breathing devices to manage OSA include the continuous positive airway pressure (CPAP), which is considered the gold standard choice, and mandibular advancement devices when CPAP cannot be tolerated or for mild to moderate OSA cases. The diagnosis of OSA is under the responsibility of the sleep medicine specialist. In presence of opioid induced CSA, special breathing devices are needed, although they are not always effective. Alternative approaches include sleep positioner to prevent supine position, acupuncture, oropharyngeal exercises, nose and jaw and bariatric surgeries and lingual nerve stimulation devices [39]. Again, phenotyping is a path that will help clinicians to select treatments with the highest potential [10].

For periodic limb movement, as described above, medications addressing its pathophysiology such as dopamine agonists and α2δ calcium channel ligands, ferritin injection and codeine are among the evidence-based choices [45, 46]. It is a common belief that using codeine in periodic limb movement-restless leg syndrome patients has low risk of addiction, a challenging topic currently under investigation [44].

Emerging therapies:

Magnetic or direct current non-invasive brain stimulation are emerging therapies for persistent pain among non-responders to usual pain or sleep treatment. Indeed, they have beneficial effects with minimal risk on chronic pain syndrome, OSA, restless leg syndrome and sleep disturbances [76, 77]. Although epilepsy is a documented risk, it rarely occurs with newer protocols. Furthermore, two recent systematic reviews and meta-analyses support that combining non-invasive brain stimulation and exercise have synergistic benefits on pain [78].

Pink noise is a new avenue that improves sleep by enhancing slow wave sleep (SWS) and also memory; yet we do not know if it is useful for sleep-pain patients [79]. Such a non-invasive and non-sleep disrupting approach is done by the application of series of brief sound (30-50dB) applied in the rise of SWS for a few seconds. The benefit of sleep application of pink noise on cognition was tested on a sleep laboratory and at home with portable devices over few nights. It needs to be coupled with electroencephalography (EEG) and intelligent algorithms to select the rise in SWS and apply the specified sound. The concept is based on the putative, but still debated, role of SWS as a concomitant biomarker of sleep disturbance in pain patients. Scoring on EEG of sleep spindles, excessive arousal, dominance of fast brain waves, overactive cyclic alternating pattern and autonomic-sympathetic over activation are among the possible putative biomarkers of sleep-pain patients [10, 80]. Sleep is a complex behavioral and physiological state, but phenotyping and targeting the dominant cause(s) is a path of future.

Final take home messages

Realistic and optimistic discussion with patients is encouraged. A series of single actions could make significant differences if we help patients to adjust their pain relief and/or sleep improvement expectations. Because poor sleep and pain are complex interrelated conditions, expectations of total relief are unrealistic. Moreover, poor sleep and pain seems to that have, in a given individual, their own personalized signature. In other words, it is different from individual to individual due to socio-psycho-biomedical phenotypes. We cannot extract the living person from interactions with the environment in which they live and work; the psychosocial influences!

The support from various health care providers (e.g. psychologist, physical therapist, social workers), diet, yoga or exercise (at reasonable intensity), seem to have additive benefits in patients suffering from putative deleterious pain/sleep and sleep/pain interactions (see Figure 7.3). The support from family and friends seems to be of great help as well.

Furthermore, acceptance of the natural day-to-day and night-to-night fluctuations in pain intensity and sleep quality, and its consequent impact, may help patients to cope with sleep and pain concomitant disturbances so as to achieve better quality of life and sleep, not only duration.

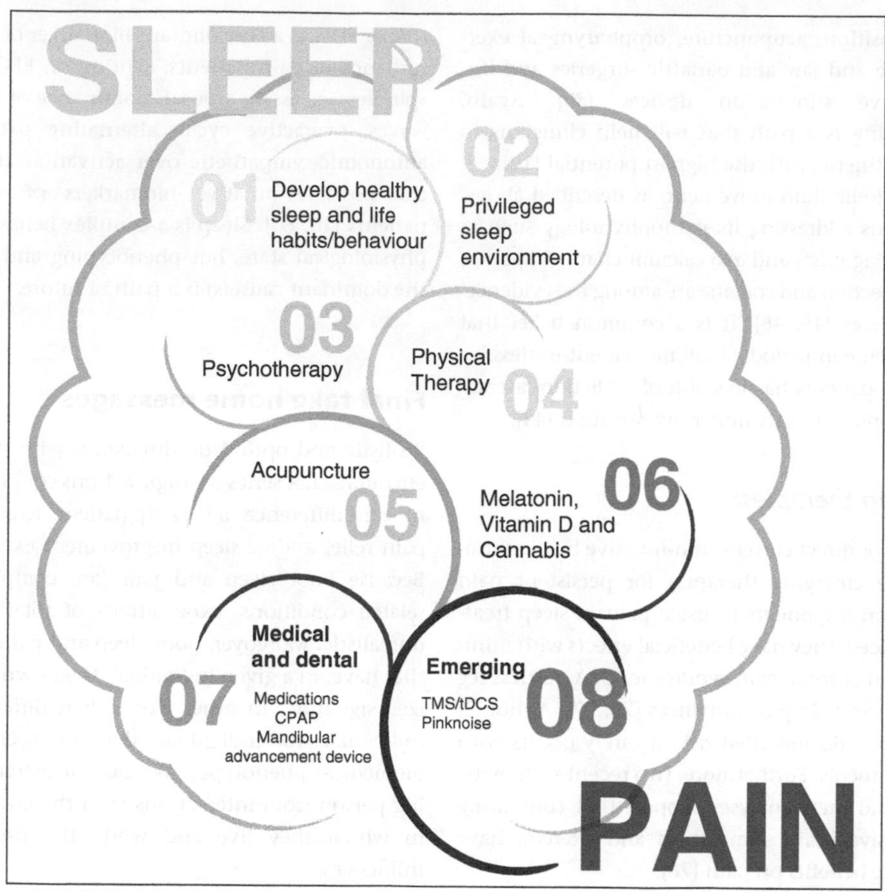

Figure 7.3 Avenues to improve the deleterious interaction of pain and poor sleep, in presence of sleep disorders such as insomnia, sleep disordered breathing (Obstructive Sleep Apnea) or periodic limb movements.

References

1 Herrero Babiloni A, De Koninck BP, Beetz G, De Beaumont L, Martel MO, Lavigne GJ. (2020) Sleep and pain: recent insights, mechanisms, and future directions in the investigation of this relationship. *Journal of neural transmission* **127(4)**:647–60.

2 Mathias JL, Cant ML, Burke ALJ. (2018) Sleep disturbances and sleep disorders in adults living with chronic pain: a meta-analysis. *Sleep Medicine* **52**:198–210.

3 Lobbezoo F, Ahlberg J, Raphael KG *et al.* (2018) International consensus on the assessment of bruxism: Report of a work in progress. *J Oral Rehabil* **45(11)**:837–44.

4 Treede RD, Rief W, Barke A *et al.* (2019) Chronic pain as a symptom or a disease: the IASP Classification of Chronic Pain for the International Classification of Diseases (ICD-11). *Pain* **160(1)**:19–27.

5 Khoury S, Chouchou F, Amzica F *et al.* (2013) Rapid EEG activity during sleep dominates in mild traumatic brain injury patients with acute pain. *Journal of Neurotrauma* **30(8)**:633–41.

6 Chauny JM, Paquet J, Carrier J *et al.* (2018) Subjective sleep quality and its etiology in the emergency department. *Cjem* **21(2)**:249–52.

7 Tang NK, Goodchild CE, Sanborn AN, Howard J, Salkovskis PM. (2012) Deciphering the temporal link between pain and sleep in a heterogeneous chronic pain patient sample: a multilevel daily process study. *Sleep* **35(5)**:75–687a.

8 Frange C, Hachul H, Hirotsu C, Tufik S, Andersen ML. (2019) Temporal analysis of chronic musculoskeletal pain and sleep in postmenopausal women. *J Clin Sleep Med* **15(2)**:223–234.

9 Palada V, Gilron I, Canlon B, Svensson CI, Kalso E. (2020) The circadian clock at the intercept of sleep and pain. *Pain* **161(5)**:894–900.

10 Herrero Babiloni A, Beetz G, Tang NKY, *et al.* (2020). Towards the endotyping of the sleep-pain interaction: a topical review on multitarget strategies based on phenotypic vulnerabilities and putative pathways. *Pain* **162(5)**:1281–8.

11 Chouchou F, Dang-Vu TT, Rainville P, Lavigne G. (2018). The role of sleep in learning placebo effects. *Int Rev Neurobiol* **139**:321–55.

12 Lavigne G, Brousseau M, Kato T *et al.* (2004) Experimental pain perception remains equally active over all sleep stages. *Pain* **110(3)**:646–55.

13 Lavigne G, Zucconi M, Castronovo C, Manzini C, Marchettini P, Smirne S. (2000) Sleep arousal response to experimental thermal stimulation during sleep in human subjects free of pain and sleep problems. *Pain* **84(2-3)**:283–90.

14 Colloca L, Barsky AJ. (2020) Placebo and nocebo effects. *The New England Journal of Medicine.* **382(6)**:54–561.

15 Rasch B, Born J. (2013) About sleep's role in memory. *Physiol Rev* **93(2)**:681–766.

16 Gatzounis R, Schrooten MGS, Crombez G, Vlaeyen JWS. (2018) Forgetting to remember? Prospective memory within the context of pain. *European Journal of Pain (London, England)* **22(3)**:14–625.

17 Oosterman JM, Derksen LC, van Wijck AJ, Veldhuijzen DS, Kessels RP. (2011) Memory functions in chronic pain: examining contributions of attention and age to test performance. *The Clinical Journal of Pain.* **27(1)**:70–5.

18 Mazza S, Perchet C, Frot M, et al. Asleep but aware? (2014) *Brain and Cognition* **87**:7–15.

19 Edwards RR, Almeida DM, Klick B, Haythornthwaite JA, Smith MT. (2008)Duration of sleep contributes to next-day pain report in the general population. *Pain* **137(1)**:202–7.

20 Haack M, Mullington JM. (2005) Sustained sleep restriction reduces emotional and physical well-being. *Pain* **119(1-3)**:56–64.

21 Smith MT, Edwards RR, McCann UD, Haythornthwaite JA. (2007) The effects of sleep deprivation on pain inhibition and spontaneous pain in women. *Sleep* **30(4)**:494–505.

22 Seminowicz DA, Remeniuk B, Krimmel SR *et al.* (2019) Pain-related nucleus accumbens function: modulation by reward and sleep disruption. *Pain* **160(5)**:1196–207.

23 Krause AJ, Prather AA, Wager TD, Lindquist MA, Walker MP. (2019) The pain of sleep loss: a brain characterization in humans. *The Journal of Neuroscience.* **39(12)**:2291–300.

24 AASM. (2014) *International Classification of Sleep Disorders.* 3rd edn.

25 Morin CM, Drake CL, Harvey AG *et al.* Insomnia disorder. *Nat Rev Dis Primers 1:15026.*

26 Ohayon MM. (2002) Epidemiology of insomnia: what we know and what we still need to learn. *Sleep Medicine Reviews* **6(2)**:97–111.

27 Morin CM, LeBlanc M, Daley M, Gregoire JP, Merette C. (2006) Epidemiology of insomnia: prevalence, self-help treatments, consultations, and determinants of help-seeking behaviors. *Sleep Medicine* **7(2)**:123–30.

28 Castro LS, Poyares D, Leger D, Bittencourt L, Tufik S. (2013) Objective prevalence of insomnia in the Sao Paulo, Brazil epidemiologic sleep study. *Annals of Neurology.* 74(**4**):537–46.

29 Kronholm E, Partonen T, Harma M *et al.* (2016) Prevalence of insomnia-related symptoms continues to increase in the Finnish working-age population. *Journal of Sleep Research.* **25(4)**:454–457.

30 Pallesen S, Sivertsen B, Nordhus IH, Bjorvatn B. (2014) A 10-year trend of insomnia prevalence in the adult Norwegian population. *Sleep Medicine* **15(2)**:173–79.

31 Smith MT, Klick B, Kozachik S *et al.* (2008) Sleep onset insomnia symptoms during hospitalization for major burn injury predict chronic pain. *Pain* **138(3)**:497–506.

32 Generaal E, Vogelzangs N, Penninx BW, Dekker J. (2017) Insomnia, leep duration, depressive symptoms, and the onset of chronic multisite musculoskeletal pain. *Sleep* **40(1)**.

33 Smith MT. (2004) Suicidal ideation in outpatients with chronic musculoskeletal pain: An exploratory study of the role of sleep onset insomnia and pain intensity. *The Clinical Journal of Pain.* **20**:111–118.

34 Berry RB QS, Abreu AR, Bibbs ML, DelRosso L, Harding SM *et al.* (2020). The AASM manual for the scoring of sleep and associated events: rules, terminology and technical specifications, version 2.6. https://aasm.org/clinical-resources/scoring-manual/. Accessed 30 June, 2020.

35 Marshansky S, Mayer P, Rizzo D, Baltzan M, Denis R, Lavigne GJ. (2018) Sleep, chronic pain, and opioid risk for apnea. *Prog Neuropsychopharmacol Biol Psychiatry* **87(Pt B)**:234–44.

36 Gomes T, Juurlink DN, Antoniou T, Mamdani MM, Paterson JM, van den Brink W. (2017) Gabapentin, opioids, and the risk of opioid-related death: A population-based nested case-control study. *PLoS Medicine* **14(10)**:e1002396.

37 Carberry JC, Amatoury J, Eckert DJ. (2018) Personalized management approach for OSA. *Chest* 153(**3**):744–55.

38 Senaratna CV, Perret JL, Lodge CJ *et al.* (2017) Prevalence of obstructive sleep apnea in the general population: A systematic review. *Sleep Medicine Reviews* **34**:70–81.

39 Lavigne GJ, Herrero Babiloni A, Beetz G *et al.* (2020) Critical issues in dental and medical management of obstructive sleep apnea. *Journal of Dental Research* **99(1)**:26–35.

40 Dewan NA, Nieto FJ, Somers VK. (2015) Intermittent hypoxemia and OSA: implications for comorbidities. *Chest* **147(1)**:266–74.

41 Smith MT, Wickwire EM, Grace EG *et al.* (2009) Sleep disorders and their association with laboratory pain sensitivity in temporomandibular joint disorder. *Sleep* **32(6)**:779–90.

42 Mubashir T, Nagappa M, Esfahanian N *et al.* (2020) Prevalence of sleep-disordered breathing in opioid users with chronic pain: a systematic review and meta-analysis. *J Clin Sleep Med* **16(6)**:961–9.

43 Piovezan RD, Kase C, Moizinho R, Tufik S, Poyares D. (2017) Gabapentin acutely increases the apnea-hypopnea index in older men: data from a randomized, double-blind, placebo-controlled study. *Journal of Sleep Research* **26(2)**:166–70.

44 Lavigne GJ, Herrero Babiloni A, Mayer P, Daoust R, Martel MO. (2020) Thoughts on the 2019 American Academy of Sleep Medicine position statement on chronic opioid therapy and sleep. *Journal of Clinical Sleep Medicine* **16(5)**:831–3.

45 Trotti LM. (2017) Restless legs syndrome and sleep-related movement disorders. *Continuum (Minneap Minn)* **23(4, Sleep Neurology)**:1005–1016.

46 Aurora RN, Kristo DA, Bista SR **et al.** (2012) The treatment of restless legs syndrome and periodic limb movement disorder in adults--an update for 2012: practice parameters with an evidence-based systematic review and meta-analyses: an American Academy of Sleep Medicine Clinical Practice Guideline. *Sleep* **35(8)**:1039–62.

47 Mayer P, Heinzer R, Lavigne G. (2016) Sleep bruxism in respiratory medicine practice. *Chest* **149(1)**:262–71.

48 Andersen ML, Araujo P, Frange C, Tufik S. (2018) Sleep disturbance and pain: a tale of two common problems. *Chest* **154(5)**:1249–59.

49 Baad-Hansen L, Thymi M, Lobbezoo F, Svensson P. (2019) To what extent is bruxism associated with musculoskeletal signs and symptoms? A systematic review. *Journal of Oral Rehabilitation* **46(9)**:845–61.

50 Cremaschi RC, Hirotsu C, Tufik S, Coelho FM. (2019) Chronic pain in narcolepsy type 1 and type 2 - an underestimated reality. *Journal of Sleep Research* **28(3)**:e12715.

51 St-Onge MP, Mikic A, Pietrolungo CE. (2016 Effects of eiet on sleep quality. *Adv Nutr.* **7(5)**:938–49.

52 Edwards BA, Bristow C, O'Driscoll DM *et al.* Assessing the impact of diet, exercise and the combination of the two as a treatment for OSA: a systematic review and meta-analysis. *Respirology (Carlton, Vic)* **24(8)**:740–51.

53 Geneen LJ, Moore RA, Clarke C, Martin D, Colvin LA, Smith BH. (2017) Physical activity and exercise for chronic pain in adults: an overview of Cochrane Reviews. *The Cochrane Database of Systematic Reviews* **4(4)**:Cd011279.

54 Kovacevic A, Mavros Y, Heisz JJ, Fiatarone Singh MA. (2018) The effect of resistance exercise on sleep: A systematic review of randomized controlled trials. *Sleep Medicine Reviews* **39**:52–68.

55 Lazaridou A, Koulouris A, Devine JK *et al.* Impact of daily yoga-based exercise on pain, catastrophizing, and sleep amongst individuals with fibromyalgia. *Journal of Pain Research*. **12**:2915–23.

56 Tang NK. (2009) Cognitive-behavioral therapy for sleep abnormalities of chronic pain patients. *Current Rheumatology Reports*. **11(6)**:451–60.

57 Nijs J, Mairesse O, Neu D *et al.* (2018) Sleep disturbances in chronic pain: neurobiology, assessment, and treatment in physical therapist practice. *Physical Therapy* **98(5)**:325–35.

58 Silva M, Lustosa TC, Arai VJ *et al.* (2019) Effects of acupuncture on obstructive sleep apnea

severity, blood pressure control and quality of life in patients with hypertension: a randomized controlled trial. *Journal of Sleep Research* **2019**:e12954.

59 Wang L, Xu J, Zhan Y, Pei J. (2020) Acupuncture for obstructive sleep apnea (OSA) in adults: a systematic review and meta-analysis. *Biomed Res Int* **2020**:6972327.

60 Yang FM, Yao L, Wang SJ *et al.* (2020) Current tracking on effectiveness and mechanisms of acupuncture therapy: a kiterature rview of high-quality studies. *Chin J Integr Med* **26(4)**:310–20.

61 Kaur T, Shyu BC. (2018) Melatonin: a new-generation therapy for reducing chronic pain and improving sleep disorder-related pain. *Advances in Experimental Medicine and Viology* **1099**:229–51.

62 Emet M, Ozcan H, Ozel L, Yayla M, Halici Z, Hacimuftuoglu A. (2016) A review of melatonin, its receptors and drugs. *Eurasian J Med* **48(2)**:135–41.

63 de Oliveira DL, Hirotsu C, Tufik S, Andersen ML. (2017) The interfaces between vitamin D, sleep and pain. *The Journal of Endocrinology* **234(1)**: R23–r36.

64 Cranford JA, Arnedt JT, Conroy DA *et al.* (2017) Prevalence and correlates of sleep-related problems in adults receiving medical cannabis for chronic pain. *Drug and Alcohol Dependence* **180**:227–33.

65 Bachhuber M, Arnsten JH, Wurm G. (2019) Use of cannabis to relieve pain and promote sleep by customers at an adult use dispensary. *J Psychoactive Drugs* **51(5)**:400–4.

66 Kuhathasan N, Dufort A, MacKillop J, Gottschalk R, Minuzzi L, Frey BN. (2019) The use of cannabinoids for sleep: A critical review on clinical trials. *Exp Clin Psychopharmacol* **27(4)**:383–401.

67 Suraev AS, Marshall NS, Vandrey R *et al.* (2020) Cannabinoid therapies in the management of sleep disorders: a systematic review of preclinical and clinical studies. *Sleep Medicine Reviews* **53**:101339.

68 Choi S, Huang BC, Gamaldo CE. (2020) Therapeutic uses of cannabis on sleep disorders and related conditions. *J Clin Neurophysiol* **37(1)**:39–49.

69 Carley DW, Prasad B, Reid KJ *et al.* (2018) Pharmacotherapy of apnea by cannabimimetic enhancement, the PACE clinical trial: effects of dronabinol in obstructive sleep apnea. *Sleep* **41(1)**.

70 Atkin T, Comai S, Gobbi G. (2018) Drugs for insomnia beyond benzodiazepines: pharmacology, clinical applications, and discovery. *Pharmacological Reviews* **70(2)**:197–245.

71 Gomes T, Greaves S, van den Brink W *et al.* (2018) Pregabalin and the risk for opioid-related death: a nested case-control study. *Annals of Internal Medicine* **169(10)**:732–34.

72 Babiloni AH, Beetz G, Bruneau A, Martel MO, Cistulli PA, Nixdorf DR, Conway JN, Lavigne G.J.(2021) Multitargeting the sleep-pain interaction with pharmacological approaches: a narrative review with suggestions on new avenues of investigation. *Sleep Medicine Reviews***59**:101459.

73 Khouzam HR. (2017) A review of trazodone use in psychiatric and medical conditions. *Postgraduate Medicine* **129(1)**:140–148.

74 Cistulli PA, Hedner J. (2019) Drug therapy for obstructive sleep apnea: from pump to pill? *Sleep Med Rev* **46**:A1–a3.

75 Taranto-Montemurro L, Messineo L, Wellman A. (2019) Targeting endotypic traits with medications for the pharmacological treatment of obstructive sleep apnea. A review of the Current Literature. *Journal of Clinical Medicine* **8(11)**.

76 Herrero Babiloni A, Bellemare A, Beetz G, *et al.* (2020) The effects of non-invasive brain stimulation on sleep disturbances among different neurological and neuropsychiatric conditions: a systematic review. *Sleep Medicine Reviews* **55**:101381.

77 Herrero Babiloni A, Guay S, Nixdorf DR, de Beaumont L, Lavigne G.(2018)Non-invasive brain stimulation in chronic orofacial pain: a systematic review. *Journal of Pain Research* **11**:1445–57.

78 Cardenas-Rojas A, Pacheco-Barrios K, Giannoni-Luza S, Rivera-Torrejon O, Fregni F. (2020) Noninvasive brain stimulation combined with exercise in chronic pain: a systematic review and meta-analysis. *Expert Rev Neurother* **20(4)**:401–12.

79 Zhou J, Liu D, Li X, Ma J, Zhang J, Fang J. (2012) Pink noise: effect on complexity synchronization of brain activity and sleep consolidation. *J Theor Biol* **306**:68–72.

80 Caravan B, Hu L, Veyg D, *et al.* (2020) Sleep spindles as a diagnostic and therapeutic target for chronic pain. *Molecular Pain* **16**: 1744806920902350.

Chapter 8

Clinical assessment in adult patients

Christine Short[1] & Mary E. Lynch[2]

[1] Associate Professor, Dalhousie University, Department of Medicine, Division of Physical Medicine and Rehabilitation; Department of Surgery, Division of Neurosurgery, Queen Elizabeth II Health Sciences Centre, Halifax, Nova Scotia, Canada
[2] Department of Anesthesia, Pain Management and Perioperative Medicine, Department of Psychiatry, Department of Pharmacology, Dalhousie University, Halifax, Nova Scotia, Canada

Pain is what the patient says it is

(Ronald Melzack, 1975)

Introduction

There is no objective imaging study or laboratory test that can measure pain; however, we can objectively measure the manifestations of pain. The patient's verbal report and behavior provide most of the information. In some cases, there is a limp or some other obvious manifestation of the pain. However, there is no hint of the pain in many cases; it is invisible to the observer. Carr *et al.* [1] have reviewed the importance of narrative in pain and the fact that the patient's description is particularly required in chronic pain because there are no specific diagnostic tests for pain; words are often all the patient has [2]. Thus, the best clinical tools in pain assessment, in cognitively intact adults, are the clinician's capacity to listen to the patient as they tell their story, careful observation and a thorough physical examination that includes a thorough neurosensory and musculoskeletal examination.

The history

It is best to start with an open-ended question, simply ask the patient to tell you about their pain. Make time for the patient to tell their story. Later you can fill in the gaps. Table 8.1 presents the key elements required in a full biopsychosocial history. In most cases, in order to obtain a full history and physical examination as well as communicating diagnosis and suggested management, the clinician will need 90–120 minutes. We realize that this length of time will not be possible in all clinical contexts, so it is reasonable to obtain this information over several appointments, depending on the clinical setting. The important thing is that the initial assessment is not complete until you have obtained all of this information. A thorough initial assessment is critical in building a good therapeutic alliance with the person experiencing pain. Without this, it will be difficult to build a successful management plan.

Patient expectations and goals

Within the first few minutes, ask the patient about their expectations or goals. Patients may not be looking for complete relief and will often surprise you by

Clinical Pain Management: A Practical Guide, Second Edition. Edited by Mary E. Lynch, Kenneth D. Craig, and Philip W. Peng.

Table 8.1 Essential elements in the history and physical examination of the patient presenting with chronic pain.

History	
Chief complaint and history of present illness	Exploring location, onset, quality, context, severity, duration, modifying factors, spontaneous/ evoked aspects and associated signs and symptoms (sleep, appetite, energy, concentration, memory, mood, libido, suicidal ideation), previous treatment for pain (include complimentary therapies), previous consultations and investigations
Functional history	Impact of pain on level of function Mobility: bed mobility, transfers, wheelchair mobility, ambulation, driving and community access and devices required Activities of daily living: e.g. bathing, toileting, dressing, eating, hygiene and grooming Instrumental activities of daily living: e.g. meal preparation, laundry, telephone use, home maintenance, child or pet care Communication issues, sexual function
Past medical and surgical history	Specific conditions: cardiopulmonary, musculoskeletal, neurological and rheumatological and Medications
Psychosocial history	Past psychiatric and addiction history Home environment and living circumstances, family and friends support system, vocational activities, finances, recreational activities, spirituality and litigation
Family history	
Review of systems	
Physical	
General medical physical examination	Cardiac Pulmonary Gastrointestinal Genital/urinary and pelvic (if applicable) Lymphatics
General neurological and mental status examination	General appearance, behavior, flow of speech, ability to participate in the history and physical exam process Orientation: most patients in an outpatient setting will be oriented to person, place and time; in an inpatient setting, questions regarding re-orientation may be more important Affect: is affect congruent with the content of the interview? Attention and concentration Thought content: is it consistent with questions posed and the context of the pain interview or is there evidence of disorganized thought, delusional thinking? Is there any unusual behavior that might suggest a perceptual abnormality such as hallucinations?
Cranial nerve	**1** Odor perception (smell) **2** Confrontation visual fields, fundi, visual acuity **3,4,6** External ocular movements, diplopia, nystagmus, pupil response **5** Jaw strength, corneal reflexes, facial sensation **7** Facial power **8** Auditory acuity (hearing) **9 &10** Dysarthria, dysphagia **11** Sternocleidomastoid and trapezius power **12** Tongue atrophy strength and fasiculations
Sensation	Light touch and pinprick Presence or absence of allodynia, hyperalgesia, cold and heat hypersensitivity

(Continued)

Table 8.1 (Continued)

Motor	Key muscles (Biceps C5–6, brachioradialis C6, triceps C7, finger flexors C8, finger abductors T1, Hip flexors L2, knee extensors L3–4, ankle dorsiflexors L4-5, ankle plantar flexors L5-S1) Strength (0 = no movement, 1 = flicker, 2 = movement with gravity eliminated, 3 = movement only against gravity, 4 = movement can be overcome by resistance, 5 = full power) Coordination Involuntary movements Tone/spasticity
Reflexes (roots)	Biceps C5–6, brachioradialis C6, triceps C7, knee extensors L3–4, ankle, ankle plantar flexors L5-S1
Musculoskeletal	
Inspection	Behavior ease of movement during the history and physical examination, symmetry edema, color change, atrophy, joint deformity, quality of skin, hair distribution
Palpation	Joint stability Range of motion (active and passive) Strength testing Bony/joint/muscles and soft tissues Include assessment of trigger points of myofascial pain

saying they are looking for strategies to control or cope better with the pain. They may also present specific goals such as a wish to walk farther, play with their grandchildren or return to work, whether this be unpaid work within the home or wage-earning work outside of the home.

Psychological history

Given the importance of psychosocial determinants of pain and related disability, enquiry into these factors is imperative. Chapter 11 presents the details of this assessment. We provide brief observations here.

When patients present with a chief complaint of chronic pain, they are usually comfortable reviewing the details of the pain. However, some patients may experience discomfort with questions along psychological lines fearing that you are suggesting that the pain is psychologically caused. Starting with a focus on the physiological aspects of the pain will ease some of these fears. A statement like, "Now that I have heard about the pain, I would like to get to know more about how this pain is affecting you and what strategies you are using to get through each day with it." This places the questions about mood and anxiety in context for the patient. You can then move into questions regarding the impact the pain has had on sleep, appetite, energy, concentration, mood and sex drive. If the patient reports depression or significant irritability of mood, this is the time to ask about suicidal ideation. You may begin to explore this by asking, "Has it ever gotten to the point where you feel that life might not be worth living? If yes,"Have you ever come close to acting on these thoughts?", "Can you tell me about it?", "What stopped you?", and "How do you feel now?"

The Columbia Suicide Severity Rating Scale (C-SSRS) is an excellent tool for assessing suicidal ideation and risk [3]. It is a questionnaire used for suicide assessment that was developed by multiple institutions, led by investigators at Columbia University with National Institute of Mental Health support. It is now available in over 140 country-specific languages and has been used in multiple settings including schools, universities military, first responders, primary care and in research trials. The full risk assessment version is 3 pages long with the initial page assessing several risk categories and protective factors. It measures severity and intensity of suicidal ideation, behaviors and lethality of suicide attempts. It also comes in a short 6 question "screener" version that allows an initial rapid assessment of imminent risk (see table 8.2). A

Table 8.2 Columbia Suicide Severity Rating Scale (C-SSRS) Screener. Used with permission from The Columbia Lighthouse Project.

	Past Month	
1. **Have you wished you were dead or wished you could go to sleep and not wake up?**		
2. **Have you actually had any thoughts about killing yourself?** If **YES** to 2, answer questions 3, 4, 5 and 6 If **NO** to 2, go directly to question 6		
3. **Have you thought about how you might do this?**		
4. **Have you had any intention of acting on these thoughts of killing yourself, as opposed to you have the thoughts but you definitely would not act on them?**	**High Risk**	
5. **Have you started to work out or worked out the details of how to kill yourself? Do you intend to carry out this plan?**	**High Risk**	
Always Ask Question 6	Life-time	Past 3 Months
6. Have you done anything, started to do anything, or prepared to do anything to end your life? *Example*: Collected pills, obtained a gun, gave away valuables, wrote a will or suicide note, held a gun but changed your mind, cut yourself, tried to hang yourself, etc.		**High Risk**

The screener can be downloaded from https://cssrs.columbia.edu/documents/clinical-practice-screener-recent/ and more information, including details regarding protocols, is available at https://cssrs.columbia.edu/the-columbia-scale-c-ssrs/cssrs-for-communities-and-healthcare/#filter=.general-use.english.

positive response to any of the items on the screener indicates the need for further assessment and care, a positive response to items 4,5 or 6 indicates the need for immediate referral to professional care.

For survivors of trauma, whether this be domestic abuse, military exposure or industrial or motor vehicle accidents, it is also important to screen for post-traumatic stress disorder (PTSD). Examples of questions to begin to explore for PTSD may include: "Have you re-experienced the accident (or other traumatic event) in any way such as recurrent distressing memories, dreams or nightmares or flashbacks?" "Do you avoid the site of the accident?" "Have you found yourself more vigilant, hyperaware or easily startled?" Examples of questions to begin to explore anxiety or panic might include: "Do you feel that you suffer from excessive anxiety or worry?" "Do you have any physical symptoms associated with this like trembling, restlessness, increased heart rate, sweating, trouble breathing?"

The risk of substance abuse or chemical dependency should be explored, especially when prescription of opioid is considered. Details of this assessment can be found in Chapter 39. The suggestions above are examples of ways to begin to explore for psychological pathology. If you find symptoms suggestive of a mood or anxiety disorder then further assessment and referral for psychological services may be required.

Personal social vocational history

An individual who has grown up in an abusive or traumatic environment will be less likely to have learned healthy coping strategies to deal with experiences such as chronic pain and will require training in healthy strategies. Also, current social circumstances including shelter, financial stress, supports and dependants are critical when understanding what the patient is dealing with and are important in planning appropriate management.

Functional impact

Level of education, ability to function, current work or disability, losses caused by pain and the patient's perspective about the future must also be assessed.

The interference items from the Brief Pain Inventory (BPI) [4] are helpful in beginning to assess functional impact and more detail regarding standardized measures are presented in Chapter 11.

Measurement of pain and screening instruments

For the measurement of pain intensity, we have found the numerical rating scale easiest for patients, "On a 0 to 10 point scale, where 0 equals no pain and 10 indicates worst possible pain, how bad is your pain?" It is helpful to ask the person over the last day what has been their worst pain out of 10, their least pain, their average pain and their pain right now (from the Brief Pain Inventory [4]). For pain quality the Short Form McGill Pain Questionnaire is excellent [5], for physical function and interference with function the BPI interference scale is highly regarded [4] and to assess health-related quality of life the SF-36 scale is widely used [6]. These are some of our favorite measures. For further detail, Chapter 4 provides a conceptual basis for psychosocial parameters of assessment and Chapter 11 provides a review of the many screening instruments available for measurement of pain. See also the chapter on evaluation of the pain patient in Bonica's Management of Pain 5th edition [7] or pain assessment in Wall and Melzack's *Textbook of Pain, 6th Edition* [8]. For a discussion regarding measurement of core domains in the assessment of pain in clinical trials, see publications by the IMMPACT[1] group [9].

Physical examination

The goal of the physical examination is to confirm any suspicions you have obtained from the history as to possible sources or generators of pain. It is important to identify reversible factors that might be contributing to pain. It is this information that will provide the foundation upon which to build your investigation and treatment plan. A brief outline is presented in Table 8.1.

The time spent during the history and physical examination has many functions. One is to build the database you need for diagnosis and treatment. The other is to continue to build a relationship of trust with the patient. With this in mind, first and foremost put the patient at ease. We always let the patient know that some of the physical examination will be uncomfortable, but it may be necessary to cause some discomfort in order to find out where the sources of pain might be. Always reassure the patient to let you know if anything is too uncomfortable so that part of the examination can be adjusted or discontinued. Lastly, make sure at all times that the patient is draped/dressed appropriately for their comfort throughout the physical examination.

Observation

The physical examination starts with observation. Much of this can be done while taking the history. Note whether the patient appears to be in distress. Unlike acute pain, most patients with chronic pain do not look distressed on the outside. Do not let this allow you to minimize the patient's suffering. Observe the individual's posture and movement during the interview. People with chronic musculoskeletal pain will often move frequently during the interview to try to find a position of comfort. We always invite them to move as they need to at the beginning of the history and physical assessment. Posture should be noted in sitting and standing positions. For example, the protracted or rolled shoulder and protruded chin is common in individuals presenting with back, neck and shoulder pain (Figure 8.1). Observe the gait. A lurch or limp may indicate a musculoskeletal (MSK) or neurologic impairment that could be contributing to pain and may be corrected or improved with treatment such physical therapy or orthotics.

Musculoskeletal examination

The musculoskeletal (MSK) examination should be detailed for regions identified as painful and should include inspection of the joint(s) and surrounding soft tissues, range of motion, palpation and special tests for that region. Limitations in range of motion

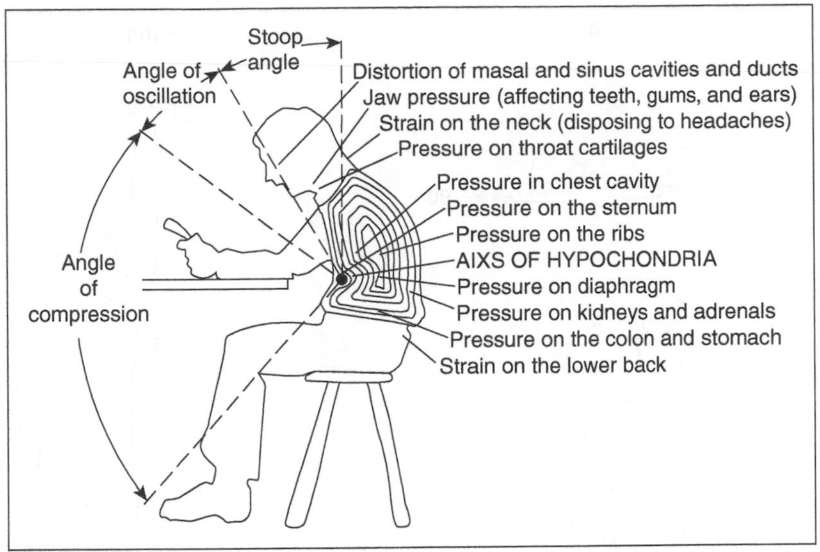

Figure 8.1 Posture theory diagram.

or MSK abnormalities may be fixed and require accommodation or flexible in which case correction may be possible. For a more detailed presentation of the MSK examination the reader is referred to MaGee [10].

Inspection

Note muscle wasting and asymmetry, which may result from disuse or neurologic impairments. Observe for swelling and redness especially around joints that are symptomatic. Note any unusual rashes or pigmentation. A quick screen of the asymptomatic joints is appropriate, followed by a more detailed review of symptomatic areas. If the patient is suspected to have sympathetically maintained pain, one should look for color, temperature and trophic changes as well as dystonia.

Range of motion

A goniometer is an inexpensive easy to use tool for assessing range of motion (ROM) (Figure 8.2). Always start with active ROM as this is within the control of the individual and the safest way to proceed. If there is restriction of ROM you can then add a gentle passive assist to the joint to see if there is any further movement. If there is restricted ROM it is important to distinguish if it is due to pain, weakness or tightness. Figure 8.3 shows ROM testing for the appendicular joints. ROM of the lumbosacral spine is best measured using Schober's test which examines the movement of the lumbosacral spine during flexion (Figure 8.4). The normal excursion should be greater than 4.5 cm. There are a wide range of published

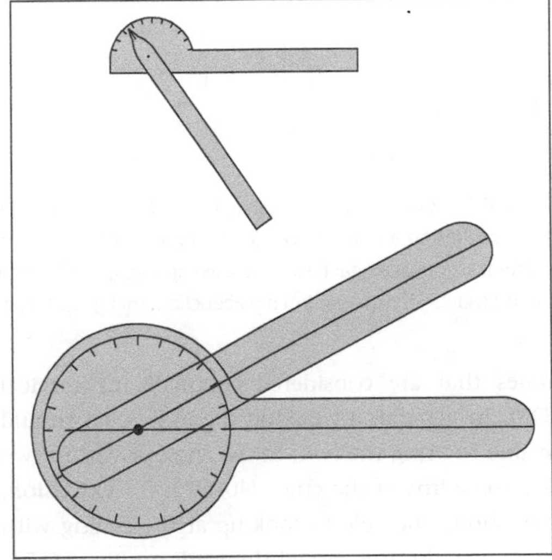

Figure 8.2 Goniometer. Reproduced from Braddom [12], with permission from Elsevier.

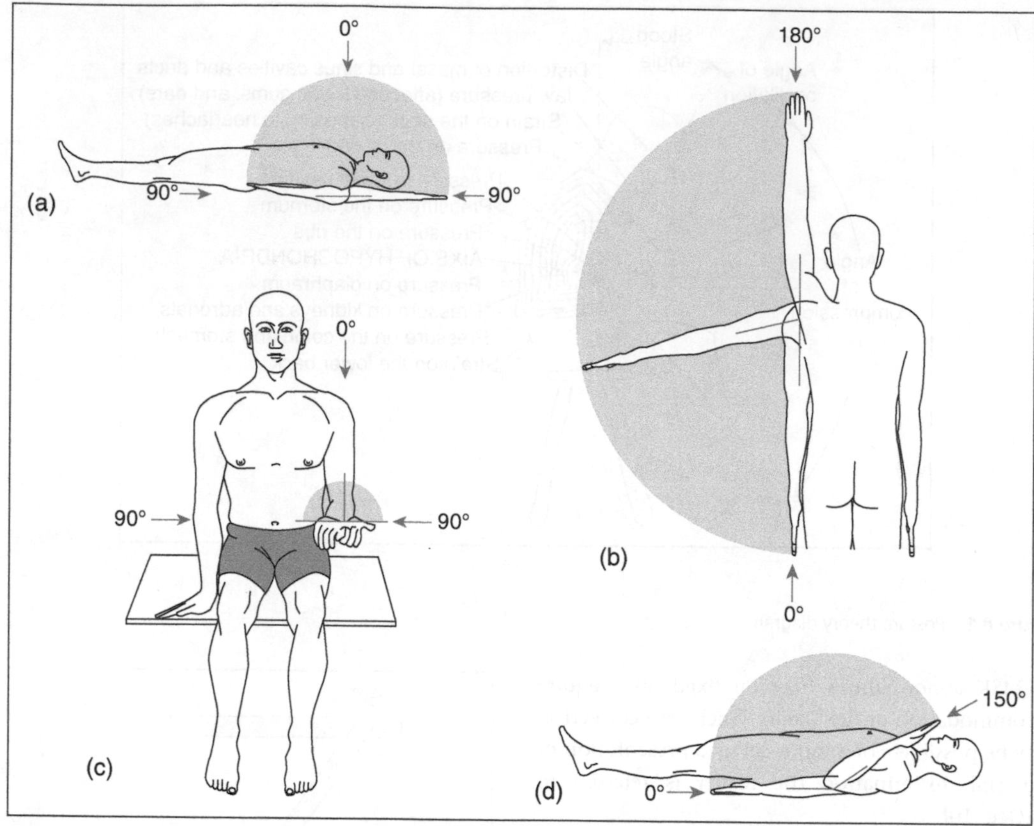

Figure 8.3 Range of motion testing for the apendicular joints. (a) Shoulder flexion; (b) shoulder abduction; (c) elbow supination; (d) elbow flexion and extension; (e) wrist adduction (30°) and abduction (20°); (f) wrist flexion and extension; (g) finger flexion; (h) metacarpophalangeal flexion; (i) knee flexion; (j) ankle dorsi (20°) and plantar (50°) flexion; (k) hip flexion; (l) hip external (45°) and internal (35°) rotation; (m) hip abduction; (n) hip adduction. Reproduced from Braddom [10], with permission from Elsevier.

values that are considered "normal" for cervical ROM. In general, for flexion the individual should be able to bring the chin to the chest or within two fingerbreadths of the chest (40–60°). For extension, they should be able to look up at the ceiling with their eyes in the straightforward position (55°). Lateral bending should be 45° to either side and lateral rotation 70–90° to the right and left (Figure 8.5).

Palpation

Palpate for swelling to define its character and note increased heat. Palpate joints and bony deformities for crepitus. Palpate soft tissues for tenderness and presence of myofascial trigger points [9]. When palpating apply firm pressure (about 4 kg of pressure or enough pressure to blanch the nail on your palpating finger). There is a difference between tender points of fibromyalgia and trigger points of myofascial pain (Chapter 30).

Special tests

There are special tests for many MSK disorders and several tests for each joint which can be quite overwhelming to the assessor (for a full list and descriptions see MaGee [19]). In most cases if you remember your basic anatomy and biomechanics then you will be able to identify the pathology. For example, if you are considering a tendonopathy as a source of ongoing pain then:

1 Palpate the tendon for tenderness;

2 Stretch or stress the tendon, trying to reproduce the clinical symptom of pain.

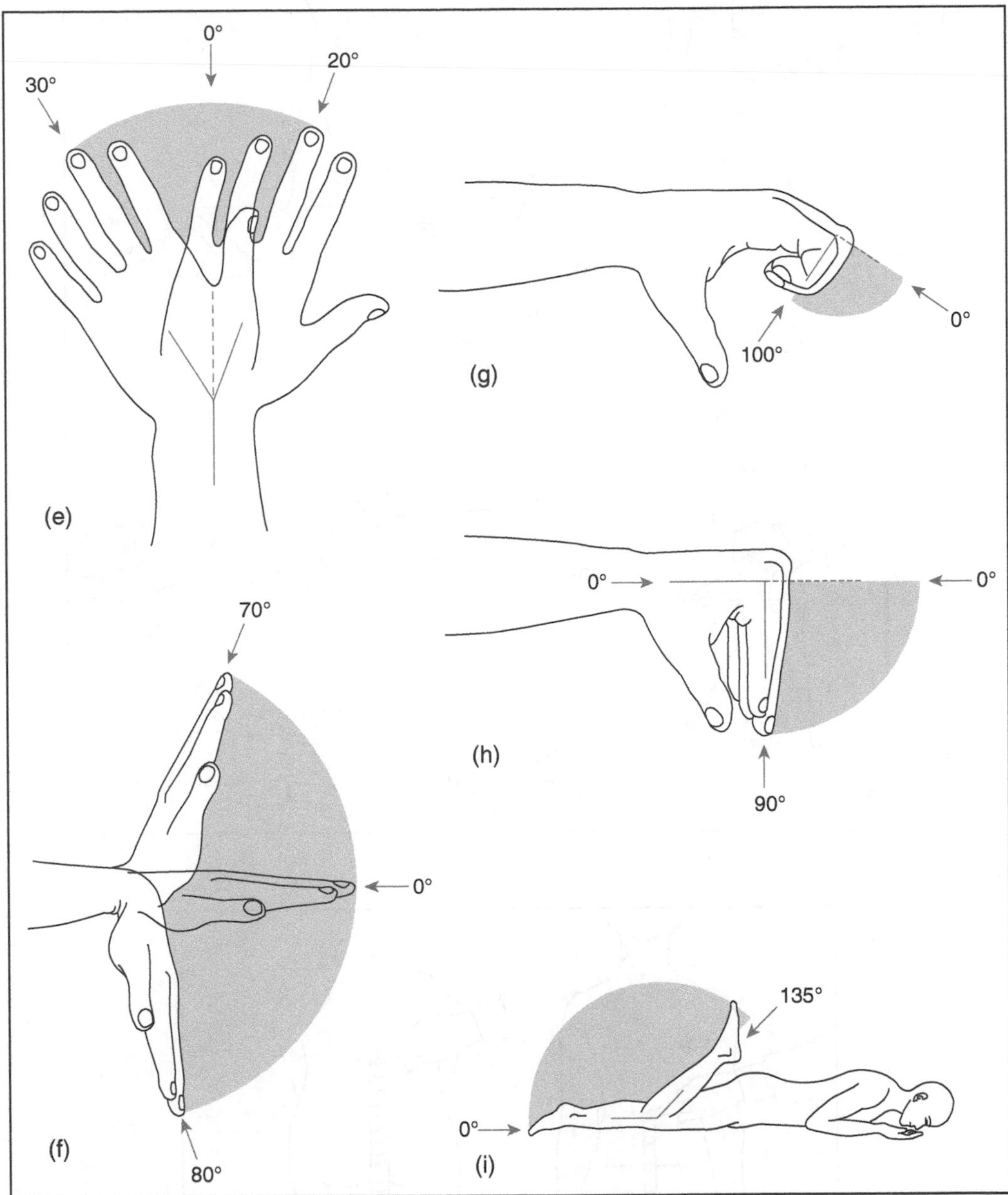

Figure 8.3 (Continued)

Neurological examination

In most patients presenting with pain a good neurological examination is also essential. Again, a general screening examination is appropriate followed by a more detailed examination of symptomatic areas.

Cranial nerves

Most of the cranial nerve assessment can be observed during the history, with later examination of vision, visual fields and oral, pharyngeal function and sensory examination of the face on the physical examination (Table 8.1).

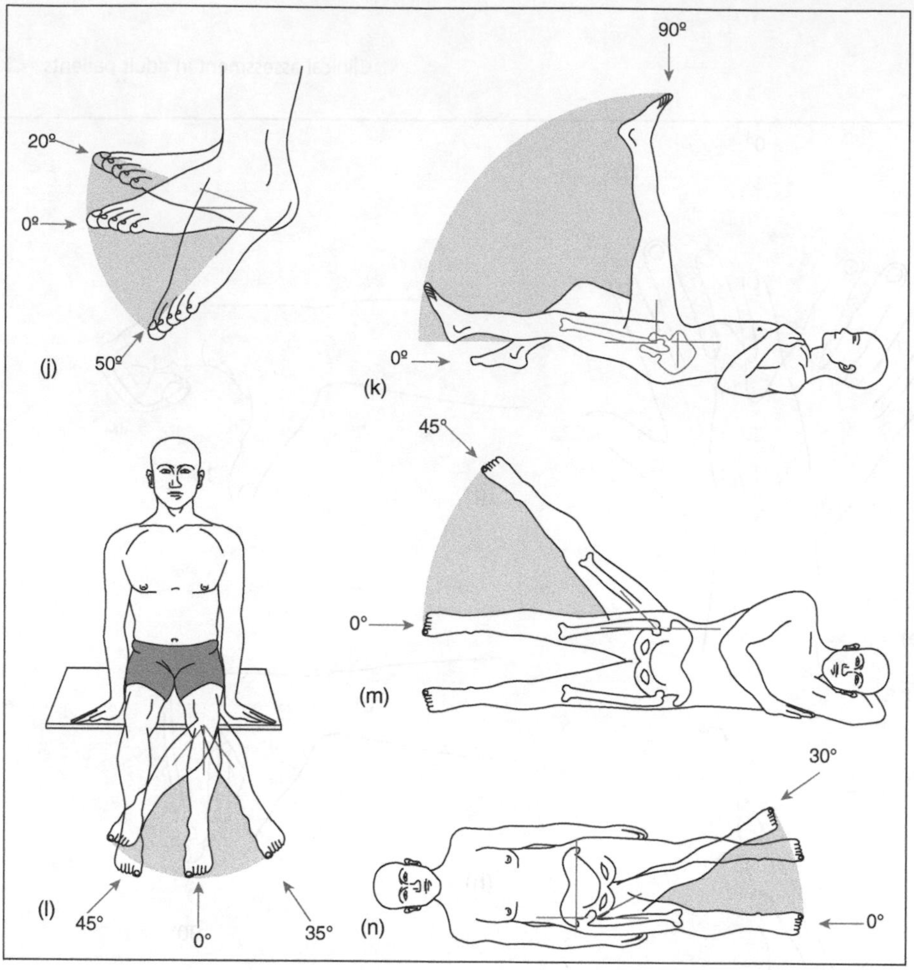

Figure 8.3 (Continued)

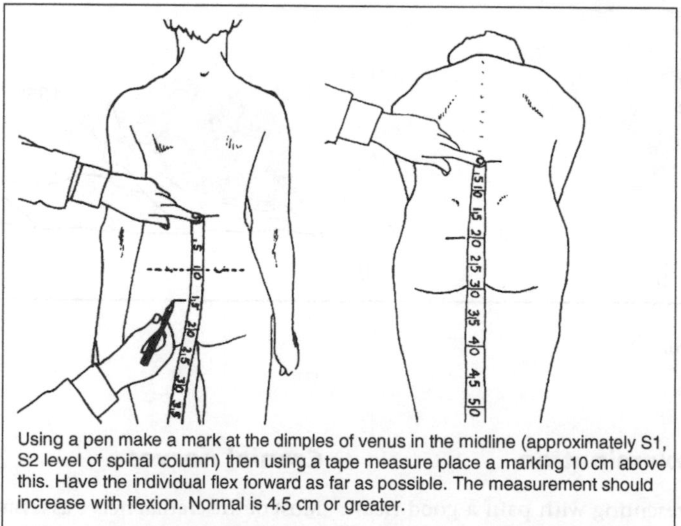

Using a pen make a mark at the dimples of venus in the midline (approximately S1, S2 level of spinal column) then using a tape measure place a marking 10 cm above this. Have the individual flex forward as far as possible. The measurement should increase with flexion. Normal is 4.5 cm or greater.

Figure 8.4 Illustration of Schober's test for range of motion of the lumbosacral spine. Using a pen make a mark at the dimples of Venus in the midline (approximately S1,S2 level of spinal column) then, using a tape measure, place a marking 10 cm above this. Have the individual flex forward as far as possible. The measurement should increase with flexion. Normal is 4.5 cm or greater. *Source*: McRae R. (1997) *Clinical Orthopaedic Examination*, 4th edn. Churchill Livingstone, New York. p. 133. Reproduced with permission from Elsevier.

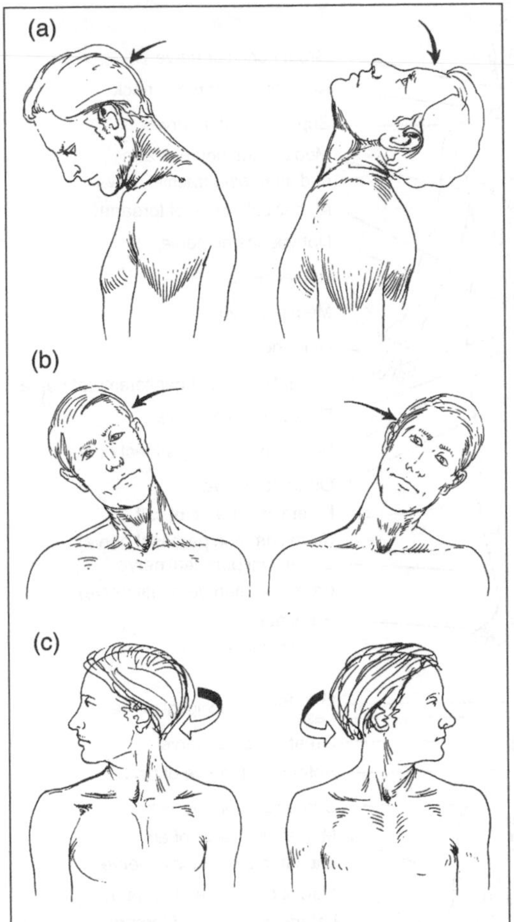

Figure 8.5 C-spine range of motion. (a) Flexion and extension; (b) lateral flexion; (c) lateral rotation. Reproduced from Hoppenfeld [14], with permission from Pearson Education.

Motor examination

Observe muscle wasting and fasiculations; a regional or radicular pattern of wasting and weakness may suggest an underlying neurological disorder. Pain can cause disuse which can lead to diminished strength and wasting. This is usually less profound than that seen with lower motor neuron damage and is not associated with fasiculations. Motor tone should be observed as normal, increased or decreased. If a region is painful, it is often difficult for the individual to relax fully and this will make assessment of tone more difficult to interpret. As much as possible, let the individual you are examining move within their range of comfort (for more detail see Braddom [12]).

Sensory examination

A good sensory examination includes an assessment of light touch and response to sharp stimulation. Regional areas of numbness are commonly associated with regional soft tissue pain especially in the presence of muscle tightness and spasm. These do not necessarily mean that there is neurological dysfunction related to the pain. Areas of sensory abnormality that follow a specific dermatome or peripheral nerve distribution suggest an underlying neurological injury or compressive neuropathy that may be potentially reversible (Figure 8.6). The presence of allodynia or hyperalgesia may suggest a component of neural sensitization and will assist in identifying whether there is a neuropathic component to the individual's pain. Further detail regarding the neurosensory examination is covered in Chapter 10.

Reflexes

The deep tendon reflexes should be described as normal, increased or decreased and assist in identifying a neurological problem involved in the pain process; note any asymmetry.

Cerebellar examination

The screening examination includes observation regarding balance, coordination, tremor and smoothness of motion during the other aspects of the physical examination.

Table 8.3 summarizes some pearls of the physical examination for chronic pain.

Conclusions

A complete biopsychosocial history followed by an appropriate physical examination will give you the diagnosis in over 90% of cases. Further investigations, where available, are used primarily to confirm your working diagnosis. Once this thorough assessment has been completed you now have the data to build a comprehensive treatment plan.

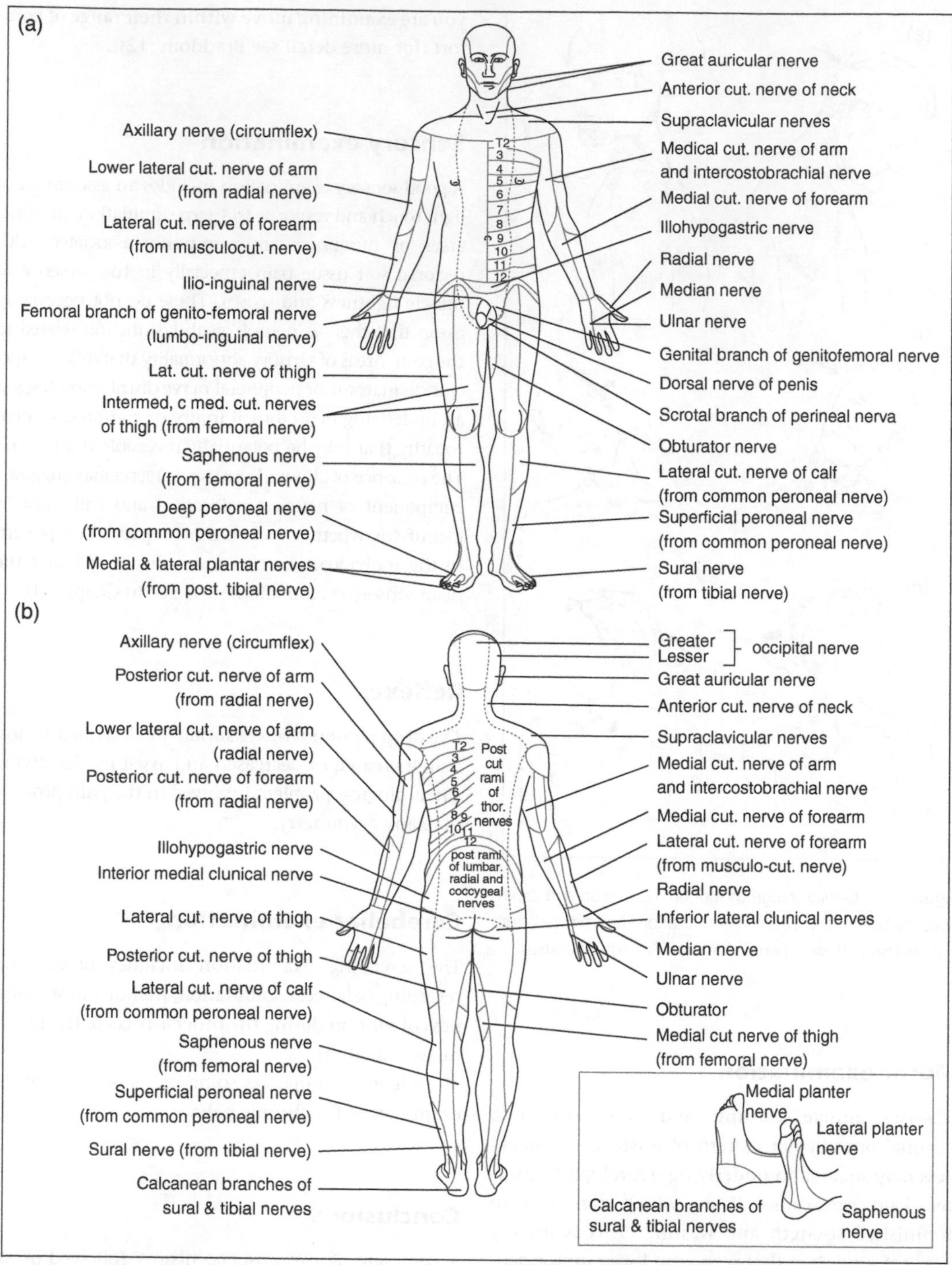

Figure 8.6 Areas of sensory abnormality that follow a specific dermatome or peripheral nerve distribution (A, B). Reproduced from Braddom [9], with permission from Elsevier.

Table 8.3 Physical examination pearls.

Presenting complaint	Examination pearl	Comments
Hip or back pain	Check for Leg Length Discrepancy (LLD), palpate GT area for signs of bursitis	LLD can change the biomechanics of the lower extremity and back and contribute to ongoing pain and dysfunction. With GT bursitis, pain often radiates into the lateral upper leg.
Back or lower extremity joint pain	Check the feet	Foot deformities like LLD put abnormal strain on the low back and lower extremity structures. This can lead to knee, hip and/or low back complaints.
Neck pain	Posture! Posture! Posture!	Even subtle poor posture can greatly increase the strain on the neck and increase discomfort.
Neck and back pain	Ask about the pillow and mattress	Proper support during sleep can alleviate a multitude of symptoms.
Neck pain	Always do a neurological screen for myelopathy	The neurologic screen for myelopathy in neck pain should include upper extremity and lower extremity strength and sensation and reflex examination. The Babinski sign may be an important sign for myelopathy.
Persistent shoulder pain	Do not forget to examine the long head of the biceps in the bicipital groove (see examining tendons above)	This is often missed when rotator cuff tendonopathy is diagnosed. Pain coming from the biceps tendon needs to be treated as well.

GT, greater trochanteric; LLD, leg length discrepancy.

References

1 Carr DB, Loeser JD, Morris DB. (2005) *Narrative, Pain, and Suffering* IASP Press, Seattle, WA.

2 Charon R. (2005) A narrative medicine for pain. In: Carr DB, Loeser JD, Morris DB, eds. *Narrative, Pain, and Suffering*. IASP Press, Seattle. pp. 29–44.

3 Posner K, Brown GK, Stanly B et al. (2011) *Am J Psychiatry* **168(12)**:1266–77.

4 Cleeland CS, Ryan KM. (1994) Pain assessment: global use of the Brief Pain Inventory. *Ann Acad Med Singapore* **23(2)**:129–38.

5 Melzack R. (1987) The short-form McGill Pain Questionnaire. *Pain* **30(2)**:191–7.

6 Ware JE Jr, Sherbourne CD. (1992) The MOS 36-item short-form health survey (SF-36). I. Conceptual framework and item selection. *Med Care* **30(6)**:473–83.

7 Ballantyne JC, Fishman SM, Rathmell JP. (2019). *Bonica's Management of Pain*. 5th edn. Lippincott Williams, & Wilkins, Philadelphia.

8 McMahon S, Koltzenburg M, Tracey I, Turk DC. (2013) *Wall & Melzack's Textbook of Pain*. 6th edn. Elsevier, Netherlands.

9 Dworkin RH, Turk DC, Farrar JT *et al.* (2005) Core outcome measures for chronic pain clinical trials: IMMPACT recommendations. *Pain* **113(1–2)**:9–19.

10 MaGee DJ. (2008) *Orthopedic Physical Assessment*, 5th edn. Saunders, St. Louis.

11 Travell JG, Simons DG. (1992) Myofascial Pain and Dysfunction Trigger Point Manual Vol.2, *The Lower Extremities*. Williams and Wilkins, Philadelphia.

12 O'Dell MW, Lin D, Singh R, Christolias GC. (2016) In: Cifu DX. *Braddom's Physical Medicine and Rehabilitation* 5th edn. Elsevier, Philadelphia.

13 American Psychiatric Association. (2013) *Diagnostic and Statistical Manual of Mental Disorders 5*. American Psychiatric Association, Washington, D.C.

14 Hoppenfeld S. (1976) *Physical Examination of the Spine and Extremities*. Appleton Century Crofts, East Norwalk.

15 Ballantyne, J. C., S. M. Fishman and J. P. Rathmell (2019). *Bonica's Management of Pain*, 5th Edn. Wolters Kluwer, Philadelphia.

16 McMahon, S., M. Koltzenburg, I. Tracey and D. Turk (2013). *Wall and Melzack's Textbook of Pain*. 6th Edn. Elsevier, Netherlands.

Part 2

Assessment of Pain

Chapter 9

Measurement and assessment of pain in pediatric patients

Jennifer N. Stinson[1,2,3]**, Kathryn A. Birnie**[4,5]**, & Petra Hroch Tiessen**[6]

[1] *Child Health Evaluation Sciences, The Hospital for Sick Children, Toronto, Ontario, Canada*

[2] *Department of Anesthesia and Pain Medicine, The Hospital for Sick Children, Toronto, Ontario, Canada*

[3] *Lawrence S. Bloomberg, Faculty of Nursing, University of Toronto, Ontario, Canada*

[4] *Department of Anesthesiology, Perioperative, and Pain Medicine, University of Calgary, Calgary, Alberta, Canada*

[5] *Alberta Children's Hospital Research Institute, Calgary, Alberta, Canada*

[6] *Department of Anesthesiology and Pain Medicine, University of Toronto, Toronto, Ontario, Canada*

Introduction

This chapter provides an overview of the assessment of pain in children from neonates to adolescents. The difference between pain assessment and pain monitoring is highlighted and the key steps in pain assessment identified. Self-report, observer-report, behavioral and physiological indicators of pain in children are reviewed. Information about commonly used pain tools is provided and the factors that need to be considered when choosing a pain assessment tool are outlined. Finally, the need for clear documentation about pain assessment and how regularly pain assessment should be undertaken are also discussed.

Comprehensive pain assessment in children

Pain in children occurs across a spectrum of conditions including everyday pains, acute injuries and medical events, recurrent or chronic pain and pain related to chronic disease. Pain assessment is the first step in the management of pain. Accurate assessment of children's pain is needed to diagnose medical conditions and to guide pain management interventions [1,2]. To treat pain effectively, ongoing monitoring of the presence and severity of pain and the child's response to treatment is essential.

Pain assessment poses many challenges in infants and children because of: (a) the subjective and complex nature of pain; (b) developmental and language limitations that preclude comprehension and self-report; and (c) dependence on others to infer pain from behavioral and physiological indicators. The important steps in assessing pain in children include:

1 recording a comprehensive pain history;

2 assessing the child's pain using a developmentally appropriate pain assessment tool; and

3 selection of an appropriate intervention [3].

Assessment should be followed by ongoing monitoring of pain, having allowed time for pain-relieving interventions to work. Parents and

Clinical Pain Management: A Practical Guide, Second Edition. Edited by Mary E. Lynch, Kenneth D. Craig, and Philip W. Peng.

significant family members know their child best and can often recognize subtle changes in manner or behavior. They have a particularly important role in pain assessment [1].

Pain measurement generally describes the quantification of pain intensity (e.g. "How much does it hurt?"). The emphasis is on the quantity, extent or degree of pain. Pain assessment is a broader concept than measurement and involves clinical judgment based on observation of the nature, significance and context of the child's pain experience [4]. Comprehensive pain assessment involves exploring the intensity of pain, location of pain, its duration, frequency, the sensory qualities (e.g. word descriptors), cognitive (e.g. perceived impact of pain on aspects of everyday life) and affective (e.g. pain unpleasantness) aspects of the pain experience [3]. Furthermore, contextual and situational factors that may influence children's perception of pain should also be explored. This exploration helps healthcare professionals to make decisions regarding the most likely cause of the pain (nociceptive, neuropathic or mixed) and to choose the most appropriate intervention(s).

Obtaining a pain history

Conducting a thorough history of the child's prior pain experiences and current pain complaints is the first step in pain assessment. Standardized pain history forms have been developed for talking with children and parents/caregivers about the pain [5]. To assess pain of relatively brief duration, instruments measuring pain intensity, location and affect are typically used. For a child with chronic pain, a more detailed pain history needs to be taken that measures the frequency, duration, time course and activity interference due to pain (Table 9.1) [2,3].

Approaches to measuring pain in children

The three approaches to measuring pain are self-report (what the child says), behavioral (how the child behaves) and physiological indicators (how the child's body reacts) [3]. These measures are used separately (unidimensional) or in combination (multidimensional or composite) in a range of pain assessment tools that are available to use in practice. The ideal would be a composite measure including self-report and one or more of these other approaches [6,7].

Children's self-report of their pain is the preferred approach and should be used with children who are able to understand and use self-report scales (e.g. 4–6 years of age and older) and are not overtly distressed [8,9]. With infants, toddlers, preverbal, nonverbal, cognitively impaired and sedated children who are unable to self-report, an appropriate behavioral or composite pain assessment tool should be used. Observer-report of the child's pain by a parent/caregiver or health professional can be used; however, it should not be considered equivalent to the child's own report as observers tend to over or underestimate the child's pain [10]. If the child is overtly distressed, no meaningful self-report can be obtained at that point in time. The child's pain can be estimated using a behavioral pain assessment tool until the child is less distressed [6].

Tools for assessing pain in children

Self-report tools

More than 60 tools have been developed for self-report of pain intensity by school-aged children and adolescents; however, only those outlined below are considered well-established with sufficient measurement properties for consideration in at least some children [8]. For a more in-depth review of self-report measures and their psychometric properties see the two reviews by Cohen *et al.* [2] and Birnie *et al.* [8].

Numerical pain scales

A numerical rating scale (NRS) consists of a range of numbers (e.g. 0–10 or 0–100) which can be represented in verbal or graphic format. Children are told that the lowest number represents no pain/hurt and the highest number represents the worst pain or hurt you could ever imagine. The child is instructed to state, circle, or record the number that best represents their level of pain intensity. Verbal 11-point NRS are the most frequently used pain intensity measure with children and are recommended for use for acute, postoperative, or chronic pain with children aged 6 or older who dis-

Table 9.1 Pain history questions for children with chronic pain and their parents/caregivers

Description of pain	**Type of pain** *Is the pain acute (e.g. postoperative pain), recurrent (e.g. headaches) or chronic (e.g. arthritis)?* **Onset of pain** *When did the pain begin? What were you doing before the pain began? Was there any initiating injury, trauma or stressors?* **Duration** *How long has the pain been present* (e.g. hours/days/weeks/months)? **Frequency** *How often is pain present? Is the pain always there or is it intermittent? Does it come and go?* **Location** *Where is the pain located? Can you point to the part of the body that hurts?* (Body outlines can be used to help children indicate where they hurt). *Does the pain go anywhere else* (e.g. radiates up or down from the site that hurts)? Pain radiation can also be indicated on body diagrams. **Intensity** *What is your pain intensity at rest? What is your pain intensity with activity?* *Over the past week what is the least pain you have had? What is the worst pain you have had? What is your usual level of pain?* **Quality of pain** School-aged children can communicate about pain in more abstract terms. *Describe the quality of your pain* (e.g. word descriptors such as sharp, dull, stabbing, burning, throbbing). Word descriptors can provide information on whether the pain is nociceptive, nociplastic, or neuropathic in nature or a combination.
Associated symptoms	*Are there any other symptoms that go along with or occur just before or immediately after the pain* (e.g. nausea, vomiting, tiredness or difficulty ambulating)? *Are there any changes in the color or temperature of the affected extremity or painful area?* (These changes most often occur in children with conditions such as complex regional pain syndromes).
Temporal or seasonal variations Impact on daily living	*Is the pain affected by changes in seasons or weather?* *Does the pain occur at certain times of the day?* *Has the pain led to changes in daily activities and/or behaviors* (e.g. sleep disturbances, change in appetite or mood, decreased physical activity, social interactions or school attendance)? *What level would the pain need to be so that you could do all your normal activities* (e.g. tolerability)? *What level would the pain need to be so that you won't be bothered by it?* (Rated on similar scale as pain intensity.) *What brings on the pain or makes the pain worse* (e.g. movement, stress, etc.)?
Pain relief measures	*What has helped to make the pain better?* *What medication have you taken to relieve your pain? If so what was the medication and did it help? Were there any side effects?* It is important to also ask about the use of physical, psychological and complementary and alternative treatments tried and how effective these methods were in relieving pain (Chapter 28). The degree of pain relief or intensity of pain after a pain-relieving treatment/intervention should be determined.

Source: Stinson J. (2009) [3]. Reproduced with permission.

play numeracy skills [8]. Verbal NRS have the advantage that they can be verbally administered without a print copy and are easy to score. A high degree of agreement is shown between verbal NRS and those presented electronically [11]. Verbal NRS now have the most evidence examining their validity and reliability of all self-report pain intensity scales with children [8].

Faces pain scales

Faces pain scales present the child with drawings or photographs of facial expressions representing increasing levels of pain intensity. The child is asked to select the picture of a face that best represents their pain intensity and their score is the number of the expression chosen. The Faces Pain Scale-Revised [12]) uses line drawings and is strongly recommended for use with children aged 7 years and older [8]. The Wong-Baker FACES Pain Rating Scale also uses line drawings. Its use is only weakly recommended as it is limited by the use of a face with tears to demonstrate the worst pain possible. This design is problematic as faces pain scales with a happy and smiling no pain face or faces with tears for most pain possible have been found to affect the pain scores recorded [13]. Therefore, faces pain scales with neutral expressions for no pain are generally recommended [13]. Other faces scales use photographs, such as the Oucher photographic, which is no longer a generally recommended tool [8]. In addition to faces scales for pain intensity, the Children's Fear Scale is a faces scale with demonstrated measurement properties that asks children to self-report their fear from not at all scared to the most scared possible [14].

Graphic rating scales

The most commonly used graphic rating scale is the Pieces of Hurt Tool (also referred to as the Poker Chip Tool). This tool consists of four red poker chips, representing a little bit of hurt (one chip) to the most hurt you could ever have (four chips). The child is asked to select the number of chips that represents his/her pain intensity and the tool is scored from 0 to 4. Although, the Pieces of Hurt Tool was originally developed for use with young preschool children, its measurement properties suggest it is weakly recommended for use with children 6 years and older [8]. It should not be used for self-report of postoperative or chronic pain. Additional drawbacks to its use include sanitizing the chips between patient use and the potential for losing chips [15].

Visual analog scales

Visual analog scales (VAS) require the child to select a point on a vertical or horizontal line where the ends of the line are defined as the extreme limits of pain intensity from no pain to worst pain possible. The child is asked to make a mark along the line to indicate the intensity of their pain. The Color Analog Scale uses gradation of color and size to reflect increases in pain intensity from small and white (no pain) to wider and deep red (most pain) [8]. The VAS is weakly recommended for children aged 6–8 years and older; whereas the CAS is recommended for children aged 8 years and older [8]. While VAS are easy to reproduce, photocopying may alter length of line and they require the extra step of measuring the line which increases the burden and likelihood for errors. Electronic versions of the VAS and CAS show good agreement with their paper-based counterparts [16].

Multidimensional pain tools

Although pain intensity is the most commonly recorded measure of a painful episode, a more comprehensive pain assessment is often necessary for children with recurrent or chronic pain. In this situation it is necessary to assess factors such as pain triggers, types of sensations that are experienced and how the pain interferes with aspects of everyday life (Table 9.1). The Bath Adolescent Pain Questionnaire (BAPQ), which has adolescent and parent versions, is a well-validated multidimensional instrument that can aid in the comprehensive assessment of chronic pain in adolescents (social functioning, physical functioning, depression, general anxiety, pain specific anxiety, family functioning and development) [17]. There are also other validated measures to assess the cognitive-affective impact of chronic pain in adolescents such as pain anxiety, pain catastrophizing and fear of pain. Some examples include the Pain Catastrophizing Scale for Children (PCS-C), Fear of Pain Questionnaire (Child FOPQ-C) and Child Pain Anxiety Symptoms Scale (CPASS-20) [18]. Finally, the Patient Reported Outcomes Measurement Information System (PROMIS®) is a National Institutes of Health initiative, created to advance the assessment of patient-reported outcomes in patients with chronic diseases [19]. The pain specific measures include: pain intensity, pain interference short form (self-report and parent proxy), PROMIS Pediatric Short form v1.0 Pain Behaviors (self-report and parent proxy) and the Pediatric Short form v2.0 Pain Quality – Affective 8a and Pediatric Short form v2.0, Pain Quality – Sensory 8a. A complete and current list of instruments can be found at www.healthmeasures.net.

Behavioral tools

The tools developed to assess pain in infants and young children generally use behavioral indicators of pain. A wide range of specific expressive behaviors indicative of pain have been identified in infants and young children: crying or vocalization; facial expressions (e.g grimacing); body movements (e.g. withdrawal of the affected limb, touching the affected area, and tensing of limbs and torso); changes in social behavior, communication, or appetite; and changes in sleep–wake state or cognitive functions [6,7,20].

Observational tools are indicated for children who are too young to understand and use self-report scales (<6 years); too distressed to use self-report scales; impaired in their cognitive or communicative abilities; restricted by bandages, surgical tape, mechanical ventilation or muscle relaxant drugs; or whose self-report ratings are considered to be minimized, exaggerated, or unrealistic due to cognitive, emotional or situational factors [6].

Physiological indicators

Neonates and children display metabolic, hormonal and physiological responses to pain, also called biomarkers [21]. These physiological reactions all indicate the activation of the sympathetic nervous system, which is part of the autonomic nervous system, and is responsible for the fight or flight response associated with stress. Physiological changes can include changes in heart rate, respiratory rate, blood pressure, oxygen saturation, sweating and dilated pupils. These indicators usually reflect stress reactions and are only loosely correlated with self-report of pain. They can occur in response to other states such as exertion, fever and anxiety or in response to medications. On their own, physiological indicators do not constitute a valid clinical pain measure for children [6]. A multidimensional or composite measure that incorporates physiological and behavioral indicators, as well as self-report, is preferred whenever possible [6, 7,20, 21]. In the near future, advances in laboratory and technical equipment as well as computer software may provide additional ways to assess pain in clinical practice by measuring physiologic changes associated with pain such as heart rate variability, intracranial pressure, skin conductance, stress hormones, cerebral oxygenation using near infrared spectroscopy (NIRS), electroencephalography (EEG), and functional magnetic resonance imaging (MRI) [21].

Pain assessment in infants

Several pain assessment tools combine behavioral and physiological indicators as well as contextual factors (e.g. gestational age, sleep–wake state) for assessing pain in neonates [21]. The Premature Infant Pain Profile (PIPP) has been the most rigorously validated of these measures [22]. Facial activity has been the most comprehensively studied behavioral pain assessment measure in neonates. It is the most reliable and consistent indicator of pain across populations and types of pain. The facial actions associated with acute pain in neonates include bulging brow, eyes squeezed tightly shut, deepening of nasolabial furrow, open lips, mouth stretched vertically and horizontally and taut tongue [7]. For a more in-depth review of the assessment of pain in neonates and infants see Stevens *et al.* [7] and Eriksson and Campbell-Yeo [21].

Pain assessment in children with intellectual and developmental disabilities (IDD)

Infants and children with cognitive impairment or developmental delay who are unable to report pain may be at greater risk for under-treatment of pain. These include children with moderate or severe cerebral palsy, neurodevelopmental disorders, severe developmental delay and autism spectrum disorders. Moreover, there is emerging evidence that children with IDD are equally sensitive or more sensitive to pain compared to their typically developing peers [23].

It is particularly difficult to accurately assess pain experienced by these children. Although many children with IDD may have the capacities to provide basic forms of self-report, self-report is best used in conjunction with other methods of assessing pain. Credible assessment can usually be obtained from the parent/caregiver or another person who knows the child well [23, 24–26]. However, proxy judgements have been shown to underestimate the pain experience of others [23,27] and may be influenced by factors other than their child's pain [23].

Parents and caregivers may report a diversity of behavioral responses to pain but the categories outlined above are common to almost all children and can provide clues to caregivers and healthcare workers that the child might be experiencing pain. The diversity of behavioral responses to pain underlines the importance of obtaining a thorough baseline history from caregivers of children with cognitive impairments.

While there are several pain assessment tools for this population, three tools have been found reliable and are well validated. These are the:

1 Non-Communicating Children's Pain Checklist–Revised (NCCPC-R [24]);

2 Revised Faces, Legs, Activity, Cry, Consolability (r-FLACC [28]);

3 Paediatric Pain Profile (PPP) [25,26] (see www.ppprofile.org.uk/).

The NCCPC-R has been used to assess acute pain (e.g. resulting from a fall), chronic pain (e.g. due to a medical condition) and postoperative pain, in neurologically impaired children. Postoperative pain has also been assessed with the r-FLACC, and the PPP has been used to assess persistent daily pain in this group of children. Synthesized data from a evidence-based review, feedback from a family-based hospital advisory board and a quality improvement study with nurses and parents caring for children with cognitive impairments supported using the r-FLACC over the PPP in practice [29]. The clinical utility of the r-FLACC has also been rated higher than other tools for neurologically impaired children, suggesting it may be more readily adopted into clinical practice [30]. In the absence of "gold standard" pain measures, consider each child as their own control and compare behavior and response to interventions against previous assessments [31]. For more detailed information about the assessment of pain in cognitively delayed children see Chapter 42 and Oberlander & Symons [32].

Other approaches for assessing pain in children

Pain diaries are another way to track pain in children with recurrent or chronic pain. While paper-based diaries have been used in clinical and research practice for decades, they are prone to recall biases and poor compliance. Real-time data collection methods using electronic hand-held devices have been developed for children with recurrent and chronic pain [33-41]. Pain-QuILT™ is one example of a web- and mobile-based tool for the visual self-report and electronic tracking of sensory pain [39]. Patients can choose from a library of pain quality 'icons' to express different types of pain, such as a 'matchstick' for 'burning pain'. Descriptive icons can be assigned a rating of intensity (0–10 NRS) and then dragged-and-dropped onto a detailed virtual body map to show pain location (See Figure 9.1). Finally, several pediatric chronic pain registries have been developed such as CHOIR at Stanford in USA [42] and Pediatric Electronic Persistent Pain Outcome Collaboration (PaedePPOC) in Australia [43]. These registries have been successfully integrated into children's pain services, yielding timely point-of-care information to support clinicians and families, and valuable data to inform quality improvement, research and future health care planning.

Choosing the right pain assessment measure

There are many reliable, valid and clinically useful pain assessment tools for assessing pain in neonates, infants [7,19], children and adolescents [2,13]. However, no easily administered, widely accepted, uniform technique exists for assessing pain for all children [3]. Perhaps the most important consideration is to choose a single set of tools for a given institution and then to use these tools consistently. Organizations should develop clinical practice guidelines that clearly outline the tools that should be used for each age group (see Figure 9.2 for an example of the clinical practice guidelines for assessing pain in children developed by the Hospital for Sick Children [44]).

Frequency of pain assessment and documentation

Effective pain management depends on regular assessment of the presence and severity of pain and the patient's response to pain management interventions. Every patient should have their pain assessed:

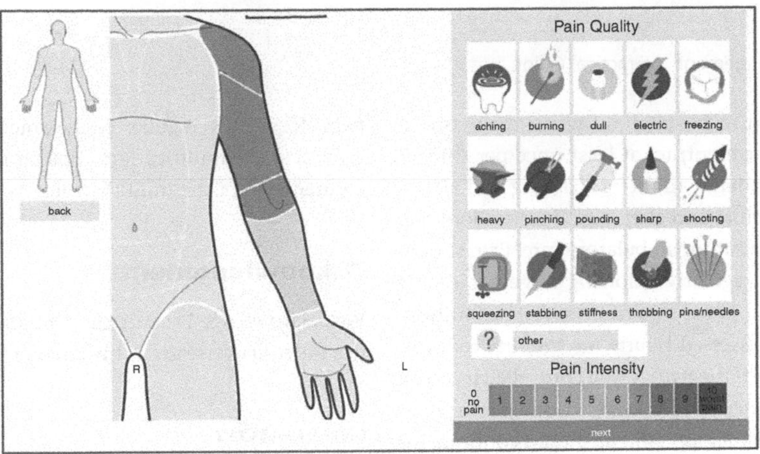

Figure 9.1 Screenshot of Pain-QuILT™

Pain Assessment: WHEN?

- On admission and once per shift
- Before/during/after invasive procedures

Pain Assessment: HOW?

Use developmentally appropriate tool

PIPP	FLACC	Pain Word Scale	FACES	Numeric Rating Scale	NCCPC
Preterm & Full Term	2 mo-7 yrs	3-7 yrs	5-12 yrs	≥ 7 yr	3–18 yrs (Non-communicative patients)

Is pain present?

No → Pain Assessment: WHEN?

Yes ↓

Pain Management: INTERVENTIONS

Pharmacological
- Apply topical anesthetic for IVs/phlebotomy
- Give analgesics regularly
- Use least invasive route (orally if possible)
- Mild pain: Acetaminophen ± NSAID
- Moderate &
- Severe pain: Acetamin*± NSAID + opioid

Ensure no contraindications exist

Physical
- Heat and/or cold (NOT for neonates)
- Massage
- Pressure
- Activity out of bed
- Swaddling (Neonate)
- Sucrose (< 2 yrs)

Psychological
- Explanation (Invasive procedure)
- Distraction
- Relaxation

Consider:
- Child Life Specialist
- Psychology/psychiatry consult for coping strategies

Reassess in 1 hour → Pain Assessment: HOW?

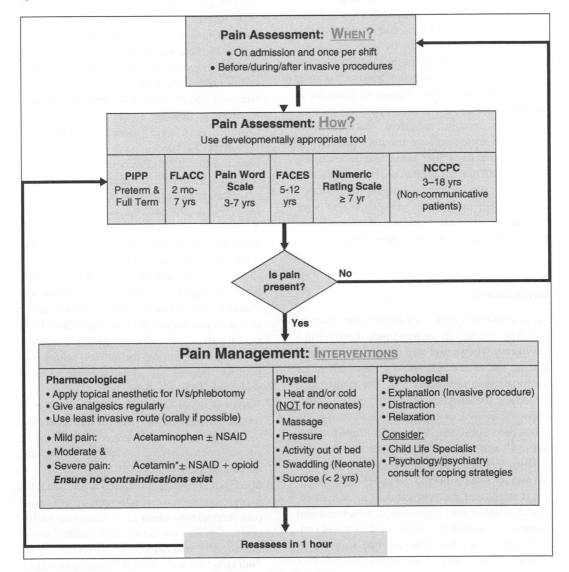

Figure 9.2 Example of an organization-specific pain assessment algorithm.

(a) on admission to hospital; (b) when they visit an emergency department; (c) at least once per shift (if they are an inpatient); (d) before, during and after a procedure; (e) before and after pain intervention; and (f) at each office visit for ambulatory care. Pain should be assessed very regularly following surgery and/or if the patient has a known painful medical condition. Pain should be assessed hourly for the first 6 hours. After this period, if the pain is well controlled it can be assessed less frequently (e.g. every 4 hours). If the pain is fluctuating, regular assessment should continue for 48–72 hours; after this period, the pain intensity will normally have peaked and be starting to subside [3,44]. Regular assessment and documentation facilitates effective treatment and communication among members of the healthcare team, patient and family. Pain is considered to be the fifth vital sign and therefore should be assessed and documented along with the other vital signs. Putting mechanisms in place that make documentation of pain easy for clinicians helps ensure consistent documentation. Standardized forms/tools for the documentation of pain allow for the initial assessment and ongoing reassessment. They can also be used for the documentation of the efficacy of pain-relieving interventions. Including pain intensity as part of the vital signs record allows for pain to be assessed, documented and taken as seriously as other vital signs [3,45].

Conclusions

Pain assessment is vital for effective pain management. The first step in assessing pain is recording a pain history. The second step in pain assessment is assessing the child's pain using a developmentally appropriate pain assessment tool. The third step is monitoring the effectiveness of the pain-relieving interventions used or implemented. Validated and reliable pain assessment tools are available for children of all ages. However, no individual tool can be broadly recommended for pain assessment in all children and across all contexts. The child's self-report of pain is considered the gold standard for those who are able to self-report. Physiological, behavioral and self-report indicators can all be used to assess children's pain. Pain should be assessed regularly to detect the presence of pain and to evaluate the effectiveness of treatments. Finally, documentation of pain facilitates regular reassessment of pain and enhances communication about a patient's pain to all members of the multidisciplinary care team.

Acknowledgments

We acknowledge Dr. Patrick McGrath as co-author of the previous version of this chapter.

References

1 Moon E, McMurtry M, McGrath PJ. (2008) Assessment of pain in children. In: Hunsley J, Mash EJ, eds. *A Guide to Assessments That Work*. Oxford University Press, New York. pp. 51–575.

2 Cohen LL, Lemanek K, Blount RL *et al.* (2008) Evidence-based assessment of pediatric pain. *J Pediatr Psychol* **33**:939–55.

3 Stinson J. (2009) Pain assessment. In: Twycross A, Bruce L, Dowden S, eds. *Managing Pain in Children: A Clinical Guide*. Wiley-Blackwell, Oxford. pp. 85–108.

4 Johnston CC. (1998) Psychometric issues in the measurement of pain. In: Finley GA, McGrath PJ, eds. *Measurement of Pain in Infants and Children*. IASP Press, Seattle, WA. pp. 5–21.

5 Acute Pain Management Guideline Panel. (1992) *Acute Pain Management in Infants, Children, and Adolescents: Operative and Medical Procedures – Quick Reference Guide for Clinicians*. AHCPR No. 92–0020. Agency for Health Care Policy and Research, Public Health Service, US Department of Health and Human Services, Rockville, MD.

6 von Baeyer C, Spagrud LJ. (2007) Systematic review of observational (behavioral) measures of pain for children and adolescents aged 3 to 18 years. *Pain* **127**:140–50.

7 Stevens BJ, Pillai Riddell RR, Oberlander TE *et al.* (2007) Assessment of pain in neonates and infants. In: Anand KJS, Stevens BJ, McGrath PJ, eds. *Pain in Neonates and Infants*, 3rd edn. Elsevier, Edinburgh. pp. 67–90.

8 Birnie KA, Hundert AS, Lalloo C *et al.* (2019) Recommendations for selection of self-report pain intensity measures in children and adolescents: a systematic review and quality assessment of measurement properties. *Pain* **160(1)**:5–18. doi: 10.1097/j.pain.0000000000001377. PMID: 30180088.

9 von Baeyer CL, Jaaniste T, Vo HLT, *et al.* (2017) Systematic Review of Self-Report Measures of Pain Intensity in 3- and 4-Year-Old Children: Bridging a Period of Rapid Cognitive Development. *J Pain* **18(9)**:1017–1026. doi: 10.1016/j.jpain.2017.03.005

10 Zhou H, Roberts P, Horgan L. (2008) Association between self-report pain ratings of child and parent, child and nurse and parent and nurse dyads: meta-analysis. *Journal of Advanced Nursing* **63(4)**:334–342. DOI: 10.1111/j.1365-2648.2008.04694.x.

11 Castarlenas E, Sánchez-Rodríguez E, Vega Rde L *et al.* (2015) Agreement between verbal and electronic versions of the numerical rating scale (NRS-11) when used to assess pain intensity in adolescents. *Clin J Pain* **31(3)**:229–34. doi: 10.1097/AJP.0000000000000104

12 Hicks CL, von Baeyer CL, Spafford PA *et al.* (2001) The Faces Pain Scale – Revised: toward a common metric in pediatric pain measurement. *Pain* **93**:173–83.

13 Stinson JN, Kavanagh T, Yamada J *et al.* (2006) Systematic review of the psychometric properties, interpretability and feasibility of self-report pain intensity measures for use in clinical trials in children and adolescents. *Pain* **125**:143–57.

14 McMurtry CM, Noel M, Chambers CT *et al.* (2011) Children's fear during procedural pain: preliminary investigation of the Children's Fear Scale. *Health Psychol* **30(6)**:780–8. doi: 10.1037/a0024817.

15 Hester N, Foster R, Kristensen K. (1990) Measurement of pain in children: generalizabil lity and validity of the pain ladder and poker chip tool. *Adv Pain Res Ther* **15**:79–84.

16 Sánchez-Rodríguez E, de la Vega R, Castarlenas E *et al.* (2015) AN APP for the Assessment of Pain Intensity: Validity Properties and Agreement of Pain Reports When Used with Young People. *Pain Med* **16**(10):1982–92. doi: 10.1111/pme.12859.

17 Eccleston E, Jordan A, McCrackena LM *et al.* (2005) The Bath Adolescent Pain Questionnaire (BAPQ): development and preliminary psychometric evaluation of an instrument to assess the impact of chronic pain on adolescents. *Pain* **118**:263–70.

18 Fisher E, Heathcote LC, Eccleston C *et al.* (2018) Assessment of pain anxiety, pain catastrophizing, and fear of pain in children and adolescents with chronic pain: A systematic review and meta-analysis. *Journal of Pediatric Psychology* **43(3)**, 314–325. https://doi.org/10.1093/jpepsy/jsx103

19 Cella D, Yount S, Rothrock N, *et al* & PROMIS Cooperative Group. (2007) The Patient-Reported Outcomes Measurement Information System (PROMIS): progress of an NIH Roadmap cooperative group during its first two years. *Med Care* **45**(5 Suppl 1):S3–S11. doi: 10.1097/01.mlr.0000258615.42478.55.

20 Duhn LJ, Medves JM. (2004) A systematic integrative review of infant pain assessment tools. *Adv Neonatal Care* **4**:126–40.

21 Eriksson M, Campbell-Yeo M. (2019) Assessment of pain in newborn infants. *Semin Fetal Neonatal Med* **24(4)**:101003. doi: 10.1016/j.siny.2019.04.003.

22 Stevens B, Johnston C, Petryshen P *et al.* (1996) Premature Infant Pain Profile: development and initial validation. *Clin J Pain* **12**:13–22.

23 Barney CC, Andersen RD, Defrin R *et al.* (2020) Challenges in pain assessment and management among individuals with intellectual and developmental disabilities. *PAIN Reports* **5(4)**:e821, doi: 10.1097/PR9.0000000000000822

24 Breau LM, McGrath PJ, Camfield C *et al.* (2002) Psychometric properties of the Non-communicating Children's Pain Checklist – Revised. *Pain* **99**:349–57.

25 Hunt A, Goldman A, Seers K *et al.* (2004). Clinical validation of the paediatric pain profile. *Developmental medicine and child neurology* **46(1)**: 9–18, doi: 10.1017/s0012162204000039

26 Hunt A, Wisbeach A, Seers K, *et al.* (2007) Development of the paediatric pain profile: Role of video analysis and saliva cortisol in validating a tool to assess pain in children with severe neurological disability. *Journal of pain and symptom management* **33(3)**: 276–289, doi: 10.1016/j.jpainsymman.2006.08.011

27 Rajasagaram U, Taylor DM, Braitberg *et al.* (2009) Paediatric pain assessment: differences between triage nurse, child and parent. *J Paediatr Child Health* **45(4)**:199–203. doi: 10.1111/j.1440-1754.2008.01454.x. PMID: 19426378.

28 Malviya S, Voepel-Lewis T, Burke C *et al.* (2006) The revised FLACC observational pain tool: improved reliability and validity for pain assessment in children with cognitive impairment, *Paediatric anaesthesia* **16(3)**: 258–265, doi: 10.1111/j.1460-9592.2005.01773.

29 Chen-Lim ML, Zarnowsky C, Green R, *et al.* (2012) Optimizing the assessment of pain in children who are cognitively impaired through the quality improvement process. *Journal of Pediatric Nursing* **27(6)**:750–759, doi:10.1016/j.pedn.2012.03.023

30 Voepel-Lewis T, Malviya S, Tait AR *et al.* (2008) A comparison of the clinical utility of pain assessment tools for children with cognitive impairment. *Anesthesia and Analgesia* **106(1)**:71–78, doi: 10.1213/01.ane.0000287680.21212.d0

31 Siden H, Oberlander T. (2008) 'Pain management for children with a developmental disability in a primary care setting', *Pain in Children: A Practical Guide for Primary Care*, Humana Press. New York NY.

32 Oberlander TF, Symons F. (2006) *Pain in Children and Adults with Developmental Disabilities*. Paul H. Brookes, Baltimore, MD.

33 Palermo TM, Valenzuela D, Stork PP. (2004) A randomized trial of electronic versus paper pain diaries in children: impact on compliance, accuracy, and acceptability, *Pain* **107(3)**:213–219, doi: 10.1016/j.pain.2003.10.005

34 Stinson J, Petroz G, Tait G *et al.* (2006) E-Ouch: Usability testing of an electronic chronic pain diary for adolescents with arthritis. *Clinical Journal of Pain* **22(3)**:295–305, doi: 10.1097/01.ajp.0000173371.54579.31

35 Stinson J, Stevens B, Feldman BM, *et al.* (2008) Construct validity of a multidimensional electronic pain diary for adolescents with arthritis. *Pain* **136(3)**:281–292, doi: 10.1016/j.pain.2007.07.002

36 Lewarndowski AS, Palermo TM, Kirchner HL *et al.* (2009) Comparing diary and retrospective reports of pain and activity restriction in children and adolescents with chronic pain conditions. *The Clinical journal of pain* **25(4)**:299–306, doi: 10.1097/AJP.0b013e3181965578

37 Connelly M, Anthony KK, Sarniak R *et al.* (2010) Parent pain responses as predictors of daily activities and mood in children with juvenile idiopathic arthritis: the utility of electronic diaries. *Journal of Pain Symptom Management* **39(3)**:579–590, doi:10.1016/j.jpainsymman.2009.07.013

38 Jacobs E, Stinson J, Duran J *et al.* (2012) Usability testing of a Smartphone for accessing a web-based e-diary for self-monitoring of pain and symptoms in sickle cell disease. *Journal of pediatric hematology/oncology* **34(5)**: 326–335, doi: 10.1097/MPH.0b-13e318257a13c

39 Lalloo C, Stinson JN, Brown SC *et al.* (2014) Pain-QuILT: Assessing clinical feasibility of a Web-based tool for the visual self-repot of pain in an interdisciplinary pediatric chronic pain clinic. *The clinical journal of pain* **30**(11): 934–943, doi: 10.1097/AJP.0000000000000049

40 Huguet A, McGrath PJ, Wheaton M *et al.* (2015) Testing the feasibility and psychometric properties of a mobile diary (myWHI) in adolescents and young adults with headaches. *JMIR mhealth and uhealth* **3(2)**, p.e39.

41 Fortier MA, Chung WW, Martinez A *et al.* (2016) Pain buddy: A novel use of m-health in the management of children's cancer pain. *Computers in Biology and Medicine* **76**, pp.202–214.

42 Bhandari RP, Feinstein AB, Huestis SE, *et al.* (2016) Pediatric-Collaborative Health Outcomes Information Registry (Peds-CHOIR): a learning health system to guide pediatric pain research and treatment. *Pain.* **157(9)**:2033–2044. doi:10.1097/j.pain.0000000000000609

43 Lord SM, Tardif HP, Kepreotes EA *et al.* (2019) The Paediatric electronic Persistent Pain Outcomes Collaboration (PaedePPOC): establishment of a binational system for benchmarking children's persistent pain services. *PAIN* **160(7)**:1572–1585. doi: 10.1097/j.pain.0000000000001548

44 The Hospital for Sick Children. (2008) *Pain Assessment and Management of the Child: Pain Assessment Policy and Pain Management Clinical Practice Guidelines*. The Hospital for Sick Children, Toronto.

45 Clinical Practice Guidelines. (2009) *The Recognition and Assessment of Acute Pain in Children: Update of Full Guideline*. Royal College of Nursing, London.

Chapter 10

Laboratory investigations, imaging and neurological assessment in pain management

Pam Squire[1] **& Misha Bačkonja**[2]

[1] *University of British Columbia, Vancouver, British Columbia, Canada*
[2] *Department of Anaesthesiology and Pain Medicine, University of Washington Medical School, Seattle, Washington, USA*

General principles

No imaging, laboratory or electrophysiological test can show pain. Pain remains a clinical diagnosis and these tests only provide additional information to complement clinical decision making. Currently, there are no clinically independent biomarkers for pain, nor can imaging or any other technique localize or characterize pain. Furthermore, chronic pain is usually a multifactorial problem. In a patient with chronic low back pain, for example, contributing factors may include degenerative joint disease, root entrapment, myofascial pain, muscle deconditioning, central sensitization and the influences of altered mood and psychosocial circumstances. For this reason, pain must be evaluated in a multidimensional context, including the medical diagnosis, or diagnoses, most directly responsible for the pain complaint, medical and psychological comorbidities and the social and occupational context [1].

Many patients present with pain that is poorly correlated with clinical findings and clinical investigations that are negative or non-diagnostic. One of the essential roles of the pain practitioner is to care for patients with either no identifiable source of pain by testing methods or sustained pain despite treatment of an identified source of pain by history and physical examination. Clinicians must recognize when the cost of further investigation exceeds diminishing returns.

Diagnostic studies provide supportive evidence for a clinical diagnosis but are not pathognomonic. Investigations must always be interpreted in the clinical context. This chapter reviews common laboratory, imaging and neurological investigations for the assessment of patients with chronic pain disorders.

Common laboratory, imaging and neurological investigations for the patient living with chronic pain

Laboratory investigations

Laboratory studies are conducted to identify disorders that could be primary or contributory causes of a chronic pain disorder. Relatively few laboratory studies contribute substantially to the diagnosis of painful conditions. Inflammatory markers may be among the most important.

Erythrocyte sedimentation rate (ESR) and C-reactive protein (CRP) are acute phase reactants that function as relatively non-specific indicators of a systemic inflammatory response. ESR is usually, but

Clinical Pain Management: A Practical Guide, Second Edition. Edited by Mary E. Lynch, Kenneth D. Craig, and Philip W. Peng.

not universally, elevated in polymyalgia rheumatica, and CRP is often elevated in this condition as well [2]. Both ESR and CRP are commonly used as markers of active rheumatoid arthritis [3]. Active inflammatory processes that consume complement can be identified by a reduction in circulating complement (C3, C4) levels. Hepatitis C antibody testing is warranted in individuals with unexplained polyarticular pain and idiopathic neuropathy, particularly if clinical or laboratory evidence of hepatic disease is present [4]

Sjögren's syndrome is an inflammatory disorder that is probably under-recognized and is commonly associated with widespread pain as well as pain from associated sensory neuropathy [5]. Dry eyes and dry mouth (sicca symptoms) are the fundamental clinical feature. Diagnostic criteria include a combination of clinical, paraclinical and laboratory parameters including autoantibodies against Ro (SS-A) and/or La (SS-B) antigens [6]. Many patients who fulfill criteria are seronegative. Nonetheless, Sjögren's antibody testing should be obtained in patients with unexplained myofascial or neuropathic pain and sicca symptoms

Vasculitides can present with unexplained pain, from diffuse aches and pains that are difficult to pinpoint to more specific pain from nerve infarction or gastrointestinal ischemia. Protoplasmic or classic staining antineutrophil cytoplasmic antibodies (p-ANCA and c-ANCA) are more specific markers of systemic vasculitides. c-ANCA is a highly sensitive marker for Wegener's granulomatosis, polyarteritis nodosa and Churg–Strauss vasculitis, whereas p-ANCA is a sensitive marker for vasculitis due to systemic lupus erythematosus, rheumatoid arthritis and Sjögren's syndrome. Vasculitis is a tissue diagnosis and must be confirmed pathologically; however, these serologic markers can be helpful in providing justification for tissue biopsy and, on occasion, therapeutic intervention pending a tissue diagnosis in the appropriate clinical setting.

There is a strong correlation between spondyloarthritis (a spectrum of conditions including ankylosing spondylitis and reactive arthritis) and HLA B27 positivity. HLA B27 testing can be very helpful in patients with an appropriate clinical syndrome, particularly if imaging studies are non-diagnostic (see below).

Many rheumatological conditions, such as rheumatoid arthritis, cause chronic multifocal or widespread pain on the basis of inflammatory joint and connective tissue disease. These are diagnosed principally on the basis of clinical criteria with laboratory support.

The following laboratory abnormalities are occasionally obtained, with little evidence of value, in chronic pain states:

1 There is, to our knowledge, no compelling evidence that evaluating thyroid function, serum cortisol or growth hormone levels is of value in the investigation of fibromyalgia [7].

2 It has been proposed that reduced levels of 1,25OH vitamin D can be responsible for a reversible widespread pain syndrome, although the evidence supporting this assertion is modest [8].

3 Creatine phosphokinase (CPK) is commonly elevated in inflammatory muscle disease, but these conditions are usually painless. CPK is normal in myofascial pain syndromes.

To date neither biomarkers for pain, such as substance P or other inflammatory cytokines, nor known genetic information (such as the role of the pain protecting haplotype for guanosine triphosphate [GTP] cyclohydrolase 1) [9], can be used as independent indicators of pain or the transition from acute to chronic pain [10].

Imaging studies

X-rays

X-rays are inexpensive, readily available in any medical facility and can provide information about the skeletal system but provide little information about soft tissues. They remain useful investigations for musculoskeletal medicine which are used as starting point to demonstrate degenerative changes in joints, pathologic fractures, diffuse idiopathic skeletal hyperostosis (DISH), scoliosis, tumors with osseous involvement or calcified tendons or cystic and sclerotic changes where tendons insert into bone.

Computed tomography scan

Computed tomography (CT) scan is a two-dimensional gray-scale representation of the relative densities of tissues usually acquired axially. CT can provide information regarding both bony structures and soft tissues. Three-dimensional reconstructions are possible as are multiplanar images that reconstruct axial slices into three-dimensional images. The main limitation of CT scanning is that it may provide a significant dose of radiation and does not visualize soft tissues as well as magnetic resonance imaging (MRI). CT scanning, often with contrast, may be the investigation of choice when MRI scanning is contraindicated.

Magnetic resonance imaging

Magnetic resonance imaging (MRI) evaluates soft tissues such as discs, tendons, ligaments, cartilage and nerve roots and is sensitive for imaging tumors. A non-contrast MRI is sufficient in the majority of cases. The addition of intravenous gadolinium allows better imaging of infection, tumor or fibrosis. MRI scans are not good for showing bony cortex architecture because bone cortex has little water content and hence appears as black on MRI scans. MRI scans can show change in marrow signal and can demonstrate bone marrow edema, a non-specific finding associated with a variety of painful conditions including insufficiency or fatigue fractures, inflammatory or ischemic disorders, degenerative conditions such as osteoarthritis, cartilage defects, tendon abnormalities and complex regional pain syndrome but this is only a surrogate marker of bony cortex architecture. MRI cannot diagnose osteoporosis but quantitative CT (QCT) scanning can be used to evaluate bone density. MRI is more sensitive than bone scan for detection of vertebral compression fractures but CT scans are the investigations of choice for demonstrating abnormalities within bone, a radiodense material.

MRI has a few important limitations. First, the strong magnetic field precludes investigation of patients with metallic fragments in the eye, pacemakers, cochlear implants or some intracranial vascular clips. Most metal placed as part of orthopedic procedures, including spine procedures, is considered permissible. Administration of gadolinium-containing MRI contrast agents should be avoided in patients with moderately or severely impaired renal function (e.g. estimated glomerular filtration rate <15–30 mL/min).

Magnetic resonance neurography and peripheral nerve evaluation

Magnetic resonance neurography (MRN) and peripheral nerve ultrasonography are emerging techniques for imaging individual peripheral nerves for identification of localized structural abnormalities, such as edema, focal entrapment or hypertrophy due to infiltration or demyelination [27,28] and can be used as a diagnostic adjunct in conditions affecting proximal nerve segments, where the value of EMG/NCS is limited.

A recent study evaluated 239 patients with sciatica who had failed to recover with standard diagnosis and treatment. Using MR neurography and an MR guided piriformis injection of local anesthetic and steroid confirmed piriformis syndrome in 67.8%. Rediagnosis was achieved in all but 4.2% [29]

Myelography and post-myelogram CT

Myelography and post-myelogram CT scanning allows visualization of bony structures and neural elements and are indicated when both are needed and MRI is contraindicated. Myelography and upright MRI scanning enable imaging of the thecal sac and emerging nerve roots while weight-bearing and/or while performing flexion–extension movements. If an infiltrative, malignant or infectious process is being considered, cerebrospinal fluid should be withdrawn for analysis during the procedure. Myelograms are done very infrequently because MRI imaging has evolved to provide the same information previously provided by myelograms.

Nuclear imaging

Nuclear imaging involves detection of gamma radiation produced either as the direct result of radioactive decay (e.g. ^{99m}Tc) or positron-electron annihilation (e.g. ^{15}O).

Bone scanning

Bone scanning uses technetium agents that affix to the bone surface by attaching to the hydroxyapatite crystals in bone and calcium crystals in mitochondria. Tracer is increased locally where there is new bone formation because these regions are hyperemic, and increased blood flow exposes the bone to more tracer over a given period of time. Bone scanning can be very sensitive but not very specific, as fractures, degenerative disease and other benign findings may also produce a positive scan and up to 40% of positive findings occur at sites that are asymptomatic. Painful lesions identified by bone scanning include malignancies, prosthetic loosening in a cemented prosthesis (a normal bone scan essentially rules out prosthetic complications), pars defects and complex regional pain syndrome (CRPS), although the yield in early CRPS is limited.

Single photon emission computed tomography

Single photon emission computed tomography (SPECT) scanning allows three-dimensional views and may improve the localization and characterization of an image. SPECT of known facet joint disease may help to predict which patients are most likely to respond to facet joint injections [11].

Positron emission tomography

Positron emission tomography (PET) scanning is based on the principle that specific radio-labeled tracers can bind to specific receptors on various tissues, and depending on which tissue and its metabolic step is being studied highly specific tracers are produced. Synthesis of tracers is technologically very involved and available only at imaging centers that specialize in nuclear imaging. PET scanning is most useful in differentiation of malignant and non-malignant lesions but otherwise has limited use in pain management. False positive results are generally due to metabolically active infectious or inflammatory lesions such as granulomas (fungal or tuberculous) or rheumatoid nodules and are more common than false negative results [12]. PET scanning will have a lower specificity in areas where these types of infection are endemic.

Combined Magnetic Resonance Imaging (MRI) and Positron emission tomography (PET) in the evaluation of neuropathy and musculoskeletal pain

Combined PET/MRI scanning is a promising tool to provide whole body quantitative multiparametric evaluation to assist in determining possible pain generators including inflammation. One technique used to identify the cause of sciatica symptoms used fluorodeoxyglucose (18F-FDG) as a tracer as it's uptake is increased in injured nerves and denervated calf muscles in rats. To overcome the poor spatial resolution of PET, patients in this study were simultaneously scanned after tracer in a PET/3TMRI scanner. In 5 of 9 patients, spinal nerve impingement due to a herniated disk was identified as a relevant lesion on the basis of both MRI morphology and high ^{18}F-FDG uptake [30].

In another patient similar scanning was able to identify a hematoma and a chronic fibrosed plantaris foot tendon with altered foot biomechanics as the cause of chronic foot pain [31].

Ultrasound

Pathological changes in soft tissues associated with pain include changes in stiffness and neovascularization. The following are evolving imaging strategies to quantitatively evaluate these parameters.

Ultrasound elastography in musculoskeletal and neuropathic pain

Elastography measures the elasticity of a specific tissue. Strain elastography compares before and after regions of interest by semiquatitatively measuring a strain ratio and comparing two areas. Shear wave elastography evaluates the change in shape in a tissue after a transverse periodic shear wave and has been used to evaluate tendons and muscles.

Shearwave elastography can demonstrate signal voids in partial thickness tendon tears and an increase in stiffness in association with thickened tendons and ligaments. In Achilles, patellar and epicondylar tendinopathy, a correlation between tendon stiffness and patient symptoms has been demonstrated.

Measuring shear strain at tissue interfaces in myofascial pain is in its infancy. It is possible to use this technology to measure the elastic properties of muscles such as the quadriceps, gastrocnemius and upper trapezius however studies documenting correlation with pain and dysfunction are limited [32].

Ultrasound with microvascular imaging with power doppler, contrast enhanced ultrasound (CEUS) and superb microvascular imaging (SMI)

Tendinopathy and synovitis are associated with an increase in local microvascularization. This was initially identified using Power Doppler but this was limited by its inability to detect low-velocity blood flow.

CEUS using second generation long lasting contrast agents can identify reduced muscle perfusion states in type 2 diabetes and systemic sclerosis. Quantitative assessment using averaged time-intensity curves within a region of interest can characterize different perfusion patterns. Pixel-based quantification of the contrast agent accurately discriminated between a number of different forms of arthritis.

Superb Microvascular Imaging (SMI) has demonstrated the ability to image small vessels with reduced motion artefact and better visualization. The improvement was found to be clinically significant when evaluated in patients with rheumatoid arthritis, lateral epicondylosis, and carpal tunnel syndrome but not in knee osteoarthritis [33].

Shearwave elastography is emerging as a tool to identify biomechanical processes, predominantly stiffness, in nerves, muscles, ligaments and tendons. Key challenges with this technology will be accounting for the different degree of stiffness in the many layers of soft tissues and using higher spatial resolution to measure individual layers rather than providing a composite.

Early evidence demonstrates shearwave elastography is able to discriminate the severity of carpal tunnel syndrome based on increased stiffness [34].

Diabetic peripheral neuropathy is associated with increased stiffness of the tibial nerve detectable using shearwave elastography [35, 36, 37].

Neurophysiological and other neurological investigations

Electromyography

Electromyography (EMG) is performed by recording spontaneous discharges of muscle cells, indicative of muscle disease or denervation, and the configuration and firing pattern of motor unit potentials, which represent the coordinated discharge of muscle cells all innervated by a common motor neuron. Nerve conduction studies (NCS) are performed by passing a depolarizing current through individual named nerves and recording the evoked nerve action potential, in the case of sensory conduction studies, or the compound muscle action potential (response from muscle) in the case of motor conduction studies. EMG/NCS is highly sensitive at addressing the following questions:

1 Is nerve of muscle disease present?
2 In the case of nerve disease, is the primary process a disorder of axons or myelin?
3 Does the condition involve motor nerves, sensory nerves, or both?
4 What is the localization of the process?

Examples of pain states that can be reliably identified by NCS/EMG include radiculopathy, plexopathy, multifocal polyneuropathy, distal symmetric polyneuropathy and sensory neuropathy.

EMG/NCS has the following limitations:

1 EMG/NCS only evaluates large myelinated axons. Because neuropathic pain is often due to disease of small myelinated Aδ and C fibers, EMG/NCS can be normal in patients whose condition principally affects these "small fibers." Approximately 30% of diabetic neuropathies can be small fiber neuropathies and will have a normal EMG/NCS [13]. Small fiber neuropathy can be assessed functionally with quantitative sensory testing and confirmed pathologically with determination of epidermal nerve fiber density (see below). Until these modalities became available, there was little awareness of the concept of small fiber neuropathy (SFN).
2 Not all nerves can be readily studied using this technique. Truncal or inguinal mononeuropathies, for example, are not readily evaluated with EMG/NCS.
3 EMG/NCS can be painful, especially in patients who have cutaneous mechanical allodynia and hyperalgesia.
4 EMG/NCS provides information about peripheral nerve physiology but not about pain. Many patients with substantial EMG/NCS evidence of neuropathy have no pain, and many patients with normal EMG/NCS studies, particularly those with SFN (see below) have neuropathic pain.

Quantitative sensory testing

Quantitative sensory testing (QST) refers to testing of sensory perception in response to standardized stimuli under conditions of psychophysical testing. The goal of testing is to quantitate both sensory loss (e.g. hypoalgesia or hypoesthesia) and sensory gain (e.g.

hyperalgesia, allodynia and hyperpathia) within small and large fiber sensory modalities. There are 4 components to QST that influence its results: stimulus, patient, instructions and the person conducting the testing. QST protocols utilize a broad range of cutaneous and deep tissue stimuli, including brush, punctate, pressure, vibration, warm, cool, painful hot and painful cold. Some stimuli, such as thermal, vibration and punctate stimuli, can be delivered in a graded fashion to allow determination of thresholds for perception of innocuous sensation or pain [14]. Pressure algometry is usually used for deep tissue testing. Stimulus intensity can also be fixed at a suprathreshold intensity, in which case the patient is asked to rate the perceived intensity of the modality in question [15]. When evaluated in conjunction with typical symptoms of neuropathic pain, demonstration of sensory loss or sensory gain is one defining feature of neuropathic pain. Some QST findings are felt to have specific mechanistic significance. For example, heat hyperalgesia is thought to reflect peripheral sensitization, while dynamic mechanical allodynia (report of pain from innocuous light brushing of the skin) is thought to reflect central sensitization. Abnormal thermal or punctate sensation can provide supportive evidence of SFN when nerve conduction studies, which evaluate large nerve fibers, are normal [16,17].Other stimuli including electrical and ischemic stimuli (such as a blood pressure cuff) are used to stimulate deeper tissues to evaluate pain modulation systems [38].

QST has several limitations at present. First, control values are limited to certain methods and body sites, and data on test–retest reproducibility are inadequate for interpretation of data across time and across centers. Second, the test is a psychophysical evaluation and therefore it is critically dependent on the instruction and training of the subject as well as the person performing QST testing. Instruction should be standardized and applied to all testing procedures. Patients who are unable (because of neurological conditions such as dementia or intoxication) or unwilling (because of psychological factors) to concentrate or for other reasons are not able to fully participate in testing will provide invalid results. For similar reasons, both patients and personnel performing the test must be adequately trained to perform the testing. The testing should be preceded by standardized instructions to subjects and performed in a designated quiet room without distractions [39].

Epidermal nerve fiber density

Epidermal nerve fiber density (ENFD) analysis is based on immunostaining a 3-mm punch biopsy of skin for PGP 9.5, a pan-neuronal marker, and quantifying the density of nerve fibers in the epidermis[40]. Epidermal nerves are the terminals of C and Aδ fibers, most of which are nociceptors. ENFD determination provides pathological confirmation of epidermal nerve fiber loss and is therefore often used to support the diagnosis of neuropathy, particularly when EMG/NCS is normal. Another strength of ENFD is that skin biopsy can be performed in sites where nerve conduction studies are not performed, such as the trunk, and results can be compared with established norms or, if none exist and the contralateral side is clinically unaffected, a control biopsy from the contralateral side of the same patient. Unfortunately, appropriate tissue processing is available in relatively few centers.

ENFD determination has proven to be a valuable tool in the diagnosis of neuropathy due to diabetes, impaired glucose tolerance and the metabolic syndrome, HIV infection and Sjögren's syndrome, among others [17–19]. Biopsy cannot differentiate between different causes of SFN.

The development of ENFD determination and, to a lesser extent, QST, is largely responsible for a revolution in neuromuscular and pain medicine. Previously, EMG/NCS was viewed by clinicians as the sine qua non of peripheral nerve diagnosis, and it was commonly assumed that patients with normal EMG/NCS did not have neuropathy. This resulted in a diagnostic and management conundrum for patients with neuropathic pain and normal EMG/NCS studies. It is now well recognized that specific features of neuropathic pain (punctate and thermal sensory deficits in combination with hyperalgesia, allodynia and hyperpathia, as well as spontaneous paresthesias and pain) in the absence of other neurological symptoms or signs are a common presentation of what is now known as small fiber neuropathy (SFN), and that EMG/NCS are normal in pure SFN [20]. This has been particularly helpful for individuals who do not have a length-dependent pattern [41].

While there is no "gold standard" for the diagnosis of SFN, it has been proposed that the diagnosis be confirmed by the presence of two of the following three findings: deficits in punctate or thermal sensation on neurological examination, abnormal ENFD and thermal QST abnormalities (Figure 10.1) [21].

Somatosensory evoked potential studies

Somatosensory evoked potential studies (SEPs) are performed by passing a depolarizing current through a peripheral nerve and recording the evoked neural response. Unlike NCS, in which recording electrodes are placed over a peripheral nerve, in SEPs recordings are made over the spine and scalp in order to record traveling and stationary waves evoked by the peripheral stimulus and thereby assess conduction through the somatosensory pathways in the central nervous system. SEPs are delayed or absent in the presence of structural or metabolic pathology in the central nervous system pathways under study. SEPs are the only physiological test of conduction through sensory pathways of the central nervous system and can be a useful procedure in selected patients with unexplained sensory symptoms and normal peripheral conduction and non-diagnostic imaging studies [22].

The principal limitation of SEPs in the context of pain evaluation is that clinically available SEPs evaluate large, myelinated fibers and the posterior column-lemniscal system, and therefore do not assess transmission in tracts critical to nociception. To overcome this limitation, several SEP techniques for assessment of the small-fiber-spinothalamic system have been developed in recent years. These include laser evoked potentials

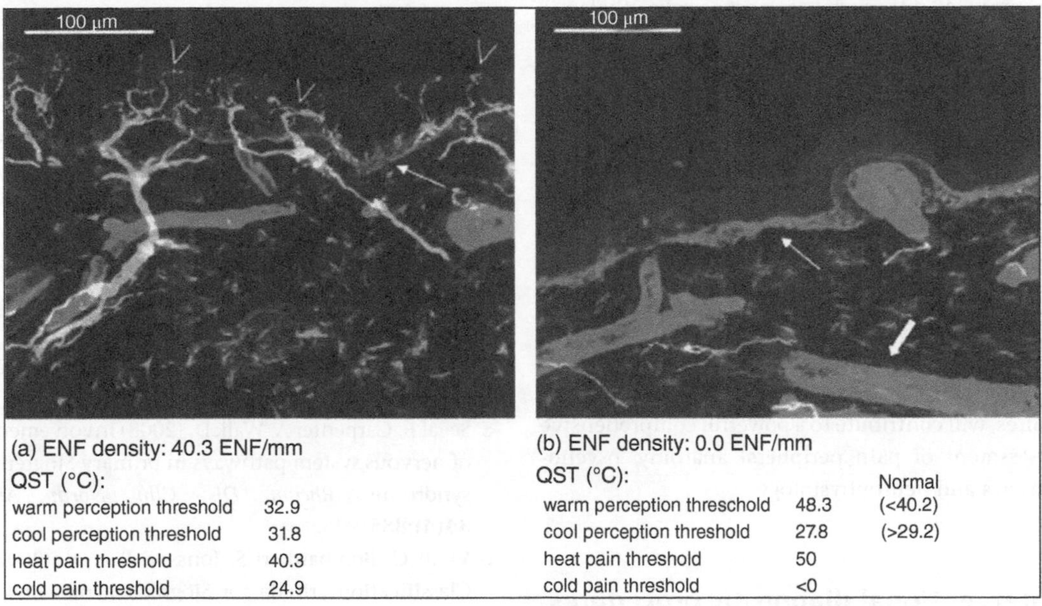

100 μm
100 μm
(a) ENF density: 40.3 ENF/mm
QST (°C):
warm perception threshold 32.9
cool perception threshold 31.8
heat pain threshold 40.3
cold pain threshold 24.9
(b) ENF density: 0.0 ENF/mm
QST (°C):
Normal
warm perception threschold 48.3 (<40.2)
cool perception threshold 27.8 (>29.2)
heat pain threshold 50
cold pain threshold <0

Figure 10.1 ENFD and QST for evaluation of neuropathic pain due to possible small fiber neuropathy. Both patients presented with spontaneous burning pain and allodynia. Nerve conduction studies and cutaneous perception of touch, vibration and position were normal in both patients. Patient A demonstrated normal threshold determination QST, normal foot ENF density and both thermal allodynia and multimodality hyperalgesia on suprathreshold QST. She has no evidence of functional or structural deficit. Her symptoms and signs suggest sensitization, but the mechanism is unknown. Patient B demonstrated elevated thermal thresholds, reduced foot ENF density and reduced mechanical and thermal perception in the foot. The diagnosis is small fiber neuropathy

Dermal and epidermal nerves are stained in white and basement membrane and blood vessels (collagen IV) are stained in gray. In (a), epidermal nerves (arrowheads) are plentiful and arise from robust subepidermal nerves. In (b), no epidermal nerves are seen and there is a paucity of dermal innervations as well. Thin arrows: epidermal basement membrane. Thick arrow: dermal arteriole. Normal ENF density is > 12.2 ENF/mm (5th percentile cutoff).

(LEPs), contact-heat evoked potentials (CHEPs) and pain-related evoked potentials (PREPs). Like SEPs, these all utilize scalp-recorded evoked potentials; the principal difference is in the nature of the stimulus. LEPs utilize a very brief laser radiant heat pulse to activate A-δ fibers. There is evidence that scalp-recorded LEP amplitudes reflect the integrity of pain processing pathways in the peripheral and central nervous system [23] and may prove useful as a surrogate marker for analgesia [24]. CHEPs use a short pulse of painful heat applied directly to the skin as the stimulus or painful stimulus. The amplitude of the CHEPs scalp-evoked response has been shown to correlate with perceived pain intensity in normal subjects [25]. More recent studies have demonstrated that LEP's and CHEPs to stimulation of a painful territory are emerging as a physiological signature of small fiber neuropathy or spinothalamic system neuropathic pain syndromes [42,43] such as post stroke thalamic pain [44].

A CHEPs device is commercially available (Medoc Ltd., Ramat Yishai, Israel). PREP use a small electrical stimulus with high current density to depolarize cutaneous afferents, and this technique has been used in studies of HIV neuropathy [26]. While these are all emerging techniques, their promise lies in their ability to assess both central and peripheral pain pathways and their putative correlation with perceived pain intensity. It is hoped that pain-evoked potentials, in combination with ENF density, QST and pain questionnaires, will contribute to a powerful comprehensive assessment of pain peripheral anatomy, psychophysics and neurophysiology.

Interventional diagnostic procedures

Diagnostic neural blockade

Diagnostic neural blockade is usually fluoroscopic, CT or ultrasound guided injections utilizing various concentrations of local anesthetics that are used to demonstrate the contribution of a particular anatomic structure (e.g., facet, nerve or disc) in the evaluation of pain. The role of diagnostic blockade in the investigation of chronic pain is discussed in detail in Chapter 19.

Conclusions

In summary, chronic pain is a biopsychosocial phenomenon and no test shows pain. Pain clinicians must be prepared to care for their patients with either no identifiable source of pain or sustained pain despite treatment for an identified source of pain.

Nonetheless, there are a number of imaging and neurological investigations as well as specific diagnostic procedures that may assist in the overall assessment of the patient presenting with chronic pain. Currently available tests have been presented along with developing technologies such as QST, ENFD, SEPs, and emerging ultrasound, MRI and PET imaging.

References

1 Backonja M, Argoff C. (2005) Neuropathic pain-definition and implications for research and therapy. *J Neuropathic Pain Symptom Palliation* **1(2)**:11–17. Available at http://www.haworthpress.com/web/JNPSP.

2 Cantini, F, Salvarani, C, Olivieri, I. (1998) Erythrocyte sedimentation rate and C-reactive protein in the diagnosis of polymyalgia rheumatica. *Ann Intern Med* **128**:873.

3 Donald F, Ward MM. (1998) Evaluative laboratory testing practices of United States rheumatologists. *Arthritis Rheum* **41**:725–9.

4 Sharara AI, Hunt CM, Hamilton JD. (1996) Hepatitis C. *Ann Intern Med* **125**:658–68.

5 Segal B, Carpenter A, Walk D. (2008) Involvement of nervous system pathways in primary Sjögren's syndrome. *Rheum Dis Clin North Am* **34(4)**:885–906.

6 Vitali C, Bombardieri S, Jonsson R *et al*. (2002) Classification criteria for Sjögren's syndrome: a revised version of the European criteria proposed by the American-European Consensus Group. *Ann Rheum Dis* **61**:554–8.

7 Geenen R, Jacobs JW, Bijlsma JW. (2002) Evaluation and management of endocrine dysfunction in fibromyalgia. *Rheum Dis Clin North Am* **8(2)**:389–404.

8 Straube S, Moore RA, Derry S. (2009) Vitamin D and chronic pain. *Pain* **141**:10–3.

9 Tegeder I, Costigan M, Griffin RS *et al*. (2006) GTP cyclohydrolase and tetrahydrobiopterin

regulate pain sensitivity and persistence. *Nat Med* **12**:1269–77.

10 Mao J. (2009) Translational pain research: achievements and challenges. *J Pain* **10(10)**: 1001–11.

11 Pneumaticos SG, Chatziioannou SN, Hipp JA *et al.* (2006) Low back pain: prediction of short-term outcome of facet joint injection with bone scintigraphy. *Radiology* **238**:693.

12 Casey KL, Bushnell MC. (2000) Pain Imaging. *IASP* Press, Seattle.

13 England JD, Gronseth GS, Franklin G *et al.* (2009) Practice Parameter: evaluation of distal symmetric polyneuropathy. Role of autonomic testing, nerve biopsy, and skin biopsy (an evidence-based review). Report of the American Academy of Neurology, American Association of Neuromuscular and Electrodiagnostic Medicine, and American Academy of Physical Medicine and Rehabilitation. *Neurology* **72(2)**: 177–84.

14 Rolke R, Magerl W, Andrews CK *et al.* (2006) Quantitative sensory testing: a comprehensive protocol for clinical trials. *Eur J Pain* **10**: 77–88.

15 Walk D, Sehgal N, Moeller-Bertram T *et al.* (2009) Quantitative sensory testing and mapping: a review of nonautomated quantitative methods for examination of the patient with neuropathic pain. *Clin J Pain* **25(7)**:632–40.

16 Hansson P, Backonja M, Bouhassira D. (2007) Usefulness and limitations of quantitative sensory testing: clinical and research application in neuropathic pain states. *Pain* **129**: 256–9.

17 Dyck PJ, Dyck PJ, Larson TS *et al.* (2000) Patterns of quantitative sensation testing of hypoesthesia and hyperalgesia are predictive of diabetic polyneuropathy: a study of three cohorts. Nerve Growth Factor Study Group. *Diabetes Care* **23**:510–7.

18 Smith AG, Rose K, Singleton JR: (2008) Idiopathic neuropathy patients are at high risk for metabolic syndrome. *J Neurol Sci* **273**:25–8.

19 Zhou L, Kitch DW, Evans SR *et al.* (2007) Correlates of epidermal nerve fiber densities in HIV-associated distal sensory polyneuropathy. *Neurology* **68**:2113–9.

20 Vlčková-Moravcová E, Bedna⊠ík J, Ladislav D *et al.* (2008) Diagnostic validity of epidermal nerve fiber densities in painful sensory neuropathies. *Muscle Nerve* **37**:50–60.

21 Devigili G, Tugnoli V, Penza P *et al.* (2008) The diagnostic criteria for small fibre neuropathy: from symptoms to neuropathology. *Brain* **131**:1912–25.

22 Walk D, Zaretskaya M, Parry GJ. (2003) Symptom duration and clinical features in painful sensory neuropathy with and without nerve conduction abnormalities. *J Neurol Sci* **214**:3–6.

23 Treede RD, Lorenz J, Baumgärtner U. (2003) Clinical usefulness of laser-evoked potentials. *Neurophysiol Clin* **33(6)**:303–14.

24 Truini A, Panuccio G, Galeotti F *et al.* (2010) Laser-evoked potentials as a tool for assessing the efficacy of antinociceptive drugs. *Eur J Pain* **14(2)**:222–5.

25 Granovsky Y, Granot M, Nir RR *et al.* (2008) Objective correlate of subjective pain perception by contact heat-evoked potentials. *J Pain* **9**:53–63.

26 Katsarava Z, Yaldizli O, Voulkoudis C *et al.* (2006) Pain related potentials by electrical stimulation of skin for detection of small-fiber neuropathy in HIV. *J Neurol* **253**:1581–4.

27 Filler A. (2009) Magnetic resonance neurography and diffusion tensor imaging: origins, history, and clinical impact of the first 50,000 cases with an assessment of efficacy and utility in a prospective 5000-patient study group. *Neurosurgery* **65**:29–43.

28 Koenig RW, Pedro MT, Heinen CPG *et al.* (2009) High-resolution ultrasonography in evaluating peripheral nerve entrapment and trauma. *Neurosurg Focus* **26(2)**:E13.

29 Filler AY, Haynes J, Jordan SE et al. (2005) Sciatica of nondisc origin and piriformis syndrome: diagnosis by magnetic resonance neurography and interventional magnetic resonance imaging with outcome study of resulting treatment. *J Neurosurg Spine* **2(2):**99–115.

30 Cipriano PW, Yoon D, Gandhi H et al. (2018) ^{18}F-FDG PET/MRI in chronic sciatica: early results revealing spinal and nonspinal abnormalities. *Nucl Med* **59(6):**967–972.

31 Cipriano PW, Yoon D, Holley D et al. (2019) Diagnosis and successful management of an unusual presentation of chronic foot pain using positron emission tomography/magnetic resonance imaging and a simple surgical procedure *Clin J Sport Med* **12(31):** e11–4.

32 Ryu J, Jeong WK. (2017) Current status of musculoskeletal application of shear wave elastography. *Ultrasonography* **36**:185–97.

33 Gitto S, Messina C, Vitale N et al. (2020) Quantitative musculoskeletal ultrasound. Semin *Musculoskelet Radiol*. **24(4):**367–74.

34 Wee TC, Simon NG. (2020) Shearwave elastography in the differentiation of carpal tunnel syndrome severity. *PM&R* **12(11):**1134-.

35 He Y, Xiang X, Zhu B-H, Qiu L. (2019) Shear wave elastography evaluation of the median and tibial nerve in diabetic peripheral neuropathy. *Quant Imaging Med Surg* **9(02):**273–82.

36 Jiang W, Huang S, Teng H, et al. (2019) Diagnostic performance of two- dimensional shear wave elastography for evaluating tibial nerve stiffness in patients with diabetic peripheral neuropathy. *Eur Radiol* **29(05):**2167–74.

37 Dikici AS, Ustabasioglu FE, Delil S, et al. (2017) Evaluation of the tibial nerve with shear-wave elastography: a potential sonographic method for the diagnosis of diabetic peripheral neuropathy. *Radiology* **282(02):**494–501.

38 Damien,J, Colloca L, Bellei-Rodriguez CE *et al.* (2018) Pain Modulation: From conditioned pain modulation to placebo and nocebo effects in experimental and clinical pain. *Int Rev Neurobiol* **139**: 255–96.

39 Getz Kelly K, Cook T, Backonja MM. (2005) Pain ratings at the threshold are necessary for quantitative sensory testing. *Muscle Nerve* **32**:179–84.

40 Kennedy WR, Wendelschafer-Crabb G, Johnson T. (1996) Quantitation of epidermal nerves in diabetic neuropathy. *Neurology* **47**:1042–8.

41 Khan S, Zhou L. (2012) Characterization of non-length-dependent small-fiber sensory neuropathy. *Muscle Nerve* **45(1):**86–91.

42 Wu SW, YC PC, et al. (2017) Biomarkers of neuropathic pain in skin nerve degeneration neuropathy: contact heat-evoked potentials as a physiological signature. *Pain* Mar **158(3):**516–25.

43 Garcia-Larrea L, Hagiwara K. (2019) Electrophysiology in diagnosis and management of neuropathic pain. *Rev Neurol* **185(1-2)**:26–37.

44 Vartiainen N, Perchet C, Magnin M *et al.* (2016) Thalamic pain: anatomical and physiological indices of prediction. *Brain* **139**:708–22.

Chapter 11

Psychological assessment of persons with chronic pain

Robert N. Jamison[1] & Kenneth D. Craig[2]

[1] *Departments of Anesthesia and Psychiatry, Brigham and Women's Hospital, Harvard Medical School, Chestnut Hill, Massachusetts, USA*
[2] *Department of Psychology, University of British Columbia, Vancouver, British Columbia, Canada*

Introduction

Psychological and social risk factors associated with greater pain severity and longevity, as well as poorer outcomes from treatment of pain, include pain chronicity, psychological distress, a history of abuse or trauma, poor social support and significant cognitive dysfunction and deficits [1, 2]. In particular, psychopathology and/or extreme emotionality have been recognized as contraindications for certain therapies [3]. Outcome studies highlight poor response to treatment among patients with psychiatric comorbidity, with this prevalent among persons with chronic pain, including comorbid opioid use disorder [4]. For example, spinal pain patients with both anxiety and depression have a 62% worse return-to-work rate than those with no psychopathology. Similarly, cognitive processes such as maladaptive beliefs and pessimistic expectations are associated with poorer functional outcomes among patients with chronic low back pain [5, 6]. Psychosocial issues typically become more important the longer pain remains a problem in the patient's life. Early psychological assessment typically provides a statement of treatment objectives that could include psychological and social issues and allows ongoing assessment to help establish treatment effectiveness.

Psychological assessment is designed to identify problematic emotional reactions, maladaptive thinking and behavior and social problems that contribute to pain and disability. Routine assessment would seem imperative [7]. When psychosocial issues are identified, treatment can be tailored to addressing these challenges in the patient's life, thereby improving the likelihood and speed of recovery and the prevention of ongoing or more severe problems [8, 9].

Components of a psychological assessment

A number of themes should be addressed during a thorough psychological assessment of a person with pain. Semi-structured clinical interviews (Table 11.1) and self-report instruments (Table 11.2) allow for assessment of the different domains of the pain experience, functional impairment and pain-related disability. While these are the most common strategies, reports from others (e.g. family members or caregivers) and evidence of performance in life situations also are of value. Selection of the strategy requires consideration of whether the measure possesses good psychometric properties [10]. The following highlights those themes that should be

Clinical Pain Management: A Practical Guide, Second Edition. Edited by Mary E. Lynch, Kenneth D. Craig, and Philip W. Peng.

assessed, with detailed assessment strategies following this account:

1 *Somatosensory qualities* of the experience, with this usually best understood through description of the severity, location and temporal characteristics of painful experiences. Individuals who use many pain descriptors and are highly pain-sensitive are at greater risk for poor long-term pain outcomes.

2 *Affective qualities* of the experience. Distressing emotional qualities of a painful experience as well as pre-existing emotional dispositions such as a mood disorder with associated anxiety, fear and depression contribute to heightened response to pain.

3 *Cognitive features*, with patterns of thinking able to exacerbate and maintain dysfunctional pain, or, on the contrary, able to facilitate coping. Catastrophizing is a set of cognitive and emotional processes encompassing magnification of pain-related stimuli, feelings of helplessness and a generally pessimistic orientation to pain outcomes. Higher catastrophizing predicts greater pain-related disability and healthcare utilization. In contrast, perceived self-efficacy, or confidence that one can deal with pain, is associated with better function and well-being

4 *Pain behavior*. There is substantial variability in the extent to which chronic pain interferes with activities of daily living or contributes to functional

Table 11.1 Categories to be addressed during an interview.

1 Pain description and history of pain onset
2 Aggravating and minimizing factors
3 Past and current treatments, including medication use
4 Daily activities: content and level
5 Relevant medical history
6 Development, education, family and employment history
7 Compensation status, engagement in litigation
8 Family and personal history of drug or alcohol abuse and substance dependence
9 Family and personal history of psychiatric disturbance and treatment
10 History of suicidal ideation and current emotional status
11 Financial and social support
12 Perceived directions for treatment

Table 11.2 Selected assessment categories and frequently used psychometric measures.

Assessment Category	Psychometric measures
1 *Psychosocial history*	Comprehensive pain questionnaire and demographic factors
	Structured clinical interview
2 *Pain intensity*	Numerical rating scales (NRS)
	Visual analog scales (VAS)
	Verbal rating scales (VRS)
	Pain drawings (PD)
3 *Mood and personality*	Patient-Reported Outcomes Information System (PROMIS) Depression
	Patient Health Questionnaire (PHQ-9)
	Hospital Anxiety and Depression Scale (HADS)
	Beck Depression Inventory (BDI-II)
	Minnesota Multiphasic Personality Inventory (MMPI)*
	Symptom Checklist 90 (SCL-90)
	Millon Behavior Health Inventory (MBHI)
	Center for Epidemiologic Studies Depression Scale (CES-D)
4 *Functional capacity and quality of life*	Short-Form Health Survey (SF-36);
	Short Form 12 (SF12)
	Multidimensional Pain Inventory (WHYMPI)
	Pain Disability Index (PDI)
5 *Pain beliefs and coping*	Coping Strategies Questionnaire (CSQ)
	Pain Catastrophizing Scale (PCS)
	Survey of Pain Attitudes (SOPA)

* See text for potential disadvantages in interpreting results in patients with chronic pain.

impairment. A careful appraisal of pain behavior through observation of patients both during and outside the examining situation can be of value, for example, when engaged in spontaneous activity in everyday situations.

5 *Personal history*. Ethnic and cultural background, family socialization, and important life experiences influence the capacity to cope with pain. A history of trauma or physical or sexual abuse can have an adverse effect on coping with pain. When significant others in a person's family have had a history of chronic or particularly severe pain, there may be a predisposition to similar patterns in the patient.

6 *Psychosocial stressors* tend to negatively impact coping and result in increased healthcare utilization. Of particular importance would be current social contexts provoking distress (e.g. with employers or family members) either directly (e.g. unemployment, social isolation) or indirectly (e.g. dysfunctional relationships) related to painful episodes.

7 *Social context of the assessment* can be very important. While clinicians must be aware of the objectives of referral sources, patients similarly are typically aware of the expectations and goals of referral agencies and those engaged in the assessment. Although the focus may be upon reducing painful distress, improving functional capacity, and reducing pain-related disability, referral sources may be interested in credibility and legitimacy of pain complaints. Patients frustrated with lack of success from treatment and hampered by financial concerns and negative experiences may react differently in assessment situations than those without such experiences or concerns.

Clinical Interviews

Informal and semi-structured interviews are core features of most clinical assessment. In addition to establishing patient/clinician relationships they ensure consistent coverage of critical information categories across patients. Table 11.1 describes basic information categories typically pursued during the initial interview.

Assessment Self-Report Measures

To standardize outcome reporting among patients with chronic pain, an international multidisciplinary panel recommended pain intensity, physical functioning, and health-related quality of life (HRQoL) as core outcome domains [11]. The Patient-Reported Outcomes Measurement Information System (PROMIS) is a highly reliable, valid, publicly available assessment tool that measures these core domains. PROMIS has been used to successfully measure pain, fatigue, depression, anxiety, sleep disturbance, physical social and sexual function, and global quality of life among chronic pain patients and is frequently used in clinical outcome studies [12-15]. Other selected assessment categories and frequently used reliable and valid psychometric measures to assess the domains mentioned above are listed in Table 11.2.

Pain intensity

A number of tools have been devised to provide a global measure of how much the person hurts, including numerical pain ratings (NRS), visual analog scales (VAS), verbal rating scales (VRS), and faces scales (i.e., depictions of graded facial displays of distress) [16], using self-monitored reliable and valid pain intensity ratings [17]. Among these self-report measures, the NRS (e.g. 0–10 or 0–100 scale), tend to be most popular among professionals because they are easy to administer and score. However, there is no evidence to suggest that VAS or VRS are any less sensitive to treatment effects. Another popular means of measuring pain intensity is the VAS, which asks the patient to mark the point on the line that best indicates present pain severity between extreme limits of pain at either end [17]. Electronic VAS diaries have been shown to be as reliable as paper measures [18]. There are a number of VRS that consist of phrases (as few as 4 or as many as 15, often ranked in order of severity from "no pain" through "mild pain", "moderate pain", and "severe pain" to "excruciating pain") chosen by the patients to describe the intensity of their pain [17]. They can be favored as they provide some qualitative information about subjective magnitude, in contrast to intensity ratings using the VAS or NRS. In addition, external validity is improved by descriptive anchors that establish the meaning of numerical values. Repeated assessment over time has a number of benefits: averaging multiple measures of pain intensity increases the reliability and validity of the assessment, reports serve as a baseline to establish whether continued treatment is needed after an appropriate trial period, and they allow assessing the overall impact of treatment for pain.Given concerns that single estimates of pain severity confound sensory, emotional, and cognitive features of the experience, the McGill Pain Questionnaire has been used to differentiate different sensory/discriminative, affective/motivational, and cognitive/appraisal qualities [19, 20]. Patients select from multiple verbal descriptors to characterize their pain on these dimensions. The current focus has been upon short forms useful in extracting a subscale of affective distress [21].

A popular assessment tool to measure the intensity and character of pain is the Brief Pain Inventory [22]. The BPI provides information about pain history, intensity, and location as well as the degree to which the pain interferes with daily activities, mood, and enjoyment of life. Scales (rated from 0 to 10) indicate the intensity of pain in general, at its worst, at its least, average pain, and pain "right now" over the past 24 hours. A figure representing the body is provided for the patient to shade the area corresponding to the location of his or her pain. Test-retest reliability for the BPI reveals correlations of 93 for worst pain, 78 for usual pain, and 59 for pain now. Numerous studies have supported the reliability and validity of the BPI for the assessment of pain among patients with chronic pain conditions. The initial validation study yielded internal consistency (Cronbach's alpha) coefficients of 85 and 88 for the intensity and interference subscales, respectively [23].

Mood and personality

Although depression, anxiety, and irritability can be a normal response to pain, individuals with chronic pain can frequently present with significant psychopathology and catastrophize about their pain, which can greatly interfere with coping and response to treatments for pain [24–26]. Up to 40% of chronic pain patients in primary care practices present with significant psychopathology. This percentage can increase to 75% in specialty pain practices [27]. Often these are individuals with a history of physical or sexual abuse, substance abuse or personality disorder. Patients with higher levels of negative affect present with more somatic complaints, have more pain, and are prone to greater utilization of medical services [28, 29].

Psychopathology and/or extreme emotionality have been seen as contraindications for certain therapies [8]. Mental health professionals continue to debate the best way to measure psychopathology and/or emotional distress in patients with chronic pain. Although most measures are helpful in ruling out severe psychiatric disturbance, unfortunately no measure can boast validity in predicting treatment outcome. A recent trend shows the PROMIS Depression [30, 31], the Patient Health Questionnaire-9 (PHQ-9) [30], the Beck Depression Inventory (BDI-II) [33] and the Hospital Anxiety and Depression Scale (HADS) [34] to be frequently included in psychological assessments of persons with chronic pain [35]. A brief description of PROMIS scales has been provided above.

The PHQ-9 is a brief, 9-item, self-report measure of depression. The BDI assesses depressive symptoms in patients with chronic pain. This 21-item self-report questionnaire measures the severity of depression and is commonly used to evaluate the outcome of treatment. It is easy to administer and score, although one limitation is the potential for misinterpretation of an elevated depression score as a result of the frequent endorsement of somatic items (e.g. fatigue, sleep disturbances and loss of sexual interest) by patients with chronic pain. The Center for Epidemiologic Studies Depression Scale (CES-D) is an additional tool for assessment of depressive symptoms in patients with pain [34]. The HADS is a 14-item scale designed to assess the presence and severity of anxious and depressive symptoms in people with medical illness—it excludes items of fatigue and sleeplessness which might be attributed to the physical disease. Seven items assess anxiety and seven items measure depression, each coded 0–3. The HADS has been used extensively in clinics and has adequate reliability and validity [34].

Measures that have been frequently used in the past to evaluate personality and emotional distress, but are less frequently used today, include the Minnesota Multiphasic Personality Inventory (MMPI-2) [37], the Symptom Checklist 90 (SCL-90-R) [38], and the Millon Behavior Health Inventory (MBHI) [39]. The MMPI is an instrument traditionally used in assessing psychopathology. This 567 true– false item measure yields a distinct profile for each patient that can predict return-to-work in males following surgical treatment. Although this test has been widely used to measure psychopathology, the profiles obtained in people living with pain can be misinterpreted because of the physical symptoms reported by these patients [38]. Patients may also dislike the test's emphasis on psychopathology.

The SCL-90 is a 90-item checklist general assessment of emotional distress that provides a global index of functioning score as well as nine subscale scores. It is a relatively brief measure including individual items that may pertain specifically to persons with chronic pain. Its disadvantages include a high correlation between subscales and the absence of validity scales to detect subtle inconsistencies in responses. The MBHI, another popular measure for assessing mood and personality among patients with pain, includes 150 true–false items and offers 20 subscales that measure: (a) styles of relating to providers; (b) psychosocial stressors; and (c) response to illness. Unlike other measures, the MBHI emphasizes medical rather than emotional concerns.

Functional Capacity

Some clinicians consider pain reduction meaningless unless accompanied by a noticeable change in function. Thus, some reliable measurement of level of activity should be used before and after the onset of therapy. Research has shown that physical impairment, defined as an objective medical condition, such as an amputation, is not very predictive of disability, which is an inability to work because of a medical impairment. Rather, beliefs about an injury predict disability and physical performance after surgery better than `pain ratings or a physical impairment' [41, 42]. Measures that can be used to assess activity level and function include the Short-Form Health Survey (SF-36) [43], the West Haven-Yale Multidimensional Pain Inventory (WHYMPI, mostly known now as the MPI) [44] and the Pain Disability Index (PDI) [45]. It is preferable to consider functional measures that are specific to the chronic pain condition being assessed (e.g., back pain patients will have different activity limitations than someone with upper extremity pain).

The SF-36, which was initially developed from the Medical Outcomes Study to survey health status, includes eight scales that measure (1) limitations in physical activities due to health problems, (2) limitations in social activities due to physical and emotional problems, (3) limitations in usual role activities due to physical health problems, (4) bodily pain, (5) general mental health, (6) limitations in usual role activities due to emotional problems, (7) vitality (energy and fatigue), and (8) general health perceptions. Although the SF-36 is a popular measure, pain patients tend to score very low (severe limitations) such that modest improvements can go undetected. An expanded measure known as the Treatment Outcomes of Pain System (TOPS) [46] that incorporates the SF-36, has been modified specifically for patients with pain to improve sensitivity and reliability of measurement of treatment outcome.

The MPI is a 56-item measure made up of 7-point rating scales. The subscales assess activity interference, perceived support, pain severity, negative mood, and perceived control. The advantage of this self-report instrument is that it was created specifically for chronic pain patients and can be useful in classifying those patients into three types: dysfunctional, interpersonally distressed, and adaptive copers [47]. Strong evidence supports the presence of these three types in the assessment of chronic pain patients [48].

Other popular functional measures include the Oswestry Disability Questionnaire [49], The Roland-Morris Functional Disability Scale [49], the Waddell Disability Instrument [50], the Functional Rating Scale [51], and the Back Pain Function Scale [52]. Kinesiophobia is the fear of pain due to movement, a potentially important factor contributing to disability among persons with chronic pain [53]. Studies have shown a connection between kinesiophobia and increased reported pain intensity and prolonged rehabilitation [53]. Thus, an assessment of kinesiophobia can be important [54]. The Tampa Scale of Kinesiophobia is a valid and reliable measure of this construct and is linked to catastrophic thinking [55, 56]. A shortened version of this measure is also available [57].

There has been a rapid increase in the use of motion sensors such as accelerometers, pedometers, heart-rate monitors and multiple-sensor devices to assess daily steps, position, and level of sleep [58]. Wearable technology that utilizes actigraphy is increasingly being used for the objective measurement of physical activity and sleep in various therapy areas, including among pain patients, as it is unintrusive and suitable for continuous tracking to allow longitudinal assessment [59]. Objective measures of movement (e.g., steps per day) have the potential of being more accurate than self-reported levels of activity since self-reports of activity level can be inaccurate and prone to recall bias. There is some preliminary evidence that activity monitors encourage increased function and correlate with improvements in mood among patients with chronic pain [60].

Pain beliefs and coping

Pain perception, beliefs about pain, and approaches to self-managing pain are important in predicting the outcome of treatment. Unrealistic or negative thoughts about an ongoing pain problem may contribute to increased pain and emotional distress, decreased functioning, a greater reliance on medication and poor outcome from surgery [61]. Certain chronic pain patients are prone to maladaptive beliefs about their condition that may not be compatible with the physical nature of their pain [62]. Patients with adequate psychological functioning exhibit a greater tendency to ignore their pain, use coping self-statements, remain active and use less medication for management of their pain [63]. Coping strategies may be defined as specific thoughts and behaviors individuals use to manage their pain or their emotional reactions to pain [64]. For example, "active" pain coping generally includes engaging in positive thinking, making encouraging self-statements, distracting one's attention from pain, undertaking as much physical activity as possible within pacing guidelines or using physical pain-reducing techniques such as relaxation exercises and stretching. Facilitating such coping strategies seems to be an important part of many non-pharmacologic treatments for chronic pain. One recent prospective study of multidisciplinary treatment revealed that patients who entered treatment with stronger personal beliefs in their ability to control pain, and those who increased their use of positive self-statements and cognitive reinterpretation of pain, showed the most substantial decreases in pain-related interference at 6 months and 18 months post-treatment [65]. Coping strategies may affect the patient's level of attentiveness to pain, the ability to persist in the face of pain, and the extent to which the patient feels entitled to be taken care of as a result of the pain.

Since efficacy expectations have been shown to influence the efforts patients will make to manage their pain, measures of self-efficacy or perceived control are useful in assessing a patient's attitude towards pain treatment [66]. Several self-report measures assess coping and pain attitudes. The frequently used tests to measure maladaptive beliefs include the Coping Strategies Questionnaire (CSQ) [67], the Pain Management Inventory (PMI) [68], the Pain Self-Efficacy Questionnaire (PSEQ) [69], the Survey of Pain Attitudes (SOPA) [70], and the Inventory of Negative Thoughts in Response to Pain (INTRP) [71]. Other instruments include the Pain Beliefs and Perceptions Inventory (PBPI) [72], and the Chronic Pain Self-Efficacy Scale (CPSS) [73].

Psychological models of chronic pain, such as the fear-avoidance model, demonstrate that the way people cognitively process their pain sensations is a strong determinant of their future pain-related behavior [74]. Catastrophizing is a central variable in the fear-avoidance model that accounts for 7–31% of the variance in pain severity [75]. In addition, pain catastrophizing creates maladaptive pain cognitions that can be a risk factor for developing depression, disability, and higher pain intensity [76, 77]. As a result, a great deal of empirical research has focused on the important concept of catastrophizing when assessing painful experiences [78–80]. While catastrophizing positively correlates with negative affect, including depression and anxiety, it also has a unique and specific influence on pain-related outcomes [81]. Overall, greater catastrophizing is associated with amplified attentional focus on pain [82–84] and serves as a risk factor for long-term pain [85–87].

The Pain Catastrophizing Scale (PCS) [88] is a well-validated, widely used, self-report measure of catastrophic thinking associated with pain. The construct of catastrophizing incorporates magnification of pain-related symptoms, rumination about pain, feelings of helplessness and pessimism about pain-related outcomes. Assessment of catastrophizing is important because it is a strong predictor for continued pain-related disability [89]. Individuals rate the extent to which they experience (when they are in pain) the thought or feeling described by each item; scores on this 13-item measure can range from 0–52 (each item is scored 0 = not at all to 4 = all the time). The PCS has good psychometric properties in pain patients and controls [90]. Pain catastrophizing has been shown to be a powerful construct in predicting poor response to treatment for pain and is an important measure of coping [26, 87].It is suspected that patients who have unrealistic beliefs and expectations about their condition are also poor candidates for pain treatment [91, 92]. Patients who have a high catastrophizing score, who endorse passive coping on the PMI, who demonstrate low self-efficacy regarding their ability to manage their pain on the PSEQ, who describe themselves as disabled by their pain on the SOPA, and who report frequent negative thoughts about their pain on the INTRP are at greatest risk for poor treatment outcome from an implanted device.

Substance use disorder assessment

With recent attention to the 'opioid crisis', healthcare providers have been challenged with the need to provide appropriate relief from pain while avoiding risks associated with use of opioids. This has contributed to greater need to employ risk assessment measures to identify those who are more predisposed to misuse of prescription opioids [93, 94]. Guidelines from healthcare organizations and regulatory institutions have strongly encouraged the used of risk assessment screening tools [95, 96]. Stressed within these guidelines is the importance of thoroughly evaluating all potential users of prescription opioids by conducting a complete social and medical history, with medical examination and a review of medical records.

There are several validated and reliable self-report screening tools that can help to assess risk of opioid misuse. Unfortunately, many of the recommended ways to assess substance use disorders (SUDs) and alcohol dependence, particularly through the criteria outlined in the Diagnostic and Statistical Manual of Mental Disorders, fifth edition (DSM-V), have not been validated with chronic pain patients [97]. These measures tend to use signs of opioid dependence and tolerance as indicators of abuse and addiction when no abuse exists.

Over the years, several screening measures have been developed that have been shown to be particularly useful in assessing risk of prescription opioid abuse among persons with chronic pain. These include the Screener and Opioid Assessment for Patients with Pain – Revised (SOAPP-R) [98-100], that is a trait measure of abuse risk. Shorter versions of this measure [101-103] and a Spanish translation exist [104]. A sister questionnaire that assesses states of abuse risk (e.g. can change over time) is the Current Opioid Misuse Measure (COMM) [105, 106]. Both the SOAPP-R and COMM have been cross-validated and have been used extensively in clinics and in research protocols [107, 108]. A shortened version of the COMM also exists [109]. Other self-report questionnaires to assess risk of opioid misuse include the Opioid Risk Tool (ORT) [110, 111], the Diagnosis, Intractability, Risk, and Efficacy (DIRE) scale [112], the Drug Use Disorders Identification Test (DUDIT) [113], the Drug Abuse Screening Test (DAST) [114, 115], the Screening Instrument for Substance Abuse Potential (SISAP) [116], the Pain Medication Questionnaire (PMQ) [117], and a single item of catastrophizing that is useful in predicting opioid misuse among chronic pain patients [118]. A systematic review by Lawrence and colleagues [119] found the SOAPP-R, COMM, and PMQ to be most valid to assess risk of problematic analgesic use among patients with chronic pain. The ORT has been popular because of its brevity (5 items) and a revised ORT that omitted the question about prior childhood sexual abuse now finds comparable opioid risk between men and women [120]. A brief checklist designed to reflect the content of a standard opioid agreement (Opioid Compliance Checklist, OCC) has also been validated and used clinically [121, 122].

Use of innovative technology to assess pain

With the rapid increase in the use of innovative technology and smartphone pain applications (apps) to track day-to-day changes [123-125] comes evidence of the benefit of pain apps designed for persons with chronic pain to assess, monitor, and communicate their status with their providers [126]. The validity and reliability of daily assessments compared with standardized questionnaires for repeated daily measures of pain and sleep have been well established [127-129]. Pain apps have been shown to be easily introduced, well tolerated and preferred to other types of diaries and information delivery platforms [60]. With more data being collected through smartphone apps there is potential for emerging metrics to identify the risk component of population health management and care coordination.

Innovative technology can be used by healthcare providers to track persons with chronic pain, engage the patients between clinic visits, and offer information and support to improve coping. There has been a rapid increase of smartphone applications (apps) used to monitor and record health data due, in part, to the increase in mobile device availability [60]. According to the Pew Research Center, about three-quarters of U.S. adults (77%) say they own a smartphone and 46% of these owners said that their smartphone is something "they could not live without" [130, 131]. Individuals living in both urban and rural communities are more than ever capable of monitoring their progress and sending information directly to their healthcare provider using sophisticated apps [132]. There is evidence that tracking real-time data using ecological momentary assessment is preferable to retrospective diary entry [133–136]. Apps using innovative time-stamped technology can be particularly helpful in tracking variations in pain intensity and other health-related symptoms between clinic visits [60, 137, 138]. Large datasets of daily pain assessment offer opportunity for employment of computer-based classification and artificial intelligence [87]. There are various available smartphone apps that target people with both noncancer and cancer-related pain [139–142]. Although many of these apps are commercially accessible, most of them (approximately 86%) have been found to lack medical professional involvement in their development [143]. Lallo and others reviewed 224 pain apps and found little evidence that healthcare professionals had been involved in creating the apps [144]. The authors also found that only 2% of the apps they reviewed incorporated interactive social support and goal setting. None of the apps that were reviewed contained the recommended five main categories of functionality; the ability to self-monitor, set goals, build skills, educate and provide social support. In a recent review, Bhattarai and others [143] examined 373 pain self-management apps; only four successfully met their inclusion criteria according to an established usability evaluation tool. In another recent review of 195 pain management apps, Portelli and Eldred [145] found only 6 apps that incorporated a specific psychological component. The authors concluded that existing pain apps were often constructed by software developers with little input from healthcare professional and pain patients. They also reported that the pain apps tended to contain minimal theoretical content for facilitating self-management or behavioral change. Unfortunately, the life expectancy of most smartphone apps is brief. Seventy five percent of users discontinue using an app within 48 hours of downloading it, and 25% of apps are discarded after the first opening [128]. Based on anonymized data points from over 125 million mobile phones, it is estimated that 80% of apps fade away in time frames as short as 72 hours and 21% use an app only once [146, 147]. Thus, app creation needs to employ patient engagement strategies that include components that enhance relationships, that motivate and engage the user, that can be adaptive to individual change, that are easy to use and can be fun and that demonstrate caring [148].

Although teletherapy using innovative technology has been studied in individuals with depression and anxiety [149], substance use disorder [150], and various chronic medical conditions [151–153], there has been less attention to the role teletherapy might play for persons with chronic pain, particularly within an online group setting. A recent systematic review [154] and controlled trial [155] showed that teletherapy and remote online CBT strategies can be effective in improving quality of life among persons with chronic pain. Software technology can enable individuals to see and interact with each other using a web-based communication system, which mirrors what would be available in an in-person meeting (e.g. Skype, WebEx, GoToMeeting, Zoom, VSee). There is some preliminary evidence that peer-to-peer patient mentoring can improve behavior and overall health [156], and electronically-based peer support interventions would appear to hold great promise for improving outcomes in a variety of conditions, including persistent pain. It is also noted that interacting 'live' with others who experience a similar condition can be extremely helpful in improving coping with pain [157].

Future directions

Psychological assessment is designed to identify problematic emotional reactions, maladaptive thinking and behavior, and social problems that contribute to pain and disability. When psychosocial issues are identified, treatment can be tailored to address these challenges in the lives of persons with chronic pain, thereby improving the likelihood and speed of recovery and prevention of ongoing or more severe problems. Rapid changes in the way healthcare services are offered have led to a need for brief, reliable, and valid measures that establish need for service and monitor efficacy of treatment. A focus on accountability and efficacy has encouraged implementation of ongoing assessment, with preference given to treatments tailored to the individual with evidence of improvement.

In light of these changes, the economic efficiency of treatment for chronic noncancer pain will be under increased scrutiny. While evidence exists for the cost-effectiveness of therapy for chronic pain, such treatment may not meet the criterion of increased benefit with limited cost. Early and ongoing psychological assessment may help in identifying those individuals who will and do benefit most from certain pain therapies. Documentation of increased level of activity and decreased healthcare utilization among certain patients as a result of pain therapy would support the continuation of pain management interventions. The role of innovative technology and web-based assessment may play an important role in addressing these needs in the future. Future exploration of the benefits of psychological assessment and use of innovative technology in the assessment and treatment of chronic pain using rigorous longitudinal randomized controlled trials are needed.

References

1 Nicholas MK, Linton SJ, Watson PJ, Main CJ., The "Decade of the Flags" Working Group. (2011) Early identification and management of psychological risk factors ("yellow flags") in patients with low back pain: a reappraisal. *Physical Therapy* **91**:737–53.

2 Mannion AF, Elfering A. (2006) Predictors of surgical outcome and their assessment. *Eur Spine J* **15**:S93–108.

3 Main CJ, Spanswick CC. (2000) *Pain Management: An Interdisciplinary Approach*. Churchill Livingstone, New York.

4 Barry DT, Cutter CJ, Beitel M, Kerns RD, Liong C, Schottenfeld RS (2016). Psychiatric disorders among patients seeking treatment for co-occurring chronic pain and opioid use disorder. *J Clin Psychia* **77**:1413–9.

5 Iles RA, Davidson M, Taylor NF. (2008) Psychosocial predictors of failure to return to work in non-chronic non-specific low back pain: a systematic review. *Occup Environ Med* **8**:507–17.

6 Celestin J, Edwards RR, Jamison RN. (2009) Pretreatment psychosocial variables as predictors of outcomes following lumbar surgery and spinal cord stimulation: a systematic review and literature synthesis. *Pain Med* **10(4)**:639–5

7 Linton SJ, Shaw WS. (2011). Impact of psychological factors in the experience of pain. *Phys Ther Rehab J* **91**;700–11.

8 Bee P, McBeth J, MacFarlane GJ, Lovell K. (2016) Managing chronic widespread pain in primary care: a qualitative study of patient perspectives and implications for treatment delivery. *BMC Musculoskelet Disord* **17(1)**:354.

9 Dansie EJ, Turk DC (2013). Assessment of patients with chronic pain. *British Journal of Anaesthesia* **111**:19–25.

10 Kushang P, Amtmann D, Jensen MP, Smith SM, Veasley C, Turk D. (2021). Clinical outcome assessment in clinical trials of chronic pain treatments. *Pain Reports* **6(1)**:e784.

11 Chiarotto A, Boers M, Deyo RA, *et al.* (2018) Core outcome measurement instruments for clinical trials in nonspecific low back pain. *Pain* **159(3)**:481–95.

12 Kendall R, Wagner B, Brodke D, *et al.* (2018) The Relationship of PROMIS Pain Interference and Physical Function Scales. *Pain Med* **19(9)**:1720–4.

13 Cook KF, Jensen SE, Schalet BD, *et al.* (2016) PROMIS measures of pain, fatigue, negative affect, physical function, and social function demonstrated clinical validity across a range of chronic conditions. *Clin Epidemiol* **73**:89–102.

14 Khutok K, Janwantanakul P, Jensen MP, Kanlayanaphotporn R. (2021) Responsiveness of the PROMIS-29 scales in individuals with chronic low back pain.*Spine (Phila Pa 1976)* **46(2)**:107–13.

15 Stone AA, Broderick JE, Junghaenel DU, Schneider S, Schwartz JE. (2016) PROMIS fatigue,

pain intensity, pain interference, pain behavior, physical function, depression, anxiety, and anger scales demonstrate ecological validity. *J Clin Epidemiol* **74**:194–206.
16 Hicks CL, von Baeyer CL, Spafford P, van Korlaar I, Goodenough B. (2001). The Faces Pain Scale—revised: toward a common metric in pediatric pain measurement. *Pain* **93**:173–83.
17 Jensen MP, Karoly P. (2011) Self-report scales and procedures for assessing pain in adults. In: Turk DC, Melzack R, eds. *Handbook of Pain Assessment 3rd* edn. Guilford Press, New York. pp. 19–41
18 Jamison RN, Gracely RH, Raymond SA *et al.* (2002) Comparative study of electronic vs. paper VAS ratings: a randomized, crossover trial using healthy volunteers. *Pain* **99(1–2)**:341–7.
19 Main CJ. (2016). Pain assessment in context: a state of the science review of the McGill Pain Questionnaire 40 years on. *Pain* **157**:1387–99.
20 Melzack R. (1975). The McGill Pain Questionnaire: major properties and scoring methods. *Pain* **1**:277–99.
21 Dworkin RH, Turk DC, Trudeau JJ, Benson C, Biondi DM, Katz NP, Kim M. (2015). Validation of the Short-form McGill Pain Questionnaire-2 (SF-MOQ-2) in acute back pain. *Journal of Pain* **16**:357–66.
22 Cleeland CS, Ryan KM. (1994). Pain assessment. Global use of the Brief Pain Inventory. *Annals, Academy of Medicine, Singapore*. **23**:129–38.
23 Tan G, Jensen MP, Thornsby JI, Shanti BF (2004). Validation of the brief pain inventory for chronic nonmalignant pain. The Journal of Pain, 5, 133–137.
24 Bair MJ, Robinson RL, Katon W, Kroenke K. (2003). Depression and pain comorbidity: a literature review. *Archives of Internal Medicine* **163**:2433–45.
25 Martel MO, Edwards RR, and Jamison RN. (2020). The relative contribution of pain and psychological factors to opioid misuse: a 6-month observational study. *American Psychologist* **75**:772–83.
26 McHugh RK, Kneeland ET, Edwards RR, Jamison RN, Weiss RD. (2020) Pain catastrophizing and distress intolerance: differential prediction of pain and emotional stress reactivity. *J Behav Med* **43(4)**:623–9.
27 Gore M, Brandenburg NA, Dukes E, Hoffman DL, Tai KS, Stacey B.J (2005) Pain severity in diabetic peripheral neuropathy is associated with patient functioning, symptom levels of anxiety and depression, and sleep. *Pain Symptom Manage* **30(4)**:374–85.
28 Holmes D. (2016) The pain drain. *Nature* **535(7611)**:S2–3.
29 Jamison RN, Edwards RR, Liu X, *et al.* (2013) Effect of negative affect on outcome of an opioid therapy trial among low back pain patients. *Pain Practice* **13**:173–81.
30 Hays RD, Spritzer KL, Schalet BD, Cella D. (2018) PROMIS-29 v2.0 profile physical and mental health summary scores. *Qual Life Res* **27(7)**:1885–91.
31 Pilkonis PA, Yu L, Dodds NE, Johnston KL, Maihoefer CC, Lawrence SM. (2014) Validation of the depression item bank from the Patient-Reported Outcomes Measurement Information System (PROMIS) in a three-month observational study. *J Psychiatr Res* **56**:112–9.
32 Ramasamy A, Martin ML, Blum SI, *et al.* (2017) Assessment of Patient-Reported Outcome Instruments to Assess Chronic Low Back Pain. *Pain Med* **18(6)**:1098–1110.
33 Beck AT, Ward CH, Mendelson M *et al.* (1961) An inventory for measuring depression. *Arch Gen Psychiatry* **4**:561–71.
34 Norton S, Cosco T, Doyle F, Done J, Sackler A. (2013). The Hospital Anxiety and Depression Scale: a meta confirmatory factor analysis. *Journal of Psychosomatic Research* **74**:74–81.
35 Smarr KL, Keefer Al. (2011) Measures of depression and depressive symptoms: Beck Depression Inventory-II (BDI-II), Center for Epidemiologic Studies Depression Scale (CES-D), Geriatric Depression Scale (GDS), Hospital Anxiety and Depression Scale (HADS), and Patient Health Questionnaire-9 (PHQ-9). *Arthritis Care Res* **63**:S454–66.
36 Radloff LS. (1977) The CES-D scale: a self-report depression scale for research in the general population. *Appl Psychol Meas* **1**:385–401.
37 Hathaway SR, McKinley JC, Butcher JN *et al.* (1989) *Minnesota Multiphasic Personality Inventory-2:Manual for Administration*. University of Minnesota Press, Minneapolis.

38 Derogatis LR, Melisaratos N. (1983) The Brief Symptom Inventory: an introductory report *Psychol Med* **13**:595–605.

39 Millon T, Green CJ, Meagher RBJ. (1979) The MBHI: a new inventory for the psychodiagnostician in medical settings. *Prof Psychol* **10**:529–39.

40 Merskey H. (1987) Pain, personality and psychosomatic complaints. In: Burrows GD, Elton D, Stanley GV, eds. *Handbook of Chronic Pain Management*. Elsevier, Amsterdam. pp. 137–46.

41 Dance C, DeBerard MS, Gunday CJ. (2016) Pain acceptance potentially mediates the relationship between pain catastrophizing and post-surgery outcomes among compensated lumbar fusion patients. *J Pain Res* **10**:65–72.

42 Turk DC, Okifuji A, Sinclair JD *et al.* (1998) Differential responses by psychosocial subgroups of fibromyalgia syndrome patients to an interdisciplinary treatment. *Arthritis Care* **11**:397–404.

43 Ware JE, Sherbourne CD. (1992) The MOS 36-item short-form health survey (SF-36). I. Conceptual framework and item selection *Med Care* **20**:473–83.

44 Kerns RD, Turk DC, Rudy TE. (1985) The West Haven-Yale Multidimensional Pain Inventory (WHYMPI). *Pain* **23**:345–56.

45 Pollard CA. (1984) Preliminary validity study of the pain disability index. *Percept Mot Skills* **59**:974.

46 Ho MJ, LaFleur J. (2004) The treatment outcomes of pain survey (TOPS): a clinical monitoring and outcomes instrument for chronic pain practice and research. *J Pain Palliat Care Pharmocother* **18**:49–59.

47 Turk DC, Rudy TE. Towards an empirically derived taxonomy of chronic pain patients: integration of psychological assessment data. J Consult Clin Psychol 1988;**56**:233–8.

48 Flor H, Turk DC. (2011) *Chronic Pain: An Integrated Biobehavioral Approach*. IASP Press, Seattle.

49 Leclaire R, Blier F, Fortin L, Proulx R. (1997) A cross-sectional study comparing the Oswestry and Roland-Morris Functional Disability scales in two populations of patients with low back pain of different levels of severity. *Spine 22*:68–71.

50 Waddell G, Main CJ. (1984) Assessment of severity in low-back disorders. *Spine* **9**:204–8.

51 Evans JH, Kagan A 2nd. (1986) The development of a functional rating scale to measure the treatment outcome of chronic spinal patients. *Spine* **11**:277–81.

52 Stratford PW, Binkley JM. (2000) A comparison study of the Back Pain Function Scale and the Roland Morris Questionnaire. *J Rheumatol* **27**:1924–36.

53 Luque-Suarez, A., Martinez-Calderon, J., Falla, D. (2019). Role of kinesiophobia on pain, disability and quality of life in people suffering from chronic musculoskeletal pain: a systematic review. *Br J Sports Med*. **53(9)**:554–9.

54 Hanel J. Owen PJ, Held, S, *et al.* (2020). Effects of exercise training on fear-avoidance in pain and pain-free populations: systematic review and meta-analysis. *Sports Med* **50(12)**:2193–207.

55 Miller MB, Roumanis MJ, Kakinami L, Dover GS. (2020) Chronic pain patients' kinesiophobia and catastrophizing are associated with activity intensity at different times of the day. *J Pain Res* **13**:273–84.

56 Vlaeyen JW, Kole-Snijders AM, Boeren RG, van Eek. (1995) Fear of movement/(re)injury in chronic low back pain and its relation to behavioral performance. *Pain* **62(3)**:363–72.

57 Woby SR, Roach NK, Urmston M, Watson PJ. (2005) Psychometric properties of the TSK-11: a shortened version of the Tampa Scale for Kinesiophobia. *Pain* **117(1–2)**:137–44.

58 Ainsworth B, Cahalin L, Buman M, Ross R. (2015) The current state of physical activity assessment tools. *Prog Cardiovasc Dis* **57(4)**:387–95.

59 Deodhar A, Gensler LS, Magrey M, *et al.* (2019) Assessing physical activity and sleep in axial spondyloarthritis: measuring the gap. *Rheumatol Ther* **6(4)**:487–501.

60 Sundararaman LV, Edwards RR, Ross EL, Jamison RN. (2017) Integration of mobile health (mHealth) technology in the treatment of chronic pain: a critical review. *Reg Anesth Pain Med* **42**:488–98.

61 Coronado RA, George SZ, Devin CJ *et al.* (2015) Pain sensitivity and pain catastrophizing are associated with persistent pain and disability after lumbar spine surgery. *Arch Phys Med Rehabil* **96**:1763–70.

62 Sinikallio S, Aalto T, Airaksinen O, *et al.* (2011) Depression is associated with a poorer outcome

of lumbar spinal stenosis surgery: a two-year perspective follow-up study. *Spine* **36**:677–682.

63 Pinto P, Maintyre T, Araujo-Soares V, *et al.* (2014) The role of pain catastrophizing in the provision of rescue analgesia by healthcare providers following major joint arthroplasty. *Pain Physician* **17**:15–524.

64 Hassett AL, Finan PH. (2016) The role of resilience in the clinical management of chronic pain. *Curr Pain Headache Rep* **20**:39.

65 de Rooij A, de Boer MR, Roorda LD, Steultjens MP, Dekker J. (2014) Cognitive mechanisms of change in multidisciplinary treatment of patients with chronic widespread pain: a prospective cohort study. *J Rehabil Med* **46**:173–80.

66 Helmerhorst GT, Vranceanu AM, Vrahas M, Smith M, Ring D. (2014) Risk factors for continued opioid use one to two months after surgery for musculoskeletal trauma. *J Bone Joint Surg Am* **19**:495–9

67 Rosenstiel AK, Keefe FJ. (1983) The use of coping strategies in chronic low back pain patients: relationship to patient characteristics and current adjustment. *Pain* **17**:33–44.

68 Brown GK, Nicassion PM, Wallston KA. (1989) Pain coping strategies and depression in rheumatoid arthritis. *J Consult Clin Psychol* **57**:652–7.

69 Lorig K, Chastain RL, Ung E *et al.* (1989) Development and evaluation of a scale to measure perceived self-efficacy in people with arthritis. *Arthritis Rheum* **32**:37–44.

70 Karoly P, Jensen MP. (1987) *Multimethod Assessment of Chronic Pain*. Pergamon Press, New York.

71 Gil K, Williams DA, Keefe FJ *et al.* (1990) The relationship of negative thoughts to pain and psychological distress. *Behav Ther* **21**:349–62.

72 Williams DA, Robinson ME, Geiser ME. (1994) Pain beliefs: assessment and utility. *Pain* **59**:71–8.

73 Anderson KO, Noel-Dowds B, Pellet RE, Edwards, WT, Peeters-Asourian C. (1995). Development and initial validation of a scale to measure self-efficacy beliefs in patients with chronic pain. *Pain* **63**:77–84.

74 Leeuw M, Goossens ME, Linton SJ, Crombez G, Boersma K, Vlaeyen JW. (2007) The fear-avoidance model of musculoskeletal pain: current state of scientific evidence. *J Behav Med* **30**:77–94.

75 Sullivan MJ, Thorn B, Haythornthwaite JA *et al.* (2001) Theoretical perspectives on the relation between catastrophizing and pain. *Clin J Pain* **17**:52–64.

76 Edwards RR, Bingham CO 3rd, Bathon J, Haythornthwaite JA. (2006) Catastrophizing and pain in arthritis, fibromyalgia, and other rheumatic diseases. *Arthritis Rheum* **55**:325–32.

77 Sullivan MJ, Stanish W, Waite H, Sullivan M, Tripp DA. (1998) Catastrophizing, pain, and disability in patients with soft-tissue injuries. *Pain* **77**:253–60.

78 Campbell CM, Kronfli T, Buenaver LF, *et al.* (2010) Situational versus dispositional measurement of catastrophizing: associations with pain responses in multiple samples. *J Pain* **11**:443–53.

79 Leung L. (2012) Pain catastrophizing: an updated review. *Indian J Psychol Med* **34**:204–17.

80 Sullivan MJ, Martel MO, Tripp D, Savard A, Crombez G. (2005) The relation between catastrophizing and the communication of pain experience. *Pain* **122**:282–8.

81 Edwards RR, Cahalan C, Mensing G, Smith M, Haythornthwaite JA. (2011) Pain, catastrophizing, and depression in the rheumatic diseases. *Nat Rev Rheumatol* **7**:216–24.

82 Crombez G, Eccleston C, Baeyens F, Eelen P. (1998) When somatic information threatens, catastrophic thinking enhances attentional interference. *Pain* **75**:187–98.

83 Crombez G, Eccleston C, Van den Broeck A, Van Houdenhove B, Goubert L. (2002) The effects of catastrophic thinking about pain on attentional interference by pain: no mediation of negative affectivity in healthy volunteers and in patients with low back pain. *Pain Res Manage* **7**:31–9.

84 Nagin DS. (2014) Group-based trajectory modeling: an overview. *Ann Nutr Metab* **65**:205–10.

85 Burton AW, Fine PG, Passik SD. (2012) Transformation of acute cancer pain to chronic cancer pain syndromes. *J Supportive Oncol* **10**:89–95.

86 Edwards RR, Bingham CO 3rd, Bathon J, Haythornthwaite JA. (2006) Catastrophizing and pain in arthritis, fibromyalgia, and other rheumatic diseases. *Arthritis Rheum* **55**:325–32.

87 Jamison RN, Xu X, Wan L, Edwards RR, Ross EL. (2019) Determining pain catastrophizing from daily pain app assessment data: role of computer-based classification. *J Pain* **20**:278–87.

88 Sullivan MJL, Bishop SR, Pivik J. (1995) The Pain Catastrophizing Scale: development and validation. *Psychol Assess* **7**:524–32.

89 Kim HJ, Park JW, Chang BS *et al.* (2015) The influence of catastrophizing on treatment outcomes after surgery for lumbar spinal stenosis. *Bone Joint J* **97**:1546–54.

90 Van Damme S, Crombez G, Bijttebier P, Goubert L, Van Houdenhove B. (2002) A confirmatory factor analysis of the Pain Catastrophizing Scale: invariant factor structure across clinical and non-clinical populations. *Pain* **96**:319–24.

91 Edwards RR, Giles J, Bingham CO *et al.* (2010) Moderators of the negative effects of catastrophizing in arthritis. *Pain Medicine* **11**:591–9.

92 Jamison RN. (2004) The role of psychological testing and diagnosis in patients with pain. In: Dworkin RH, Breitbart WS, eds. *Psychosocial Aspects of Pain: A Handbook for Health Care Providers*. IASP Pres, Seattle. pp. 117–137.

93 Darnall BD, Stacey BR, Chou R. (2012) Medical and psychological risks and consequences of long-term opioid therapy in women: risks and consequences of long-term opioid use in women. *Pain Med* **13**:1181–211.

94 Kahan M, Wilson L, Mailis-Gagnon A, Srivastava A, National Opioid Use Guideline Group. (2011) Canadian guideline for safe and effective use of opioids for chronic noncancer pain: clinical summary for family physicians. Part 2: special populations. *Can Fam Phys* **57**:1269–76.

95 Chou R, Fanciullo GJ, Fine P *et al.* (2009) Clinical guidelines for the use of chronic opioid therapy in noncancer pain. *J Pain* **10**:113–30.

96 Furlan AD, Reardon R, Weppler C. (2010) Opioids for chronic noncancer pain: a new Canadian practice guideline. *CMAJ* **182**:923–30.

97 First M. Spitzer RL, Gibbon M. Williams JBW. (2012) Structured Clinical Interview for DSM-IV® Axis I Disorders (SCID-I), Clinician Version, Administration Booklet. American Psychiatric Publishing, Washington, D.C.Butler SF, Budman SH, Fernandez K, Jamison RN. (2004) Validation of a screener and opioid assessment measure for patients with chronic pain. *Pain* **112**:65–75.

98 Butler SF, Fernandez K, Benoit C *et al.* (2008) Validation of the revised Screener and Opioid Assessment for Patients with Pain (SOAPP-R). *J Pain* **9**:360–72.

99 Butler SF, Budman SH, Fernandez KC *et al.* (2009) Cross-validation of a screener to predict opioid misuse in chronic pain patients. *J Addict Med* **3**:66–73.

100 Black RA, McCaffrey SM, Villapiano A, Jamison RN, Butler SF. (2018) Development and validation of an eight-item brief form of the SOAPP-R (SOAPP-8). *Pain Med* **19**:1982–7.

101 Finkelman MD, Kulich RJ, Zacharoff KL. (2015) Shortening the Screener and Opioid Assessment for Patients with Pain-Revised (SOAPP-R): a proof-of-principle study for customized computer-based testing. *Pain Med* **16**:2344–56.

102 Finkelman MD, Jamison RN, Kulich RJ. (2017) Cross-validation of short forms of the Screener and Opioid Assessment for Patients with Pain-Revised (SOAPP-R). *Drug Alcohol Depend* **178**:94–100.

103 Butler SF, Zacharoff KL, Budman SH, *et al.* (2013) Spanish translation and linguistic validation of the Screener and Opioid Assessment for Patients with Pain Revised (SOAPP-R). *Pain Med* **14**:1032–8.

104 Butler SF, Budman SH, Fernandez KC *et al.* (2007) Development and validation of the Current Opioid Misuse Measure. *Pain* **130**:144–56.

105 Butler SF, Budman SH, Fanciullo GJ, Jamison R. (2010) Cross-validation of the Current Opioid Misuse Measure (COMM) to monitor chronic pain patients on opioid therapy. *Clin J Pain* **26**:770–6.

106 Weiner SG, Horton LC, Green TC *et al.* (2016) A comparison of an opioid abuse screening tool and prescription drug monitoring data in the emergency department. *Drug Alcohol Depend* **159**:152–7.

107 Varney SM, Perez CA, Araña AA *et al.* (2018) Detecting aberrant opioid behavior in the emergency department: a prospective study using the screener and Opioid Assessment for Patients with Pain-Revised (SOAPP®-R), Current Opioid Misuse Measure (COMM)™, and provider gestalt. *Intern Emerg Med* **13**:1239–47.

108 McCaffrey SA, Black RA, Villapiano AJ *et al*; Development of a Brief Version of the Current Opioid Misuse Measure (COMM): The COMM-9. *Pain Med* **20**:113–8.

109 Webster LR, Webster RM. (2005) Predicting aberrant behaviors in opioid-treated patients: preliminary validation of the Opioid Risk Tool. *Pain Med* **6(6)**:432–42.

110 Webster LR, Dove B. (2007) Avoiding Opioid Abuse While Managing Pain: A Guide for Practitioners. Sunrise River Press, North Branch.

111 Belgrade MJ, Schamber CD, Lindgren BR. (2006) The DIRE score: predicting outcomes of opioid prescribing for chronic pain. *J Pain* **7**:671–81.

112 Hildebrand M. (2015) The psychometric properties of the Drug Use Disorders Identification Test (DUDIT): a review of recent research. *J Subst Abuse Treat* **53**:52–9.

113 Tiet QQ, Leyva YE, Moos RH *et al*. (2017) Diagnostic accuracy of a two-item Drug Abuse Screening Test (DAST-2). *Addict Behav* **74**:112–117.

114 Giguère CÉ, Potvin S. (2017) The Drug Abuse Screening Test preserves its excellent psychometric properties in psychiatric patients evaluated in an emergency setting. *Addict Behav* **64**:165–70.

115 Coambs RB, Jarry JL, Santhiapillai AS *et al*. (1996) The SISAP: a new screening instrument for identifying potential opioid abusers in the management of chronic malignant pain within general medical practice. *Pain Res Manage* **1**:155–62.

116 Holmes CP, Gatchel RJ, Adams LL *et al*. (2006) An opioid screening instrument: long-term evaluation of the utility of the Pain Medication Questionnaire. *Pain Pract* **6**:77–88.

117 Lutz J, Gross R, Long D *et al*. (2017) Predicting risk for opioid misuse in chronic pain with a single-item measure of catastrophic thinking. *J Am Board Fam Med* **30**:828–31.

118 Lawrence R, Mogford D, Colvin L. (2017) Systematic review to determine which validated measurement tools can be used to assess risk of problematic analgesic use in patients with chronic pain. *Br J Anaesth* **119**:1092–109.

119 Cheatle MD, Compton PA, Dhingra L *et al*. (2019) Development of the revised Opioid Risk Tool to predict opioid use disorder in patients with chronic nonmalignant pain. *J Pain* **20**:842–51.

120 Jamison RN, Martel MO, Edwards RR, Qian, J, Sheehan, KA, Ross, EL. (2014) Validation of a brief opioid compliance checklist for patients with chronic pain. *J Pain* **15**:1092–101.

121 Jamison RN, Martel MO, Huang CC *et al*; (2016) Efficacy of the Opioid Compliance Checklist to monitor chronic pain patients receiving opioid therapy in primary care. *J Pain* **17**:414–23.

122 Alexander JC, Joshi GP. (2016) Smartphone applications for chronic pain management: a critical appraisal. *J Pain Res* **9**:731–4.

123 Anderson, K., Burford, O., Emmerton, L. (2016). Mobile health apps to facilitate self-care: A qualitative study of user experiences. *PLoS One* **11**:e0156164.

124 Vardeh D, Edwards RR, Jamison, RN, Eccleston C. (2013) There's an app for that: mobile technology is a new advantage in managing chronic pain. *Pain: Clin Updates* **21**:1–7.

125 Jamison RN, Mei A, Ross EL. (2018) Longitudinal trial of a smartphone pain app for chronic pain patients: predictors of compliance and satisfaction. *J Telemed Telecare* **24**:93–100.

126 Jamison RN, Jurcik D, Edwards RR, Huang CC, Ross EL. (2017) A pilot comparison of a smartphone app with or without 2-way messaging among chronic pain patients: who benefits from a pain app? *Clin J Pain* **33**:676–86.

127 Reynoldson C, Stones C, Allsop M, *et al*. (2014) Assessing the quality and usability of smartphone apps for pain self-management. *Pain Med* **15**:898–909.

128 Whitehead L, Seaton P. (2016) Effectiveness of self-management mobile phone and tablet apps in long-term condition management: a systematic review. *J Med Internet Res* **18**:e97.

129 Smith A. (2015) U.S. smartphone use in 2015. Pew Research Center. Available at http://www.pewinternet.org/2015/04/01/us-smartphone-use-in-2015. Accessed on 8th September 2021.

130 Rainie L, Perrin A. (2018) Ten facts about smartphones as the iPhone turns 10. The Pew Research Center. Available at http://www.pewresearch.org/fact-tank/2017/06/28/10-facts-about-smartphones. Accessed on 8th September 2021.

131 Singh K, Bates D, Drouin K *et al*. (2016) Developing a framework for evaluating the

patient engagement, quality, and safety of mobile health applications. Issue Brief (Commonwealth Fund) 5:1–1 http://www.commonwealthfund.org/publications/issue-briefs/2016/feb/evaluating-mobile-health-apps. Accessed on 8th September 2021.

132 Blumenthal S, Somashekar G. (2016) Advancing health with information technology in the 21st century. The Huffington Post. Available at http://www.huffingtonpost.com/susan-blumenthal/advancing-health-with-inf_b_7968190.html. Accessed on 8th September 2021.

133 Jamison RN, Raymond SA, Levine JG, Slawsby EA, Nedeljkovic SS, Katz NP. (2001) Electronic diaries for monitoring chronic pain: 1-year validation study. *Pain* **91**:277–85.

134 Jamison RN, Gracely RH, Raymond SA *et al.* (2002) Comparative study of electronic vs. paper VAS ratings: a randomized, crossover trial utilizing healthy volunteers. *Pain* **99**:341–47.

135 Palermo TM, Valenzuela D. Stork PP. (2004) A randomized trial of electronic versus paper pain diaries in children: impact on compliance, accuracy, and acceptability. *Pain* **107**:213–9.

136 Stone AA, Broderick JE. (2007) Real-time data collection for pain: appraisal and current status. *Pain Med* **8**:S85–S93.

137 Heron KE, Smyth JM. (2010) Ecological momentary interventions: incorporating mobile technology into psychosocial and health behaviour treatments. *Br J Health Psychol* **15**:1–39.

138 Hundert AS, Huguet A, McGrath PJ *et al.* (2014) Commercially available mobile phone headache diary apps: a systematic review. *JMIR Mhealth Uhealth* **2**:e36.

139 Stinson JN, Jibb LA, Nguyen C *et al.* (2013) Development and testing of a multidimensional iPhone pain assessment application for adolescents with cancer. *J Med Internet Res* **15**:e51.

140 Reynoldson C, Stones C, Allsop M *et al.* (2014) Assessing the quality and usability of smartphone apps for pain self-management. *Pain Med* **15**:898–909.

141 Vega R, Roset R, Castarlenas E *et al.* (2014) Development and testing of painometer: a smartphone app to assess pain intensity. *J Pain* **15**:1001–7.

142 Bhattarai P, Newton-John T, Phillips JL. (2018) Quality and usability of arthritic pain self-management apps for older adults: a systematic review. *Pain Med* **19**:471–84.

143 Lallo C. Jibb LA, Rivera J *et al.* (2015) "There's a pain app for that": review of patient-targeted smartphone applications for pain management. *Clin J Pain* **31**:557–63.

144 Portellli P, Eldred C. (2016) A quality review of smartphone applications for the management of pain. *Br J of Pain* **10**:135–140.

145 Perro J. (2018) Mobile apps: what's a good retention rate? Available at http://info.localytics.com/blog/mobile-apps-whats-a-good-retention-rate?_ga=2.90317082.1607914945.1575073756-556096695.1575073756. Accessed on 8th September 2021.

146 Jain A, Chen A. New data shows losing 80% of mobile users is normal, and why the best apps do better. Available at http://andrewchen.co/new-data-shows-why-losing-80-of-your-mobile-users-is-normal-and-that-the-best-apps-do. Accessed on 8th September 2021.

147 Ross EL, Jamison RN, Nicholls L, Perry BM, Nolen KD. (2020) Clinical integration of a smartphone pain app for patients with chronic pain: retrospective analysis of predictors of benefits and patient engagement between clinic visits. *J Med Internet Res* **22(4)**:e16939.

148 Mathiasen K, Riper H, Andersen TE *et al.* (2018) Guided internet-based cognitive behavioral therapy for adult depression and anxiety in routine secondary care: observational study. *J Med Internet Res* **20**:e10927.

149 Lin LA, Casteel D, Shigekawa E *et al.* (2019) Telemedicine-delivered treatment interventions for substance use disorders: a systematic review. *J Subst Abuse Treat* **101**:38–49.

150 Weymann N, Dirmaier J, von Wolff A *et al.* (2015) Effectiveness of a web based tailored interactive health communication application for patients with type 2 diabetes or low back pain *J Med Internet Res* **17**:e53.

151 Kosse RC, Bouvy ML, Belitser SV *et al.* (2019) Effective engaging of adolescent asthma patients with mobile health-supporting medication adherence. *JMIR Mhealth Uhealth* **7**:e12411.

152 Hanlon P, Daines L, Campbell C *et al.* (2017) Telehealth interventions to support self-management of long-term conditions: a

systematic metareview of diabetes, heart failure, asthma, chronic obstructive pulmonary disease, and cancer. *J Med Internet Res* **19**:e172.

153 Mariano TY, Wan L, Edwards RR, Jamison RN. (2019) Online teletherapy for chronic pain: a systematic review. *J Telemed Telecare* **2**:1–14.

154 Mariano TY, Wan L, Edwards RR, Lazaridou A, Ross EL, Jamison RN. (2019) Online group pain management for chronic pain: preliminary results of a novel treatment approach to teletherapy. *J Telemed Telecare* **27(4)**:209–16.

155 Long JA, Jahnle EC, Richardson DM *et al.* (2012) Peer mentoring and financial incentives to improve glucose control in African American veterans: a randomized trial. *Ann Intern Med* **156**:416–24.

156 Thompson M, Vowles KE, Sowden G *et al.* (2018) A qualitative analysis of patient-identified adaptive behavior changes following interdisciplinary Acceptance and Commitment Therapy for chronic pain. *Eur J Pain* **22**:989–1001.

Part 3

Management

Chapter 12

Introduction to management

Mary E. Lynch

Department of Anesthesia, Pain Management and Perioperative Medicine, Department of Psychiatry, Department of Pharmacology, Dalhousie University, Halifax, Nova Scotia, Canada

Overview

All pain management should take place within the context of a biopsychosocial approach where the role of the clinician is to assist the patient in becoming an active participant in their own healthcare. The following chapters address in detail pain management from different biological, psychological and social perspectives, with the interest in this chapter focusing on integration of the approaches so as to assure all facets of care are addressed. The principles of healthful living and therapeutic exercise should be a part of every patient's care. In addition, most people living with pain will benefit from strategies for relaxation along with cognitive approaches to deal with the pain day to day. Details of treatment approaches are presented in the following chapters. This chapter provides an overview of the four steps needed in the management of pain (Table 12.1).

Start with the basics

Step 1: Listen

Pain management begins the minute you start to listen

The importance of facilitating the patient's narrative was reviewed in Chapter 8. This is a therapeutic way to collect information as there "is the need of ill people to tell their stories, in order to construct new maps and new perceptions of their relationship to the world" [1]. The Stone Center Study Group on Women with Chronic Illness and Disability state that "Giving voice to one's experience with illness is courageous" and note that courage can inspire growth [2]. In this way the pain management begins the minute you start to listen.

Step 2: Communicate the diagnosis clearly

Establish and communicate the diagnosis

In determining optimal pain management, one must first establish the diagnosis as far as possible. As presented in more detail in previous chapters, chronic pain may or may not have a definitive explanation in tissue pathology. In the former case, the pain and related disability may result from a sustained sensory abnormality occurring as a result of ongoing peripheral pathology, such as chronic inflammation. It may also be autonomous and independent of the trigger that initiated it as in post-traumatic or post-surgical neuropathic pain. Thus, patients may present with nociceptive pain (pain due to tissue damage), neuropathic pain (pain due to pathology in neural systems) or a combination. When there is no identifiable medical or biological explanation, the biopsychosocial model encourages a stronger emphasis on psychophysiological and social explanations of functional symptoms [3]. In addressing management, it is important to consider both

Clinical Pain Management: A Practical Guide, Second Edition. Edited by Mary E. Lynch, Kenneth D. Craig, and Philip W. Peng.

Table 12.1 The four steps of good pain management.

Step 1: *Listen*
Narrative or telling one's story of pain is therapeutic: pain management begins the minute you start to listen
Step 2: *Communicate the diagnosis clearly*
In order to come to terms with a chronic pain diagnosis, understanding regarding the cause along with an active plan for management is essential
Step 3: *Review healthful living*
Proper nutrition
Quit smoking
Balance of activities and rest
Good sleep hygiene
Exercise program within pain tolerance
Step 4: *Consider pain reduction treatment options in biological, psychological and social domains*
Medical
Pharmacotherapy
Neuromodulation
Surgery
Psychological: assure psychosocial issues are identified and addressed in management
Physical and rehabilitation

disease-based (e.g. diabetic neuropathy, lumbar radiculopathy, cervical sprain) and mechanistic (e.g. nociceptive, inflammatory, neuropathic) aspects of the pain. It is also important to reassure the patient as to the reality of their experience even when there is not an identifiable etiology. One must also consider comorbidities (e.g. medical, psychiatric or substance use disorders), as well as additional aspects relating to the consequences of pain and disability and the state of the patient's overall health (e.g. psychosocial issues, metabolic and circadian factors, deconditioning) all of which will influence the experience of pain. For this reason, all management should take place within a holistic active participatory context.

You must communicate the diagnosis to the patient in clear unambiguous terms. In most cases the pain will have come on in the context of illness or injury and will have persisted beyond the time where healing should have taken place. The presence of allodynia or hyperalgesia may support a diagnosis of a neuropathic pain. In this case it is appropriate to explain that the nerves that convey pain-related information are alive and can be changed after injury such that they become sensitized or "stuck in the on" position like a light switch that cannot be turned off. The patient may have been previously diagnosed with Crohn's disease or recurrent renal stones and suffering from pain in the absence of a documented Crohn's exacerbation or presenting with pain that persists between renal stones. In this case it is important to explain to the patient that they are probably suffering from visceral hyperalgesia [4] or neuropathic pain in the gut. When one is unable to make a specific diagnosis, it is important to explain that cancer and other structural pathologies have been ruled out, that you believe the patient is in pain and support them in developing a plan for management. There are many excellent self-help books about pain as well as resources online that assist with this explanation. Examples include Explain Pain Butler [5] written for patients and Explain Pain Supercharged Moseley [6] written for clinicians.

As you discuss the diagnosis, be as precise as possible. Avoid the term chronic pain syndrome. As described by Merskey over two decades ago, this term "encourages the practitioner to neglect the responsibility for establishing the precise contribution of physical and psychological problems to the overall state of the patient. It is much better to make two diagnoses and estimate their importance" [7]. In this case, one might make a diagnosis of lumbar radiculopathy or post-surgical neuropathic pain complicated by depression, anxiety or grief. There may also be a component of grief related to job loss complicated by significant financial stress. Explain all of this to the patient along with the importance of addressing all in treatment.

It is unusual for there to be no explanation for the pain. In most cases there will be an identifiable precipitating event or series of events that will assist with the diagnosis, along with physical findings such as postural or muscular asymmetries, sensory abnormalities or abnormalities on palpation. However, in some cases it may be difficult to establish a diagnosis. If this is the case, it is important to remember that medically unexplained pain is not caused by psychopathology [8-10]. The biopsychosocial explanations needed are developed elsewhere in this volume. The therapeutic process in patients with medically unexplained symptoms depends on a process of negotiation which requires dialog [11]. As with all patients, the therapeutic process thrives within an atmosphere of trust between healthcare professional and patient. Clear direct communication is critical. It is best to acknowledge that we as health professionals cannot explain everything, that we have ruled out serious illness such as cancer, inflammatory arthritis and other possibilities and that we are going to assist the patient with management of their pain to the best of our ability. The multidisciplinary approach to pain management supported in this volume encourages utilizing the resources of other healthcare professionals when appropriate. Patients report a high level of satisfaction with pain care even when the pain remains and research has suggested this is related to the patient–provider relationship and their appreciation for the providers mere voicing of interest in adequate pain treatment [12,13].

Step 3: Review healthful living

Pain management is a joint effort

Emphasize that pain management must involve a joint effort where the patient will have to do their part in managing their own pain. As healthcare professionals we will do everything we can do to reduce the pain where possible but there are key steps the patient must take to reduce pain and improve health.

There is growing support that self-management approaches are efficacious and cost effective in chronic diseases including pain. Self-management is reviewed in more detail in Chapter 25. Here, it is emphasized that all clinicians, regardless of background or setting, should review the basics of healthful living. People living with pain are as heterogeneous as the general population so for some there will already be an understanding of the need to live a healthy lifestyle. For others it will take some time for them to "get it." Patients need to understand that it is important to "live right" now that they have pain. This includes proper nutrition, quitting tobacco smoking, pacing activities, adequate sleep or down time and a basic exercise program. Nutrition and exercise are reviewed in Chapters 14 and 15, respectively. The majority of people living with chronic pain report problems with sleep, Chapter 7 provides further detail on the interaction between pain and sleep and approaches to management. The importance of quitting smoking is obvious with regards to general health but what many patients may not know is that chronic exposure to nicotine increases the chances of neural sensitization and they may be making their pain worse. In addition, it is well established that chronic smoking exacerbates autoimmune disease including rheumatoid arthritis [14], Crohn's disease [15] and multiple sclerosis [16], which often present with severe pain.

Step 4: Consider pain reduction treatment options in biological, psychological and social domains

Medical: pharmacological, interventional and surgical

In some cases, patients may benefit from medical approaches including medications, interventional therapies such as injection or surgical approaches.

Pharmacotherapy

There are several chapters reviewing the key groups of medication helpful in the management of chronic pain. The order in which these medications may be trialed may vary depending on the underlying mechanisms of pain or the patient's response. A reasonable approach is described below.

Once the physician has established the working diagnosis and has identified that analgesic medication is necessary, the usual approach is to start with a non-opioid analgesic such as a NSAID or acetaminophen for mild to moderate pain. If this is inadequate, and if there is an element of sleep loss, the next step is to add an antidepressant with analgesic qualities. If there is a component of neuropathic pain, then a trial of one of the anticonvulsant analgesic agents is appropriate. If these steps are inadequate, then a trial of an opioid analgesic may be added. Cannabinoids and topical agents may also be appropriate as single agents or in combination. In an individual patient, one or several mechanisms may be at play in the etiology of the pain and more than one agent may be necessary for pain control. Details regarding pharmacotherapy with each category of agent as well as combination pharmacotherapy are reviewed in Chapters 16- 21. There is also significant individual variation in response to medications. For this reason, it is important to take an individual approach to each patient and adjust dosage according to treatment response while minimizing side effects.

Interventional and surgical therapies

In properly selected patients, diagnostic or therapeutic blocks, neuromodulation or surgical approaches may be appropriate. The details regarding these approaches and appropriate indications are presented in Chapters 22-24.

Exercise management and physical strengthening

Pain will often lead to decreased movement, postural asymmetry, loss of strength and eventually deconditioning. This will lead to additional problems complicating the patient's original pain condition and must be addressed. Approaches offered through physiotherapy and rehabilitation programs are reviewed in Chapter 15.

Psychological therapies

The assessment and management of psychosocial aspects of pain are critical in assisting the patient presenting with pain (Chapters 11, 26 and 27). Chapter 27 reviews the fact that psychosocial variables such as catastrophic thinking and fear of movement are significant determinants of persistent pain and disability and response to all forms of treatment. Psychological and self-management interventions (Chapters 25 and 26) have demonstrable effectiveness in painful distress and pain-related disability.

Complementary therapies and integrative healthcare

Many patients seek relief through complementary therapies such as acupuncture, Qigong, massage, osteopathy and other complementary therapeutic approaches. The field of "integrative medicine," using a combination of conventional medical approaches along with the complementary therapies, has application in pain management. The growing research regarding an integrative approach has been reviewed in Chapter 28.

Conclusions

The 4 steps to good pain management include listening, communication of the diagnosis in clear terms the patient can understand, review of healthy living, self management and offering appropriate pain reduction options. Where the diagnosis is unclear after appropriate investigation, it is important to assure the patient there is no serious medical pathology and review basic pain pathophysiology. Reassure the patient you believe they are in pain and use a biopsychosocial approach where the role of the clinician is to assist the patient in becoming an active participant in their own healthcare using treatments presented in the following chapters.

References

1 Frank A. (1995) *The Wounded Storyteller*. University of Chicago Press, Chicago.

2 Reid-Cunningham M, Snyder-Grant D, Stein K *et al.* (1999) *Women with Chronic Illness: Overcoming Disconnection.* Stone Center Work in Progress Paper **80**:1–8.

3 Williams SE, Smith CA, Bruehl SB *et al.* (2009) Medical evaluation of children with chronic abdominal pain: impact of diagnosis, physician practice orientation, and maternal trait anxiety and mother's response to evaluation. *Pain* **146**:283–92.

4 Gebhart GF. (1995) *Visceral Pain*. IASP Press, Seattle.

5 Butler, D. S. and G. L. Moseley (2013). Explain Pain, 2nd edn. NOI Group Publications, Adelaide.

6 Moseley, G. L. and D. S. Butler (2017). Explain Pain Supercharged. NOI Group Publishers, Adelaide.

7 Merskey H. (1989) Psychiatry and chronic pain. *Can J Psychiatry* **34**:329–35.

8 Crombez G, Beirens K, Van Damme S *et al.* (2009) The unbearable lightness of somatization: a systematic review of the concept of somatisation in empirical studies of pain. *Pain* **145**:31–5.

9 Gagliese L, Katz J. (2000) Medically unexplained pain is not caused by psychopathology. *Pain Res Manag* **5**:251–7.

10 Merskey H. (2009) Somatization: or another God that failed. *Pain* **145**:4–5.

11 Kirmayer LJ, Groleau D, Looper KJ *et al.* (2004) Explaining medically unexplained symptoms. *Can J Psychiatry* **49**:663–72.

12 Dawson R, Spross JA, Jablonski ES *et al.* (2002) Probing the paradox of patients' satisfaction with inadequate pain management. *J Pain Symptom Manag* **23**:211–20.

13 Carr DB. (2009) What does pain hurt? *IASP Pain Clinical Updates* **XVII(3)**:1–6.

14 Baka Z, Buzás E, Nagy G. (2009) Rheumatoid arthritis and smoking: putting the pieces together. *Arthritis Res Ther* **11(4)**:238.

15 Cosnes J, Carbonnel F, Carrat F *et al.* (1999) Effects of current and former cigarette smoking on clinical course of Crohn's disease. *Aliment Pharmacol Ther* **13(**11**)**:1403–**11**.

16 Healy BC, En A, Guttman CR *et al.* (2009) Smoking and disease progression in multiple sclerosis. *Arch Neurol* **66**:858–64.

Chapter 13

Managing chronic pain in primary care

Sarah E.E. Mills[1] & Blair H. Smith[1]

[1] *University of Dundee, Scotland, UK*

Introduction

Chronic pain is a common, complex and distressing problem, with wide-ranging impacts on the individual, family, society and health service [1]. While chronic pain is often experienced as a sequela of injury or disease, it is not simply a symptom of other medical conditions but a distinct clinical entity, with its own medical definition and system of nomenclature [2–5].

Pain is a complex biopsychosocial phenomenon which presents as "*An unpleasant sensory and emotional experience associated with, or resembling that associated with, actual or potential tissue damage* [6]. Chronic pain is pain that persists past the normal time in which healing would have been expected to occur; for most types of pain the transition from acute and chronic pain occurs after three months' duration [2]. Unlike the management of acute pain, where the emphasis is on resolving the underlying cause, in chronic pain the emphasis is on managing the pain, addressing the effects of the pain and maximizing individual's functional ability and quality of life [7].

Chronic pain has profound and diverse personal, social and psychological impacts, as well as economic consequences. The study 'Pain in Europe' found that the average duration for chronic pain was at least 7 years and that 1 in 6 people with chronic pain reported that their pain was sometimes so bad that they wanted to die [8]. The Global Burden of Disease (GBD) Study 2017 demonstrated that the high prominence of pain and pain-related diseases are the leading causes of disability and disease burden in the world [9]. It is estimated that 40–60% of people living with chronic pain have inadequate pain management [10, 11].

Chronic pain affects one-third to one-half of the UK population [1]. Among people living with chronic pain, 10–14% have moderate to severe disabling chronic pain [1]. The majority of people with chronic pain contact their general (family) practitioner (GP)[12]; 10–15% of the population present to their GP due to chronic pain [13]. Patients with chronic pain are 1.5 times more likely to visit their primary care physician than those without chronic pain and 22% to 50% of GP consultations are related to pain [14]. Primary care delivers the overwhelming majority of pain-related medical input; with only a small proportion, estimated at 0.3% to 2% of those with chronic pain, being seen each year in a pain clinic [14].

This chapter aims to address the management of chronic pain in primary care and takes as its starting point that all reasonable attempts to investigate and treat modifiable causes of pain have been made.

Management of Chronic Pain in Primary Care

The goal of treating chronic pain is to support the patient to live as well as possible, with the maximum quality of life, in spite of their chronic pain. This

Clinical Pain Management: A Practical Guide, Second Edition. Edited by Mary E. Lynch, Kenneth D. Craig, and Philip W. Peng.

support can be considered in two primary categories: drug and non-drug (including self-management) interventions.

Chronic pain treatment must take into account an evaluation of the severity, impact and type of pain experienced [15]. Because of the complex biopsychosocial nature of chronic pain and the constrained time and resources available, the assessment and management of chronic pain in primary care can be challenging [16].

Initial assessment of people with chronic pain follows the standard consultation model of history taking and examination and should ideally include a history of the pain, functional assessment, behavioral health assessment, evaluation of other comorbidities, physical examination, imaging/diagnostic tests and other relevant tests [17]. Identifying and addressing the social challenges faced by patients with chronic pain, particularly with regards to the impact on relationships, employment and roles, is an important part of a holistic chronic pain assessment. Realistically, given the time constraints inherent to the primary care consultation, a full chronic pain assessment may well take place over a number of consultations. Pain severity can be evaluated in terms of pain intensity, pain-related distress and functional impairment [18].

Agreeing Shared Treatment Goals

Evaluating patient-reported outcomes is an important part of a comprehensive chronic pain assessment [19]. It can be beneficial for clinicians and patients to discuss and agree on treatment goals for chronic pain when reviewing or initiating treatment [17, 20]. Patients with chronic pain may be initially resistant to a shift in therapeutic goals from 'pain elimination' to 'functional improvement' however, it is vital to have such conversations during pain management in primary care, to ensure that the clinician and patient both have a common treatment goal [7]. Unrealistic treatment expectations can be a major barrier to achieving good management of chronic pain in primary care [20]. Achieving a reduction in pain intensity of 30–50% is generally considered to be a successful outcome [21], though success may also come from improving quality of life and function with minimal change in actual pain intensity. Evaluating treatments and interventions against this standard can help clinicians and patients to assess and contextualize their relative successes appropriately [7]. Clinicians should ensure that patients are aware from the outset that achieving complete freedom from pain is an unusual outcome [22].

Relevant Guidelines for Assessing and Managing Chronic Pain

Many guidelines for assessment and management of chronic pain are directly relevant to primary care. Key chronic pain guidelines exist in many countries, including Australia [23], Canada [8, 24, 25], Germany (26), the United Kingdom [15, 27, 28], the United States of America [8, 29–31] and internationally [32–35]. The Scottish Intercollegiate Guideline Network (SIGN) Guideline, published in 2013 and updated in 2019, is a particularly appropriate tool for primary care physicians and makes a number of helpful recommendations for primary care physicians, a summary of which can be found in Table 13.1 [15]. This was the first, and remains the only, comprehensive evidence-based guideline aimed at non-specialists at managing chronic pain [15].

Drug Interventions

There is good evidence for the limited benefit of pharmaceutical interventions in many chronic pain conditions with 40–50% of patients obtaining some benefit. Detailed discussion of pharmacological management is beyond the scope of this chapter, but can be found in the cited guidelines above and elsewhere in this volume. While prescribing is one of the main responsibilities of any physician, it should not be the sole focus of a management plan. Furthermore, clinicians should engage patients in regular review of their prescribing to ensure that prescribed medications are optimized (effectiveness, adverse effects), rather than allowing prolonged issuing of repeat prescriptions without review.

It is important to assess and reassess chronic pain management and to ensure that each new treatment is given a long enough trial at a high enough dose (if tolerated) before moving on to other treatments. It is important to ensure that potentially effective treatments are not discarded because of an incomplete

Table 13.1 Summary of some of the key recommendations for chronic pain management made in the Scottish Intercollegiate Guideline Network (SIGN) guideline, *Management of Chronic Pain* [15].

Assessment
Physicians should identify pain type, severity, functional impact and context for all patients with chronic pain. A patient-centered compassionate approach is likely to yield the most successful outcome for pain management. Referral to secondary care should be considered if: non-specialist management is failing, chronic pain is poorly controlled, there is significant distress and/or where specific specialist intervention or assessment is considered.
Supported self-management
Self-management can be effective in managing chronic pain. Its use should be considered in early stages in chronic pain. Patients should be able to access self-help resources at any stage of their treatment.
Pharmacological therapies
Assessments of pharmacological therapies for people with chronic pain should occur at least yearly. The guideline makes specific recommendation about the use of different medications for different kinds of chronic pain. Specialist advice or referral to secondary care should be considered for patients on >50mg/day morphine equivalent dose. Physicians should look for signs of abuse, addiction or other harms in patients using strong opioids. A combination of different analgesics should be considered for patients with neuropathic pain.
Psychologically based interventions
Referral to pain management programs should be considered. Patients should be made aware that the aim of such programs is to improve coping skills and quality of life, rather than alleviate pain itself.
Physical therapies
Exercise or exercise therapies are recommended, in any form, for patients with chronic pain. All patients with chronic pain should be encouraged to stay active. Supervised exercise sessions and targeted physical activity interventions should be used where possible.
Complementary Therapies
Acupuncture should be considered for some people with chronic pain.
*Note – this list is not comprehensive; there are 55 recommendations are included in this Guideline

trial of treatment. Inappropriate timing or dose of drugs, poor medication compliance and unreasonable patient expectations for treatment can lead to the premature abandonment of potentially useful treatments.

The majority of people with chronic pain take analgesic medication. A large-scale survey in Sweden found that almost half of all people with chronic pain were taking non-prescription analgesics, including non-steroidal anti-inflammatory drugs (NSAIDs) (55%), paracetamol (acetaminophen) (43%) and weak opioids (13%). They found that two-thirds of people with chronic pain were taking prescription analgesics, including NSAIDs (44%), weak opioids (23%), paracetamol (18%) and strong opioids (5%) [11].

With any type of chronic pain, paracetamol (acetaminophen) is generally the first drug of choice because of its good tolerability and efficacy [36, 37]. However, recent systematic reviews found that paracetamol was no more effective than placebo in chronic pain conditions [38, 39]. Any additional analgesic agents should be selected to target the type of pain, generally categorized into either 'nociceptive' or 'neuropathic'. Nociceptive pain is traditionally associated with damage to tissues and is often due to historical trauma or injury, while neuropathic pain arises as a result of an injury (including disease or lesions) to the somatosensory system [40]. People with chronic pain may have mixed pain aetiology with both nociceptive and neuropathic elements and may therefore require a multimodal prescribing approach.

Neuropathic pain should be treated with appropriate neuromodulator analgesia, in a progression through tricyclic antidepressants, then gabapentin, then pregabalin [41]. In patients who have pain that is very localized, or where the use of neuromodulator analgesic is contraindicated or ineffective, consideration should be given to topical preparations, including lidocaine and capsaicin. When dealing with neuropathic pain opioids can sometimes be of benefit; however, while tramadol can be initiated in primary care, it is recommended that morphine only be initiated for neuropathic pain by secondary care physicians [41]. Any person who requires strong opioids for neuropathic pain should be considered for referral to secondary care pain management services.

If treatment of nociceptive pain is initiated with paracetamol, this could be augmented, as appropriate and providing there are no contra-indications, with nonsteroidal anti-inflammatory drugs (NSAIDs), such as ibuprofen and naproxen [37]. When considering using NSAIDs, clinicians must take into account patients' age, comorbidities (including asthma, chronic kidney disease and risk of GI bleeding). Inappropriate NSAID prescribing for patients with chronic pain is common and poses an urgent patient safety risk [42]. Topical NSAIDs, such as ibuprofen gel, can be used effectively in many causes of chronic pain and have better safety than oral NSAIDs and comparable efficacy; however, they are not recommended for all types of pain [43]. Opioids have increasingly become a mainstay of the treatment for nociceptive pain; however, their risks of dependence, overdose, misuse, abuse, diversion, adverse events (e.g. falls) and death, when compared to other analgesics, mean they should be used with extreme caution [37, 44]. The SIGN guideline for chronic pain recommends that, "All patients receiving opioid doses of >50 mg/day morphine equivalent should be reviewed regularly (at least annually) to detect emerging harms and consider ongoing effectiveness. Pain specialist advice or review should be sought at doses >90 mg/day morphine equivalent" [15]. When reviewing patients' use of opioids, clinicians should bear in mind that there is no evidence for their effectiveness in long-term use, but that there is evidence for the above risks of potentially serious harms. The risk of clinical dependence and addiction means that once patients have been started on opioids it can be challenging to discontinue their use [29]. Patients on regular opioids should receive early reviews of any newly-prescribed medication and a full medical review at least annually [15]. In patients where there is a history of misuse or abuse of prescription or non-prescription drugs or other substances, opioid prescribing may be best to be limited to initiation specialist pain clinics only.

Chronic pain condition-specific treatments may be appropriate, depending on the nature of the painful condition, e.g., the use of triptans in patients with chronic migraine, or carbamazepine for trigeminal neuralgia. In situations where pathology-specific medications are used, it is important to ensure that appropriate treatment is initiated and that a sufficient length of time is given to trial each treatment before patients are referred to secondary care.

Patients should have their analgesia reviewed at each assessment, in order to titrate medications to their maximum effective or tolerated dose, to assess the level of symptom relief and adverse effects produced by any given medication and to discontinue any medication that is not proving to be effective or tolerated in minimizing symptom burden. Because patients' analgesia requirements will change over time, regular reviews are required in order to ensure that therapy is optimized and continues to be appropriate and that side-effects are identified and treated appropriately.

Non-Drug Interventions

Non-drug approaches to improving symptoms in people living with chronic pain are a vital part of the holistic patient-centered approach to pain management. Such approaches frequently call upon the wider primary care multidisciplinary team and can be delivered by GPs, nurses, practice staff, physiotherapists, occupational therapists, pharmacists, psychologists, counselors, behavioral therapists, social workers and complementary therapists. In order to select appropriate non-drug treatments, it is important to tailor non-drug management plans both to the patient and to the local area. A GP's knowledge of the patient's motivation, health beliefs, personal circumstances and of local services and referral pathways is essential in optimizing non-drug treatment [45]. Though the evidence base for non-drug treatments is often limited, it is increasing rapidly. It is important to note that for such interventions, an absence of evidence for effectiveness is not the same as evidence of absence of effectiveness.

Psychological Approaches

Psychological approaches are generally proven to be of benefit in chronic pain, however do not all transfer directly to primary care. They include pain management programs, unidisciplinary education, behavioral therapies, cognitive behavioral therapy (CBT) and acceptance and commitment therapy (ACT) [15].

Access to psychological approaches is difficult and evidence is limited in primary care. In managing chronic pain, physicians should remember that there is a common co-occurrence of depression and chronic pain and both need to be managed in order to achieve improvement in either [46].

Interventions based on CBT can be used in primary care either alone, as an adjunct to drug interventions, or as part of a comprehensive pain management program (PMP). There is evidence that primary-care based CBT interventions result in improved measures of disability, reduced pain intensity, reduced depression and better quality of life one year after intervention than those receiving standard care for chronic pain [47]. See elsewhere in this volume for details on these approaches.

Self-Management

Self-management encompasses any activity which "enhances function, improves mood and decreases pain" by targeting and challenging the "emotional, cognitive and behavioral responses to pain" [48]. It includes an individual's approaches and changes to lifestyle, daily activities and attitudes to re-formulate the conception of pain and its impact on life. One important component of self-management can be receiving a 'chronic pain' diagnosis from a healthcare professional, as this can be the first step in helping people 'thrive' (live well with chronic pain)[49]. Self-management tools, such as self-management programs and electronic delivery including online resources, can be effective to complement other drug and non-drug therapies [15]. One example is The Pain Toolkit (http://www.paintoolkit.org). Self-management has been shown to be both effective and potentially cost-effective in improving pain among an older adult population [50]. In a review of patients with chronic pain, many felt that discussions about self-management occurred too late or not at all during their experience of chronic pain [51]. Again, self-management approaches are described in more details elsewhere in this volume.

Mindfulness, is a self-management approach aimed at developing positive reactions to mental and physical processes which contribute to dysfunctional behavior and emotional distress. Research suggests that practising mindfulness is associated with improved patient-centered outcomes, reduced pain catastrophizing, improved physical functioning and reduced utilization of health-care [52, 53]. There are multiple web-based resources for mindfulness.

Physiotherapy and Exercise

Strong evidence, underpinned by national and international guidelines, supports physical activity as a safe and effective intervention for all people with chronic pain [15, 54, 55]. There is insufficient evidence to recommend any particular type [54, 56]. Activity levels are often guided by patient preferences, beliefs and access to facilities.

For musculoskeletal pain, physiotherapy is beneficial in reducing pain intensity and improving physical function [57]. There is evidence that adding motivational interventions to traditional physiotherapy confers additional benefits in terms of increasing physical activity and patient adherence to physiotherapy exercises [58].

Peripheral Nervous System Stimulation

Trans-cutaneous Electronic Nerve Simulation (TENS) is a simple pain relief treatment which uses electrodes placed on the skin to deliver recurrent stimulation to neurons and which has some evidence of benefit in treating chronic pain [15, 59]. Overall evidence, though, is weak, and more research is needed [60].

Complementary Therapies

Complementary and Alternative Medicine (CAM) includes such diverse practices as acupuncture, aromatherapy, biofeedback, chiropractic medicine, diet therapy, herbalism, homeopathy, hypnosis, massage therapy, meditation, naturopathy, osteopathic manipulative therapy and reflexology. CAM is frequently used within the community of people with chronic pain; one study found that over

70% of patients with chronic pain had used complementary therapies; others found that people with chronic pain using CAM had high levels of patient satisfaction [61–63].

CAM is a very heterogeneous category; some approaches have no formal qualification, regulation or training and have little to no evidence supporting their effectiveness. However, other approaches, including the manual therapies of chiropractic and osteopathy, have formal degree qualifications, national regulatory bodies and an expanding evidence base in published literature [15, 64].

Few primary care practitioners are qualified to provide these treatments; however, patients are likely to ask their advice. Perhaps the best advice to give to patients is to be aware of the limited evidence and if they choose to use complementary therapies only to use registered practitioners.

However, it is important for physicians to be aware of what CAM therapies their patients are accessing, in order to have a holistic view of their care and to be aware of any potential implications on medical care, for example with respect to drug interactions with herbal medicines.

Pain-Management Programs (PMPs)

Pain Management Programs (PMPs) are based on combined psychological and behavioral approaches and combine patient education and practice sessions aimed at helping people with chronic pain to manage their pain and everyday activities better [65]. PMPs have been shown to be effective interventions in both primary and secondary care [66], with benefits including reduction in medication usage and lower healthcare utilization [66, 67]. However, because access to PMPs is geographically variable and often very restricted, their utility in primary care may be relatively limited.

Referral to specialist pain clinic

Referral to a pain specialist clinic should be considered in some cases. There are a number of reasons for which a GP should consider referral to secondary care; broad reasons for referral are shown in Table 13.2.

Some patients attend secondary and/or tertiary pain management services with high expectations that their pain will be cured; this expectation is often unrealistic and can lead to a breakdown in the therapeutic relationship. It is important that the GP establish with the patient at the time of referral to secondary care that they are being referred for management of their pain rather than further investigation of underlying cause, or for 'cure'.

Table 13.2 Broad reasons for referral to secondary care pain services.

- Inadequate pain control achieved despite treatment according to the above principles
- Complex presentation, requiring specialist, multi-disciplinary assessment and resources
- Consideration of specialist interventions (spinal cord stimulation, nerve block or strong opioids)
- Access to a specialist interdisciplinary team and/or pain management program
- Specific patient request (for reassurance or "second opinion")
- Confirmation that all reasonable approaches have already been explored

The aims of secondary care pain services include helping the patient towards an improved understanding of why they have chronic pain and what external influences worsen their chronic pain. They should also be helped to develop a self-management plan and a crisis plan for managing exacerbations of their chronic pain. Patients usually continue to attend their GP while under the management of a secondary care pain clinic and a collaborative approach to pain management between primary and secondary care should be adopted.

Conclusions

Chronic pain is a common problem and the majority of patients with chronic pain are managed in primary care. GPs therefore require adequate evidence, training and resources to assess and manage chronic pain in a primary care setting. There are now high-quality guidelines available and a growing evidence base for holistically managing chronic pain, including pharmacological and non-pharmacological interventions. However, further education, research and resources targeted at primary care management of chronic pain are required to ensure that the care being delivered is as efficient, effective and evidence-based as possible. Good communication within the primary care team, and between physicians in primary and secondary/tertiary care, can maximize the effectiveness of chronic pain management strategies.

References

1 Fayaz A, Croft P, Langford R, Donaldson J, Jones G. (2016) Prevalence of chronic pain in the UK: a systematic review and meta-analysis of population studies. *BMJ Open* **6(6)**:e010364.

2 IASP. (1986) Classification of chronic pain. Descriptions of chronic pain syndromes and definitions of pain terms. *Pain Suppl* 3:S1–226.

3 Tracey I, Bushnell M. (2009) How neuroimaging studies have challenged us to rethink: is chronic pain a disease? *J Pain* **10(11)**:1113–20.

4 World Health Organization. (2018). ICD-11 International Classification of Diseases for Mortality and Morbidity Statistics. Available from https://icd.who.int/browse11_2018-06/l-m/en#!. Accessed on 15th September 2021.

5 Treede R-D, Rief W, Barke A *et al.* (2019) Chronic pain as a symptom or a disease: the IASP Classification of Chronic Pain for the International Classification of Diseases (ICD-11). *Pain* **160(1)**:19–27.

6 Raja SN, Carr DB, Cohen M *et al.* (2020). The revised International Association for the Study of Pain definition of pain: concepts, challenges, and compromises. *Pain* 161**(9)**:1976–82.

7 Schneiderhan J, Clauw D, Schwenk TL. (2017) Primary care of patients with chronic pain. JAMA **317(23)**:2367–8.

8 Busse JW, Craigie S, Juurlink DN *et al.* (2017) Guideline for opioid therapy and chronic non-cancer pain. *CMAJ* **189(18)**:E659–E66.

9 James S. (2018) Global, regional, and national incidence, prevalence, and years lived with disability for 354 diseases and injuries for 195 countries and territories, 1990-2017: a systematic analysis for the Global Burden of Disease Study 2017. *Lancet (London, England)* **392**:1789–858.

10 Breivik H, Collett B, Ventafridda V, Cohen R, Gallacher D. (2006) Survey of chronic pain in Europe: Prevalence, impact on daily life, and treatment. *European Journal of Pain* **10(4)**:287–333.

11 Breivik H. (2012) A major challenge for a generous welfare system: a heavy socio-economic burden of chronic pain conditions in Sweden - and how to meet this challenge. *European Journal of Pain (London, England)* **16(2)**:167.

12 Green LA FG, Yawn BP *et al.* (2001) The ecology of medical care revisited. *N Engl J Med* **344**:2021–5.

13 McQuay HJ KE, Moore RA, eds.(2008) *Epidemiology of Chronic Pain*. IASP Press, Seattle.

14 Smith BH, Fors EA, Korwisi B *et al.* (2019) The IASP classification of chronic pain for ICD-11: applicability in primary care. *Pain* **160(1)**:83–7.

15 Scottish Intercollegiate Guidelines Network (SIGN). (2019) SIGN 136. Management of Chronic Pain. Health Improvement Scotland, Edinburgh. https://www.sign.ac.uk/assets/sign136.pdf. Accessed on 27th Feb 2022.

16 Smith BH, Torrance N. (2011) Management of chronic pain in primary care. Current Opinion in Supportive and Palliative Care. **5(2)**:137–42.

17 Thies KM, Anderson D, Beals-Reid C. (2019) Project ECHO Chronic Pain. *Journal of Continuing Education in the Health Professions* **39(3)**: 194–200.

18 Lim JA, Choi SH, Lee WJ *et al.*(2018) Cognitive-behavioral therapy for patients with chronic pain: implications of gender differences in empathy. *Medicine* **97(23)**:e10867.

19 Langford DJ, Tauben DJ, Sturgeon JA, Godfrey DS, Sullivan MD, Doorenbos AZ. (2018) Treat the patient, not the pain: using a multidimensional assessment tool to facilitate patient-centered chronic pain care. *Journal of General Internal Medicine* **33(8)**:1235–8.

20 Provensano D, Khalid K, Giannetti V. (2018) Evaluation of primary care physician chronic pain management practice patterns. *Pain Physician* **21**:E593–E602.

21 Dworkin RH, Turk DC, Wyrwich KW *et al.* (2008) Interpreting the clinical importance of treatment outcomes in chronic pain clinical trials: IMMPACT recommendations. *Journal of Pain* **9(2)**:105–21.

22 Mills SEE, Nicolson KP, Smith BH. (2019) Chronic pain: a review of its epidemiology and associated factors in population-based studies. *British Journal of Anaesthesia*. **123(2)**:e273–e83.

23 Royal Australian College of General Practioners. (2015) Prescribing drugs of dependence in generalpPractice: clinical governance framework. Royal Australian College of General Practitioners. Available at https://www.racgp.org.au/FSDEDEV/media/documents/Clinical%20Resources/Guidelines/Drugs%20of%20dependence/Prescribing-drugs-of-dependence-in-general-practice-Part-A.pdf. Accessed on 30th March 2020.

24 Moulin DE, Clark AJ, Gilron I *et al.* (2007) Pharmacological management of chronic neuropathic pain - consensus statement and guidelines

from the Canadian Pain Society. *Pain Research & Management* **12(1)**:13–21.

25 Kahan M, Mailis-Gagnon A, Wilson L, Srivastava A. (2011) Canadian guideline for safe and effective use of opioids for chronic noncancer pain clinical summary for family physicians. Part 1: general population. *J Can Fam Physician* **57(12)**:1257–66.

26 O'Brien T, Christrup LL, Drewes AM *et al.* (2017) European Pain Federation position paper on appropriate opioid use in chronic pain management. *Eur J Pain* **21(1)**:3–19.

27 NICE NIfHaCE. (2013) Neuropathic pain – pharmacological management. NICE clinical guideline 173. November 2013. Available at https://www.nice.org.uk/guidance/cg173/evidence/full-guideline-pdf-4840898221.

28 Centre for Clinical Practice at NICE (UK). 2013. Neuropathic Pain: The Pharmacological Management of Neuropathic Pain in Adults in Non-specialist Settings [Internet]. London: National Institute for Health and Care Excellence, (UK); (NICE Clinical Guidelines, No. 173). Available at https://www.ncbi.nlm.nih.gov/books/NBK266257/.

29 Chou R, Fanciullo GJ, Fine PG *et al.* (2009) Clinical guidelines for the use of chronic opioid therapy in chronic noncancer pain. *The Journal of Pain* **10(2)**:113–30.

30 Bates D, Schultheis BC, Hanes MC *et al.* (2019) A comprehensive algorithm for anagement of neuropathic pain. *Pain Med* **20(**Suppl 1**)**:S2–S12.

31 Dowell D, Haegerich T, Chou R. (2016) CDC guideline for prescribing opioids for chronic pain - United States. MMWR Recomm Rep. **18(65)**:1–49.

32 Finnerup NB, Attal N, Haroutounian S et al. (2015) Pharmacotherapy for neuropathic pain in adults: a systematic review and meta-analysis. *Lancet Neurology* **14(2)**:162–73.

33 Centre for Clinical Practice at NICE (UK). 2014. Osteoarthritis: care and management]. London: National Institute for Health and Care Excellence, (UK); (NICE Clinical Guidelines, No. 177.) Available at https://www.nice.org.uk/guidance/cg177/resources/osteoarthritis-care-and-management-pdf-35109757272517.

34 Abdulla A, Adams N, Bone M et al. (2013). Guidance on the management of pain in older people. *Age Ageing* **42** Suppl 1:i1–57.

35 Opioids for persistent pain: summary of guidance on good practice from the British Pain Society. *Br J Pain.* 6(1):9–10. doi:10.1177/2049463712436536 (2012).

36 Ventafridda V, Saita L, Ripamonti C, De Conno F (1985) WHO guidelines for the use of analgesics in cancer pain. I*nternational Journal of Tissue Reactions* 7(1):93–6.

37 Stanos S, Brodsky M, Argoff C *et al.* (2016) Rethinking chronic pain in a primary care setting. *Postgrad Med.* **128(5)**:502–15.

38 Machado GC, Maher CG, Ferreira PH et al. (2015) Efficacy and safety of paracetamol for spinal pain and osteoarthritis: systematic review and meta-analysis of randomised placebo controlled trials. *BMJ* **350**:h1225.

39 Wiffen PJ, Knaggs R, Derry S, Cole P, Phillips T, Moore RA. Paracetamol (acetaminophen) with or without codeine or dihydrocodeine for neuropathic pain in adults. The Cochrane Database of Systematic Reviews. **12**:CD012227.

40 Finnerup NB, Haroutounian S, Kamerman P *et al.* (2016) Neuropathic pain: an updated grading system for research and clinical practice. *Pain 157***(8)**:1599–606.

41 Centre for Clinical Practice at NICE (UK) (2013) Neuropathic pain - pharmacological management. London: National Institute for Health and Care Excellence, (UK); (NICE Clinical Guidelines, No. 173). Available at https://www.nice.org.uk/guidance/cg173/evidence/full-guideline-pdf-4840898221.

42 Ussai S, Miceli L, Pisa FE et al. (2015) Impact of potential inappropriate NSAIDs use in chronic pain. *Drug Design, Development and Therapy* **9**:2073–7.

43 Haroutiunian S, Drennan DA, Lipman AG. (2010) Topical NSAID therapy for musculoskeletal pain. *Pain Medicine.* **11(4)**:535–49.

44 Brinksman S. (2018) Opioids and chronic pain in primary care. The British Journal of General Practice **68(**675**)**:454–5.

45 Seal K, Becker W, Tighe J, Li Y, Rife T. (2017) Managing chronic pain in primary care: it really does take a village. *Journal of General Internal Medicine* **32(8)**:931–4.

46 Dobscha S, Corson K, Perrin N *et al.* (2009) Collaborative care for chronic pain in primary care: a cluster randomized trial. *JAMA* **301(12)**:1242–52.

47 Lamb SE, Hansen Z, Lall R et al. (2010) Group cognitive behavioural treatment for low-back

pain in primary care: a randomised controlled trial and cost-effectiveness analysis. *The Lancet* **375**(9718):916–23.

48 Cameron PSC. (2012) The need to define chronic pain self-management. *Journal of Pain Management* **5(3)**:231–6.

49 Wijma AJ, van Wilgen CP, Meeus M, Nijs J. (2016) Clinical biopsychosocial physiotherapy assessment of patients with chronic pain: the first step in pain neuroscience education. *Physiother Theory Pract* **32(5)**:368–84.

50 Boyers D, McNamee P, Clarke A *et al.* (2013) Cost-effectiveness of self-management methods for the treatment of chronic pain in an aging adult population: a systematic review of the literature. *Clinical Journal of Pain* **29(4)**:366–75.

51 Gordon K, Rice H, Allcock N *et al.* (2017) Barriers to self-management of chronic pain in primary care: a qualitative focus group study. *The British Journal of General Practice* **67(**656**)**:e209–e17.

52 Bawa FL, Mercer SW, Atherton RJ *et al.* Clague F, Keen A, Scott NW, et al. Does mindfulness improve outcomes in patients with chronic pain? Systematic review and meta-analysis. *The British Journal of General Practice*2015;65(635):e387–400.

53 Toye F, Andrews J, Barker K et al. (2013) Patients' experiences of chronic non-malignant musculoskeletal pain: a qualitative systematic review. *British Journal of General Practice* **63(**617**)**:e829–e41.

54 Geneen L, Moore R, Clarke C, Martin D, Colvin L, Smith B. (2017) Physical activity and exercise for chronic pain in adults: an overview of Cochrane Reviews. *Cochrane Database of Systematic Reviews* **4(4)**:CD011279.**(4)**.

55 Rausch Osthoff A-K, Niedermann K, Braun J *et al.* (2018) 2018 EULAR recommendations for physical activity in people with inflammatory arthritis and osteoarthritis. *Annals of the Rheumatic Diseases* **77(9)**:1251–60.

56 Parreira P, Heymans MW, van Tulder MW et al. (2017) Back schools for chronic non-specific low back pain. [Review]. *Cochrane Database of Systematic Reviews* **8(8)**:CD011674.

57 Magalhaes MO, Muzi LH, Comachio J *et al.* (2015) The short-term effects of graded activity versus physiotherapy in patients with chronic low back pain: a randomized controlled trial. *Manual Therapy* **20(4)**:603–9.

58 McGrane N, Galvin R, Cusack T, Stokes E. (2015) Addition of motivational interventions to exercise and traditional physiotherapy: a review and meta-analysis. *Physiotherapy* **101(1)**:1–12.

59 Loh J, Gulati A. (2015) The use of transcutaneous electrical nerve stimulation (TENS) in a major cancer center for the treatment of severe cancer-related pain and associated disability. *Pain Medicine* **16(6)**:1204–10.

60 Gibson W, Wand B, Meads C, Catley M, O'Connell N. (2019) Transcutaneous electrical nerve stimulation (TENS) for chronic pain - an overview of Cochrane Reviews. *Cochrane Database of Systematic Reviews 2019***4(4)**:CD011890.

61 Pannek J, Pannek-Rademacher S, Wollner J. (2015) Use of complementary and alternative medicine in persons with spinal cord injury in Switzerland: a survey study. *Spinal Cord* **53(7)**:569–72.

62 Haetzman M, Elliott AM, Smith BH, Hannaford P, Chambers WA. (2003) Chronic pain and the use of conventional and alternative therapy. *Family Practice* **20(2)**:147–54.

63 Cosio D, Lin EH. (2015) Effects of a pain education program in Complementary and Alternative Medicine treatment utilization at a VA medical center. *Complementary Therapies in Medicine* **23(3)**:413–22.

64 Rubinstein SM, van Middelkoop M, Assendelft WJJ, de Boer MR, van Tulder MW. (2011) Spinal manipulative therapy for chronic low-back pain an update of a Cochrane Review. *Spine* **36(13)**:E825–E46.

65 British Pain Society (BPS). Participant Information for Pain Management Programmes. 2018. Available at https://www.britishpainsociety.org/static/uploads/resources/files/pmp2013_main_FINAL_v6.pdf. Accessed on 7th September 2021.

66 AlMazrou SH, Elliott RA, Knaggs RD, AlAujan SS. (2020) Cost-effectiveness of pain management services for chronic low back pain: a systematic review of published studies. *BMC Health Serv Res* **20(1)**:194.

67 Westman A, Linton SJ, Öhrvik J, Wahlén P, Leppert J. (2008) Do psychosocial factors predict disability and health at a 3-year follow-up for patients with non-acute musculoskeletal pain?: A validation of the Örebro Musculoskeletal Pain Screening Questionnaire. *European Journal of Pain* **12(5)**:641–9.

Chapter 14

Medical nutrition therapy for chronic pain management

Andrea Glenn[1], Meaghan Kavanagh[1], Laura Bockus-Thorne[2], Lauren McNeill[3], Vesanto Melina[4], David Jenkins[1], & Shannan Grant[2,5]

[1] *Department of Nutritional Sciences, University of Toronto, Toronto, Ontario, Canada*
[2] *Department of Applied Human Nutrition, Mount Saint Vincent Hospital, Halifax, Nova Scotia, Canada*
[3] *Tasting to Thrive, Toronto, Ontario, Canada*
[4] *Nutrispeak, Vancouver, British Columbia, Canada*
[5] *Departments of Pediatrics and Obstetrics and Gynaecology, IWK Health Centre, Halifax, Nova Scotia, Canada*

Introduction

Nutrition is a cornerstone in the management of a number of chronic diseases, including cardiovascular disease (CVD) and type 2 diabetes [1]. Most commonly, pain management programs have included physical, psychosocial and medical interventions, but not nutritional interventions [2, 3] other than general recommendations to achieve and maintain a "healthy weight" to help manage chronic non-cancer pain [4]. This lack of focus on nutrition is despite evidence that patients with chronic pain have been shown to have lower diet quality and may consume diets higher in calories, fat and added sugars and lower in fruits and vegetables compared to the recommended Canadian dietary guidelines [5, 6]. Moreover, people with chronic pain have been found to choose animal-based sources of protein more often, which is also not in agreement with current dietary guidelines that recommend choosing protein that comes from plants more often [5, 6].

Diet has been identified as one of the highest care priorities for people with chronic non-cancer pain [7]. Moreover, there are physiological and metabolic data indicating patients living with chronic pain can benefit from nutrition intervention [8]. These data are promising, but limited. What is clear, however, is that current evidence supports shared decision-making [9]. Shared decision making is rooted in patient-focused care, described as approaching medical care with the feelings, mental health, perceptions and expectations of the patient in mind [10]. Commonly found in nursing literature, person-centered care takes this concept a step further, keeping the patient at the center of care, but recognizing all people working within organizations and communities, have their own needs, biases, strengths and limitations. This approach to language also aims to actively avoid victimization and hierarchical patient-provider dynamics [10].

There is emerging evidence that diet may play an important role in chronic pain management, particularly through regulating inflammatory pathways [11]. Many patients with chronic pain have elevated levels of pro-inflammatory markers, such as C-reactive protein (CRP), tumor necrosis factor

Clinical Pain Management: A Practical Guide, Second Edition. Edited by Mary E. Lynch, Kenneth D. Craig, and Philip W. Peng.

(TNF)-alpha, and interleukin (IL)-6, that can be reduced through diet [12, 13]. Undesirable alterations in the microbiome have also been documented in patients with chronic pain and/or depression, through the "microbiota-gut-brain" axis and have been associated with several chronic diseases [14]. The microbiome may provide another mechanism in which diet can positively influence outcomes in chronic pain, through promoting the development of a more diverse and stable microbiota [15]. For instance, plant-based dietary patterns, such as vegan and vegetarian diets, have been found to beneficially modulate the microbiome [15]. Most of the evidence to date in the area of diet and chronic pain management relates to pain measurement scales and inflammation.

Current literature exploring the role of diet and chronic pain

Peer-reviewed literature exploring the role between diet and chronic pain is heterogeneous and fragmentary, including a diversity of study designs, methods, interventions, outcomes, and patient populations and therefore limiting a health care team's access to high quality evidence. Systematic reviews and meta-analyses on diet and pain are lacking due to the inability to combine the different interventions together to determine their overall effect on pain outcomes. Moreover, much of this research has also focused on supplements/natural health products, such as omega-3 fatty acids (Table 14.1), rather than on whole foods and dietary patterns, which are the key focus of current chronic disease management clinical practice guidelines [1]. Table 14.1 highlights some potential nutrients that may be of concern for people living with chronic pain that should be assessed with the onset of treatment and throughout the care process.

Dietary patterns have, however, shown promise for various chronic pain conditions [8]. Most of the evidence on specific dietary patterns in chronic pain includes plant-based diets: (1) vegetarian diets that may include dairy and eggs but no meat, poultry or fish, (2) vegan diets which include no animal products or (3) dietary patterns that are mostly-plant based (i.e. a traditional Mediterranean diet that allows small amounts of meat, poultry, fish, dairy and eggs, but mostly consists of plant foods). The evidence for these dietary patterns is summarized in the following section.

Plant-based dietary patterns and pain

Using a systematic review approach, two trained and experienced reviewers (AG and MK) identified 14 intervention studies on plant-based dietary patterns and chronic pain [16–29]. The most common chronic pain condition that was investigated was rheumatoid arthritis [16, 22, 23, 25–28]. Other chronic pain conditions that were examined included: fibromyalgia [17, 21, 24], migraines [18], general chronic pain [29], osteoarthritis [20], and diabetic neuropathy [19]. The plant-based dietary pattern interventions varied considerably between the studies identified, however, all the diets shared common characteristics of being high in fiber, plant-based proteins, fruit, vegetables, nuts, and whole grains. Two studies assessed vegetarian diets [16, 29] and three studies assessed a whole foods low-fat plant-based diet (i.e. vegan) [19, 20, 26]. The remaining studies included a vegetarian dietary pattern with additional interventions such as a fasting period, raw foods only, or a gluten-free diet. Most studies were conducted over 15 years ago, with nine of the 14 being published before 2005 [16, 17, 21, 23–28]. The average length of the studies was 4.7 months, and the most common way to assess pain was through quantification of patient report using standardized tools. Thirteen of the studies assessed pain using a visual analogue pain scale (VAS), which is frequently used in standard care [30], while Towery et al. used a numeric pain rating scale [29]. Other questionnaires were used to measure additional health outcomes, such as the Health Assessment Questionnaire (HAQ) and the Short Form Health Survey (SF-36), both of which also include a VAS pain scale. Overall, 11 of the 14 studies found the plant-based diet interventions improved pain and related health outcomes. Two of the higher-quality studies, Hafström et al [23] and Clinton et al [20], included a randomized controlled trial (RCT) design, and are described in more detail below.

Hafström et al. investigated a gluten-free vegan diet over nine months in 66 patients with rheumatoid arthritis compared to the non-vegan control diet [23]. The gluten-free aspect of the diet counselled patients to replace gluten-containing foods with

Table 14.1 Potential nutrients of concern for people living with chronic pain

Nutrient	Rationale for Concern	Mechanisms	Sources (Foods and Supplements)
Magnesium	• Magnesium has been suggested as an important nutrient for chronic pain conditions [62] • This mineral is "probably effective" for **migraine prevention** [63] • While evidence in other types of chronic pain (i.e. complex regional pain syndrome and refractory chronic low back pain) exists, more research is needed [64]	• Anti-inflammatory and analgesic effects • Main mechanism is through blocking the N-methyl-D-aspartate (NMDA) receptor	• Nuts, seeds, whole grains, and legumes (beans, peas, lentils and soy foods) • Magnesium is a central mineral in the chlorophyll molecule, therefore, leafy greens are a good source • Supplementation may be considered as many patients do not consume enough magnesium-rich foods in their regular diet
Omega-3 Fatty Acids	• The Western diet provides relatively high intakes of omega-6 fatty acids along with low levels of omega-3 fatty acids • By increasing intakes of omega-3 fatty acids or omega-3 to omega-6 ratio, it is possible to decrease the production of omega-6 metabolites which may contribute to inflammation and immune dysregulation • Evidence suggests that omega-3 polyunsaturated fatty acid supplementation can reduce arthritic pain, especially in those with **rheumatoid arthritis** [65] • Fish oil was found to improve **osteoarthritis**-related pain in overweight adults [66]	• The essential omega-3 fatty acid alpha-linolenic acid (ALA) is an essential omega-3 fatty acid and can be converted into eicosapentaenoic acid (EPA) and docosahexaenoic acid (DHA) within the body, although the conversion is low • All compete for the same enzyme for elongation, thus relatively high intakes of omega-6 fatty acids reduce the already low conversion rate of ALA to long chain EPA and DHA	• ALA is found in walnuts, hempseeds, chia seeds and ground flaxseeds • EPA and DHA are mostly found in fish, however, the actual sources are other marine sources, such as algae • Algae-based supplements may be used for some patients • Fish oil has been a major commercial source of EPA and DHA, however, their original sources (algae), are available and may have additional health benefits

Vitamin D	• Deficiency is common in patients with chronic pain • Association between low levels of serum vitamin D (25-hydroxyvitamin D3) and higher pain intensity have been found [67]	• The role of vitamin D in chronic pain is not fully understood, however, this vitamin has immunoregulation and anti-inflammatory effects • High serum vitamin D associated with lower levels of inflammatory markers such as CRP	Vitamin D is found in: • Fortified foods such as non-dairy and dairy milks and margarines • Oily fish (sardines, salmon, herring etc.) • Some egg yolks • Sun-dried or UV-exposed mushrooms • Supplements are recommended for those residing in latitudes far from the equator, in urban areas with smog, those who get little sun exposure and in countries where fortification is less common (such as Europe)
Vitamin B12 (cyanocobalamin)	• Deficiency can lead to sensory symptoms or unexplained chronic pain • Deficiency is common in chronic pain populations (found to be present in 10% of people living with chronic pain) • Supplements have been shown to improve various pain conditions, such as **diabetic neuropathy** and **lower back pain**	• Major role in nervous system functioning • Co-factor in myelin formation, required for methylation of the myelin basic protein which makes up the myelin sheath around nerves	• Supplementation is recommended for those with gastrointestinal diseases, those who follow a vegetarian or vegan diet, and for those over the age of 50 years • Patients on PPIs, histamine H2-receptor antagonists or metformin are at higher risk of deficiency
Fiber	• Low fiber intake is common in the general Canadian population and in those with chronic pain [5] • Opioid-induced-constipation has been reported in 41–81% of patients receiving opioids [52, 68]	• Fiber improves bowel movements and weight management, and helps contribute to a healthy microbiome • Short-chain fatty acids are produced from soluble fiber fermentation with key roles in regulating host metabolism	• Fiber sources include fruits, vegetables, legumes and whole grains • Increase in water intake along with high fiber foods and supplements is important • Increase in fiber through plant foods and specific foods such as bran and prunes can help avoid opioid-induced constipation • Patients should be counseled to start eating a high fiber diet **prior** to starting opioids • Fiber supplementation should be started at the same time as opioid prescription

whole grains such as buckwheat and millet. The primary outcome of the study was change in patients' signs and symptoms of rheumatoid arthritis, measured by the American College of Rheumatology response criteria (ACR20) [23, 31]. After nine months, significant improvements in pain and the number of tender and swollen joints were found in patients randomized to the vegan group compared to the control group [23]. It is important to note that the gluten-free diet aspect of this study is not essential to improve chronic pain or inflammatory outcomes [16, 18–20, 26], unless the patient has diagnosed gluten sensitivity or celiac disease. Gluten-free diets can be more expensive, may be lacking in certain micronutrients (such as iron), and some gluten-free grains are of higher glycemic index [32–34], therefore, these diets should only be recommended when medically necessary and in consultation with a Registered Dietitian. Clinton et al [20] investigated a whole-foods plant-based diet (i.e. vegan) over six weeks in 40 patients with osteoarthritis compared to a control group who maintained their usual diet [20]. The primary outcome of the study was change in both pain and physical function. Significant improvements in both pain and physical function were found in the vegan group compared to the control group.

In addition to this evidence, other mostly plant-based dietary patterns, such as the Mediterranean (Med) Diet, have also been explored as medical nutrition therapy for patients with rheumatoid arthritis [35]. For example, a randomized controlled trial investigated the effects of a Med diet over 12 weeks in 51 patients with rheumatoid arthritis [36]. The Med Diet significantly improved pain and related outcomes such as disease activity (i.e. joint tenderness and swelling), physical function and quality of life when compared to a standard Western control diet. These plant-based diet interventions have been described in a recent systematic review and meta-analysis [8]. However, more research is needed to make stronger conclusions on the role of nutrition in chronic pain. As discussed, the diets investigated in chronic pain management are diverse and heterogeneous, however, the overall collection of evidence for plant-based dietary patterns is promising, especially given the breadth of evidence in support of plant-based diets in other chronic diseases, for many of which pain is often a symptom.

Specific foods for chronic pain management and inflammation

Many specific foods have been studied for their role in chronic pain and inflammation. Table 14.2 highlights some of these specific foods that have been linked to outcomes in people living with chronic pain or have been found to have anti-inflammatory or pro-inflammatory effects.

Dietary patterns for common pain comorbidities

Medical diagnoses for chronic diseases, including obesity, type 2 diabetes (T2DM) and CVD have been linked with chronic pain [37]. For example, rates of overweight and obesity have been found to be higher in those with chronic pain compared to the general population [7], although several factors are likely impacting this finding. For instance, undesired weight gain can be the result of chronic pain's impact on one's ability to shop, cook and exercise. That said, evidence implies chronic pain may be caused or exacerbated by overweight and obesity. Counseling patients on maintaining a healthy weight is often part of standard pain management, with particular evidence for those with osteoarthritis or joint pain [4]. This approach is not in agreement with recent clinical practice guidelines for the prevention and management of obesity (as a chronic disease), which is now focused on behavior-based interventions rather than on weight management or weight loss as a goal of treatment [38]. It is now well-accepted that some people can carry "extra weight" without health issues [39]. This shift away from weight loss and towards improving behaviors, such as diet, physical activity, smoking cessation and stress management, has been shown to improve evidence-based outcomes (such as glycemic control, blood lipids, blood pressure and risk of CVD and T2DM) [40, 41]. This focus on behavior may also be particularly relevant in chronic pain conditions, as many people who have chronic pain also have nutrition-related comorbidities such as hypertension, T2DM and CVD [7]. While weight loss may be beneficial for some people living with chronic pain, success in weight loss, particularly long-term, is not always possible, necessary or desired by patients [42]. It is important for healthcare providers and patients

Table 14.2 Foods to choose more or less often for chronic pain management

Food Group	Foods to Choose More often	Foods to Choose Less Often
Fruits & Vegetables [11]	All fruits and vegetables are healthy options, but ones of special note include: **Fruit**: apples, berries, citrus fruit, grapes, olives, tomatoes **Vegetables**: cruciferous vegetables (broccoli, cauliflower, cabbage, kale, Brussel sprouts, etc.)	**Not applicable**
Protein Foods [11]	**Legumes**: such as beans, peas and lentils, and particularly soybeans/tofu/tempeh/other soy products **Nuts and seeds:** such as almonds, pistachios and walnuts, sunflower seeds and pumpkin seeds **Dairy and soy:** yogurt/probiotic yogurt, and low-fat dairy/cheese, soymilk **Fatty fish**: such as mackerel, salmon, sardines, tuna **Eggs** **Lean poultry:** skin removed	**Red meat:** such as beef, pork and lamb **Processed meats:** such as sausages, ham, bacon, salami, hot dogs, smoked meat, cold cuts, etc.
Grains & Starches [11]	**Whole grains:** such as millet, oats, amaranth, quinoa, barley, bulgur, whole grain breads, whole grain pasta, brown rice, etc.	**High glycemic index foods and refined grains:** such as foods that are ultra-processed or high in added sugars, products made from white flour, white rice, crackers, etc.
Oils/Fats [11]	**Omega-3 fatty acids**: eicosapentaenoic acid (EPA) & docosahexaenoic acid (DHA) from fatty fish and fish oils, and plant-based sources, such as seaweed and algae, and alpha-linolenic acid (ALA) sources like walnuts, and ground flax, chia and hemp seeds **Monounsaturated fatty acids:** such as avocado/avocado oil, canola oil, olive oil, peanut oil, sesame oil	**High saturated fat sources**: such as butter, palm oil **Omega-6 fatty acids**: such as corn oil, safflower oil, soybean oil, sunflower oil. These oils do not need to be avoided, however, a higher ratio of omega-3 to omega-6 fatty acids is more desirable for inflammation, therefore, recommendation of omega-3 sources is important
Other [11]	**Water**: adequate hydration **Dark chocolate**: > 70% cocoa solids	**Sugar-sweetened beverages**: such as soda, fruit drinks or beverages **Sweets**: such as pastries, cookies and candies **Fried foods**: such as French fries, potato chips, other fried foods

to have a firm understanding of adiposity-based chronic disease, body diversity and behavior change theory and practice if embarking on lifestyle support, as many of these behaviors are intersectional [38]. For example, many patients can have multiple sociodemographic, genetic and other factors that impact their risk for chronic disease, some of which cannot be changed or would be difficult to change due to pain impacting their daily activities. Focusing on behavior change should include readiness assessment, evidence-based counseling techniques and SMART goals when appropriate [43]. For example, using Table 14.2, patients may be able to change some of the foods they eat that fall under the "choose less often" category with foods under the "choose more often" category. This modification could include a simple swap of a high-glycemic refined grain (i.e. white rice) to a low-glycemic index whole grain (i.e. quinoa) at their meal. Another example could include swapping red meat for a plant-based protein (such as legumes, like lentils or soy).

Although some believe weight loss is the main mechanism by which plant-based dietary patterns may improve pain outcomes, other researchers have found that weight reduction did not correlate with improvements in measures of pain or function [44]. Although warranting further investigation, the mechanisms behind why plant-based dietary patterns improve pain outcomes may be related to improvement of underlying conditions such as inflammation, the microbiome and other evidence-based health outcomes (i.e. glycemic control, cholesterol, etc-). It is well documented that inflammation is typically high in both chronic pain [12] and cardiometabolic disease [45]. Therefore, dietary recommendations for T2DM and CVD may also be beneficial for people living with chronic pain. Dietary patterns that are beneficial for cardiometabolic disease and inflammation can be found in Table 14.3. With exceptions for vegetarian, vegan and Mediterranean diets, as discussed previously, these diets do not have direct evidence for chronic pain management. However, an important connection between these dietary patterns is that they are all largely plant-based and high in fiber, with high intakes of fruit, vegetables, legumes, nuts and whole grains. In general, plant-based dietary patterns often consist of lower intakes of saturated fat, added

Table 14.3 Dietary patterns recommended for cardiometabolic disease prevention and management

Dietary Pattern	Description of the Diet
Vegan diet[1] [69-71]	Devoid of all animal products
Vegetarian diet[1] [70, 71]	Contains no meat, fish, or poultry, includes dairy and/or eggs
Mediterranean diet [72, 73]	Traditional way of eating in countries along the Mediterranean Sea. The diet is high in fruits and vegetables, whole grains, legumes, nuts, and olive oil
Low glycemic index (GI) diet [74, 75]	A dietary pattern that focuses on consuming carbohydrate-containing foods that have a low GI (the GI is a scale that ranks carbohydrate-containing foods by how much they raise blood glucose compared to a standard food)
Portfolio diet[1] [76]	Originally developed to lower low-density lipoprotein (LDL) cholesterol. The diet is low in saturated fat and cholesterol and emphasizes plant protein (mainly soy), nuts, viscous fiber sources (such as psyllium, oats and barley), plant sterols, and heart healthy oils (olive, canola, avocado, soy, etc.)
Dietary approaches to stop hypertension (DASH) diet [77]	Originally developed to treat high blood pressure. The diet emphasizes fruits, vegetables, low-fat dairy, whole grains, nuts and legumes, and limits red and processed meats, sugary foods and sodium
Nordic diet [78]	Traditional way of eating in the Nordic countries. The diet is rich in rich in root vegetables, cabbage, fish, rye bread, oats, berries, apples and pears

[1] See Davis B, Melina V. (2014). Becoming Vegan: Comprehensive Eduction. Book Publishing Company, Summertown. This book is a fully referenced, 611-page book written by two registered dieticans and geared to health professionals and those wanting in-depth information) that covers every aspect of plant-based eating. It includes material on rheumatoid and osteoarthritis, diabetes and peripheral neuropathy, the Portfolio diet, chronic diseases, pain control and essential fatty acids.

sugars[nd caloric intake compared to typical Western diets that include more animal products, making the former more in line with dietary recommendations for healthy eating [6, 46].

Other Nutrition Considerations

Medications and nutrition

Patients with chronic pain may be prescribed medications that can interfere with nutrient absorption and cause nutrient depletion and other unwanted side effects that may impact their diet. Such common medications include nonsteroidal anti-inflammatory drugs (NSAIDs), antidepressants, anticonvulsants, opioids and cannabinoids. Medical nutrition assessment includes pharmacotherapy and complementary/integrative medicine use (including prescription and over-the counter medications, and herbal and natural health products), with particular attention to food-drug interactions. In agreement with interdisciplinary practice guidelines, clinicians should collaborate with Registered Dietitians to ensure an appropriate comprehensive assessment is completed and any side effects from medications, natural health products and cannabinoids are assessed, monitored and evaluated. Four examples of pharmacological treatments that would be relevant to nutrition assessment include:

1 NSAIDs: Aspirin may deplete vitamin C levels [47] and cause gastric mucosal injury, which can impact dietary intake. Patients may benefit from vitamin C supplementation [48]. The microbiome may also be negatively impacted by proton-pump inhibitors (PPIs) typically prescribed for preventing or treating NSAID-induced damage [49].

2 Antidepressants: Patients taking selective serotonin reuptake inhibitors (SSRIs) may have an increased risk of osteoporosis [50]. Calcium and vitamin D supplementation may be necessary. Some antidepressants increase fatigue and impact appetite, leading to impacts on diet quality and nutritional risk [51].

3 Opioids: Constipation is one of the most common side-effects from opioid use [52]. Treatment can include a high-fiber diet (see Table 14.1), increased fluid intake and increased physical activity started with onset of treatment. Registered Dietitians can work closely with patients to ensure fibers and foods are selected that satisfy evidence-based approaches to treatment of constipation, the patients' preferences, adverse reactions to food and sensitivities and to avoid micronutrient depletion.

4 Cannabinoids: May increase appetite [53], which may lead to increased intake. Data on this patient population indicate higher intake of ultra-processed, calorie dense foods in comparison to the general population, which leads to the assumption that cannabinoids may increase intake of these foods. Despite this concern, there is insufficient evidence to conclude that the increase in appetite from cannabinoids causes weight gain in this patient population [54].

Chronic pain and food behaviors

As highlighted above, the role of nutrition in chronic pain management has focused on weight loss. Nevertheless, after reviewing the literature, it is clear that dietary choices, weight and chronic pain are strongly linked. For example, individuals with chronic pain may consume ultra-processed and fast foods due to their convenience or use these foods as a means of comfort for their pain [55]. Another study found that patients with chronic pain reported that they commonly experience hedonic hunger triggered by physical pain, and/or emotional or binge-eating in response to pain [56]. Other studies have found that pain severity was associated with higher intakes of added sugars and fat [57]. Diet and chronic pain are much more complex than simply cravings for comfort food, and the pain itself may be why some patients are not eating according to national dietary guidelines.

People with chronic pain may also have other food-related issues, such as difficulty cooking, opening food packaging, and changes in appetite related to their pain or other life circumstances. For example, many individuals with chronic pain experience depression, social isolation and mobility issues [37]. These factors can contribute to poor appetite and/or impaired nutritional intake. Results from observational studies comparing the nutritional intake of patients with chronic pain (i.e. chronic musculoskeletal pain and fibromyalgia) to those without chronic pain have found that people living with chronic pain have lower intakes of total calories, protein and certain micronutrients (such as calcium, zinc, magnesium, vitamin D and vitamin A) [58–60]. This impaired nutritional intake can lead to malnutrition, which is of particular concern for elderly patients. Patients with chronic pain may therefore benefit from malnutrition screening and nutrition risk assessment.

Importance of equity, diversity, inclusion and accessibility when providing care

Patients' values and preferences should always be considered when providing nutrition recommendations. Patient-centered approaches include the consideration that chronic pain is personal and subjective. As discussed in the section on dietary patterns for common pain comorbidities, solely focusing on weight loss for managing chronic pain is not evidence-based, may not be accessible for all people living with chronic pain (i.e. those with mobility issues) and may increase risk for disordered eating behaviors or eating disorders. Clinicians need to consider barriers to adherence to diet, including: the cost of food, food intolerances or allergies, gastrointestinal side effects, culinary skills, pain affecting dietary habits, mobility and cultural and environmental considerations. A Registered Dietitian can work with the team and patient to find a dietary pattern that can result in long-term adherence while improving chronic pain and other health outcomes.

Overall, chronic pain can negatively impact a patient's culinary skills, eating habits and diet quality. Clinicians should ask their patients about food shopping, preparation and consumption habits and refer patients to the appropriate healthcare provider to assist with any food-related concerns as needed (i.e. Registered Dietitians, Mental Health Specialists/ Psychologists, Occupational Therapists, Social Workers).

Conclusions

Based on the current literature, there is promising evidence that plant-based dietary patterns (i.e. vegan, vegetarian or Mediterranean) can be beneficial for chronic pain management, possibly due to the anti-inflammatory effects of these diets. However, more rigorous and high-quality randomized controlled trials are needed to confirm these findings. Many people with chronic pain also experience other nutrition-related comorbidities (obesity, CVD and T2DM). Thus, diets centered on fruits, vegetables, whole grains, nuts, healthy oils and plant protein and that minimize foods high in saturated fat (i.e. red and processed meats, butter, etc.), added sugars and refined grains, are generally beneficial and recommended, as highlighted in Tables 14.2 and 14.3.

Given the strong links between diet and health outcomes applicable to people living with chronic pain, patients should frequently undergo nutritional assessment and counseling. This nutritional assessment should be initiated early on in their treatment. For this to happen effectively, pain clinics need to have nutrition included in their screening procedures (e.g. malnutrition screening). Multiple tools are available to assess for malnutrition, such as the Canadian Nutrition Screening Tool (CNST) [61]. Each tool has been designed for a specific population and setting, and only some can be administered by non-dietitians. For example, the CNST does not need to be administered by a nutrition professional and is an easy and simple tool that can be administered by several healthcare providers if a Registered Dietitian is not available. However, the inclusion of Registered Dietitians to the interprofessional pain team is recommended to support patient self-management in nutrition.

References

1 Anderson TJ, Grégoire J, Pearson GJ *et al.* (2016) 2016 Canadian Cardiovascular Society Guidelines for the Management of Dyslipidemia for the Prevention of Cardiovascular Disease in the Adult. *Canadian Journal of Cardiology* **32(11)**:1263–82.

2 Busse JW, Craigie S, Juurlink DN *et al.* (2017) Guideline for opioid therapy and chronic non-cancer pain. *Canadian Medical Association Journal* 189**(18)**:E659.

3 CADTH. Non-pharmacological methods for managing chronic pain: preventive methods 2020. Available at www.cadth.ca/sites/default/files/tools/Chronic%20Pain/Clinician%20Resources/National%20versions/clinician_summary_preventive_FINAL.pdf. Accessed on 3rd December 2020.

4 CADTH. Body weight modification interventions for chronic non-cancer pain: a review of clinical effectiveness 2020. Available athttps://www.cadth.

ca/body-weight-modification-interventions-chronic-non-cancer-pain-review-clinical-effectiveness. Accessed on 3rd December 2020.

5 Meleger AL, Froude CK, Walker J, 3rd. (2014) Nutrition and eating behavior in patients with chronic pain receiving long-term opioid therapy. *PM R* **6(1)**:7–12.e1.

6 Health Canada. Canada's Food Guide 2019. Available at https://food-guide.canada.ca/en/. Accessed on 3rd December 2020.

7 Brain K, Burrows T, Rollo ME, Hayes C, Hodson FJ, Collins CE. (2017) Population characteristics in a tertiary pain service cohort experiencing chronic non-cancer pain: weight status, comorbidities, and patient goals. *Healthcare (Basel)* **5(2)**.28.

8 Brain K, Burrows TL, Rollo ME *et al.* (2019) A systematic review and meta-analysis of nutrition interventions for chronic noncancer pain. *J Hum Nutr Diet* **32(2)**:198–225.

9 Satterfield JM, Spring B, Brownson RC *et al.* (2009) Toward a transdisciplinary model of evidence-based practice. *Milbank Q* **87(2)**:368–90.

10 McCormack B, Borg M, Cardiff S *et al.* (2015) Person-centredness - the 'state' of the art. *Int Pract Dev J* **5**:1–15.

11 Rondanelli M, Faliva MA, Miccono A *et al.* (2018) Food pyramid for subjects with chronic pain: foods and dietary constituents as anti-inflammatory and antioxidant agents. *Nutr Res Rev* **31(1)**:131–51.

12 Zhang J-M, An J. (2007) Cytokines, inflammation, and pain. *Int Anesthesiol Clin* **45(2)**:27–37.

13 Eichelmann F, Schwingshackl L, Fedirko V, Aleksandrova K. (2016) Effect of plant-based diets on obesity-related inflammatory profiles: a systematic review and meta-analysis of intervention trials. *Obesity Reviews* **17(11)**:1067–79.

14 Li S, Hua D, Wang Q *et al.* (2020 The role of bacteria and its derived metabolites in chronic pain and depression: recent findings and research progress. *Int J Neuropsychopharmacol* **23(1)**:26–41.

15 Tomova A, Bukovsky I, Rembert E *et al.* (2019) The effects of vegetarian and vegan diets on gut microbiota. *Front Nutr* **6**:47.

16 Adam O, Beringer C, Kless T *et al.* (2003) Anti-inflammatory effects of a low arachidonic acid diet and fish oil in patients with rheumatoid arthritis. *Rheumatology International* **23(1)**: 27–36.

17 Azad KA, Alam MN, Haq SA *et al.* (2000) Vegetarian diet in the treatment of fibromyalgia. *Bangladesh Med Res Counc Bull* **26(2)**:41–7.

18 Bunner AE, Agarwal U, Gonzales JF, Valente F, Barnard ND. (2014) Nutrition intervention for migraine: a randomized crossover trial. *J Headache Pain* **15(1)**:69.

19 Bunner AE, Wells CL, Gonzales J, Agarwal U, Bayat E, Barnard ND. (2015) A dietary intervention for chronic diabetic neuropathy pain: a randomized controlled pilot study. *Nutrition & Diabetes* **5(5)**:e158–e.

20 Clinton CM, O'Brien S, Law J, Renier CM, Wendt MR. (2015) Whole-foods, plant-based diet alleviates the symptoms of osteoarthritis. *Arthritis* **2015**:708152.

21 Donaldson MS, Speight N, Loomis S. (2001) Fibromyalgia syndrome improved using a mostly raw vegetarian diet: an observational study. *BMC Complement Altern Med* **1**:7.

22 Elkan AC, Sjöberg B, Kolsrud B, Ringertz B, Hafström I, Frostegård J. (2008) Gluten-free vegan diet induces decreased LDL and oxidized LDL levels and raised atheroprotective natural antibodies against phosphorylcholine in patients with rheumatoid arthritis: a randomized study. *Arthritis Res Ther* **10(2)**:R34.

23 Hafström I, Ringertz B, Spångberg A *et al.* (2001) A vegan diet free of gluten improves the signs and symptoms of rheumatoid arthritis: the effects on arthritis correlate with a reduction in antibodies to food antigens. *Rheumatology (Oxford)* **40(10)**:1175–9.

24 Kaartinen K, Lammi K, Hypen M, Nenonen M, Hanninen O, Rauma AL. (2000) Vegan diet alleviates fibromyalgia symptoms. *Scand J Rheumatol* **29(5)**:308–13.

25 Kjeldsen-Kragh J, Haugen M, Borchgrevink CF *et al.* (1991) Controlled trial of fasting and one-year vegetarian diet in rheumatoid arthritis. *Lancet* **338(8772)**:899–902.

26 McDougall J, Bruce B, Spiller G, Westerdahl J, McDougall M. (2002) Effects of a very low-fat, vegan diet in subjects with rheumatoid arthritis. *J Altern Complement Med* **8(1)**:71–5.

27 Nenonen MT, Helve TA, Rauma AL, Hänninen OO. (1998) Uncooked, lactobacilli-rich, vegan food and rheumatoid arthritis. *Br J Rheumatol* **37(3)**:274–81.

28 Sköldstam L, Larsson L, Lindström FD. (1979) Effect of fasting and lactovegetarian diet on rheumatoid arthritis. *Scand J Rheumatol* **8(4)**:249–55.

29 Towery P, Guffey JS, Doerflein C, Stroup K, Saucedo S, Taylor J. (2018) Chronic musculoskeletal pain and function improve with a plant-based diet. *Complement Ther Med* **40**:64–9.

30 Pain BC Society. Assessment Tools & Clinical Guidelines 2020 [Available at https://www.painbc.ca/health-professionals/assessment-tools. Accessed on 3rd December 2020.

31 Felson DT, Anderson JJ, Boers M *et al.* (1996) American College of Rheumatology. Preliminary definition of improvement in rheumatoid arthritis. *Arthritis Rheum* **38(6)**:727–35.

32 Atkinson FS, Foster-Powell K, Brand-Miller JC. (2008) International tables of glycemic index and glycemic load values: 2008. *Diabetes Care* **31(12)**:2281.

33 Jamieson JA, Gougeon L. (2017) Gluten-free foods in rural maritime provinces: limited availability, high price, and low iron content. *Can J Diet Pract Res* **78(4)**:192–6.

34 Jenkins DJ, Thorne MJ, Wolever TM, Jenkins AL, Rao AV, Thompson LU. (1987) The effect of starch-protein interaction in wheat on the glycemic response and rate of in vitro digestion. *Am J Clin Nutr* **45(5)**:946–51.

35 Forsyth C, Kouvari M, D'Cunha NM *et al.* (2018) The effects of the Mediterranean diet on rheumatoid arthritis prevention and treatment: a systematic review of human prospective studies. *Rheumatol Int* **38(5)**:737–47.

36 Sköldstam L, Hagfors L, Johansson G. (2003) An experimental study of a Mediterranean diet intervention for patients with rheumatoid arthritis. *Ann Rheum Dis* **62(3)**:208–14.

37 van Hecke O, Hocking LJ, Torrance N *et al.* (2017) Chronic pain, depression and cardiovascular disease linked through a shared genetic predisposition: analysis of a family-based cohort and twin study. *PLoS ONE* **12(2)**:e0170653.

38 Wharton S, Lau DCW, Vallis M *et al.* (2020) Obesity in adults: a clinical practice guideline. *Canadian Medical Association Journal* **192(31)**:E875.

39 Bombak A. (2014) Obesity, health at every size, and public health policy. *Am J Public Health* **104(2)**:e60–7.

40 Mozaffarian D, Kamineni A, Carnethon M, Djoussé L, Mukamal KJ, Siscovick D. (2009) Lifestyle risk factors and new-onset diabetes mellitus in older adults: the Cardiovascular Health Study. *Archives of Internal Medicine* **169(8)**:798–807.

41 Chiuve SE, Rexrode KM, Spiegelman D, Logroscino G, Manson JE, Rimm EB. (2008) Primary prevention of stroke by healthy lifestyle. *Circulation* **118(9)**:947–54.

42 Hafekost K, Lawrence D, Mitrou F, O'Sullivan TA, Zubrick SR. (2013) Tackling overweight and obesity: does the public health message match the science? *BMC Med* **11**:41.

43 Filoramo MA. (2007) Improving goal setting and goal attainment in patients with chronic noncancer pain. *Pain Management Nursing* **8(2)**:96–101.

44 Sköldstam L, Brudin L, Hagfors L, Johansson G. (2005) Weight reduction is not a major reason for improvement in rheumatoid arthritis from lacto-vegetarian, vegan or Mediterranean diets. *Nutrition Journal* **4**:15.

45 Blake GJ, Ridker PM. (2002) Inflammatory biomarkers and cardiovascular risk prediction. *J Intern Med* **252(4)**:283–94.

46 Clarys P, Deriemaeker P, Huybrechts I, Hebbelinck M, Mullie P. (2013) Dietary pattern analysis: a comparison between matched vegetarian and omnivorous subjects. *Nutr J* **12**:82.

47 Konturek PC, Kania J, Hahn EG, Konturek JW. (2006) Ascorbic acid attenuates aspirin-induced gastric damage: role of inducible nitric oxide synthase. *J Physiol Pharmacol* **57 Suppl 5**:125–36.

48 Patel V, Fisher M, Voelker M, Gessner U. (2012) Gastrointestinal effects of the addition of ascorbic acid to aspirin. *Pain Pract* **12(6)**:476–84.

49 Blackler RW, Gemici B, Manko A, Wallace JL. (2014) NSAID-gastroenteropathy: new aspects of pathogenesis and prevention. *Curr Opin Pharmacol* **19**:11–6.

50 Eom CS, Lee HK, Ye S, Park SM, Cho KH. (2012) Use of selective serotonin reuptake inhibitors and risk of fracture: a systematic review and meta-analysis. *J Bone Miner Res* **27(5)**:1186–95.

51 Riediger C, Schuster T, Barlinn K, Maier S, Weitz J, Siepmann T. (2017) Adverse effects of antidepressants for chronic pain: a systematic review and meta-analysis. *Frontiers in Neurology* **8**:307.

52 Bell TJ, Panchal SJ, Miaskowski C, Bolge SC, Milanova T, Williamson R. (2009) The prevalence, severity, and impact of opioid-induced bowel dysfunction: results of a US and European Patient Survey (PROBE 1). *Pain Med* **10(1)**:35–42.

53 Kirkham TC. (2009) Cannabinoids and appetite: food craving and food pleasure. *Int Rev Psychiatry* **21(2)**:163–71.

54 Meier MH, Caspi A, Cerdá M *et al.* (2016) Associations between cannabis use and physical health problems in early midlife: a longitudinal comparison of persistent cannabis vs tobacco users. *JAMA Psychiatry* **73(7)**:731–40.

55 Vandenkerkhof EG, Macdonald HM, Jones GT, Power C, Macfarlane GJ. (2011) Diet, lifestyle and chronic widespread pain: results from the 1958 British Birth Cohort Study. *Pain Res Manag* **16(2)**:87–92.

56 Janke AE, Kozak AT. (2012) "The more pain I have, the more I want to eat": obesity in the context of chronic pain. *Obesity (Silver Spring)* **20(10)**:2027–34.

57 Choi KW, Somers TJ, Babyak MA, Sikkema KJ, Blumenthal JA, Keefe FJ. (2014) The relationship between pain and eating among overweight and obese individuals with osteoarthritis: an ecological momentary study. *Pain Research & Management* **19(6)**:e159–e63.

58 Batista ED, Andretta A, de Miranda RC, Nehring J, Dos Santos Paiva E, Schieferdecker ME. (2016) Food intake assessment and quality of life in women with fibromyalgia. *Rev Bras Reumatol Engl Ed* **56(2)**:105–10.

59 Zick SM, Murphy SL, Colacino J. (2020) Association of chronic spinal pain with diet quality. *Pain Rep* **5(5)**:e837.

60 Kianifard T, Chopra A. (2018) In the absence of specific advice, what do patients eat and avoid? Results from a community based diet study in patients suffering from rheumatoid arthritis (RA) with a focus on potassium. *Clinical Nutrition ESPEN* **28**:214–21.

61 Nutrition Care in Canada. Canadian Nutrition Screening Tool (CNST) 2014 Available at http://www.nutritioncareincanada.ca/sites/default/uploads/files/CNST.pdf. Accessed on 3rd December 2020.

62 Kirkland AE, Sarlo GL, Holton KF. (2018) The role of magnesium in neurological disorders. *Nutrients* **10(6)**:730.

63 Silberstein SD, Holland S, Freitag F, Dodick DW, Argoff C, Ashman E. (2012) Evidence-based guideline update: pharmacologic treatment for episodic migraine prevention in adults. *Neurology* **78(17)**:1337.

64 Banerjee S, Jones S. (2017) Magnesium as an Alternative or Adjunct to Opioids for Migraine and Chronic Pain: A Review of the Clinical Effectiveness and Guidelines. Canadian Agency for Drugs and Technologies in Health, Ottawa.

65 Senftleber NK, Nielsen SM, Andersen JR *et al.* (2017) Marine oil supplements for arthritis pain: a systematic review and meta-analysis of randomized trials. *Nutrients* **9(1)**:42.

66 Kuszewski JC, Wong RHX, Howe PRC. (2020) Fish oil supplementation reduces osteoarthritis-specific pain in older adults with overweight/obesity. *Rheumatology Advances in Practice* 4**(2)**.

67 von Känel R, Müller-Hartmannsgruber V, Kokinogenis G, Egloff N. (2014) Vitamin D and central hypersensitivity in patients with chronic pain. *Pain Med* **15(9)**:1609–18.

68 Kalso E, Edwards JE, Moore RA, McQuay HJ. (2004) Opioids in chronic non-cancer pain: systematic review of efficacy and safety. *Pain* **112(3)**:372–80.

69 Le LT, Sabaté J. (2014) Beyond meatless, the health effects of vegan diets: findings from the Adventist cohorts. *Nutrients* **6(6)**:2131–47.

70 Viguiliouk E, Kendall CW, Kahleová H *et al.* (2019) Effect of vegetarian dietary patterns on cardiometabolic risk factors in diabetes: A systematic review and meta-analysis of randomized controlled trials. *Clin Nutr* **38(3)**:1133–45.

71 Glenn AJ, Viguiliouk E, Seider M *et al.* (2019) Relation of vegetarian dietary patterns with major cardiovascular outcomes: a systematic review and meta-analysis of prospective cohort studies. *Front Nutr* **6**:80.

72 Becerra-Tomás N, Blanco Mejía S *et al.* (2020) Mediterranean diet, cardiovascular disease and mortality in diabetes: A systematic review and meta-analysis of prospective cohort studies and randomized clinical trials. *Crit Rev Food Sci Nutr* **60(7)**:1207–27.

73 Estruch R, Ros E, Salas-Salvadó J *et al.* (2018) Primary prevention of cardiovascular disease with a Mediterranean diet supplemented with extra-virgin olive oil or nuts. *New England Journal of Medicine* **378(25)**:e34.

74 Livesey G, Taylor R, Livesey HF *et al.* (2019) Dietary glycemic index and load and the risk of type 2 diabetes: a systematic review and updated meta-analyses of prospective cohort studies. *Nutrients* **11(6)**.

75 Livesey G, Livesey H. (2019) Coronary heart disease and dietary carbohydrate, glycemic index, and glycemic load: dose-response meta-analyses of prospective cohort studies. *Mayo Clin Proc Innov Qual Outcomes* **3(1)**:52–69.

76 Chiavaroli L, Nishi SK, Khan TA *et al.* (2018) Portfolio dietary pattern and cardiovascular disease: a systematic review and meta-analysis of controlled trials. *Prog Cardiovasc Dis* **61(1)**:43–53.

77 Chiavaroli L, Viguiliouk E, Nishi SK *et al.* (2019) DASH dietary pattern and cardiometabolic outcomes: an umbrella review of systematic reviews and meta-analyses. *Nutrients* **11(2)**.

78 Ramezani-Jolfaie N, Mohammadi M, Salehi-Abargouei A. (2019) The effect of healthy Nordic diet on cardio-metabolic markers: a systematic review and meta-analysis of randomized controlled clinical trials. *Eur J Nutr* **58(6)**:2159–74.

Chapter 15

Physical therapy and rehabilitation

David M. Walton[1] & Timothy H. Wideman[2]

[1] *School of Physical Therapy, Western University, London, Ontario, Canada*
[2] *School of Physical and Occupational Therapy, McGill University, Montréal, Canada*

Pain and Physical Therapies

Physical therapists have long been focused on helping patients manage pain and engage in a satisfactory life trajectory. For the purposes of this chapter, physical therapy will be defined as a collective of non-pharmaceutical and non-surgical interventions. These are most commonly delivered by physical therapists / physiotherapists, but some or all may be delivered by other rehabilitation or movement-based professionals depending on local regulatory and service delivery frameworks. This chapter, an update to the prior work of Simmonds and Wideman in the first edition of this book, will not describe all possible physical therapy approaches to pain management but instead provide an overview of common frameworks, strategies, and intended outcomes of such interventions.

Physical therapy for pain has evolved over time, from a historical focus on pathomechanical understandings of pain to more contemporary biopsychosocial frameworks. Arguably the most widely-recognized health framework in physical therapy is the International Classification of Functioning, Disability, and Health (ICF) [1]. Notably for physical therapists, the ICF model recognizes that disablement and pain are influenced by sets of variables unique to each person, including predisposing risk factors, intra-individual factors (e.g. biology, lifestyle), psychosocial attributes (e.g. anxieties, fears, and coping skills) and extra-individual physical and social factors (e.g. support networks, socioeconomic status) that can affect the presence or severity of disability. As such, similar lumbar structural pathology might be barely noticed or a minor inconvenience in one person while the same type of pathology can lead to pain, distress, and significant disablement in another. Self-management and patient empowerment in managing their own pain are common hallmarks of physical therapy treatment strategies.

Perhaps one of the most notable shifts in physical therapy practice over the previous 10-15 years has been increased recognition of non-specific effects of many interventions. For example, Fuentes and colleagues [2] conducted a randomized, single blind trial of the effect of transcutaneous electrical nerve stimulation (TENS) in chronic low back pain in which both the intervention (active vs. sham TENS) and interpersonal context (limited vs. enhanced therapeutic alliance) were manipulated. Their results showed that both active and sham TENS were nearly twice as effective under the enhanced therapeutic alliance condition. When interpreted in light of a growing body of observational research showing little to no association between findings of structural pathology and pain [3,4], physical therapy has seen a shift away from highly-specific movement-based therapies to adopt more non-specific interventions that integrate person-centered biology, psychology, and socio-contextual factors into treatment decisions.

Clinical Pain Management: A Practical Guide, Second Edition. Edited by Mary E. Lynch, Kenneth D. Craig, and Philip W. Peng.

Clinical assessment

With the increasing respect for individual person-centric influences on pain and on the likelihood of successful rehabilitation, comprehensive assessment and evaluation of the patient's pain experience is a key component to targeted physical therapy. Much of this has been described in Chapters 8-11 of this book so need not be repeated here, other than to reinforce that good assessment prioritizes the patient's narrative as the closest thing to a 'gold standard' of pain currently available [5]. To this end, many physical therapy training programs have seen progressive movement towards emphasizing competencies that facilitate effective partnerships and alliances [6].

Mechanistic or phenotypic classifications of pain drivers have also seen increasing adoption by physical therapists. This information can be obtained through direct questioning and patient narratives, supplemented by questionnaires, medical diagnostics where appropriate, and clinical tests of physical function. This knowledge provides the therapist with an understanding of what modifiable factors (physical, psychological and/or social) should be targeted to positively impact pain, function and social participation.

Patient Self-report Tools

Several standardized self-report assessment measures may be used by physical therapists to measure pain, beliefs, disability and quality of life. The measures range from simple one-dimensional questionnaires that take a few seconds to complete, to complex multidimensional questionnaires that can sample a wide range of activities, thoughts and interference with social roles. Survey research has found that the most commonly used patient-reported outcome (PRO) is the simple 0-10 Numeric Pain Rating Scale (NPRS) [7]. While simple, quick, and useful as an omnibus indicator of current pain intensity, it is a non-specific tool that provides little guidance for clinical decisions. Other longer but potentially more informative measures include the Brief Pain Inventory (BPI) [8] and Pain Disability Index (PDI) [9] as generic interference scales, and region-specific tools such as the Neck Disability Index [10], Oswestry Disability Index [11], Lower Extremity Functional Scale [12] or Disabilities of the Arm, Shoulder, and Hand (DASH) scales [13]. These are intended to measure how much pain or related symptoms interfere with activity or sense of well-being. It should be noted that activity interference questions are rarely calibrated to an external criterion standard (e.g. a rating of '5' on a question of walking interference does not discriminate between walking from bed to bathroom or a long community walk), but many tools have published population-based reference norms against which individual patient scores can be compared to estimate the level of disability. These highly standardized tools can be supplemented by more patient-centered tools, such as the Patient Specific Functional Scale [14] or the Canadian Occupational Performance Measure [15] that allow patients to endorse personally-important functions. More psychologically-oriented tools, such as the Pain Catastrophizing Scale [16] or the Tampa Scale for Kinesiophobia [17], are increasingly used as prognostic or treatment modification tools, with practice frameworks evolving to better integrate their use in physical therapy.

Physical performance tests

Unlike self-report, which are based on patient perceptions, physical therapists will also use standardized performance tests to provide more quantitative information on physical ability (e.g. time, distance, strength or range of motion). While usually administered under clinically controlled conditions, when considered alongside responses to PROs and patient narrative they can provide a more comprehensive view of pain and resultant interference. Common tests include active range of motion through goniometry, timed-up-and-go, six-minute walk test, balance tasks (e.g. the star excursion [18] or Berg Balance [19] tests), and fine motor dexterity tests, among a host of others. Each source of information moves clinician and patient towards a shared understanding of the drivers of the pain experience, associated movement abilities and difficulties, and towards intervention decisions.

Other Clinical Tests

The suite of tools available to physical therapists has evolved alongside the increasing recognition of the complexities of pain. Alternative or complementary tests include measures of joint position sense error (JPSE) [20], two-point discrimination (2PD) [21], laterality recognition (measuring time and error when judging whether an image is of the left or right side of the body) [22], postural sway [23], smoothness (or 'jerk') of movement [24], and a suite of quantitative sensory tests (QST). The most common QST protocol currently in practice is measurement of pressure pain detection threshold (PPDT) through algometry. This is a psychophysical metric of mechanical pain sensitivity, most commonly tested through a handheld algometer with a 1cm^2 rubber tip applied to the skin over top of the painful region. The pain threshold is that force (pressure) at which the patient indicates the sensation has changed from pressure to pain. The average of two or three repetitions has been found to provide good reliability in clinical settings [25], and can be an indicator of local or widespread hyperalgesia / sensitization when tested over different body regions. [26] PPDT is also a common test stimulus when exploring the phenomena of conditioned pain modulation [27] or exercise-induced hyperalgesia [28], both potentially providing additional clues as to the best initial approach to managing pain and improving patient function.

Synthesizing Assessment Findings with Treatment Planning

When working with patients for whom pain is a primary complaint, physical therapists have different options based on pain acuity.

Acute pain: Physical therapists have traditionally focused on facilitating tissue healing in the acute stage of injury or pain. However, available research does not offer compelling evidence that intervention based on tissue 'stages of healing' leads to more rapid recovery.[29, 30] More recently, prognostic screening tools have been published that allow clinicians to identify the most likely recovery trajectories for patients with acute pain. Such tools exist for acute low back pain [31], acute traumatic neck pain [32], and mixed region acute pain [33, 34]. These can be used to identify those patients in the acute stage of injury that may be at greatest risk of persistent problems. A 'prognosis-based' approach to acute pain management is seeing increasing support in the literature [35, 36]. Accordingly, a reasonable approach to managing acute musculoskeletal pain is to use prognostic tools to predict outcome, identify modifiable factors in those deemed high risk of non-recovery and intervene early to prevent chronic problems, while taking a more arm's-length approach to those deemed low risk.

Chronic Pain: In the chronic pain stage, the focus shifts from prognosis to managing primary pain drivers identified through the comprehensive assessment strategies described earlier and optimizing quality of life. Critical to achieving a successful outcomes is establishing *what* a successful outcome will be for each patient. Commonly these are resumption of some aspect of lost prior life activities, social roles or general symptom reduction and ease of life, but these should not be assumed to be the only acceptable outcomes for all people. Through discussion and reflection, clinicians hear patient concerns, fears, and desires and work with them to calibrate expectations, establish milestones of improvement, and build person-centric intervention strategies.

Treatment approaches

Described below are common treatment approaches employed by physical therapists for management of pain. Intended as an overview, readers should remember that *nothing works for everyone, though everything will work for someone.*

Reassurance, activity-encouragement and education

While not all patients will need formal pain education, a common role of the physical therapist is to identify unhelpful or inaccurate beliefs and provide advice and education in a patient-centered fashion. Education commonly attempts to validate and demystify the patient's experiences of pain and help establish realistic and achievable expectations. Prior research has shown that people in pain tend to prioritize pathomechanical or biomedical explanations for pain [37] while related research suggests that strong beliefs in such explanations may contribute to beliefs that pain is associated with tissue fragility or damage, increasing experiences of fear and disablement [38,39]. Patients may benefit from reassurance from an expert that movement is safe and important for healthy tissues, and that it can facilitate pain reduction and contribute to a sense of control over pain.

Pain-related education can take many forms, and the optimal mode should be established by first understanding the knowledge base from which the patient is starting, their values, preferred learning style, and the purpose or outcomes expected as a result of the intervention. If delivered in an insensitive, patronizing, paternalistic, or generic way attempts at education can have the opposite effect – leading to further feelings of stigma or shame if the impression is that the therapist is blaming the patient for 'thinking wrong'. For those who are likely to benefit from education, options range from informational pamphlets or infographics, through streaming online video sites, websites, blogs, podcasts, books, group classes, to personally-tailored one-on-one educational sessions. An emerging competency for physical therapists lies in review and critical appraisal of these sources for their trustworthiness and relevance for different patients.

A formalized type of education, commonly referred to as *pain neuroscience education* (PNE), usually follows a curriculum that can be tailored to the patient and is delivered in a direct one-to-one fashion. Drawn from principles of cognitive therapy, this type of education covers a range of topics, from the function of peripheral tissues and nerves, through to cortical neuroplasticity and biopsychosocial interactions in the experience of pain. Evidence is mounting to suggest that when delivered in the right way, to the right patient, at the right time, PNE can significantly reduce feelings of fear and distress about pain, improve range of motion, strength, and self-efficacy [40]. Interestingly, that same evidence suggests that of all the effects of good PNE, its smallest effect is on pain severity itself, providing a sound reminder that pain, distress, and disability are related but distinct constructs.

Biophysical modalities

Physical therapists are skilled in application of several biophysical modalities that involve different forms of energy transferred to targeted tissues. Their intended therapeutic effects commonly involve one or more of: pain reduction, muscle relaxation, increased soft-tissue extensibility, increased blood circulation, inflammation reduction or stimulation of tissue healing. Commonly used biophysical agents for physical therapy management of pain include thermotherapy (heat/cold application) and transcutaneous electrical nerve stimulation (TENS) while less common modalities include low-intensity laser light therapy (LILT), shortwave diathermy (SWD), therapeutic ultrasound, and extracorporeal shockwave therapy (ESWT). Occasionally some biophysical modalities will be used in conjunction with topical creams, such as steroid-based or non-steroidal anti-inflammatory (NSAID) creams.

The empirical evidence base to support many biophysical agents in managing pain is conflicting. For example, systematic reviews of effectiveness of TENS have been recently published for conditions such as neuropathic pain[41], primary dysmenorrhea [42], fibromyalgia [43], and chronic pain in general [44]. In all such cases, the results indicate a small but significant effect of TENS (about 1 point on a 0-10 NPRS) over sham TENS, but no evidence of benefit over other interventions. A consistent finding across reviews is the generally low quality of evidence in the primary trials and inconsistencies in reporting of application and dosing, leading most review groups to report no or very low confidence in the results. However, more recent well-designed trials are emerging that indicate differential effects of TENS for pain based on intended outcome. For example, Dailey and colleagues found that a 4-week trial of home-use TENS was significantly more effective in reducing *movement-evoked pain* (rather than pain at rest) compared to sham or no TENS controls in women with fibromyalgia [45].

The evidence base for other biophysical modalities in chronic pain management reveals similar limitations to interpretation. Findings of small or no effect have been reported in recent reviews on the effectiveness of therapeutic ultrasound for chronic low back pain [46] and cryotherapy (ice) for pain from knee osteoarthritis [47]. ESWT currently enjoys a stronger body of evidence, though in highly specific conditions such as chronic pelvic pain syndrome in men [48], chronic plantar fasciitis [49], and chronic calcific tendinitis of the shoulder [50]. Both ESWT and LILT may have a small but significant beneficial effect on tenosynovitis conditions of the hand and wrist. [51]

While benefit may be limited, cost and risk of adverse outcomes are also low with proportionately low barriers to implementation. For example, the ability to apply these modalities independently at home can be empowering for the patient and may be useful as a safety net when engaging in activity reintegration. On the other hand, the explanations often used to describe the mechanisms of these modalities can reinforce beliefs in tissue-based damage, vulnerability, and fear of movement or reinjury. Therapists should engage with their patients to better understand their beliefs and expectations about pain and the mechanisms of biophysical modalities before suggesting a course of treatment. Like education, modalities are best viewed as part of a larger multimodal intervention plan, rather than a stand-alone treatment strategy.

Manual Therapies

The manual therapies represent a loosely defined collection of hands-on diagnostic and interventional techniques applied to the surface of the body. Techniques range in intensity from light touch through to high-velocity, low-amplitude thrust often called 'manipulation'. The intended purpose of manual therapies is commonly described as 'normalizing' the biomechanical relationships of targeted joint, nerve, muscle or connective tissue structures. Proposed mechanisms include effects on elastic properties or elongation of tissue, reduced local inflammation, or breaking tissue adhesions. More contemporary conceptualizations of mechanisms have shifted to more non-specific effects. These include neurophysiological effects on tonic or phasic nerve conduction, awareness of and support to painful or neglected body regions or even the documented effects of supportive direct manual contact between people [52]. Notably for chronic pain conditions, it is unlikely that pain can be fully explained by abnormal biomechanics in a particular tissue, however that does not mean manual therapies no longer hold value in these cases when applied judiciously and with clear aims.

Like education and biophysical modalities, evidence to support manual therapy as a stand-alone intervention for pain is sparse. However, a stronger body of evidence exists to support combinations of manual therapy and exercise as effective interventions for neck or low back pain. [53,54] As reporting of parameters of manual therapies in most such studies is unclear or ambiguous, the therapist must make decisions about the location, direction, duration, frequency, and vigor of manual interventions when deemed appropriate. Adverse events may be frequent especially with more vigorous techniques, but these are usually limited to transient and mild to moderate increases in pain. However, more serious adverse events have been reported, most commonly following upper cervical manipulations that may result in vertebrobasilar dissection, stroke, and even death [55]. The other most notable risk is similar to that of biophysical modalities, in that depending on how the mechanisms of action are described to the patient, the perceived need for manual therapy could reinforce unhelpful beliefs that tissues are vulnerable or that a simple cure is available when it is not. Again, physical therapists use their best judgement when deciding on the suitability of such techniques for patients.

Physical activity

A considerable body of evidence suggests that those with pain who remain physically active tend to enjoy better long-term outcomes. However, causation is often difficult to prove; it is unclear whether increased physical activity improves pain, or if those who feel better equipped to manage their pain engage in more physical activity. Nonetheless, there is at least biological rationale for the benefits of physical activity and exercise in improving functional capacity in people with chronic pain.

More difficult to establish are the precise parameters of physical activity that should be encouraged. Becoming a familiar refrain, several reviews and meta-analyses have lamented the lack of detail reported in many clinical trials regarding types of exercise, or the frequency, duration, intensity, and context that would allow clear guidelines to be endorsed [39,56]. Accordingly, physical therapists often rely on empirical evidence, clinical experience, creativity, and patient values in helping their patients identify meaningful, targeted, and engaging activity or exercise protocols. Not all exercises are built the same. It is important to explore what 'exercise' means to a patient as well as the goal of exercise. Physical therapists should have the knowledge and clinical reasoning to create an exercise program that is tailored to the patient's goals, abilities, and available resources (e.g. time, environment, equipment). By taking this approach physical therapists are increasingly leveraging principles of behavior change to create exercise programs that reward progress, with clear milestones and indicators of improvement. Eventually the progression of exercise and activity can progress from a conscious pursuit to eventually fading into an automatic way of 'being in one's body' as other life pursuits take priority. [57]

Behavioral psychology principles in physical therapy

Physical therapy training programs are increasingly adopting aspects of behavioral psychology into their curricula. Effective behavioral interventions like exercise are facilitated by considering these frameworks and concepts, and physical therapists are exploring these ideas in their interventions.

The intervention strategy known broadly as cognitive behavior therapy (CBT) is informing physical therapy interventions in interesting ways. Describing a wide range of strategies, in its broadest sense CBT is focused on challenging maladaptive thoughts and beliefs about pain and restructuring those towards healthier behaviors that allow patients to be more fully engaged with life. CBT strategies for pain are described in Chapter 26 and approaches to fear of movement in Chapter 27. There is a growing body of evidence to indicate that physical therapists can be trained to deliver 'psychologically-informed physical therapy' [58], and many of the educational and exercise interventions described previously in this chapter may function through a mechanism of challenging and changing maladaptive beliefs about pain (e.g. the belief that pain always signals tissue damage). Thought monitoring, graded exposure to feared activities, and stress management strategies have all shown evidence of improved functional outcomes [8,59] that have been adapted for use in physical therapy approaches to pain management [36].

Another approach borrowed from psychology that has recently seen increased use by physical therapists is Motivational Interviewing [60] (MI). MI has been adopted for its application to many of the challenges physical therapists face when working towards behavior change in patients. MI is useful for identifying and mitigating barriers or obstacles to engagement, rolling with resistance, overcoming ambivalence and helping patients form their own arguments in favor of adopting the new behavior. In this way MI can be useful to guide patients as they move through stages of change, from precontemplation to action and maintenance. While first described in the early 1980s, MI is relatively new to physical therapists and trained practitioners are currently working on the best approaches to integrate this largely psychological technique into traditional physical therapy strategies.

New or Alternative Interventions

While biophysical modalities, education, manual therapies and exercise/activity are longstanding cornerstones of physical therapy practice, alternative interventions are being adopted. Among others, these include use of digital technologies (e.g. wearable sensors or trackers), virtual reality, mindfulness-based meditation and awareness strategies, and acupuncture or 'dry needling' techniques.

Illusions and sensory distortions are also being used with promising effect by physical therapists managing pain. One such approach has been dubbed 'Graded Motor Imagery' (GMI) [61]. This involves a series of progressive cognitive challenges and manipulations, starting with laterality recognition (in which patients are tasked with quickly deciding whether an image is of a right or left hand), to imagined movements (e.g. imagine your affected hand closing or opening), through mirror box therapy. In mirror box therapy, the patient places the affected hand (or residual limb in the case of phantom limb pain) behind an opaque mirror and their unaffected hand on the table surface in front of the mirror, equidistant to the hidden affected hand. By visually attending to the reflected image of the unaffected hand, the patient is seeing a visual illusion of their unaffected hand occupying the space on the visual field normally reserved for the affected hand. By being coached through different movements, patients use the affected hand as much as possible while mimicking the movements with the unaffected hand, resulting in a visual illusion that the affected hand is moving with ease. The mirror box approach has been adapted to feet, entire arms and other body regions, with most evidence of effectiveness in central pain conditions[62,63]. More recently, virtual and augmented reality technologies are able to provide visual images of fully intact or functioning limbs in a 3D environment and preliminary evidence indicates promise for helping those with intractable pain find some, albeit often temporary, relief [64].

There are several other intervention strategies that physical therapists may employ, including workplace modifications, aquatic therapy and deep tissue release techniques, though we have described the most common ones. As of the end of 2020, forced by the COVID-19 pandemic, physical therapists have adapted to provide many of their services through distance-based 'telerehabilitation' platforms. These have the advantage of optimizing access for those who are unable to attend in person and are leading to new ways of thinking about physical therapy.

Summary

Maintaining or improving personal physical mobility is an important outcome for many people in pain. Physical therapists partner with their patients to assist them in overcoming functional impairments and help the patient to manage pain within their personal environment. Physical therapists are an important part of interprofessional teams who assist people presenting with complex pain problems, using their unique domain of knowledge about the body and movement in partnership with other disciplines. Together the aim is to improve quality of life and function with the goal of removing barriers to experiences of satisfaction and hope.

References

1 World Health Organization. (2001) *International Classification of Functioning, Disability and Health.* World Health Organization, Geneva.

2 Fuentes J, Armijo-Olivo S, Funabashi M *et al.* (2014). Enhanced therapeutic alliance modulates pain intensity and muscle pain sensitivity in patients with chronic low back pain: an experimental controlled study. *Phys Ther* **94(4)**:477–99.

3 Ranson CA, Kerslake RW, Burnett AF, Batt ME, Abdi S. (2005) Magnetic resonance imaging of the lumbar spine in asymptomatic professional fast bowlers in cricket. *J Bone Joint Surg Br* **87**:1111–6.

4 Takatalo J, Karppinen J, Niinimaki J *et al.* (2011) Does lumbar disc degeneration on MRI associate with low back symptom severity in young Finnish adults? *Spine (Phila Pa 1976)* **36(25)**:2180–9.

5 Wideman TH, Edwards RR, Walton DM, Martel MO, Hudon A, Seminowicz DA. (2019) The multimodal assessment model of pain. *Clin J Pain* **35**:212–21.

6 Wideman TH, Miller J, Bostick G, Thomas A, Bussières A. (2018) Advancing pain education in Canadian physiotherapy programmes: Results of a consensus-generating workshop. *Physiother Canada* **70**:24–33.

7 Macdermid JC, Walton DM, Cote P, Santaguida PL, Gross A, Carlesso L, ICON. (2013) Use of outcome measures in managing neck pain: an international multidisciplinary survey. *Open Orthop J* **7**:506–20.

8 Boersma K, Linton S, Overmeer T, Jansson M, Vlaeyen J, de Jong J. (2004) Lowering fear-avoidance and enhancing function through exposure in vivo. *A multiple baseline study across six patients with back pain. Pain* **108**:8–16.

9 Tait RC, Pollard CA, Margolis RB, Duckro PN, Krause SJ. (1987) The Pain Disability Index: psychometric and validity data. *Arch Phys Med Rehabil* **68**:438–41.

10 Vernon H, Mior S. (1991) The Neck Disability Index: a study of reliability and validity. *J Manipulative Physiol Ther* **14**:409–415.

11 Fairbank JC, Pynsent PB. (2000) The Oswestry Disability Index. *Spine (Phila Pa 1976)* **25**:2940–52; discussion 2952.

12 Binkley JM, Stratford PW, Lott SA, Riddle DL. (1999) The Lower Extremity Functional Scale (LEFS): scale development, measurement properties, and clinical application. North American Orthopaedic Rehabilitation Research Network. *Phys Ther* **79**:371–83.

13 Hudak PL, Amadio PC, Bombardier C. (1996) Development of an upper extremity outcome measure: the DASH (disabilities of the arm, shoulder and hand) [corrected]. The Upper Extremity Collaborative Group (UECG). *Am J Ind Med* **29**:602–8.

14 Westaway MD, Stratford PW, Binkley JM. (1998) The patient-specific functional scale: validation of its use in persons with neck dysfunction. *J Orthop Sports Phys Ther* **27**:331–8.

15 Law M, Baptiste S, McColl MA, Opzoomer A, Polatajko H, Pollock N. (1990) The Canadian Occupational Performance Measure: An outcome measure for occupational therapy. *Can J Occup Ther* **57**:82–7.

16 Sullivan MJL, Bishop SR, Pivik J. (1995) The Pain Catastrophizing Scale: development and validation. *Psychol Assess* **7**:524–532.

17 Roelofs J, Sluiter JK, Frings-Dresen MH *et al.* (2007) Fear of movement and (re)injury in chronic musculoskeletal pain: Evidence for an invariant two-factor model of the Tampa Scale for Kinesiophobia across pain diagnoses and Dutch, Swedish, and Canadian samples. *Pain* **131**:181–90.

18 Gribble PA, Hertel J, Plisky P. (2012) Using the star excursion balance test to assess dynamic postural-control deficits and outcomes in lower extremity injury: A literature and systematic review. *J Athl Train* **47**:339–57.

19 Berg K. (1989) Balance and its measure in the elderly: a review. *Physiother Canada* **41**:240.

20 de Vries J, Ischebeck BK, Voogt LP *et al.* (2015) Joint position sense error in people with neck pain: A systematic review. *Man Ther* **20**:736–44.

21 Ehrenbrusthoff K, Ryan CG, Grüneberg C, Martin DJ. (2018) A systematic review and meta-analysis of the reliability and validity of sensorimotor measurement instruments in people with chronic low back pain. *Musculoskelet Sci Pract* **35**:73–83.

22 Reinersmann A, Haarmeyer GS, Blankenburg M *et al.* (2010) Left is where the L is right. Significantly delayed reaction time in limb laterality recognition in both CRPS and phantom limb pain patients. *Neurosci Lett* **486**:240–5.

23 Field S, Treleaven J, Jull G. (2008) Standing balance: a comparison between idiopathic and whiplash-induced neck pain. *Man Ther* **13**:183–91.

24 Zhou Y, Loh E, Dickey JP, Walton DM, Trejos AL. (2018) Development of the circumduction metric for identification of cervical motion impairment. *J Rehabil Assist Technol Eng* **5**:205566831877798.

25 Walton DM, MacDermid JC, Nielson W, Teasell RW, Chiasson M, Brown L. (2011) Reliability, standard error, and minimum detectable change of clinical pressure pain threshold testing in people with and without acute neck pain. *J Orthop Sports Phys Ther* **41**:644–50.

26 Lluch E, Nijs J, Courtney CA *et al.* (2018) Clinical descriptors for the recognition of central sensitization pain in patients with knee osteoarthritis. *Disabil Rehabil* **40**:2836–45.

27 Martel MO, Wasan AD, Edwards RR. (2013) Sex differences in the stability of conditioned pain modulation (CPM) among patients with chronic pain. *Pain Med* **4**:1757–68.

28 Wideman TH, Finan PH, Edwards RR *et al.* (2014). Increased sensitivity to physical activity among individuals with knee osteoarthritis: relation to pain outcomes, psychological factors, and responses to quantitative sensory testing. *Pain* **155**:703–11.

29 Foster NE, Anema JR, Cherkin D *et al.* (2018) Prevention and treatment of low back pain: evidence, challenges, and promising directions. *Lancet* **391**:2368–83.

30 Teasell RWW, McClure JAA, Walton D et al. (2010) A research synthesis of therapeutic interventions for whiplash-associated disorder (WAD): part 4 - noninvasive interventions for chronic WAD. *Pain Res Manag* **15**:313–22.

31 Hill J, Lewis M, Papageorgiou AC, Dziedzic K, Croft P. (2004) Predicting persistent neck pain: a 1-year follow-up of a population cohort. *Spine (Phila Pa 1976)* **29**:1648–54.

32 Ritchie C, Hendrikz J, Kenardy J, Sterling M. (2013) Derivation of a clinical prediction rule to identify both chronic moderate/severe disability and full recovery following whiplash injury. *Pain* **154**:2198–206.

33 Hockings RL, McAuley JH, Maher CG. (2008) A systematic review of the predictive ability of the Orebro Musculoskeletal Pain Questionnaire. *Spine (Phila Pa 1976)* **33**:E494–E500.

34 Walton DM, Krebs D, Moulden D *et al.* (2016) The traumatic injuries distress scale: A new tool that quantifies distress and has predictive validity with patient-reported outcomes. *J Orthop Sports Phys Ther* **46**(**10**:920–8.

35 Hill JC, Dunn KM, Main CJ, Hay EM. (2010) Subgrouping low back pain: a comparison of the

STarT Back Tool with the Orebro Musculoskeletal Pain Screening Questionnaire. *Eur J Pain* **14**:83–89.

36 Sterling M, Smeets R, Keijzers G, Warren J, Kenardy J. (2018) Physiotherapist-delivered stress inoculation training integrated with exercise versus physiotherapy exercise alone for acute whiplash-associated disorder (StressModex): a randomised controlled trial of a combined psychological/physical intervention. *Br J Sports Med* **53(19)**:1240–7.

37 Setchell J, Costa N, Ferreira M, Makovey J, Nielsen M, Hodges PW. (2017) Individuals' explanations for their persistent or recurrent low back pain: A cross-sectional survey. *BMC Musculoskelet Disord* **18(1)**:466.

38 Grotle M, Vollestad NK, Veierod MB, Brox JI. (2004) Fear-avoidance beliefs and distress in relation to disability in acute and chronic low back pain. *Pain* **112**:343–52.

39 Shaw WS, Huang YH. (2005) Concerns and expectations about returning to work with low back pain: Identifying themes from focus groups and semi-structured interviews. *Disabil Rehabil* **27**:1269–81.

40 Moseley GL, Nicholas MK, Hodges PW. (2004) A randomized controlled trial of intensive neurophysiology education in chronic low back pain. *Clin J Pain* **20**:324–30.

41 Gibson W, Wand BM, O'Connell NE. (2017) Transcutaneous electrical nerve stimulation (TENS) for neuropathic pain in adults. *Cochrane Database Syst Rev* **9(9)**:CD011976.

42 Arik MI, Kiloatar H, Aslan B, Icelli M. (2020) The effect of tens for pain relief in women with primary dysmenorrhea: A systematic review and meta-analysis. Explore **2541**. Online ahead of print.

43 Arienti C. (2019) Is transcutaneous electrical nerve stimulation (TENS) effective in adults with fibromyalgia? A Cochrane Review summary with commentary. *J Musculoskelet Neuronal Interact* **19**:250–2.

44 Gibson W, Wand BM, Meads C, Catley MJ, O'Connell NE. (2019) Transcutaneous electrical nerve stimulation (TENS) for chronic pain - an overview of Cochrane Reviews. *Cochrane Database Syst Rev* **4(4)**:CD011090.

45 Dailey DL, Vance CGT, Rakel BA, Zimmerman MB, Embree J, Merriwether EN, Geasland KM, Chimenti R, Williams JM, Golchha M, Crofford LJ, Sluka KA. (2020) Transcutaneous electrical nerve stimulation reduces movement-evoked pain and fatigue: a randomized, controlled trial. *Arthritis Rheumatol* **72**:824–36.

46 Ebadi S, Henschke N, Forogh B et al. (2020) Therapeutic ultrasound for chronic low back pain. *Cochrane Database Syst Rev* **7(7)**:CD009169.

47 Dantas LO, Moreira R de FC, Norde FM, Mendes Silva Serrao PR, Alburquerque-Sendín F, Salvini TF. (2019) The effects of cryotherapy on pain and function in individuals with knee osteoarthritis: a systematic review of randomized controlled trials. *Clin Rehabil* **33**:1310–19.

48 Yuan P, Ma D, Zhang Y *et al.* (2019) Efficacy of low-intensity extracorporeal shock wave therapy for the treatment of chronic prostatitis/chronic pelvic pain syndrome: A systematic review and meta-analysis. *Neurourol Urodyn* **38**:1457–66.

49 Sun K, Zhou H, Jiang W. (2020) Extracorporeal shock wave therapy versus other therapeutic methods for chronic plantar fasciitis. *Foot Ankle Surg* **26**:33–8.

50 Wu YC, Tsai WC, Tu YK, Yu TY. (2017) Comparative effectiveness of nonoperative treatments for chronic calcific tendinitis of the shoulder: a systematic review and network meta-analysis of randomized controlled trials. *Arch Phys Med Rehabil* **98:1678**-92.e6.

51 Ferrara PE, Codazza S, Cerulli S, Maccauro G, Ferriero G, Ronconi G. (2020) Physical modalities for the conservative treatment of wrist and hand's tenosynovitis: A systematic review. *Semin Arthritis Rheum* **50**:1280–90.

52 Ditzen B, Neumann ID, Bodenmann G *et al.* (2007) Effects of different kinds of couple interaction on cortisol and heart rate responses to stress in women. *Psychoneuroendocrinology* **32**:565–74.

53 Geisser ME, Wiggert EA, Haig AJ, Colwell MO. (2005) A randomized, controlled trial of manual therapy and specific adjuvant exercise for chronic low back pain. *Clin J Pain* **21**:463–70.

54 Miller J, Gross A, D'Sylva J *et al.* (2010) Manual therapy and exercise for neck pain: A systematic review. *Man Ther* **15(4)**:334–54.

55 Ernst E. (2007) Adverse effects of spinal manipulation: a systematic review. *J R Soc Med* **100**:330–8.

56 Gross AR, Paquin JP, Dupont G *et al.* (2016) Exercises for mechanical neck disorders: A Cochrane review update. *Man Ther* **24**:25–45.

57 Leder D. (1990) *The Absent Body*. University of Chicago Press, Chicago. Available at https://press.uchicago.edu/ucp/books/book/chicago/A/bo3622735.html. Accessed Dec 17 2020.

58 Lentz TA, Beneciuk JM, Bialosky JE *et al.* (2016) Development of a yellow flag assessment tool for orthopaedic physical therapists: results from the optimal screening for prediction of referral and outcome (OSPRO) Cohort. *J Orthop Sports Phys Ther* **46**:327–43.

59 Ong AD, Zautra AJ, Reid MC. (2010) Psychological resilience predicts decreases in pain catastrophizing through positive emotions. *Psychol Aging* **25**:516–23.

60 Miller WR, Rollnick S. (2002 *Motivational Interviewing: Preparing People for Change*. Guilford Press, New York.

61 Moseley GL. (2004) Graded motor imagery is effective for long-standing complex regional pain syndrome: a randomised controlled trial. *Pain* **108**:192–8.

62 Campo-Prieto P, Rodríguez-Fuentes G. (2018) Effectiveness of mirror therapy in phantom limb pain: a literature review. *Neurologia* **S0213**-4852(**18**)30201–9. Online ahead of print.

63 Méndez-Rebolledo G, Gatica-Rojas V, Torres-Cueco R, Albornoz-Verdugo M, Guzmán-Muñoz E. (2017) Update on the effects of graded motor imagery and mirror therapy on complex regional pain syndrome type 1: A systematic review. *J Back Musculoskelet Rehabil* **30**:441–449.

64 Tong X, Wang X, Cai Y *et al.* (2020) "I dreamed of my hands and arms moving again": a case series investigating the effect of immersive virtual reality on phantom limb pain alleviation. *Front Neurol* **11**:876.

Part 4

Pharmacotherapy

Chapter 16

Antidepressant analgesics in the management of chronic pain

Katharine N. Gurba[1] **& Simon Haroutounian**[1]

[1] *Washington University Pain Center and Department of Anesthesiology, Washington University School of Medicine, St. Louis, Missouri, USA*

Introduction

Antidepressants are important analgesic adjuncts in the treatment of chronic non-cancer pain. This chapter is based on systematic reviews of high-quality randomized clinical trials of antidepressant agents in multiple chronic non-cancer pain conditions [1-9].

Three classes of antidepressant agents have been widely tested for efficacy in chronic pain: tricyclic antidepressants (TCAs), serotonin-norepinephrine reuptake inhibitors (SNRIs) and selective serotonin reuptake inhibitors (SSRIs). Currently, several TCAs and SNRIs are FDA-approved for treatment of chronic pain.

TCAs currently in common clinical use include amitriptyline, nortriptyline, imipramine and desipramine. Additionally, there are also closely-related tetracyclic antidepressant medications, mirtazapine and maprotiline. The first TCA, imipramine, was approved for treatment of depression in 1959 [10]. Within two years, publications also reported efficacy in myalgia, facial pain and headache. TCAs are now considered first-line treatment in several chronic pain conditions. TCAs act at multiple molecular targets; they inhibit presynaptic serotonin and norepinephrine reuptake transporters and block additional targets including voltage-gated sodium channels [11], adrenergic α1 and α2 receptors, histamine H1 receptors and muscarinic receptors [10]. Each of these receptor targets has been associated with increased pain or neuronal hypersensitivity [12], and the non-selective mechanisms of TCAs may contribute to analgesic efficacy in multiple conditions. However, due to this broad pharmacologic profile, TCAs are often associated with multiple side effects including xerostomia, urinary retention, orthostasis and sedation. Therefore, interest grew in developing antidepressants with fewer side effects.

Emerging evidence on the monoamine hypothesis of depression in the 1960s suggested that low serotonin levels played a role in major depressive disorder [13,14]. Consequently, pharmaceutical companies focused efforts on developing inhibitors of the serotonin reuptake transporter, culminating in the approval of fluoxetine in 1987. Other SSRIs tested in chronic pain include sertraline, paroxetine, citalopram and escitalopram. Several small trials found that SSRIs were more effective than placebo in conditions including diabetic peripheral neuropathy, headache and somatoform disorder; however, a 2016 narrative review concluded that a meta-analysis of SSRI chronic pain trials was impossible due to trial heterogeneity, quality and risk of bias [15].

Serotonin-norepinephrine reuptake inhibitors, developed shortly after SSRIs, proved more efficacious in treatment of chronic pain. This pharmacologic class includes the medications duloxetine,

Clinical Pain Management: A Practical Guide, Second Edition. Edited by Mary E. Lynch, Kenneth D. Craig, and Philip W. Peng.

venlafaxine, desvenlafaxine and milnacipran. Their most common side effects include nausea, constipation, fatigue and xerostomia. However, these effects often tend to abate with continuing therapy [16].

Pharmacological mechanisms

There is well-established, complex interplay between pain and emotion. However, trials have clearly demonstrated that the analgesic effects of antidepressants are not solely due to their effects on mood [17]. Additionally, analgesic effects tend to occur more quickly and at lower doses than antidepressant effects [18]. One important analgesic mechanism seems to involve modulation of ascending pain signals by central monoaminergic pathways [12,19,20]. Descending noradrenergic pathways arise from the locus coeruleus and project to the spinal cord. Norepinephrine (NE) binds to multiple subtypes of adrenoreceptors, but inhibitory α2 receptors have been most commonly implicated for pain modulation. Of note, these receptors are also highly expressed in brain regions important for pain processing, including periaqueductal gray, rostral ventromedial medulla (RVM), thalamus, prefrontal cortex and amygdala.

Central serotonergic pain modulation is rather complex. Descending projections from the RVM evoke spinal release of serotonin (5-HT), which can inhibit or facilitate pain signaling depending on which 5-HT receptor is activated. Preclinical research suggests that 5-HT1 receptor subtypes, which are Gi/Go coupled G-protein coupled receptors (GPCRs), may inhibit nociceptive pathways. Conversely, 5-HT2 receptors (which are Gq-coupled GPCRs) and 5-HT3 receptors (which are cation channels) may facilitate nociceptive pathways.

TCAs share a tricyclic chemical structure and can be divided to secondary amines and tertiary amines, depending the on the number of methyl (-CH3) groups on the side chain nitrogen. Secondary amine TCAs (nortriptyline, desipramine) result from the demethylation of tertiary amines (amitriptyline and imipramine, respectively), and typically have higher affinity to norepinephrine transporter than to serotonin transporter. In tertiary amines, this ratio is reversed. In addition, secondary amines have lower affinity to muscarinic acetylcholine receptors and thus have a lower likelihood of anticholinergic side effects, especially at low doses. There are some differences among tertiary amine TCAs as well. The affinity of imipramine to block histaminergic H1 receptors, for example, is lower than of amitriptyline [21]; therefore, it might be less sedating.

TCAs are metabolized by the hepatic cytochrome P450 (CYP450) system. Tertiary amine TCAs can be metabolized by multiple CYP450 systems (e.g., CYP1A2, CYP2C19 and CYP2D6). Desipramine and nortriptyline are metabolized almost exclusively by CYP2D6, and thus may be substantially affected by genetic polymorphisms of the CYP2D6 enzyme [21]. All TCAs have excellent oral bioavailability, and have long enough plasma elimination half-lives to allow once-daily administration.

The analgesic mechanism of SNRIs is assumed to be similar to that of TCAs in terms of serotonin and norepinephrine reuptake inhibition, but both venlafaxine and duloxetine have very low affinity to cholinergic, adrenergic and histaminergic receptors. In addition, venlafaxine is more selective to the serotonin transporter in lower doses.

Safety profile

Tricyclic antidepressants

Common side effects of TCAs include drowsiness, dry mouth, urinary retention, constipation, weight gain and orthostatic hypotension [9]. Other effects can include increased intraocular pressure, increased risks of falls in elderly, palpitations, QT prolongation and arrhythmias at high doses. TCAs should not be combined with other QT-prolonging drugs. They should be used with caution when combined with other serotonergic agents to minimize the risk of serotonin syndrome [22] and in epileptic patients as TCAs can reduce the threshold for seizures [23].

Serotonin-norepinephrine reuptake inhibitors

The most common side effects of SNRIs include nausea, drowsiness and dizziness. Gastrointestinal side effects such as constipation, diarrhea and dry mouth are often reported[9]. SNRIs, similar to SSRIs, may affect the effects of serotonin on platelets, and increase the risk of bleeding, particularly in the GI tract in patients on chronic anticoagulant or antiplatelet therapy[24]. Venlafaxine may also cause sweating, weight loss, and headaches. Hypertension has been reported in 3–13% of subjects, especially with high doses of 375 mg/day [25].

Chronic pain conditions

Neuropathic pain

Neuropathic pain is defined as pain caused by a lesion or disease of the somatosensory nervous system. Most antidepressant pain research has focused on neuropathic pain, and both TCAs and SNRIs are considered first-line agents in multiple neuropathic pain conditions. Current IASP Neuropathic Pain Special interest group (NeuPSIG) guidelines regarding pharmacologic treatment of neuropathic pain were updated based on a systematic review and meta-analysis of randomized controlled trials published (or unpublished but with results available) between 1966 and 2014 [1]. Subjects' diagnoses included post-herpetic neuralgia, diabetic and non-diabetic painful polyneuropathy (DPPN, PPN), post-amputation pain, post-traumatic or post-surgical neuropathic pain (including plexus avulsion and complex regional pain syndrome type II), central post-stroke pain (CPSP), spinal cord injury (SCI) pain and multiple sclerosis (MS)-associated pain. Studies included in the meta-analysis were randomized, double-blind, placebo- or first-line drug-controlled trials with a parallel group or crossover design, at least ten patients per group and a primary outcome measure of neuropathic pain intensity. For each antidepressant class, the authors calculated the number needed to treat (NNT) for 50% pain intensity reduction (or 30% pain reduction, or at least moderate pain relief) and number needed to harm (NNH) for one patient to drop out of the study due to adverse effects.

Fifteen studies of tricyclic antidepressants were included in the meta-analysis: nine with amitriptyline (75–150 mg), two with desipramine alone (25–250 mg), one with nortriptyline alone (100 mg), one with nortriptyline and desipramine (160 mg), one with maprotiline (75 mg) and one with imipramine (150 mg). The majority of studies focused on painful polyneuropathy (seven studies) or post-herpetic neuralgia (three studies). One study focused on each of: central post-stroke pain, spinal cord injury, peripheral nerve injury, painful radiculopathy and multiple sclerosis. All studies demonstrated analgesic effects except two: amitriptyline 100 mg was ineffective for HIV-associated neuropathy and nortriptyline 100 mg was ineffective for painful radiculopathy. Overall, these studies provided moderate-quality evidence for efficacy of tricyclic antidepressants in most studied neuropathic pain conditions, with a combined NNT of 3.6 and NNH of 13.4. There was no apparent dose-response effect. Ultimately, TCAs were strongly recommended as first-line treatment.

Ten studies of SNRIs were included in this meta-analysis: seven with duloxetine (40–120 mg), two with venlafaxine (150–225 mg) and one with desvenlafaxine (50–400 mg). Again, most studies focused on subjects with DPPN, while one focused on mixed PPN and one on multiple sclerosis. Duloxetine and venlafaxine were efficacious in all included studies, while desvenlafaxine results were unavailable. Of note, two studies included in the systematic review but excluded from meta-analysis showed no benefit of venlafaxine over placebo in peripheral nerve injury or mixed neuropathic pain conditions. Overall, the studies included in this meta-analysis provided high-quality evidence for SNRI efficacy in neuropathic pain, with a combined NNT of 6.4 and NNH of 11.8. Therefore, SNRIs were also recommended as first-line agents in neuropathic pain.

Several placebo-controlled randomized controlled trials (RCTs) of SNRIs in neuropathic pain have been conducted since 2014. Both duloxetine and (to a lesser extent) venlafaxine reduced pain associated with chemotherapy-induced peripheral neuropathy [26]. Duloxetine was effective in patients with chronic low back pain and concomitant radicular pain [27]. Two other studies found that duloxetine improved DPPN [28,29], and a systematic review concluded that 84% of reviewed studies supported use of duloxetine as a first-line agent [16].

With regard to SSRIs, only two studies qualified for inclusion in the systematic review. Fluoxetine (40 mg) was ineffective in treatment of diabetic painful peripheral neuropathy, whereas escitalopram (20 mg) was effective in treatment of mixed painful peripheral neuropathy, with a NNT of 5.1.

Fibromyalgia

Fibromyalgia is characterized by widespread, persistent musculoskeletal pain of unclear etiology, often associated with other nonspecific symptoms such as fatigue and difficulty with sleep and cognition [30,31]. Antidepressants are often prescribed for fibromyalgia, and the SNRIs duloxetine and milnacipran are among the few FDA-approved medications for this condition. However, individual studies and even meta-analyses vary widely in their conclusions regarding efficacy. In fact, a recent systematic review and meta-analysis examining pharmacologic and non-pharmacologic therapies for pain and quality of life in fibromyalgia found only a "small and non-clinically important association for antidepressants and pain reduction in the medium term" [32].

Historically, amitriptyline has been a common treatment for fibromyalgia. Objectively, however, only poor-quality evidence supports its use. Based on four placebo-controlled studies using amitriptyline 25–50 mg, substantial (>50%) pain relief occurred in 36% of patients taking amitriptyline and 11% of patients taking placebo, producing a NNT of 4.1. With regard to adverse events, NNH for any adverse event was 3.3, but there was no difference between amitriptyline and placebo in study withdrawals due to adverse events [3].

The tetracyclic antidepressant mirtazapine has also been evaluated in fibromyalgia. A systematic review identified only three qualified studies; within these, there was some benefit for moderate (>30%) but not substantial (>50%) pain relief. However, side effects (notably somnolence, weight gain, and elevated alanine aminotransferase) were significantly more common with mirtazapine than placebo [33].

A systematic review evaluated the efficacy of SSRIs in fibromyalgia [34]. The included studies used citalopram, fluoxetine and paroxetine. The authors concluded that the only unbiased evidence for superiority to placebo was for treatment of depression in patients with fibromyalgia. However, it should be noted that more patients reported >30% pain relief with SSRI (32.6%) than placebo (22.8%). Similarly, more patients considered themselves to be much or very much improved overall in the SSRI groups (29.8%) compared to placebo groups (16%).

Duloxetine has been studied extensively as a treatment for fibromyalgia symptoms including pain; it has been shown to significantly reduce overall, moderate (>30%), and substantial (>50%) pain [35]. In the most recent systematic review on this topic from the Cochrane collaboration, both duloxetine and milnacipran were significantly, albeit slightly, more likely than placebo to produce both >50% and >30% pain reduction. There was no significant difference between the two drugs on these measures. Combined NNT was 11 and NNH (withdrawal from study due to adverse event) was 14, with the most common adverse events being nausea and drowsiness [2].

Milnacipran appears to produce similar results, consistently providing moderate pain relief to a minority of subjects with fibromyalgia. Specifically, in a systematic review of studies using milnacipran 100 mg daily, moderate pain relief (>30%) occurred in 40% of subjects taking milnacipran and 30% of subjects taking placebo. Similarly, substantial pain relief (>50%) occurred in 26% of subjects taking milnacipran and 17% of subjects taking placebo [36]. Comparable pain relief but more adverse effects and withdrawals occurred in subjects taking 200 mg daily. As such, this review calculated a NNT of 9–10 and NNH (withdrawal due to adverse event) of 14 for the 100 mg dose and 7 for the 200 mg dose.

Headache

Migraine

Tricyclic antidepressants, particularly amitriptyline, are a mainstay in migraine prophylaxis. Multiple meta-analyses have concluded that TCA treatment is associated with a significant reduction in headache burden, and that this effect increases over treatment time [37,38]. In fact, network meta-analyses have suggested that amitriptyline (60–100 mg) is superior to medications from multiple classes [38] for migraine prophylaxis.

Systematic reviews and meta-analyses have reached mixed conclusions regarding the efficacy of SSRIs and SNRIs in migraine prophylaxis. In general, it seems that SSRIs have no or minimal effect on migraine frequency or severity. Serotonin-norepinephrine reuptake inhibitors, particularly venlafaxine, may decrease headache frequency compared to placebo. However, there is no convincing evidence that either class is more effective than amitriptyline [6.7.39].

Tension-type headache

Compared to placebo, amitriptyline also reduced tension-type headache frequency and analgesic consumption, with the effect increasing over study duration up to 24 weeks follow-up. However, amitriptyline did not improve quality of life, headache severity or headache duration [39]. The few studies conducted using tetracyclic antidepressants did not find a significant effect for any outcome measure.

Similar to results for migraine, SSRIs and SNRIs do not appear to reduce the frequency, intensity or duration of tension-type headache compared to placebo or amitriptyline. In fact, patients treated with SSRIs used significantly more analgesic rescue medication compared to patients treated with TCAs [40].

Low back pain

Antidepressants are not standard treatment for axial low back pain (LBP), but many studies have been conducted with mixed results. Patients with a history of > 3 months axial low back pain randomized to amitriptyline (25 mg daily) did not have lower pain intensity than those randomized to active placebo (benztropine), but they did have significantly lower disability ratings after six months of treatment [40].

Studies comparing TCAs with SSRIs suggested that noradrenergic actions of TCAs may be more important than serotonergic mechanisms for LBP. Patients with a history of chronic LBP experienced significantly greater reduction in pain intensity compared to placebo with maprotiline (a tetracyclic antidepressant with strong noradrenergic effects) but not paroxetine [41]. Similarly, another group of patients with chronic LBP demonstrated significant reductions in pain with low-dose desipramine but not fluoxetine [42]. However, a more recent study found no benefit of desipramine, cognitive behavioral therapy, or their combination in chronic LBP [43].

There may be a role for SNRIs, particularly duloxetine, in treatment of chronic LBP. In patients with*out* depression, radiation of pain past the thigh, spinal stenosis, or more than one lumbar surgery, duloxetine (60–120 mg daily) was associated with statistically significant improvements in pain severity and physical function compared to patients receiving placebo [44].

A recent systematic review examined the efficacy of multiple drug classes, including TCAs and duloxetine, for chronic LBP. Of note, the analysis included patients with psychiatric comorbidities and radicular symptoms, but excluded patients with comorbid cervicothoracic or sacroiliac pain and patients awaiting surgery. This review concluded that TCAs were not an effective monotherapy for LBP, but duloxetine was associated with improvements in both pain and disability [8].

Osteoarthritis

Tricyclic antidepressants are not recommended by major orthopedic/rheumatologic societies to treat hip or knee osteoarthritis (OA) [45]. There is only one double-blind RCT of TCAs in OA; this recently-published study concluded that nortriptyline (25–100 mg) did not produce clinically significant pain reduction in knee OA after 14 weeks of treatment [46].

However, several recent trials have found that duloxetine is effective in osteoarthritis. These were summarized in a recent systematic review and meta-analysis [5]. The five studies eligible for meta-analysis all found a moderate but statistically significant benefit in knee osteoarthritis (OA). Remarkably, the effect sizes were comparable to those reported for prescription NSAIDs. Another recent systematic review and meta-analysis [47] was more equivocal, concluding that "a clinically important effect [of SNRIs] cannot be excluded for osteoarthritis" [47]. Of note, a post-hoc analysis of placebo-controlled duloxetine RCTs in knee OA and chronic LBP suggested that analgesia from duloxetine usually occurs early in treatment [48].

Children and adolescents

Significantly fewer studies have examined the efficacy of antidepressants in pediatric chronic noncancer pain. A Cochrane review of the available data [49] found no effect in any of the included studies. This review encompassed four studies comprising 272 participants between 6–18 years of age. The participants had conditions including chronic neuropathic pain, complex regional pain syndrome

(CRPS) type 1, irritable bowel syndrome (IBS) and functional abdominal pain or functional dyspepsia. Pre-specified primary outcomes were pain reduction ≥30%, pain reduction ≥50% and patient global impression of change much/very much improved. Unfortunately, these outcomes were not reported in the included studies. One study compared gabapentin to amitriptyline for treatment of CRPS or neuropathic pain; both drugs improved sleep quality, and there was no statistically significant difference between the treatment groups. The other three studies included in the 2017 Cochrane review examined abdominal pain (IBS, functional abdominal pain). An updated Cochrane review in 2021 focused solely on antidepressants for functional abdominal pain [50], but included only the same three studies as the 2017 review. Two of these compared amitriptyline to placebo, while one compared citalopram to placebo. No statistically significant difference in pain intensity was reported in any study.

Summary

In conclusion, there is a large body of literature examining the effects of antidepressants in adult chronic non-cancer pain. Systematic reviews and meta-analyses support the use of TCAs for headache disorders and various neuropathic pain conditions, but not for chronic low back pain (Table 16.1). Evidence is equivocal for TCA use in fibromyalgia. Only one RCT has investigated TCA use for osteoarthritis with negative results. SNRIs, particularly duloxetine, are effective for fibromyalgia, neuropathic pain, and osteoarthritis, but not chronic LBP. Systematic reviews have concluded that venlafaxine can be effective for headaches, but not superior to amitriptyline. SSRIs appear to be less useful, with only single RCTs showing any efficacy in neuropathic pain and chronic low back pain. Systematic reviews and meta-analyses concluded that SSRIs are ineffective for fibromyalgia or headache.

Table 16.1 Summary of antidepressant efficacy in common chronic pain conditions.

	TCAs			SNRIs			SSRIs		
	Systematic review & Meta-analysis	**Single RCTs**	**Open label studies**	**Systematic review & Meta-analysis**	**Single RCTs**	**Open label studies**	**Systematic review & Meta-analysis**	**Single RCTs**	**Open label studies**
Neuropathic pain	Y[1]			Y[1]			I[1]		
Fibromyalgia	I[3,33]			Y[35]			N[34]		
Headaches	Y[38,39]			N[6,7]			N[6,7]		
Low Back Pain	N[8]			N[47]			-	N[41,42], Y[51]	
Osteoarthritis	-	N[46]		Y[5], I[47]			-	-	-

Y = benefit over placebo and/or standard treatment; N = no benefit over placebo and/or standard treatment; I = inconclusive benefit; - = no studies

References

1 Finnerup NB, Attal N, Haroutounian S *et al.* (2015) Pharmacotherapy for neuropathic pain in adults: a systematic review and meta-analysis. *The Lancet Neurology* **14**:162–73.

2 Welsch P, Üçeyler N, Klose P, Walitt B, Häuser W. (2018) Serotonin and noradrenaline reuptake inhibitors (SNRIs) for fibromyalgia. *Cochrane Database of Systematic Reviews* **2(2)**:CD010292.

3 Moore RA, Derry S, Aldington D, Cole P, Wiffen PJ. (2015). Amitriptyline for fibromyalgia in adults. *Cochrane Database of Systematic Reviews* **2015(7)**:CD011824.

4 Moore RA, Derry S, Aldington D, Cole P, Wiffen PJ. (2015) Amitriptyline for neuropathic pain in adults. *Cochrane Database of Systematic Reviews* **2015(7)**:CD008242.

5 Osani, M. C. & Bannuru, R. R. (2019) Efficacy and safety of duloxetine in osteoarthritis: a systematic review and meta-analysis. *Korean J Intern Med* **34**:966–73.

6 Banzi R, Cusi C, Randazzo C, Sterzi R, Tedesco D, Moja L. (2015) Selective serotonin reuptake

inhibitors (SSRIs) and serotonin-norepinephrine reuptake inhibitors (SNRIs) for the prevention of migraine in adults. *Cochrane Database of Systematic Reviews* **4(4)**:CD002919.

7 Wang F, Wang J, Cao Y, Xu Z. (2020) Serotonin–norepinephrine reuptake inhibitors for the prevention of migraine and vestibular migraine: a systematic review and meta-analysis. *Reg Anesth Pain Med* **45**:323–30.

8 Migliorini F, Maffuli N, Eschweiler J et al. (2021) The pharmacological management of chronic lower back pain. *Expert Opinion on Pharmacotherapy* **22**:109–19.

9 Riediger C, Schuster T, Barlinn K, Maier S, Weitz J, Siepmann T. (2017) Adverse effects of antidepressants for chronic pain: a systematic review and meta-analysis. *Front. Neurol.* **8**:307.

10 Hillhouse TM, Porter JH. (2015) A brief history of the development of antidepressant drugs: from monoamines to glutamate. *Experimental and Clinical Psychopharmacology* **23**:1–21.

11 Lee Y-C, Chen P-P. (2010 A review of SSRIs and SNRIs in neuropathic pain. *Expert Opinion on Pharmacotherapy* **11**:2813–25.

12 Bravo L, Llorca-Torralba M, Berrocoso E, Micó JA. (2019) Monoamines as drug targets in chronic pain: focusing on neuropathic pain. *Front. Neurosci.* **13**:1268.

13 Schildkraut, J. J. (1967) The catecholamine hypothesis of affective disorders. A review of supporting evidence. *Int J Psychiatry* **4**:203–217.

14 Schildkraut JJ, Kety SS. (1967) Biogenic amines and emotion. *Science* **156**:21–37.

15 Patetsos E, Horjales-Araujo E. (2016) Treating chronic pain with SSRIs: what do we know? *Pain Research and Management* **2016**:1–17.

16 Rodrigues-Amorim D, Olivares JM, Spuch C, Rivera-Baltanás T (2020) A systematic review of efficacy, safety, and tolerability of duloxetine. *Front. Psychiatry* **11**:554899.

17 Obata H. (2017) Analgesic mechanisms of antidepressants for neuropathic pain. *IJMS* **18**:2483.

18 Mika J, Zychowska M, Makuch W, Rojewska E, Przewlocka B. (2013) Neuronal and immunological basis of action of antidepressants in chronic pain - clinical and experimental studies. *Pharmacol Rep* **65**:1611–21.

19 Bannister K, Dickenson AH. (2016) What do monoamines do in pain modulation? *Current Opinion in Supportive and Palliative Care* **10**: 143–8.

20 Kremer M, Yalcin I, Goumon I, *et al.* (2018) A dual noradrenergic mechanism for the relief of neuropathic allodynia by the antidepressant drugs duloxetine and amitriptyline. *J. Neurosci.* **38**:9934–54.

21 Gillman PK. (2007) Tricyclic antidepressant pharmacology and therapeutic drug interactions updated: TCAs: pharmacology and interactions. *British Journal of Pharmacology* **151**:737–48.

22 Francescangeli J, Karamchandani K, Powell M, Bonavia A.(2019) The serotonin syndrome: from molecular mechanisms to clinical practice. *IJMS* **20**:2288.

23 Montgomery SA. (2005) Antidepressants and seizures: emphasis on newer agents and clinical implications. *International Journal of Clinical Practice* **59**:1435–40. (2005).

24 Bixby AL, VandenBerg A, Bostwick JR. (2019) Clinical management of bleeding risk with antidepressants. *Ann Pharmacother* **53**:186–94.

25 Thase ME. (1998) Effects of venlafaxine on blood pressure: a meta-analysis of original data from 3744 depressed patients. *J Clin Psychiatry* **59(10)**:502–8.

26 Farshchian N, Alavi A, Heydarheydari S, Moradian N. (2018) Comparative study of the effects of venlafaxine and duloxetine on chemotherapy-induced peripheral neuropathy. *Cancer Chemother Pharmacol* **82**: 787–93.

27 Schukro RP, Oehmke MJm Geroldinger A, *et al.* (2016) Efficacy of duloxetine in chronic low back pain with a neuropathic component: a randomized, double-blind, placebo-controlled trial. *Anesthesiology* **124(1)**:150–8.

28 Gao Y, Guo X, Han P *et al.* (2015) Treatment of patients with diabetic peripheral neuropathic pain in China: a double-blind randomised trial of duloxetine vs. placebo. *Int J Clin Pract* **69**: 957–66.

29 Yasuda H, Hotta N, Kasuga M *et al.* (2016) Efficacy and safety of 40 mg or 60 mg duloxetine in Japanese adults with diabetic neuropathic pain: results from a randomized, 52-week, open-label study. *J Diabetes Invest* **7(1)**:100–8.

30 Galvez-Sánchez CM, Reyes del Paso GA. (2020) Diagnostic criteria for fibromyalgia: critical review and future perspectives. *JCM* **9**:1219.

31 Wolfe F, Clauw D, Fitzcharles M-A, *et al.* (2010) The American College of Rheumatology preliminary diagnostic criteria for fibromyalgia and measurement of symptom severity. *Arthritis Care Res* **62(5)**:600–10.

32 Mascarenhas RO, Souza MB, Oliviera MX *et al.* (2020) Association of therapies with reduced pain and improved quality of life in patients with fibromyalgia: a systematic review and meta-analysis. *JAMA Intern Med* **181(1)**:104–12.

33 Welsch P, Bernardy K, Derry S, Moore RA, Häuser W. (2018) Mirtazapine for fibromyalgia in adults. *Cochrane Database of Systematic Reviews* **8(8)**: CD012708.

34 Walitt B, Urrútia G, Nishishinya MB, Cantrell SE, Häuser W. (2015) Selective serotonin reuptake inhibitors for fibromyalgia syndrome. *Cochrane DatabaseofSystematicReviews* **2015(6)**:CD011735.

35 Lian Y-N, Wang Y, Zhang Y, Yang C-X. (2020) Duloxetine for pain in fibromyalgia in adults: a systematic review and a meta-analysis. *International Journal of Neuroscience* **130**:71–82.

36 Cording M, Derry S, Phillips T, Moore RA, Wiffen PJ. (2015) Milnacipran for pain in fibromyalgia in adults. *Cochrane Database of Systematic Reviews* **2015(10)**:CD008244.

37 Xu X, Liu Y, Dong M, Zou D, Wei Y. (2017) Tricyclic antidepressants for preventing migraine in adults: *Medicine* **96(22)**:e6989.

38 Jackson JL, Cogbill E, Santana-Davila R *et al.* (2015) A comparative effectiveness meta-analysis of drugs for the prophylaxis of migraine headache. *PLoS ONE* **10**:e0130733.

39 Jackson JL, Mancuso JM, Nickoloff S, Bernstein R, Kay C. (2017) Tricyclic and tetracyclic antidepressants for the prevention of frequent episodic or chronic tension-type headache in adults: a systematic review and meta-analysis. *J Gen Intern Med* **32**:1351–8.

40 Urquhart DM, Wluka AE, van Tulder M *et al.* (2018) Efficacy of low-dose amitriptyline for chronic low back pain: a randomized clinical trial. *JAMA Intern Med* **178**:1474.

41 Atkinson HJ, Slater MA, Wahlgren DR *et al.* (1999) Effects of noradrenergic and serotonergic antidepressants on chronic low back pain intensity. *Pain* **83(2)**:137–45.

42 Atkinson JH, Slater MA, Capparelli EV *et al.* (2007) Efficacy of noradrenergic and serotonergic antidepressants in chronic back pain: a preliminary concentration-controlled trial. *Journal of Clinical Psychopharmacology* **27**:135–42.

43 Gould HM, Atkinson JH, Chircop-Rollick T *et al.* (2020) A randomized placebo-controlled trial of desipramine, cognitive behavioral therapy, and active placebo therapy for low back pain. *Pain* **161**:1341–9.

44 Skljarevski V, Desaiah D, Liu-Seifert H *et al.* (2010) Efficacy and safety of duloxetine in patients with chronic low back pain. *Spine* **35(13)**:E578–85.

45 Katz JN, Arant KR, Loeser RF.(2021) Diagnosis and treatment of hip and knee osteoarthritis: a review. *JAMA* **325**:568.

46 Hudson B, Williman JA, Stamp LK *et al.* (2021) Nortriptyline for pain in knee osteoarthritis in general practice: a double blind randomised controlled trial. *Br J Gen Pract* **71(708)**:e538–46.

47 Ferreira GE, McLachlan AJ, Lin C-WC *et al.* (2021) Efficacy and safety of antidepressants for the treatment of back pain and osteoarthritis: systematic review and meta-analysis. *BMJ* **372**:m4825.

48 Williamson OD, Schrorer M, Ruff DD *et al.* (2014) Onset of response with duloxetine treatment in patients with osteoarthritis knee pain and chronic low back pain: a post hoc analysis of placebo-controlled trials. *Clinical Therapeutics* **36**:544–51.

49 Cooper TE, Heathcote LC, Clinch J *et al.* (2017) Antidepressants for chronic non-cancer pain in children and adolescents. *Cochrane Database Syst Rev* **8(8)**:CD012535.

50 de Bruijn CMA, Rexwinkel R, Gordon M, Benninga M, Tabbers MM. (2021) Antidepressants for functional abdominal pain disorders in children and adolescents. *Cochrane Database of Systematic Reviews* **2(2)**:CD00813.

51 Dickens C, Jayson M, Sutton C, Creed F. (2000) The relationship between pain and depression in a trial using paroxetine in sufferers of chronic low back pain. *Psychosomatics* **41**:490–9.

Chapter 17

Anticonvulsants in the management of chronic pain

Malin Carmland[1,2], Troels Staehelin Jensen[1,2], & Nanna Brix Finnerup[1,2]

[1] *Danish Pain Research Center, Aarhus University, Aarhus, Denmark*
[2] *Department of Neurology, Aarhus University Hospital, Aarhus, Denmark*

Introduction

Anticonvulsants, also called antiepileptic drugs (AED), were primarily introduced for the treatment of epilepsy. Many AEDs have pharmacological actions that can interfere with the processes involved in neuronal hyperexcitability either by decreasing excitatory or increasing inhibitory transmission, thereby exerting a neuronal depressant effect. This may explain why some AEDs are effective in bipolar mood disorders and chronic pain conditions, which may share complex pathophysiological mechanisms manifest in different areas of the nervous system.

Chronic pain is defined as pain that persists or recurs for more than 3 months and can be divided according to etiology [1]. Nociceptive pain, including inflammatory pain, is pain arising from activation of nociceptors, while neuropathic pain is defined as pain arising as pain caused by a lesion or disease of the somatosensory system [2]. A group of pain conditions, which among others include fibromyalgia, temporomandibular disorders and irritable bowel syndrome, do not fall into these two categories of pain. The underlying mechanisms in these pain syndromes are unknown, and in the new ICD-11 classification, they are classified as primary pain [1]. As reviewed in previous chapters, pharmacotherapy for chronic pain should take place within the context of a multidisciplinary approach that addresses biopsychosocial aspects and begins with a review of active healthful strategies and treatments with the least potential for harm.

This chapter reviews AEDs for the treatment of chronic neuropathic pain, migraine and fibromyalgia.

Antiepileptics in chronic pain: mechanisms of action

Until the beginning of 1990, there were around 7-8 AEDs on the market. These first-generation drugs are now accompanied by several second- and third- generation AEDs. Some have been tested in pain conditions, but far from all. The exact mechanisms by which AEDs relieve chronic pain are not known. Several mechanisms of action may be involved in altering neurotransmission by exerting a neuronal depressant effect in pain pathways [3]. This way, AEDs may attenuate the neuronal hyperexcitability, peripheral and central sensitization and ectopic activity, which are likely the responsible mechanisms underlying chronic pain conditions. These mechanisms of action include modulation of ion channels (sodium, calcium and potassium channels), augmentation of inhibitory effects (particularly by potentiating the inhibitory neurotransmitter gamma-aminobutyric acid [GABA]) and suppression of abnormal neuronal excitability such as inhibition of glutamate receptors or suppression of neurotransmitter release (Table 17.1).

Clinical Pain Management: A Practical Guide, Second Edition. Edited by Mary E. Lynch, Kenneth D. Craig, and Philip W. Peng.

Table 17.1 Main mechanism of action, common side effects and precautions of commonly used anticonvulsants for chronic pain.

Drug	Main mechanism of action	Side effects and precautions*
Carbamazepine	Sodium channel blockade	Somnolence, dizziness, ataxia, hyponatremia, leukopenia, nausea, vomiting, dermatological reactions/rash Precautions: cardiac insufficiency, previous or current haematological disease, concomitant treatment with anticholinergic medications, risk of suicidal thoughts/behaviour
Oxcarbazepine	Sodium channel blockade	Fatigue, headache, nausea, vomiting, dizziness, somnolence, diplopia, hyponatremia, potential for dermatological and anaphylactic reactions (acute onset) Precautions: Cardiac insufficiency, decreased liver or kidney function, risk of suicidal thoughts/ behaviour
Lamotrigine	Sodium channel blockade	Headache, rash, pain, fatigue, diarrhea, nausea, dry mouth, vomiting, irritability, somnolence, dizziness, tremor Precautions: potential dermatologic reactions, risk of suicidal thoughts/behaviour
Lacosamide	Sodium channel blockade	Nausea, headache, dizziness, diplopia Precautions: cardiac rhythm disorders, severe cardiac disease, 2nd or 3rd degree AV block is a contraindication, risk of suicidal thoughts/ behaviour
Pregabalin	Calcium channel blockade	Headache, somnolence, dizziness Precautions: severe chronic cardiac insufficiency, decreased kidney function (dose reduction), risk of suicidal thoughts/behaviour and abuse
Gabapentin incl. gabapentin ER/enacarbil	Calcium channel blockade (α2δ –unit)	Fever, fatigue, ataxia, dizziness, somnolence, viral infections, sedation, ataxia, dizziness, somnolence Precautions: decreased kidney function (dose reduction), risk of suicidal thoughts/behaviour and abuse
Valproate	Increased GABA inhibition, decreased glutamate excitation, sodium channel blockade	Nausea, tremor Precautions: Potential hepatotoxicity, control haematological parameters
Topiramate	Sodium and calcium channel blockade, increased GABA inhibition, decreased glutamate excitation	Fatigue, weight loss, diarrhoea, nausea, nasopharyngitis, depression, somnolence, paraesthesia, dizziness Precautions: reduced liver function, risk of suicidal thoughts/behaviour
Levetiracetam	Calcium channel blockade (binds to a synaptic vesicle protein SV2A)	Rhinitis, somnolence, headache Precautions: Reduced kidney and liver function (dose reduction)

GABA, γ-aminobutyric acid. *For full list of side effects and precautions, please refer to official summary of product characteristics.

The AEDs carbamazepine (first generation), oxcarbazepine and lamotrigine (both second generation) primarily act by blocking sodium channels. Changes in sodium channels are involved in neuropathic pain conditions [4]. Slowing of the recovery rate of voltage-gated sodium channels and inhibition of sustained high-frequency repetitive firing will stabilize membranes and reduce neuronal excitability in the peripheral and central nervous systems. A newer third-generation AED, lacosamide, enhances the slow inactivation of voltage-gated sodium channels and inhibits the collapsing response mediator protein 2 (CRMP-2), which may have a disease modifying role in pain signaling.

Valproate is a first-generation AED with a wide range of actions including potentiation of GABAergic functions, reduction in excitatory amino acids, sodium channel and glutamate receptor functions, modulation of potassium and calcium homeostasis, and enhancement of serotonergic neurotransmission [3].

Gabapentin and pregabalin are members of second-generation AEDs. They are structural derivatives of the inhibitory neurotransmitter GABA, but in spite of their name, do not appear to act through the GABAergic neurotransmitter system. The predominant mechanism of action is thought to be through its presynaptic binding to the $\alpha_2\delta$-1 and 2 subunits of voltage-gated calcium channels. These are expressed at different levels in the brain, e.g. locus coeruleus and amygdala both involved in nociception and pain processing, as well as in the spinal cord and peripheral nerves. The result is reduced excitatory transmitter release from these tissues, which may explain the anticonvulsant, analgesic and anxiolytic activity [5, 6].

Topiramate is another new-generation AED, which modulates sodium channels but also enhances GABAergic transmission and inhibits glutamate receptors.

Levetiracetam binds to the synaptic vesicle protein SV2A and interferes with vesicle exocytosis, thus impeding nerve conduction across synapses.

Both the first-generation AEDs phenytoin, valproate and carbamazepine and the newer AEDs lamotrigine, pregabalin, gabapentin, lacosamide, topiramate and levetiracetam have a range of actions that may interfere with mechanisms involved in chronic pain. Yet not all AEDs seem to be effective in relieving chronic pain. The three main pain conditions where AEDs have a role in treatment or prevention are neuropathic pain, migraine and fibromyalgia (Table 17.2).

AEDs in neuropathic pain

Neuropathic pain is a heterogeneous group of chronic pain conditions arising from lesions of the peripheral or central nervous systems. Common neuropathic pain conditions include painful diabetic polyneuropathy, post-herpetic neuralgia, trigeminal neuralgia, phantom pain, pain following

Table 17.2 Anticonvulsant drugs with documented efficacy (consistent outcome in Class I randomized double-blind controlled trials), possible efficacy (owing to inadequate or conflicting data) and evidence for no efficacy in neuropathic pain, trigeminal neuralgia, migraine prophylaxis and fibromyalgia.

Pain condition	Documented efficacy	Possible efficacy	Probably no efficacy
Neuropathic pain	Gabapentin Pregabalin	Topiramate Carbamazepine Oxcarbazepine Lacosamide Lamotrigine	Levetiracetam Valproate
Trigeminal neuralgia	Carbamazepine Oxcarbazepine	Lamotrigine	
Migraine prophylaxis	Valproate Topiramate	Gabapentin Carbamazepine	Lamotrigine Tiagabine Oxcarbazepine
Fibromyalgia	Pregabalin	Gabapentin	

peripheral nerve injury and central pain following stroke, spinal cord injury and multiple sclerosis. The various symptoms of neuropathic pain do not seem to be strongly correlated to the underlying etiology. The pain may be spontaneous and/or evoked with allodynia to cold, warmth or touch. Pain descriptors include burning, pins and needles, squeezing and shooting and freezing pain [4].

Gabapentin and pregabalin have a well-documented efficacy in various neuropathic pain conditions, including painful polyneuropathy, post-herpetic neuralgia and central pain. They are considered first-line drug choices together with tricyclic antidepressants and serotonin noradrenaline reuptake inhibitors [7]. A meta-analysis and systematic review found that pregabalin and gabapentin had an NNT of 7.7 (6.5-9.4) and 6.3 (5.0-8.3), respectively. For pregabalin, there was a dose response gradient [7].

Carbamazepine is the mainstay of treatment for trigeminal neuralgia, but the evidence is sparse [8]. Randomized controlled trials have documented comparable analgesic effects between oxcarbazepine and carbamazepine in trigeminal neuralgia [8,9]. The role of carbamazepine and oxcarbazepine in other neuropathic pain conditions is still unclear because of conflicting results from a limited number of randomized controlled trials [7]. A recent study in peripheral neuropathic pain found that oxcarbamazepine was effective in patients with the so-called irritable nociceptor phenotype (i.e. patients with preserved thermal sensation and evoked pain) [10]. Further studies are needed to confirm if oxcarbazepine should be recommended for specific phenotypes of neuropathic pain.

For other AEDs listed in table 17.2, there are inconclusive results in clinical trials and are therefore not part of either first, second- or third-line recommendations for the treatment of neuropathic pain [7]. The most recently studied AED, lacosamide, may have some effect in painful diabetic neuropathy [7], but studies have failed to prove its efficacy, maybe partly due to large placebo responses. A more recent small trial found that lacosamide had a significant effect on pain in $Na_v1.7$-related small fiber neuropathy and was generally well tolerated [11]. There is no or little evidence for efficacy of valproate, which is also associated with serious adverse events and valproate is therefore not, recommended for neuropathic pain [7]. Levetiracetam, despite some promising results from experimental animal and open-label trials, failed to find an effect in randomized placebo-controlled trials. There is weak recommendation against the use of levetiracetam for neuropathic pain [7].

AEDs in migraine

Migraine is a common disorder characterized by episodic attacks of headache, with or without aura. In patients with migraine who experience a low frequency of attacks, avoidance of factors that trigger the migraine may be sufficient. First choice for acute pharmacological treatment is simple analgesics like paracetamol or NSAID's combined with an agent to reduce nausea. The next step in the acute treatment of migraine attacks is the use of triptans. It is important to distinguish between tension type headache and migraine attack in the pharmacological treatment. In a subgroup of patients, who experience more frequent and/or severe attacks, preventive therapy is needed [12]. Preventive treatment of migraine can be introduced if migraine attacks are > 3/months or if control of individual migraine attacks is insufficient.

The most commonly used drugs for preventive treatment are the antihypertension medications (propanolol, metoprolol, candersatan), or the AEDs (valproate, topiramate) More recently, monoclonal antibodies towards targets in the calcitonin gene related peptide (CGRP) pathway has shown to be effective in preventing attacks of migraine. The effect of gabapentin is conflicting [12]. It is classified as probably effective as a third-line drug of choice based on one placebo-controlled trial. Lamotrigine did not reduce the frequency of migraine attacks but may be effective in reducing the frequency of migraine auras. There is sparse evidence of the effect of carbamazepine, oxcarbazepine, levetiracetam and zonisamide [12,13].

AEDs in fibromyalgia

Fibromyalgia is a chronic pain condition in which the symptoms are widespread pain, with muscle tender points, fatigue, and sleep disturbances, along with an impaired quality of life.

There are two recent Cochrane reviews assessing the efficacy of pregabalin (2016) and gabapentin (2017) on pain in fibromyalgia [14,15]. For gabapentin, only one study was found eligible for inclusion. It found an effect of gabapentin, but this needs to be confirmed in other trials [14].

The meta-analysis for pregabalin included eight studies. It showed that pregabalin in doses of 300-600 mg daily was effective in pain relief with an NNT for 30% pain reduction for pregabalin 600 mg daily of 9.4 (6.2-19). Pain reduction was accompanied by improvements on other symptoms seen in fibromyalgia, and improvements on quality of life. Adverse events were more common in the treatment group compared to placebo, and included dizziness, somnolence, weight-gain and peripheral edema. Withdrawals where about 10% more common for those who received pregabalin compared to placebo [15]. The findings were supported in a more recent evidence-based review, which also concluded that pregabalin is effective for relieving pain in fibromyalgia [16]. Pregabalin can be considered for the treatment of pain and sleep disturbances, but clinicians should consider comorbidities, and the treatment should be multidisciplinary. Pregabalin has been approved for the treatment of fibromyalgia by the US Food and Drug Administration (FDA), but not by the European Medicines Agency (EMEA).

Other AEDs

Zonisamide acts on sodium and calcium channels and is sometimes used for refractory chronic pain. The treatment carries a risk of serious dermatological and hematological reactions. The role of phenytoin and clonazepam as therapeutic options are limited because other safer anticonvulsants are now available with better side effect profiles.

Other new AEDs such as the GABA-inhibitors tiagabine and vigabatrin (risk of retinal toxicity), and felbamate (multiple mechanism of actions, risk of aplastic anemia and hepatic failure) have not been tested in pain conditions. In general, several of the newer AEDs influence neuronal excitability and some pathways involved in pain processing and might in theory have a role in relieving pain. Their practical significance is however yet to be established in clinical trials.

Safety and dosing

Gabapentin and pregabalin have no pharmacokinetic drug–drug interactions, low incidence of life-threatening side effects and no contraindications except for known hypersensitivity. The most common side effects are dose-related dizziness, somnolence and headache, which may resolve in some. Other side effects include dry mouth, asthenia, blurred vision, ataxia, peripheral edema and weight gain not limited to patients with edema. Adverse events have usually been mild or moderate, but not all patients tolerate these drugs. Caution should be used when given with opioids due to the risk of CNS depression. Over the past few years, there has been an increase in reports of abuse and misuse of these drugs. Gabapentin should be initiated at a dosage of 300 mg/day and then increased slowly up to 1800–3600 mg/day according to patient response and side effects [14]. Pregabalin is usually started at 75 mg once or twice daily and may be increased up to a final dosage of 600 mg/day in two or three divided doses, there is a dose-response function with better effects on higher doses [7].

Oxcarbazepine is reported to have a better side effect profile than carbamazepine but is associated with dizziness, tiredness, nausea and headache, ataxia, blurred vision and hyponatremia. From a starting dosage of 600 mg/day, oxcarbazepine may be increased by 150–300 mg every other day to 1500–3000 mg/day.

Side effects associated with the use of lamotrigine include dizziness, ataxia, diplopia, somnolence and nausea. The most concerning side effects are rash and other potentially life-threatening hypersensitivity reactions. Slow dose escalation is recommended to minimize the risk of serious hypersensitivity reactions. The final dosage in the treatment of neuropathic pain is 200–400 mg/day in two divided doses.

Lacosamide is associated with dizziness, somnolence, nausea, tremor and headache. Caution is advised in patients with cardiac conduction disorders or severe cardiac diseases. A final dosage of 400 mg/day seems to be the optimal balance between side effects and pain relief in neuropathic pain [11].

Side effects to topiramate include sedation, weight loss, renal calculi, dizziness, ataxia, psychomotor slowing and cognitive difficulties. The recommended daily dosage of topiramate for prophylactic treatment of migraine is 25–100 mg/ day given in two divided doses with a starting dose of 15–25 mg at bedtime.

Side effects to valproate treatment include weight gain, nausea, tremor, hair loss and rare idiosyncratic reactions. Valproate for prophylactic treatment of migraine can be started at 250– 500 mg/day and increased up to 500–1800 mg/day.

Finding the drug that will produce the best possible pain relief for the individual patient may require administration of several of the mentioned drugs as monotherapy over many periods. Steady-state concentration of the anticonvulsant is obtained within days after reaching target dosage (e.g. 4–8 days for topiramate), although the maximal effect may not yet be achieved.

In some cases, polytherapy may be favorable, especially with a combination of drugs with different modes of action. Special attention to dosage is required when polytherapy is initiated because several of the anticonvulsants increase the clearance of each other (e.g. carbamazepine, phenytoin, lamotrigine, tiagabine and topiramate) with a marked reduction of plasma concentration as a result. Thus, a dose increase of each administered drug may be necessary. In contrast, concomitant administration of lamotrigine and valproic acid results in decreased elimination, and the half-life of lamotrigine may be more than doubled.

Conclusions

AEDs are often used in the treatment of neuropathic pain, fibromyalgia and migraine prophylaxis. As we have few treatments that influence the underlying pathology in these pain conditions, drugs such as anticonvulsants and antidepressants, which may suppress the neuronal hyperexcitability, are often used as symptomatic treatment.

Currently, we know little about which patients will benefit from treatment with an anticonvulsant. While some patients will show a moderate to good effect, others will show no effect. Large trials are needed to further understand and evaluate a possible relationship between the symptomatology and presumed underlying mechanisms and efficacy from different drugs with different mechanisms. Using sensory phenotyping and genetic analysis, for example to detect mutations in sodium channels [14], might be helpful to predict which drug, based on its mechanism of action, will be preferable, and to avoid a trial-and error process. In addition, we need more studies to evaluate the long-term efficacy and safety of anticonvulsants in various chronic pain conditions.

References

1 Treede RD, Rief W, Barke A.z *et al.* (2019) Chronic pain as a symptom or a disease: the IASP Classification of Chronic Pain for the International Classification of Diseases (ICD-11). *Pain* **160**:19–27.

2 Jensen TS, Baron R, Haanpaa M *et al.* (2011) A new definition of neuropathic pain. *Pain* **152**:2204–5.

3 Dickenson AH, Matthews EA, Suzuki R. (2002) Neurobiology of neuropathic pain: mode of action of anticonvulsants. *European Journal of Pain* **6 Suppl A**:51–60.

4 Colloca L, Ludman T, Bouhassira D *et al.* (2017) Neuropathic pain. *Nature Reviews Disease Primers* **3**:17002.

5 Patel R, Dickenson AH. (2016) Mechanisms of the gabapentinoids and alpha 2 delta-1 calcium channel subunit in neuropathic pain. *Pharmacology research & perspectives* **4**,:e00205.

6 Kremer M, Salvat E, Muller A *et al.* (2016) Antidepressants and gabapentinoids in neuropathic pain: Mechanistic insights. *Neuroscience* **338**:183–206.

7 Finnerup NB, Attal N, Haroutounian S *et al.* (2015) Pharmacotherapy for neuropathic pain in adults: a systematic review and meta-analysis. *The Lancet Neurology* **14**:162–73.

8 Di Stefano G, Truini A, Cruccu G. (2018) Current and Innovative Pharmacological Options to Treat Typical and Atypical Trigeminal Neuralgia. *Drugs* **78**:1433–42.

9 Bendtsen L, Zakrzewska JM, Abbott J *et al.* (2019) European Academy of Neurology guideline on trigeminal neuralgia. *Eur J Neurol* **26**:831–849.

10 Demant DT, Lund K, Vollert J *et al.* (2014) The effect of oxcarbazepine in peripheral neuropathic pain depends on pain phenotype: a ran-

domised, double-blind, placebo-controlled phenotype-stratified study. *Pain* **155**:2263–73.

11 de Greef BTA, Hoeijmakers JGJ, Geerts M *et al.* (2019) Lacosamide in patients with Nav1.7 mutations-related small fibre neuropathy: a randomized controlled trial. *Brain* **142**:263–275.

12 Dodick DW. Migraine. (2018) *Lancet* **391**:1315–1330.

13 Parikh SK, Silberstein SD (2019) Current status of antiepileptic drugs as preventive migraine therapy. *Curr Treat Options Neurol* **21**:16.

14 Cooper TE, Derry S, Wiffen PJ *et al.* (2017) Gabapentin for fibromyalgia pain in adults. *Cochrane Database of Systematic Reviews* **1**(1):CD012188.

15 Derry S, Cording M, Wiffen PJ *et al.* (2016) Pregabalin for pain in fibromyalgia in adults. *Cochrane Database of Systematic Reviews* **9**(9):CD011790.

16 Arnold LM, Choy E, Clauw DJ *et al.* (2018) An evidence-based review of pregabalin for the treatment of fibromyalgia. *Current Medical Research and Opinion* **34**:1397–409.

Chapter 18

Opioids

Andrea D. Furlan[1,2,3] & Laura Murphy[1,4,5]

[1] *KITE, Toronto Rehabilitation Institute, University Health Network, Toronto, Ontario, Canada*
[2] *Division of Physical Medicine & Rehabilitation, Department of Medicine, Faculty of Medicine, University of Toronto, Toronto, Ontario, Canada*
[3] *Institute for Work & Health, Toronto, Ontario, Canada*
[4] *Department of Pharmacy, University Health Network, Toronto, Ontario, Canada*
[5] *Leslie Dan Faculty of Pharmacy, University of Toronto, Toronto, Ontario, Canada*

We acknowledge Dawn A. Sparks & Gilbert Fanciullo as authors of the previous version of this chapter.

Introduction

Opioids are front-line treatment in the management of acute and cancer pain. In chronic pain, they are behind other non-pharmacological options and are a third-line pharmacological option, but not appropriate for all situations. The role of opioids in the management of chronic pain has been more controversial and recently impacted by an emerging global opioid crisis, mostly documented in North America, Germany and Australia [1, 2]. In this context, the scientific and clinical communities in these countries have developed guidelines regarding the use of opioids in chronic pain [3-6]. These guidelines have some variation and the Canadian guideline has been referenced here for purposes of illustration [3]. With increased awareness of risks and harms associated with opioids, actions have been taken by government, regulatory bodies and some clinicians [7]. These actions have unfortunately led to unintended consequences for people living with pain who were using opioids as part of their overall pain management [7, 8]. This illustrates the importance of maintaining access to appropriate and safe use of opioids for patients with chronic pain while balancing individual and societal harms.

The aim of this chapter is to review the pharmacology and physiology of opioids, as well as to provide rationale from which to base clinical decision-making when using opioids in the management of patients with chronic pain.

Pharmacology

Opioids activate the endogenous opioid receptors in the body. Opioids available for clinical use include both naturally occurring substances (e.g. morphine or codeine), synthetic substances (e.g. methadone, fentanyl) and semi-synthetic substances (e.g. oxycodone and hydromorphone). Opioid receptors and endogenous opioids or peptides (e.g. endorphins, enkephalins, dynorphins) form an intricate neurotransmitter arrangement known as the endogenous opioid system. The opioid receptors are found within the cellular membranes and are comprised of numerous glycoproteins. Opioid receptors belong to a superfamily of guanine (G) protein-coupled receptors [9, 10]. These G proteins act as second messengers and assist in regulating cell activities.

Clinical Pain Management: A Practical Guide, Second Edition. Edited by Mary E. Lynch, Kenneth D. Craig, and Philip W. Peng.

Table 18.1 Opioid receptors and physiological effects

Receptor	Location	Physiological effects
MOP	Brain, spinal cord, peripheral nociceptors in the gastrointestinal tract, others. induce reactions at the supraspinal level	Analgesia, euphoria, respiratory depression, emesis, immune suppression
DOP	Peripheral nociceptors, spinal cord, brain	Analgesia, immune stimulation, respiratory depression
KOP	Peripheral nociceptors brain, spinal cord	Analgesia, sedation, dysphoria, diuresis, miosis
NOP (ORL-1)	Peripheral nociceptors, brain, spinal cord	Hyperalgesia, sedation, pain responses, physical tolerance to MOP agonists

DOP= delta opioid receptor; KOP=kappa opioid receptor; MOP=mu opioid receptor; NOP= nociception orphanin FQ peptide receptor; ORL-1= opioid-receptor-like receptor 1.

There are multiple opioid receptor subtypes: mu (MOP), delta (DOP) kappa (KOP) and the nociception orphanin FQ peptide receptor (NOP), initially named the opioid-receptor-like receptor 1 (ORL-1) [9, 10]. Table 18.1 [11] outlines opioid receptor distribution and physiological effects. Most opioids can be classified by their action and affinity at the receptor. They can be classified as full agonists (e.g. codeine, fentanyl, heroin, hydromorphone, morphine, oxycodone, tramadol), partial agonists (e.g. buprenorphine) or antagonists (e.g. naloxone, naltrexone). Partial agonists are able to compete with a full agonist, such as morphine, by lowering its efficacy when acting at the same receptor. Some opioids have mixed agonist–antagonist activity (e.g. buprenorphine, pentazocine). In general, agonists selective for MOP or DOP receptors are analgesic and rewarding, whereas KOP agonists are dysphoric. There are no clinically available selective drugs available that work via DOP, KOP, or NOP receptors.

Opioid receptors vary widely in their distribution between individuals. On a cellular level, receptors are located in both presynaptic and postsynaptic positions. The dorsal horn of the spinal cord, medulla oblongata, thalamus and cortex are involved in ascending pain transmission whereas the periaqueductal gray matter, nucleus raphe magnus and ventral medulla utilize the descending pain pathways, all of which possess opioid receptors. These receptors are activated by endogenous opioids as well as exogenous opioids and, in turn, modify nociceptive transmission, modulation and perception. Activation of opioid receptors leads to closing of voltage sensitive calcium channels, stimulation of potassium efflux and hyperpolarization of the nerve and reduction of cyclic adenosine monophosphate (cAMP) production via inhibition of adenylyl cyclase, resulting in reduced neuronal cell excitability [9]. This action also inhibits the transmission of nerve impulses along with inhibition of excitatory neurotransmitter release [9].

Clinicians should consider pharmacological properties, routes of administration and formulations available and potency of opioids. The type of pain that responds better to opioids are acute nociceptive and neuropathic pain. There is controversy in using opioids to treat nociplastic chronic pain, defined as pain arising from altered nocicepton [12], because opioids are implicated in inducing paradoxical hyperalgesia [13], which can be a complicating factor. Opioid potency is generally described in comparison to morphine. Hydromorphone, for example is 5 times more potent than morphine, and oxycodone is 1.5 times more potent. An oral opioid conversion table from the Canadian Guideline for Opioids for Chronic Non-cancer Pain, is provided as Table 18.2. It also includes equivalent doses per day for threshold morphine equivalent doses (MED) described in the Canadian guideline. There is variability in opioid equivalence calculations, particularly for buprenorphine, methadone and from fentanyl transdermal to other oral opioid formulations [14]. Side effect profiles may also be considered in selection of the appropriate opioid. Differences exist depending on opioid receptor activity and other mechanisms of action. For example, morphine should be prescribed with caution to people with impaired kidney function, and tramadol can lead to

Table 18.2 Oral opioid conversion table

Opioids	To convert to oral morphine equivalent, multiply by:	To convert from oral morphine, multiply by:	50 MED equivalent dose	90 MED equivalent dose
Codeine	0.15 (0.1-0.2)	6.67	334mg/day	600mg/day
Hydromorphone	5	0.2	10mg/day	18mg/day
Morphine	1	1	50mg/day	90mg/day
Oxycodone	1.5	1	33mg/day	60mg/day
Tapentadol	0.3-0.4	2.5-3.33	160mg/day	300mg/day
Tramadol	0.1-0.2	6	300mg/day	540* mg/day

MED=Milligram morphine equivalent dose.

* The maximum recommended daily dose of tramadol is 300mg-400mg depending on the formulation.

Source: Busse JW. The 2017 Canadian Guideline for Opioids for Chronic Non-Cancer Pain. Hamilton (ON): McMasterUniversity; 2017. Reproduced with permission of CMA Joule Inc.

serotonin syndrome in combination with other serotonergic medications. The potential for pharmacodynamic drug interactions is present across the opioid class of medications, in particular with central nervous system depressants such as benzodiazepines, gabapentinoids and alcohol, which in combination increase risk of respiratory depression and death [15-18].

Opioids vary in their pharmacokinetics, i.e. absorption, distribution, metabolism and elimination from the body. Opioids are well absorbed when administered orally, however their onset and duration of action depend on numerous factors including lipid solubility, protein binding, ionization state, molecular size and membrane physiochemical properties. Differences in opioid metabolism in the liver also have clinical implications. As an example, morphine and hydromorphone undergo metabolism through glucuronidation and are therefore unlikely to have pharmacokinetic drug interactions. Morphine and hydromorphone are converted to active metabolites and excreted in the urine. In the presence of renal impairment, a morphine metabolite has significant risk of accumulation and toxicity.

Codeine, tramadol and tapentadol are considered less potent opioids; codeine and tramadol are approximately 6 times less potent than morphine, tapentadol is 3 times less potent [19]. Pharmacokinetic differences within the population may have significant impact on the efficacy and safety of codeine and tramadol, both prodrugs. Codeine must be metabolized to morphine by the cytochrome P450 system in the liver, specifically CYP2D6. There are high levels of polymorphism in the population for CYP2D6, impacting many people's ability to convert it to its active metabolite. Tramadol is a dual action analgesic blocking reuptake of norepinephrine and serotonin as well as acting as a full agonist MOP receptors. It has low affinity for opioid receptors, but similar to codeine, tramadol is also converted by CYP2D6 to a MOP full agonist, O-desmethyl tramadol with a higher binding affinity, and so is affected in a similar way by the polymorphism in the population [20]. Tapentadol also has a dual mechanism of action, in addition to activity as a MOP receptor agonist with less affinity than morphine, and it also inhibits norepinephrine reuptake. Tapentadol exerts effects without a pharmacologically active metabolite.

Fentanyl is a potent MOP receptor agonist, 100 times more potent than morphine. It is available as a transdermal formulation for use in chronic pain [21]. A rule of thumb for morphine to fentanyl conversion is that 2 mg of oral morphine is approximately equivalent to 1 mcg/hour transdermal fentanyl patch [22]. When switching to or from fentanyl patches, conservative dosing is suggested because of the range of inter-individual absorption from the patch and equianalgesic ratio with oral opioids. Attention to timing related to patch application and removal is also important in this switch [22]. Dose titration and tapering are limited by availability of patch strengths.

Methadone is a MOP receptor agonist and N-methyl-D aspartate (NMDA) antagonist. Its analgesic duration of action is approximately 6–8 hours, as a result of being highly lipophilic and having a long elimination half-life. It is important for clinicians to be familiar with the unique pharmacokinetics of methadone [23]. There is considerable inter-individual variation in estimates of oral bioavailability and elimination half-life. The oral bioavailability of methadone is different at treatment initiation compared to later on in treatment when the individual is stable on the methadone dose. This may be explained by autoinduction of methadone metabolism, which predominantly occurs by the cytochrome P450 3A4 enzyme system. The approximate morphine:methadone equivalence ratio fluctuates with increasing doses. Methadone is relatively more potent at higher dose. Thus, at morphine dosage of less than 100 mg/day the approximate equivalence ratio of morphine to methadone is 4:1; at dosage between 100 and 300 mg MED per day it becomes 8:1 and at morphine dosage greater than 300 mg/day the ratio is between 12:1 and 20:1. These ratios are intended only as a guideline. Repeated dosing and accumulation of opioids at the receptor as well as their efficacy at the receptor can alter the analgesic interval and the dosing regimen needed.

Many pharmacokinetic interactions with methadone occur through the involvement of the hepatic P450 system, and have the potential to possibly increase or decrease methadone's effects, requiring clinical assessment and potentially dose adjustment if these medications are started and stopped. In addition to CYP 3A4, methadone is also metabolized to a lesser extent by CYP1A2, 2B6, 2C8, 2C9, 2C19, and 2D6 enzymes, and is also a weak inhibitor of CYP 2D6, drugs involved in these systems have the potential to interact.

Buprenorphine is a partial agonist at the MOP and NOP receptors, and a weak KOP receptor antagonist and DOP receptor agonist. For pain, it is used as a transdermal patch [24], and for opioid use disorder it is available as a sublingual formulation in combination with naloxone, and as an injection for subcutaneous use. It is important to note that the classification of buprenorphine as a partial agonist does not translate to partial analgesic effects [25]. Its complex receptor interactions have the potential for other beneficial effects; it has been shown to effectively reduce depressive symptoms in patients unresponsive to conventional antidepressants [26], however these effects require further study.

Buprenorphine is metabolized by the cytochrome P450 3A4 system, therefore medications that inhibit or induce this enzyme system have the potential to interact.

Naltrexone is a non-selective opioid antagonist. Used for management of alcohol or opioid use disorders at doses of 50mg daily, naltrexone competes with and displaces opioid from the receptors, reversing their effects. Blockade of the opioid receptors reduces dopamine levels and associated alcohol cravings, reducing the reward or pleasure of drinking alcohol [27]. In low-doses, ranging from 1-5mg, naltrexone acts as a glial modulator with antagonism at Toll-like receptor 4, ultimately reducing TNF-α and interferon-β synthesis [28]. There is emerging evidence that low-dose naltrexone may have benefits in selected pain conditions. Small clinical trials have demonstrated that low-dose naltrexone may reduce pain in people with fibromyalgia [29, 30], and there are published case reports describing low-dose naltrexone improves symptoms of complex regional pain syndrome [31].

Naloxone is also a competitive MOP selective antagonist, used clinically for the reversal of opioid overdose. Due to extensive first-pass metabolism, it is not typically administered orally, instead, intravenous, intramuscular, or intranasal administration is common.

Pharmacogenomic testing is also emerging to provide additional information to guide clinicians in their selection of opioids for patients [32, 33].

Patient selection and risk stratification

Current literature has identified that most people with chronic pain will not benefit from long term opioids and for many the side effects will lead to treatment withdrawal, however there is a small subgroup in the range of 20% who may experience a meaningful amelioration in pain intensity as well as mental quality of life, but only 8% improve physical quality of life [34, 35]. The challenge for clinicians is to identify when it is appropriate to introduce a trial of opioid since existing evidence has not identified predictors of opioid effectiveness [36].

Proper patient selection is critical and requires a thorough evaluation and a comprehensive risk–benefit assessment. This will include a full biopsychosocial assessment and physical examination as well as an evaluation of risks related to potential adverse effects or development of problematic drug-related behaviors. Patients should be screened for personal and family history of substance use disorders and issues related to mental health and past trauma. Potential benefits such as reduction in pain and improvement in function are expected to be modest for chronic pain, and should be weighed against risks [19, 37, 38]. Potential adverse effects and long-term complications of opioids are displayed in Table 18.3 [39]. Defined therapeutic goals for each patient should be discussed and documented prior to initiation of therapy. Further discussion regarding risk stratification and management can be found in Chapter 39.

Initial treatment with opioids should be regarded as a trial lasting several weeks to a few months to determine if continued treatment is warranted. The decision to proceed with long-term opioid therapy should be made together with the patient only after careful deliberation and education about potential risks and benefits, including a plan of how opioids may be tapered or discontinued if appropriate. The opioid trial model can be especially useful in helping patients define their goals of treatment before treatment and creating a measurable target on which to prospectively base continued use of opioids. Outcomes to consider include progress towards meeting agreed upon therapeutic goals (e.g. pain relief, improvement in function), adverse effects, changes in mental health conditions and the presence or absence of drug-related behaviors, opioid use disorder or diversion. If patients do not meet their predefined goals then the trial of opioid has not been therapeutic and the opioid should be tapered and discontinued. Figure 18.1 presents an approach to the use of opioids for chronic pain.

Table 18.3 Adverse effects and long-term complications of opioids.

Adverse effects and long-term complications
Respiratory depression
Constipation
Nausea or vomiting
Sedation or clouded mentation
Pruritis
Myoclonus
Sphincter of Odi spasm
Hormonal changes (hypogonadism, hypocortisolism)
Immune modulation
Sleep apnea
Tolerance
Abnormal pain sensitivity (hyperalgesia, allodynia)
Falls, Fractures
Opioid use disorder
Dose dependent-risk of mortality

Opioid selection, dosing and titration should be individualized according to the patient's health status, age and previous exposure to opioids. Older patients and those with comorbid medical conditions should be treated with lower doses and titrated more slowly to avoid the risks of adverse effects. Immediate release opioids are preferred for initiating treatment because of their shorter half-life, they may have a lower risk of inadvertent overdose. Long-acting oral opioid formulations are available in many countries for oxycodone, morphine, hydromorphone, tapentadol, tramadol and codeine. Comparisons of long-acting versus short-acting opioids have not found significantly better pain relief [40], nor less consumption of rescue analgesia, improved quality of sleep, or improved physical function [41]. Pharmacokinetic characteristics of immediate release opioids contribute to abuse liability [42]. Short time to peak drug concentration and higher maximum drug concentrations have been shown to be important determinants of positive subjective and reinforcing effects of opioids [42]. Thus, it was expected that long-acting formulations would have a lower abuse liability than immediate-release formulations but there is limited evidence to support this. This potential advantage has been overshadowed by the availability of long-acting products at higher strengths than short-acting products which are prone to tampering (crushing and chewing and snorting or injecting), to produce immediate effects. Co-prescribing of take-home naloxone kits and appropriate training for people using opioids and their close contacts is recommended [43].

The treatment of pain including the use of opioids in patients with a current or past substance use disorder or aberrant drug-related behaviors is discussed in Chapter 39.

Monitoring and management

Monitoring of patients using opioids as part of their management for chronic non-cancer pain should be an interprofessional responsibility, particularly by healthcare professionals prescribing and dispensing these medications. Regular repeated evaluations are recommended for most patients monthly, and at a minimum every 3 months for those using opioids long-term, to reassess progress with therapeutic goals and adverse effects. Patients with higher risk or whose doses are being titrated or tapered may need

Screening and risk stratification
Comprehensive evaluation establishing diagnosis
Confirm inadequacy of non-opioid and non-pharmacological treatments
Complete thorough risk stratification assessment
Establish treatment goals and emphasize trial parameters
Ensure that the balance of risk and benefit favors treatment
Explain benefits, risks, trial and monitoring policies
Obtain written, signed pain management plan
Obtain urine toxicology specimen
Therapeutic trial (up to 8 weeks)
Start therapy at low standard dose and increase dose as tolerated to achieve acceptable analgesia
Individualize doses and titration scheme
Consider repeating urine toxicology testing
Discontinue opioid if trial targets not achieved
Continue treatment if trial targets are achieved without significant side effects
Stable phase; maintain stable dose
Require patient to pick up prescriptions at the pharmacy in person monthly
Assess and document patient's pain relief, functional ability, side effects, behaviors, urine results, quality of life, prescription monitoring program reviews
Treat side effects
Test urine toxicology at least annually in low risk patients
Treatment successful
Pain relief that improves well-being, progress toward goals, improved function and/or improved quality of life
Continue stable dose
Dose escalation
Exclude or identify disease progression
Hospitalize, if necessary
Repeat therapeutic trial phase
Aim to reach new stable dose
Obtain urine toxicology specimen
Treatment failed
Criteria for failure: failure to maintain trial goals, evidence of addiction, abuse, misuse, diversion and/or non-compliance
Wean and discontinue therapy
Dose escalation failed
Consider opioid rotation:
Switch opioid and start at lower dose or wean and discontinue therapy
Restart opioid after period of abstinence if necessary

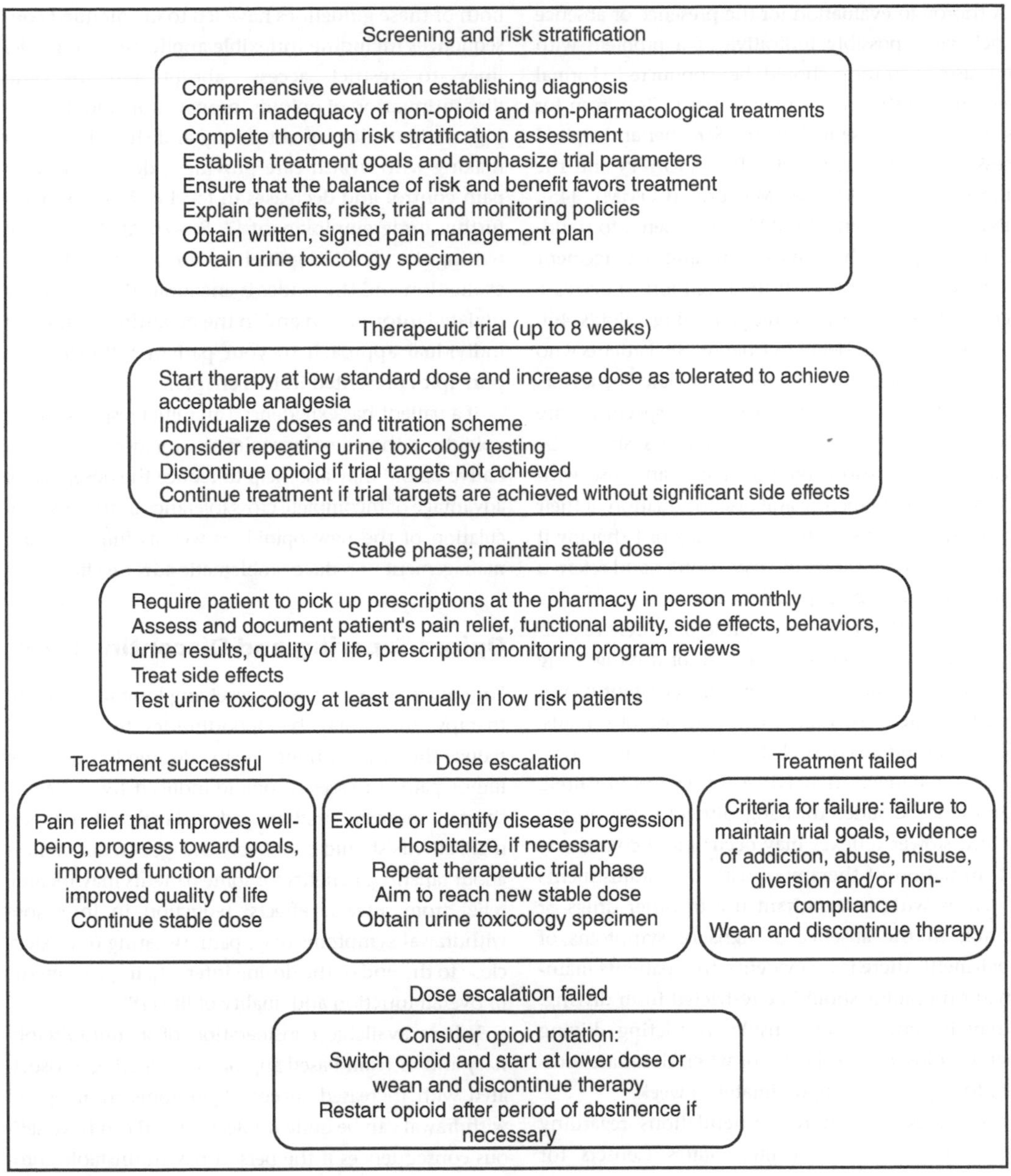

Figure 18.1 Approach to the use of opioids in the management of chronic non-terminal pain.

more frequent monitoring, and potentially weekly or daily dispensing of their medication by the pharmacist. Validated tools are recommended at baseline and for ongoing monitoring, such as the Brief Pain Inventory [44]. The Brief Pain inventory includes measures of pain intensity and interference items (i.e. general activity, mood, ability to walk and perform normal work, relations with other people, sleep and enjoyment of life). It is a valid measure of the interference of pain with physical functioning that has been studied in diverse chronic pain conditions in multiple countries. Patients who do not meet therapeutic goals or who have serious adverse effects from their opioids should be considered for opioid rotation, tapering and discontinuation of their therapy [3].

A thorough evaluation for the presence or absence of behaviors possibly indicative of a problem with drug use aberrancy should be conducted. Formal screening questionnaires may be used. To screen for opioid misuse, these include the Screener and Opioid Assessment for Patients with Pain (SOAPP) and the Current Opioid Misuse Measure (COMM) [45]. Universal precautions should be considered to standardize the approach to assessment and management of opioid-related risks with the intention to decrease stigma for people with chronic pain using opioids [46]. This is discussed in detail in Chapter 39. Patients who engage in repeated problematic drug-related behaviors and/or patients whose urine toxicology specimens are inconsistent with reported use of drugs should be engaged in discussion about their substance use, with consideration of tapering and discontinuation of their opioid therapy or switch to opioid agonist therapy if they meet criteria for opioid use disorder and referred to addiction medicine specialist care.

There is little evidence to guide providers regarding counseling patients on the risk of driving using opioids. There may be transient or persistent cognitive impairment associated with the use of opioids. Patients should be counseled not to drive or perform potentially dangerous activities if they feel impaired. Somnolence, clouded thinking, difficulty concentrating and slower reflexes may occur more commonly with initiation of therapy or with dose adjustments as well as with concomitant use of other drugs or alcohol. In the absence of signs or symptoms of impairment, there is no evidence that patients maintained on opioids should be restricted from driving. It may be prudent to consider restricting driving when opioids are first begun or when doses are escalated for a period of approximately a week.

Guidelines vary in recommendations regarding dose restrictions. The United States Centers for Disease Control and Prevention (CDC) and Canadian guidelines have indicated that doses should not exceed 50 mg of morphine equivalent dose (MED) with a recommended top dose of 90 mg MED for patients starting opioid therapy long-term, while German Pain Society guidelines mention a maximum dose of 120 mg MED [3-5]. In the US and Canada the guidelines suggest that if a patient's opioid regimens is above this threshold, a trial of opioid taper is recommended to the lowest effective dose, which may include discontinuation. Unfortunately, both of these guidelines have led to unintended consequences including inflexible application of guidelines to restrict access, abrupt tapering and discontinuation of opioids, propagation and deepening of stigma, loss of autonomy and shared decision making with health care providers, deterioration of pain control and decreases in level of function with further underemployment [7, 8, 47]. At the time of writing the US CDC guidelines are receiving further evaluation and the reader is encouraged to watch for updated information and in the meantime to take an individual approach to your patient following the principles presented in this chapter.

If a patient has experienced an initial response to an opioid and then develops tolerance rotation to an alternative opioid may also help to reduce the dose, taking advantage of incomplete cross tolerance in the dose calculation of the new opioid, as well as improve pain management or reduce problematic adverse effects.

Opioid Tapering and Discontinuation

For people who have been receiving long-term opioid therapy, there may be opportunities to taper and reduce the dose without causing decline in quality of life or pain. In cases of opioid-induced hyperalgesia, the pain intensity might be reduced with opioid tapering. Patients should be actively engaged in discussions about tapering. Benefits for some patients may include relief from adverse effects, reduction in inter-dose withdrawal symptoms (e.g., pain, sweating or anxiety close to the end of the dosing interval), improvements in overall function and quality of life [48].

Where available consideration of a multidisciplinary and/or team-based approach to tapering is associated with increased success. Symptoms from opioid withdrawal can be quite unpleasant and can have serious consequences if the person has an unstable coronary artery disease, unstable depression, or during pregnancy. Although there is expert guidance available to guide tapering plans and to address frequently asked questions, evidence is still lacking about the best method and efficacy [49]. One method of tapering is to consolidate the opioid regimen and substitute with an alternative long-acting opioid. A slow wean with a reduction of 10% of dosage every 2–4 weeks is suggested. The taper may be paused or slowed as needed, most clinicians would agree that the speed of the taper at the beginning rarely predicts the pace at the end.

Patients who have been on opioids for a long time or are highly anxious may benefit from a more gradual taper. An opioid tapering template may be helpful to guide clinicians and patients to create an individualized tapering schedule [51]. Though rapid tapering may sometimes be warranted for example, patient preference or when there is a significant imminent risk of overdose. A 25% reduction is unlikely to precipitate severe symptoms of withdrawal, however, rapid tapers should only be carried out in a medically supervised environment, where withdrawal can be managed.

Opioid use During Pregnancy

Opioid use during pregnancy may be associated with risks to the mother and the fetus [52]. These risks include pre-term birth [53] and neonatal opioid withdrawal syndrome [54]. Management of opioid use during pregnancy must be done with clinical expertise and caution, since abrupt discontinuation of opioids leading to opioid withdrawal has been associated with miscarriage and premature labor [52]. Clinicians should screen women who are pregnant for opioid use and opioid use disorder and counsel minimal or no use of opioids during pregnancy whenever feasible. If a woman using opioids long-term is planning a pregnancy, it is recommended that they attempt to taper and discontinue if possible. Pregnant women with an opioid use disorder should be offered timely access to opioid agonist therapy, both buprenorphine/naloxone and methadone are safe and have been associated with improved outcomes [52, 55].

Conclusions

This chapter reviews an approach for the clinician to prescribing opioids for chronic non-cancer pain. Patient selection, including appropriate assessment of pain, assessment of opioid-related risks including opioid use disorder and careful dose titration are key elements in conducting an opioid trial in patients with chronic pain. Ongoing careful monitoring and shared decision making are important for optimizing outcomes.

References

1 Häuser W, Schug S, Furlan AD. (2017) The opioid epidemic and national guidelines for opioid therapy for chronic noncancer pain: a perspective from different continents. *Pain Reports* **2(3)**:e599.

2 *International Narcotic Control Board (INCB) Narcotic Drugs: estimated world requirements for 2020, statistics for 2018. United Nations Publication Report No: E/INCB/2019/2.* https://www.incb.org/incb/en/narcotic-drugs/Technical_Reports/2019/narcotic-drugs-technical-report-2019.html. Accessed November 1, 2021.

3 Busse JW, Craigie S, Juurlink DN *et al.* (2017) Guideline for opioid therapy and chronic noncancer pain. *CMAJ* **189(18)**:E659–E66.

4 Dowell D, Haegerich TM, Chou R. (2016). CDC Guideline for Prescribing Opioids for Chronic Pain - United States, 2016. *MMWR Recomm Rep* **65(1)**:1–49.

5 Petzke F, Bock F, Hüppe M *et al.* (2020) Long-term opioid therapy for chronic noncancer pain: second update of the German guidelines. *Pain Reports* **5(5)**.

6 *Faculty of Pain Medicine, Australian and New Zealand College of Anaesthetists (FPMANZCA). Statement regarding the use of opioid analgesics in patients with chronic non-cancer pain.* Available at https://www.anzca.edu.au/getattachment/7d7d2619-6736-4d8e-876e-6f9b2b45c435/PS01(PM)-Statement-regarding-the-use-of-opioid-analgesics-in-patients-with-chronic-non-cancer-pain Accessed March 17, 2021.

7 Antoniou T, Ala-Leppilampi K, Shearer D, Parsons JA, Tadrous M, Gomes T. (2019) "Like being put on an ice floe and shoved away": A qualitative study of the impacts of opioid-related policy changes on people who take opioids. *Int J Drug Policy* **66**:15–22.

8 Dassieu L, Heino L, Develey É *et al.* (2021) "They think you're trying to get the drug": Qualitative investigation of chronic pain patients' health care experiences during the opioid overdose epidemic in Canada. *Canadian Journal of Pain* **15(1)**:66–80.

9 McDonald J, Lambert DG. (2005) Opioid receptors. *Continuing Education in Anaesthesia Critical Care & Pain* **5(1)**:22–5.

10 Waldhoer M, Bartlett SE, Whistler JL. (2004) Opioid receptors. *Annu Rev Biochem* **73**:953–90.

11 Vallejo R, Barkin RL, Wang VC. (2011) Pharmacology of opioids in the treatment of

chronic pain syndromes. *Pain Physician* **14(4)**: E343–60.

12 Aydede M, Shriver, A. (2018) Recently introduced definition of "nociplastic pain" by the International Association for the Study of Pain needs better formulation. *Pain* **159(6)**:1176–7.

13 Yi P, Pryzbylkowski, P. (2015) Opioid Induced Hyperalgesia. *Pain Med***16 Suppl 1**:S32–6.

14 Pereira J, Lawlor P, Vigano A *et al.* (2001) Equianalgesic dose ratios for opioids: a critical review and proposals for long-term dosing. *J Pain Symptom Manag* **22(2)**:672–87.

15 Gomes T, Juurlink DN, Antoniou T, Mamdami MM, Paterson JM, van den Brink W. (2017) Gabapentin, opioids, and the risk of opioid-related death: A population-based nested case-control study. *PLoS Med* **14(10)**:e1002396.

16 Gomes T, Khuu W, Craiovan D *et al.* (2018) Comparing the contribution of prescribed opioids to opioid-related hospitalizations across Canada: A multi-jurisdictional cross-sectional study. *Drug Alcohol Depend* **191**:86–90.

17 Jones CM, Paulozzi LJ, Mack KA. (2010) Alcohol involvement in opioid pain reliever and benzodiazepine drug abuse-related emergency department visits and drug-related deaths - United States, 2010. *MMWR Morb Mortal Wkly Rep, 2014* **63(40)**:881–5.

18 Sun EC, Dixit A, Humphreys K, Darnall BD, Baker LC, Mackey S. (2017) Association between concurrent use of prescription opioids and benzodiazepines and overdose: retrospective analysis. *BMJ* **356**:760.

19 Busse J, ed. (2017) *The 2017 Canadian guideline for opioids for chronic non-cancer pain. McMaster University, Hamilton.* Available at https://app.magicapp.org/#/guideline/8nyb0E. Accessed November 1, 2021.

20 Miotto K, Cho AK, Khalil MA, Blanco K, Sasaki JD, Rawson R. (2017) Trends in tramadol: pharmacology, metabolism, and misuse. *Anesthesia & Analgesia* **124(1)**:44–51.

21 Canadian Pharmacists Association. (2016) *[updated 2020 11 308]. Opioids [CPhA monograph].* Available at http://www.myrxtx.ca. Accessed November 1, 2021.

22 McPherson ML. (2010) *Demystifying Opioid Conversion Calculations. American Society of Health-System Pharmacists*, Inc., Bethesda.

23 Lugo RA, Satterfield KL, Kern SE. (2005) Pharmacokinetics of methadone. *J Pain Palliat Care Pharmacother* **19(4)**:13–24.

24 Canadian Pharmacists Association. (2016) [updated 2016 08 06; cited 2017 12 03]. *BuTrans® [product monograph].* Available at http://www.e-cps.ca or http://www.myrxtx.ca. Accesssed December 3, 2017.

25 Webster L, Gudin J, Raffa RB *et al.* (2020) Understanding buprenorphine for use in chronic pain: expert opinion. *Pain Med* **21(4)**:714–23.

26 Serafini G, Adavastro G, Canepa G *et al.* (2018) The efficacy of buprenorphine in major depression, treatment-resistant depression and suicidal behavior: a systematic review. *Int J Mol Sci* **19(8)**:2410.

27 Anton RF, Myrick H, Baros AM *et al.* (2009) Efficacy of a combination of flumazenil and gabapentin in the treatment of alcohol dependence: relationship to alcohol withdrawal symptoms. *J Clin Psychopharmacol* **29(4)**:334–42.

28 Toljan K, Vrooman, B. (2018) Low-dose naltrexone (LDN)-review of therapeutic utilization. *Medical Sciences (Basel, Switzerland)* **6(4)**:82.

29 Younger J, Mackey, S. (2009) Fibromyalgia symptoms are reduced by low-dose naltrexone: a pilot study. *Pain Med* **10(4)**:663–72.

30 Younger J, Noor N, McCue R, Mackey S. (2013) Low-dose naltrexone for the treatment of fibromyalgia: findings of a small, randomized, double-blind, placebo-controlled, counterbalanced, crossover trial assessing daily pain levels. *Arthritis Rheum* **65(2)**:529–38.

31 Chopra P,. Cooper, MS. (2013) Treatment of complex regional pain syndrome (CRPS) using low dose naltrexone (LDN). *Journal of Neuroimmune Pharmacology: The Official Journal of the Society on NeuroImmune Pharmacology* **8(3)**:470–6.

32 Ting S, Schug, S. (2016) The pharmacogenomics of pain management: prospects for personalized medicine. *Journal of Pain Research.* **9**:49–56.

33 Kaye AD, Garcia AJ, Hall OM *et al.* (2019) Update on the pharmacogenomics of pain management. *Pharmacogenomics and Personalized Medicine* **12**:125–43.

34 Saïdi H, Pagé MG, Boulanger A, Ware MA, Choinière M. (2018) Effectiveness of long-term opioid therapy among chronic non-cancer pain

patients attending multidisciplinary pain treatment clinics: A Quebec Pain Registry study. *Canadian Journal of Pain* **2(1)**:113–24.

35 Moulin DE, Clark JA, Gordon A *et al.* (2015) Long-term outcome of the management of chronic neuropathic pain: a prospective observational study. *J Pain* **16(9)**:852–61.

36 Kaboré JL, Saïdi H, Dassieu L, Choinière M, Pagé GM. (2020) Predictors of long-term opioid effectiveness in patients with chronic non-cancer pain attending multidisciplinary pain treatment clinics: a Quebec Pain Registry study. *Pain Pract* **20(6)**:588–99.

37 Furlan AD, Sandoval JA, Mailis-Gagnon A, Tunks E. (2006) Opioids for chronic noncancer pain: a meta-analysis of effectiveness and side effects. *CMAJ* **174(11)**:1589–94.

38 Furlan A, Chaparro LE, Irvin E, Mailis-Gagnon A. (2011) A comparison between enriched and non-enriched enrollment randomized withdrawal trials of opioids for chronic noncancer pain. *Pain Research & Management: the Yournal of the Canadian Pain Society = journal de la societe canadienne pour le traitement de la douleur.* **16(5)**:337–51.

39 Voon P, Karamouzian M, Kerr, T. (2017) Chronic pain and opioid misuse: a review of reviews. *Substance Abuse Treatment, Prevention, and Policy* **12(1)**:36.

40 Rauck RL. (2009) What is the case for prescribing long-acting opioids over short-acting opioids for patients with chronic pain? A critical review. *Pain Pract* **9(6)**:468–79.

41 Pedersen L, Borchgrevink PC, Riphagen II, Fredheim OMS. (2014) Long- or short-acting opioids for chronic non-malignant pain? A qualitative systematic review. *Acta Anaesthesiol Scand* **58(4)**:390–401.

42 Gudin JA. (2013) Assessment of extended-release opioid analgesics for the treatment of chronic pain. *J Pain Palliat Care Pharmacother* **27(1)**:49–61.

43 Tsuyuki RT, Arora V, Barnes M *et al.* (2020) Canadian national consensus guidelines for naloxone prescribing by pharmacists. *Canadian Pharmacists Journal / Revue des Pharmaciens du Canada* **153(6)**:347–51.

44 Cleeland CS. (2009) *The Brief Pain Inventory User Guide. Available at* https://www.mdanderson.org/documents/Departments-and-Divisions/Symptom-Research/BPI_UserGuide.pdf. *Accessed November 21, 2017.*

45 Lawrence R, Mogford D, Colvin, L. (2017) Systematic review to determine which validated measurement tools can be used to assess risk of problematic analgesic use in patients with chronic pain. *Br J Anaesth* **119(6)**1092–109.

46 Gourlay DL, Heit HA, Almahrezi, A. (2005) Universal precautions in pain medicine: a rational approach to the treatment of chronic pain. *Pain Med* **6(2)**:107–12.

47 Dassieu L, Kaboré J-L, Choinière M, Arruda N, Roy É. (2019) Chronic pain management among people who use drugs: A health policy challenge in the context of the opioid crisis. *Int J Drug Policy* **71**:150–6.

48 Frank JW, Lovejoy TI, Becker WC *et al.* (2017) Patient outcomes in dose reduction or discontinuation of long-term opioid therapy: a systematic review. *Ann Intern Med* **167(3)**:181–91.

49 Murphy L, Babaei-Rad R, Bunna D *et al.* (2018) Guidance on opioid tapering in the context of chronic pain: Evidence, practical advice and frequently asked questions. *Can Pharm J (Ott)* **151(2)**:114–20.

50 Kahan M, Mailis-Gagnon A, Wilson L, Srivastava A. (2011) Canadian guideline for safe and effective use of opioids for chronic noncancer pain. *Canadian Family Physician* **57**:1257–66.

51 Regier L. (2017) *Opioid Tapering Template.*, RxFiles https://www.rxfiles.ca/rxfiles/uploads/documents/Opioid-Tapering-Newsletter-Compilation.pdf. Accessed November 1, 2021.

52 Committee on Obstetric Practice American Society of Addiction Medicine (2017) Committee Opinion No. 711: Opioid Use and Opioid Use Disorder in Pregnancy. *Obstet Gynecol* **130(2)**: e81–e94.

53 Corsi DJ, Hsu H, Fell DB, Wen SW, Walker M. (2020) Association of maternal opioid use in pregnancy with adverse perinatal outcomes in Ontario, Canada, from 2012 to 2018. *JAMA Network Open* **3(7)**: e208256.

54 Patrick SW, Barfield WD, Poindexter BB. (2020) Neonatal ppioid withdrawal syndrome. *Pediatrics* **146(5)**:e2020029074.

55 Ambasta A, Malebranche M. (2019) Opioid use disorder in pregnancy. *Canadian Medical Association Journal* **191(38)**:E1057.

Chapter 19

Topical analgesics

Oli Abate Fulas & Terence J. Coderre

Department of Anesthesia and Alan Edwards Centre for Research on Pain, McGill University, Montréal, Québec, Canada

Introduction

Topical analgesics are local treatments applied to the skin or mucous membranes that alleviate pain by acting on the underlying soft tissue and peripheral nerve endings [1]. After penetrating the surface of application, these agents act on varying targets in the local tissue and sensory nerve terminals to reduce the induction and transmission of pain signal to the central nervous system (CNS). Topically applied analgesics are used to treat acute pain conditions due to wounds, ulcers, muscle aches, sprains and strains [2]. They are also recommended for the treatment of chronic pain due to osteoarthritis, neuropathic pain and complex regional pain syndrome [3–5].

Topical analgesic formulations are available in the form of solutions, ointments, creams, gels, foams, sprays, patches or plaster. The constitution of topical preparations determines their ability to penetrate the relatively impermeable epidermal skin, more specifically the stratum corneum, which is the lipophilic outermost layer of the epidermis. Topical formulations with active ingredients of greater lipophilicity and lower molecular weight can more efficiently permeate the skin to reach their local targets. New approaches to enhancing skin penetration are being developed with permeability enhancers like liposomes, lecithin organogels, flexible vesicles and nanocarriers [1]. Microemulsions and nanoemulsions have also been developed to enhance skin flux through the solubilization of lipophilic and low molecular weight active ingredients [1]. Another fundamental determinant of topical delivery is the physical status of the skin as determined by age, sex hormones, skin type and integrity [6]. Additionally, the concentration of active ingredients in topical formulations, frequency of administration and duration of exposure to the agents all factor into the delivery and effectiveness of topical treatments [6].

Analgesics applied on the skin can be purposed for either topical or transdermal drug delivery. While topical analgesics cross the skin barrier to act on the local tissue with little systemic uptake, transdermal analgesics act on remote targets, usually the CNS, after being absorbed directly into the systemic circulation, bypassing gastrointestinal absorption and hepatic first-pass metabolism. The serum therapeutic level achieved with the transdermal route is comparable to other systemic routes as is the frequency of side effects and drug-drug interactions associated with it. Topical analgesics, in contrast, feature optimal delivery of therapeutic local drug levels for pain-relieving peripheral effects and minimal risk of adverse effects (See Table 19.1).

Topical analgesics in current clinical and experimental use fall into categories that: (1) block sensory inputs; (2) activate peripheral inhibitory mechanisms; (3) target peripheral source of underling pathology; (4) are multifunctional topical combinations; and (5) those primarily intended for mucosal pain conditions. (See Table 19.2 for the mostly commonly used topical agents).

Clinical Pain Management: A Practical Guide, Second Edition. Edited by Mary E. Lynch, Kenneth D. Craig, and Philip W. Peng.

Topical therapeutics that block sensory input

Local anesthetics

Topical local anesthetic formulations mostly contain lidocaine with the seldom additions of prilocaine or tetracaine. These local anesthetics are neuronal membrane stabilizers that inhibit the frequency of opening of voltage-gated sodium channels to impair the propagation of sensory input. They can specifically block ectopic discharge from regenerating nerve fibers in which sodium channels are upregulated. They additionally act on keratinocytes, endothelial and immune cells to inhibit the release of inflammatory mediators.

Table 19.1 The benefits and shortcomings of topically delivered analgesics

Benefits	Shortcomings
Steady and therapeutic tissue concentrations achieved with minimal systemic distribution	Optimal molecular size and physicochemical properties required for efficient dermal penetration
Bioavailability unaffected by gastrointestinal absorption and hepatic first-pass effect	Bioavailability affected by variations in skin permeability and local drug metabolism
Greater patient compliance, not precluded by factors that impair oral administration	Limited use in disease states that alter dermal absorptive properties

Lidocaine is available as 5% gel, cream and patch and 8% spray. The 5% lidocaine patch is registered for first line use in post-herpetic neuralgia (PHN). The patch, worn for 12 hours in every 24 hours, also provides protection against dynamic allodynia due to mechanical stimulation. At this dose, topical lidocaine also alleviates post-surgical neuropathy, carpal tunnel syndrome and diabetic- and cancer-related neuropathies. In a randomized-control trial (RCT) on patients with focal peripheral neuropathy of varying etiologies, the 5% lidocaine patch has produced 50% relief from ongoing pain with a number needed to treat (NNT) of 4.4 (95% CI 2.5–17.5) after 7 days of administration. This efficacy was found to be comparable to other systemic agents like gabapentin and tricyclic antidepressants (TCAs) [7]. The analgesic effects of topical lidocaine depend on peripheral actions as only 3% of the drug penetrates the systemic circulation. Its long-term use in localized neuropathic pain provides sustained pain relief causing only reversible erythema and no systemic side effects [8].

Other topical local anesthetics are available as combinations of lidocaine with tetracaine (cream, 7% each), lidocaine with tetracaine (self-heating patch, 70 mg each) and lidocaine with prilocaine

Table 19.2 Common topical analgesics with their mechanism of action and indications.

Topical Agent	Mechanism of Action	Clinical/Experimental Use	NNT (95% CI)
Local Anesthetics 5% Lidocaine patch	Suppress activity of voltage-gated Na^+ channels on sensory afferents	PHN, PDN	4.4 (2.5 - 17.5) [7]
Capsaicinoids 8% Capsaicin patch	Overstimulate & desensitize TRPV1 channels on sensory afferents	PHN, PDN, HIV-neuropathy	10 (6.3 - 28) [15]
NSAIDs e.g. Diclofenac gel	Suppress inflammation through COX inhibition	Soft tissue injury (strains, sprains)	1.8 (1.5 - 2.1) [26]
		osteoarthritis, rheumatism, back pain	9.8 (7.1 - 16) [27]
Nitrates	Release NO for vasodilation	PDN	4 (2 - 7) [36]
Clonidine (0.1% gel)	Block of NE-mediated vasoconstriction & reduce nociceptor hyperexcitability	PDN	8.88 (4.3 - 50) [31]

NNT, number needed to treat; CI, confidence interval; PHN, post-herpetic neuralgia; PDN, painful diabetic neuropathy, TRPV1, transient receptor potential vanilloid-1; HIV, human immunodeficiency virus; NSAIDs, non-steroidal antinflammatory drugs; COX, cyclooxygenase; NE, norepinephrine.

(EMLA cream, 2.5% each). These preparations are commonly used to treat patients with acute pain. Topical EMLA cream alleviates pain due to facial and perineal lacerations [9, 10]. The cream is also effective in reducing wound-related pain associated with chronic leg ulcers [11].

Capsaicinoids

The capsaicinoids act by binding to the transient receptor potential vanilloid 1 (TRPV1), a non-selective cation permeable transduction channel expressed on nociceptors. While this binding causes an initial activation with the release of neuropeptides, repeated application of capsaicin or single exposure to high concentrations of capsaicin causes over-stimulation followed by desensitization of TRPV1, depletion of neuropeptides and a reversible degeneration of sensory terminals. The outcome is a defunctionalization of nociceptors that results in analgesia.

Capsaicin and its synthetic cis isomer, zucapsaicin, have been clinically used as topical preparations for the alleviation of pain. Low-concentration (0.025–0.075 %) capsaicin creams, gels and patches are available over the counter for the treatment of localized neuropathic pain but have shown little effect beyond that found with placebo treatments [12]. Recent recommendations have conditionally approved low dose topical capsaicin for the treatment of knee osteoarthritis [13]. According to a current meta-analysis, the 0.025% cream used four times a day produces clinically meaningful alleviation of pain in these patients (effect size: 0.41, 95% CI 0.17–0.64) [14].

The high-concentration (8%) capsaicin patch has analgesic effects in PHN, neuropathic back pain, human immunodeficiency virus (HIV)-neuropathy, painful diabetic neuropathy (PDN), cancer-related and post-traumatic neuropathy. In a recent systematic review, a single treatment with 8% capsaicin patch produced significant pain relief in postherpetic neuralgia at 2 to 12 weeks with NNT to obtain 30% pain reduction of 10 (95% CI 6.3–28) [15]. Similarly, the patch produced analgesia in painful HIV-neuropathy that lasted 2 to 12 weeks with NNT of 11 (95% CI 6.2–47) for a 30% reduction in pain intensity. The studies included used a low dose (0.04%) capsaicin patch as their control-treatment to prevent unblinding as topical application of capsaicin causes transient erythema and burning sensations. Patients with mixed localized neuropathic pain have been shown to get greater relief from allodynia with 8% capsaicin patch as compared to oral pregabalin [16].

While low concentration formulations of capsaicin need repeated administration to produce an effect, a single application of the 8% capsaicin patch for 30–60 mins produces analgesic effects lasting for up to 3 months [15]. Local reactions like burning pain, erythema, swelling and pruritus that occur after the topical treatment are more frequent and severe with these high concentration patches. This is the reason behind the recommendations for obtaining the 8% capsaicin patch treatment in the presence of a health care professional. The adverse effects are managed with pre-treatment using local anesthetics or cooling after patch application. Even at low concentrations capsaicin has been found to cause a reversible degeneration of sensory and autonomic intraepidermal nerve fibers (IENFs) [17].

Zucapsaicin is a synthetic *cis* isomer of capsaicin with a similar mechanism of action but fewer adverse local reactions. The 0.075% zucapsaicin (civamide) cream has been found to effectively alleviate pain and physical function in patients with knee osteoarthritis in a 12-week long multicenter RCT [18]. No measurable systemic absorption of the drug was detected and local reactions like burning and rash occurred in 5% of the patients. In the same study, an open-label, 12-month long-term continuation of treatment with 0.075% zucapsaicin produced a 34% reduction of osteoarthritic pain score from baseline.

Topical therapeutics that activate inhibitory systems

Topical opioids

Cutaneous and mucosal sensory nerve endings express opioid receptors and their expression is upregulated in pathological painful conditions [19]. When activated, opioid receptors inhibit adenylyl cyclase and modulate ion channels to result in the dampening of pain transmission in nociceptors. There is some evidence for the analgesic efficacy of topical opioids in malignant and non-malignant skin ulcers and oropharyngeal mucositis as observed from small RCTs [20]. In the studies, gel formulations of morphine and diamorphine alleviated pain in patients with pressure ulcers in palliative care.

Topical cannabinoids

Cannabinoid receptors are present on peripheral nerve terminals, keratinocytes and immune cells in the skin [21]. Their activation inhibits cutaneous nociceptors by affecting the activities of adenylate cyclase, mitogen-activated protein kinase and various ion channels [21]. There is preliminary evidence for the topical analgesic use of cannabinoids in neuropathic pain. In patients with symptomatic peripheral neuropathy of varying etiologies, an RCT assessing topical treatment with cannabidiol oil administered for 4 weeks produced significant reduction in pain [22]. Similarly, a four-week-long topical treatment with a cream containing the cannabinoid receptor agonist N-palmitoylethanolamine has alleviated pain in patients with postherpetic neuralgia enrolled into an open-label trial [23].

Moreover, topical cannabidiol has been reported to reduce pain and promote healing in a case series of pediatric patients with the blistering skin disorder, epidermolysis bullosa [24]. Similarly, topical application of medical cannabis produced pain reduction of greater than 30% in a prospective case series of patients with pyoderma gangrenosum, an ulcerative inflammatory skin condition that produces an intense and opioid-resistant pain [25].

Topical analgesics that target peripheral sources of pathology

NSAIDs

Nonsteroidal anti-inflammatory drugs (NSAIDs) produce anti-inflammatory and analgesic effects through the reversible inhibition of cyclooxygenase-(COX) dependent metabolism of arachidonic acid into various inflammatory mediators that include prostaglandins and prostacyclin. Topical NSAIDs dampen the sensitization of peripheral nociceptors by such inflammatory mediators that are the source of pathology in acute and chronic inflammatory and musculoskeletal pain.

Several topical NSAID preparations have demonstrated efficacy in acute pain conditions like join strains, sprains and overuse injuries. In a recent systematic review and metanalysis, topical diclofenac gel (1.2–2.3%) (Emulgel) produced a 50% reduction in acute musculoskeletal pain with an NNT of 1.8 (95% CI 1.5–2.1) [26]. For topical ibuprofen gel, the NNT was 3.9 (95% CI 2.7–6.7) and that of topical ketoprofen gel 2.5 (95% CI 2.0–3.4). The treatments were given at least once daily for up to seven days and NNT calculations for each of the topical preparations included 2–5 RCTs with 240–350 participants in studies of moderate to high quality. A slightly lower efficacy was reported for plaster preparations of diclofenac and ketoprofen in patients with acute musculoskeletal pain with an NNT ranging between 3.2 and 8.2. In these studies, the topical use of NSAIDs has been associated with mild and transient local irritation with erythema and pruritis but not at a higher frequency than their placebo counterparts. Systemic adverse effects are rare, as plasma concentrations of NSAIDs after topical administration is less than 5% of the level attained through systemic routes [26].

In chronic musculoskeletal pain, specifically knee osteoarthritis, topical administration of diclofenac and ketoprofen produces analgesia. In this group of patients, at least 50% reduction in pain has been achieved after 6 to 12 weeks of treatment with topical diclofenac gel or solution yielding an NNT of 9.8 (95% CI 7.1–16) whereas that of topical ketoprofen gel was 6.9 (95% CI 5.4–9.3). These values come from a metanalysis in a recent Cochrane systematic review that included 4–6 moderate quality trials with greater than 5,000 patients [27]. The efficacy of topical NSAIDs is also being explored in non-musculoskeletal chronic pain conditions. A RCT in a small cohort of patients with PHN and complex regional pain syndrome (CRPS) showed that a 1.5% topical solution of diclofenac produced a significant improvement in self-reported pain [28].

Clonidine

Clonidine is a presynaptic α_2-adrenergic agonist used as an antihypertensive agent that also has analgesic effects when administered topically [29]. Its analgesic mechanisms may involve alleviating microvascular dysfunction through the inhibition of vasoconstrictive norepinephrine (NE) released from peripheral sympathetic terminals innervating the microvasculature. It may also reduce nociceptor hyperexcitability by direct activation of its α_2-adrenergic and I_2-imidazoline receptors [30].

Topical clonidine produces improvement in PDN as demonstrated by a metanalysis of two studies that resulted in a NNT of 8.88 (95% CI 4.3–50) to obtain a 30% reduction in pain [31]. The studies, that involved close to 350 patients, examined the analgesic effect of 0.1–0.2% clonidine gel applied to both feet 2–3 times daily for 8–12 weeks. The existing limited evidence for the efficacy of topical clonidine in PDN has so far led to recommendations for the use of the drug in situations where alternate treatment options have been exhausted due to inefficacy, contraindications and side effects. Topical clonidine produces none of the undesirable adverse effects like dry mouth, sedation and hypotension that occur with its systemic administration [31].

Nitrates

Nitrates like glyceryl trinitrate (GTN) and isosorbide dinitrate are agents that are locally metabolized to release nitric oxide (NO) and produce vasodilation by increasing guanylate cyclase levels in the vascular smooth muscle [32]. Ischemic pain conditions are known to benefit from treatment with nitrates [33]. There is some evidence for the analgesic effects of topical nitrates in pain conditions like CRPS, PDN and musculoskeletal pain due to tendinopathies [34–36]. GTN spray given for 4 weeks produced a significant reduction in pain scores as compared to placebo in a group of 50 patients with PDN enrolled in a cross-over double-blind RCT. The NNT was calculated to be 4 (95% CI 2–7) [36]. Similarly, the use of topical GTN patches in patients with acute shoulder tendinopathies reduced pain intensity, though its long-term benefit could not be ascertained [35]. Headaches are a common side effect of systemic absorption of nitrates and can potentially follow topical treatment with GTN.

Topical combinations

Topical combinations of analgesics create room for greater efficacy due to their potential to impact multiple pathological processes. One of the most studied topical analgesic combination for chronic pain is composed of the antidepressant amitriptyline and the NMDA receptor antagonist ketamine. While amitriptyline has multiple peripheral effects including actions on opioid, cholinergic, histaminergic and adenosine receptors, as well as various ion channels, ketamine primarily blocks the glutaminergic N-methyl-D-aspartate (NMDA) receptors with additional actions on calcium channels and cholinergic, monoaminergic and opioid receptors. RCTs that investigated the singular use of either agent for the treatment of chronic pain conditions like neuropathic pain has produced mixed results giving no consistent indication for their analgesic efficacy [37, 38].

A 2-week long treatment with the topical combination of amitriptyline 2% and ketamine 1% has produced a 33% reduction in average daily pain in a RCT of patients with PHN [39]. A double-blind RCT that compared this topical combination to oral gabapentin in PHN has revealed that 4 weeks of treatment with either of these agents produced comparable pain-relieving effects with no significant difference in analgesic efficacy [39]. Similarly, a combination of ketamine (1.5%) and amitriptyline (3%) with the addition of baclofen (0.75%) in pluronic lecithin organogel has improved symptoms of tingling, cramping and burning pain in the hands of patients with chemotherapy-induced painful neuropathy in a double-blind RCT [40].

Topical therapeutics for mucosal tissue

Painful pathologies of mucosal tissues are particularly amenable to topical analgesics, given the relative ease for drug absorption at these sites. Oral mucositis after chemotherapy is commonly treated with topical morphine mouth rinse (0.1–0.2%) and gel (0.1 %) [20]. Orofacial neuropathic pain, pulpitis and chemotherapy-induced mucositis have also been effectively treated with oral (lozenge, gum, mouthwash, gel, etc.) therapies, including 0.01–0.25% capsaicin, 2% amitriptyline, 0.2% topical clonidine and 5% ketamine [41]. Topical steroids in the form of pastes, ointments and mouthwashes have been observed to relieve pain due to aphthous ulcers [42]. Local anesthetics gels and creams have also demonstrated efficacy in relieving mild to moderate pain due to oral mucosal lesions caused by trauma and ulceration [42].

For pain pathologies in the rectal, genital and perineal areas that include vulvodynia, proctodynia and pudendal neuralgia, analgesia has been achieved with the topical agents 1–2.5% amitriptyline (alone or combined with other agents), 2–6% gabapentin and 2% ketamine [41].

Current advancements in topical analgesics

Research efforts in the development of effective topical therapeutics for acute and chronic pain are still ongoing. New topical formulations of local anesthetics, NSAIDs and capsaicin with improved constitution and dosing are being investigated in clinical trials for different pain conditions. More interestingly, novel therapeutics like funapide (XEN402), a selective NaV1.7/1.8 channel antagonist, are being investigated for the treatment of PHN.

Another potential for advancement in the repertoire of topical analgesics can come through the utilization of analgesic combinations in the form of co-drugs, drug-drug salts, co-crystals and ionic liquids. These preparations are made by pairing multi-targeted analgesic agents based on not only therapeutic complementarity, but also physicochemical properties so better solubility and bioavailability are achieved. While co-drugs are conjugates typically bound together by covalent chemical bonds, drug-drug salts, co-crystals and hydrates are crystalline compounds of two or more active drugs, linked by ionic or hydrogen bonds. Ionic liquids are salts in the liquid form. The synthesis of such analgesic combinations has been reported and constitutes agents with local anesthetic, anti-inflammatory, antidepressant and opioid activities. Some examples are lidocaine-ibuprofen, lidocaine-etodolac, lidocaine-aspirin, aspirin-tramadol and celecoxib-tramadol all pending investigations as topical analgesic formulations [43,44].

Acknowledgements

T.J.C. has received grant support from CIHR, NSERC, FRQS-QPRN and the Louise and Alan Edwards Foundation. O.A.F. received studentships from the Louise and Alan Edwards Foundation and the MUHC Research Institute.

References

1 Stanos SS. (2020) Topical analgesics. *Phys Med Rehabil Clinic N Am* **31(2)**:233–44.

2 Derry S, Conaghan P, Da Silva JAP, Wiffen PJ, Moore A. (2016) Topical NSAIDs for chronic musculoskeletal pain in adults. *Cochrane Database Syst Rev* **4(4)**:CD007400.

3 National Clinical Guideline Centre (UK). (2014) Osteoarthritis: Care and Management in Adults. London: National Institute for Health and Care Excellence (UK); (NICE Clinical Guidelines, No. 177.) Available at https://www.nice.org.uk/guidance/cg177/resources/osteoarthritis-care-and-management-pdf-35109757272517.

4 Harden RN, Oaklander AL, Burton AW *et al.* (2013) Complex regional pain syndrome: practical diagnostic and treatment guidelines, 4th edn. *Pain Med* **14(2)**:180–229.

5 Finnerup NB, Attal N, Harotounian S *et al.* (2105) Pharmacotherapy for neuropathic pain in adults: a systematic review and meta-analysis. *Lancet Neurol* **14(2):** 162–73.

6 Tverdohleb T, Candido KD, Knezevic NN. (2019) Topical medications. In *Pain: A Review Guide*, Abd-Elsayed, A., eds. Springer International Publishing: Cham, pp. 293–6.

7 Davies PS, Galer BS. (2004) Review of lidocaine patch 5% studies in the treatment of postherpetic neuralgia. *Drugs* **64(9)**:937–47.

8 Wilhelm IR, Tzabazis A, Likar R, Sittl R, Griessinger N. (2010) Long-term treatment of neuropathic pain with a 5% lidocaine medicated plaster. *Eur J Anaesthesiol (EJA)* **27(2)**:169–73.

9 Park SW, Oh TS, Choi JW *et al.* (2015) Topical EMLA cream as a pretreatment for facial lacerations. *Arch Plast Surg* **42(1)**:28–33.

10 Abbas AM, Mohamed AA, Mattar OM *et al.* (2020) Lidocaine-prilocaine cream versus local infiltration anesthesia in pain relief during repair of perineal trauma after vaginal delivery: a systematic review and meta-analysis. *J Matern Fetal Neonatal Med* **33(6)**:1064–71.

11 Purcell A, Buckley T, King J, Moyle W, Marshall AP. (2020) Topical analgesic and local anesthetic

agents for pain associated with chronic leg ulcers: A systematic review. *Adv Skin Wound Care* **33(5)**:240–51.

12 Derry S, Moore RA. (2012) Topical capsaicin (low concentration) for chronic neuropathic pain in adults. *Cochrane Database Syst Rev* **2012(9)**:CD010111.

13 Kolasinski SL, Neogi T, Hochberg MC *et al*. (2020) American College of Rheumatology/Arthritis Foundation guideline for the management of osteoarthritis of the hand, hip, and knee. *Arthritis Rheumatol* **72(2)**:220–33.

14 Persson M, Stocks J, Walsh DA, Doherty M, Zhang W. (2018) The relative efficacy of topical non-steroidal anti-inflammatory drugs and capsaicin in osteoarthritis: a network meta-analysis of randomised controlled trials. *Osteoarthritis Cartilage* **26(12)**:1575–82.

15 Derry S, Rice AS, Cole P, Tan T, Moore AW. (2017) Topical capsaicin (high concentration) for chronic neuropathic pain in adults. *Cochrane Database Syst Rev* **1(1)**:CD007393.

16 Cruccu G, Nurmikko T, Ernault E, Riaz FK, McBride WT, Haanpää M. (2018) Superiority of capsaicin 8% patch versus oral pregabalin on dynamic mechanical allodynia in patients with peripheral neuropathic pain. *Eur J Pain* **22(4)**:700–6.

17 Nolano M, Simone DA, Wendelschafer-Crabb G, Johnson T, Hazen E, Kennedy WR. (1999) Topical capsaicin in humans: parallel loss of epidermal nerve fibers and pain sensation. *Pain* **81(1-2)**:135–45.

18 Schnitzer TJ, Pelletier J-P, Haselwood DM *et al*. (2012) Civamide cream 0.075% in patients with osteoarthritis of the knee: A 12-week randomized controlled clinical trial with a longterm extension. *J Rheumatol* **39(3)**:610–20.

19 Bigliardi PL, Tobin DJ, Gaveriaux-Ruff C, Bigliardi-Qi M, (2009) Opioids and the skin – where do we stand? *Exp Dermatol* **18(5)**:424–30.

20 LeBon B, Zeppetella G, Higginson IJ. (2009) Effectiveness of topical administration of opioids in palliative care: A systematic review. *J Pain Sympt Manage* **37(5)**:913–7.

21 Guindon J, Beaulieu P. (2009) The role of the endogenous cannabinoid system in peripheral analgesia. *Curr Mol Pharmacol* **2(1)**:134–9.

22 Xu DH, Cullen BD, Tang M, Fang Y. (2020) The effectiveness of topical cannabidiol oil in symptomatic relief of peripheral neuropathy of the lower extremities. *Curr Pharm Biotechnol* **21(5)**:390–402.

23 Phan NQ, Siepmann D, Gralow I, Ständer S. (2010) Adjuvant topical therapy with a cannabinoid receptor agonist in facial postherpetic neuralgia. *J Deutsch Dermatol Gesellschaft* **8(2)**:88–91.

24 Chelliah MP, Zinn Z, Khuu P *et al*. (2018) Self-initiated use of topical cannabidiol oil for epidermolysis bullosa. *Ped Dermatol* **35(4)**:e224–7.

25 Maida V, Corban J. (2007) Topical medical cannabis: A new treatment for wound pain - three cases of pyoderma gangrenosum. *J Pain Sympt Manage* **54(5)**:732–6.

26 Derry S, Moore RA, Gaskell H, McIntyre M, Wiffen PJ. (2015) Topical NSAIDs for acute musculoskeletal pain in adults. *Cochrane Database Syst Rev* **2015(6)**:CD007402.

27 Derry S, Wiffen PJ, Kalso EA *et al*. (2017) Topical analgesics for acute and chronic pain in adults - an overview of Cochrane Reviews. *Cochrane Database Syst Rev* **5(5)**:CD008609.

28 Ahmed SU, Zhang Y, Chen L *et al*. (2015) Effect of 1.5% topical diclofenac on clinical neuropathic pain. *Anesthesiology* **123(1)**:191–8.

29 Sawynok J. (2003) Topical and peripherally acting analgesics. *Pharmacol Rev* **55(1)**:1–20.

30 Khan ZP, Ferguson CN, Jones RM. (1999) Alpha-2 and imidazoline receptor agonists, their pharmacology and therapeutic role. *Anaesthesia* **54**: pp. 146–165.

31 Wrzosek A, Woron J, Dobrogowski J *et al*. (2015) Topical clonidine for neuropathic pain. *Cochrane Database Syst Rev* **8**:CD010967.

32 Mitchell JA, Ali F, Bailey L *et al*. (2008) Role of nitric oxide and prostacyclin as vasoactive hormones released by the endothelium. *Exp Physiol* **93**: pp. 141–147.

33 Nossaman VE, Nossaman BD, Kadowitz PJ. (2010) Nitrates and nitrites in the treatment of ischemic cardiac disease. *Cardiol Rev* **18**: pp. 190–197.

34 Groeneweg G, Niehof S, Wesseldijk F *et al*. (2008) Vasodilative effect of isosorbide dinitrate ointment in complex regional pain syndrome type 1. *Clin. J. Pain* **24**: pp. 89–92.

35 Cumpston M, Johnston RV, Wengier L *et al*. (2009) Topical glyceryl trinitrate for rotator cuff disease. *Cochrane Database Syst Rev* **3**:CD006355.

36 Agrawal RP, Choudhary R, Sharma P *et al.* (2007) Glyceryl trinitrate spray in the management of painful diabetic neuropathy: a randomized double blind placebo controlled cross-over study. *Diabetes Res Clin Pract* **77**: pp. 161–167.

37 Thompson DF, Brooks KG. (2015) Systematic review of topical amitriptyline for the treatment of neuropathic pain. *J Clin Pharm Ther* **40**: pp. 496–503.

38 Kopsky DJ, Keppel Hesselink JM *et al.* (2015) Analgesic effects of topical ketamine. *Minerva Anestesiol* **81**: pp. 440–449.

39 Sawynok J, Zinger C. (2016) Topical amitriptyline and ketamine for post-herpetic neuralgia and other forms of neuropathic pain. *Expert Opin Pharmacother* **17**: pp. 601–609.

40 Barton DL, Wos EJ, Qin R *et al.* (2011) A double-blind, placebo-controlled trial of a topical treatment for chemotherapy-induced peripheral neuropathy: NCCTG trial N06CA. *Supportive Care in Cancer: Official Journal of the Multinational Association of Supportive Care in Cancer* **19**: pp. 833–841.

41 Coderre TJ. (2018) Topical drug therapeutics for neuropathic pain. *Expert Opin Pharmacother* **19**: pp. 1211–1220.

42 Robertson JJ. (2016) Managing pharyngeal and oral mucosal pain. *Curr Emerg Hosp Med Rep* **4**: pp. 57–65.

43 Gascon N, Almansa C, Merlos M *et al.* (2019) Co-crystal of tramadol-celecoxib: preclinical and clinical evaluation of a novel analgesic. *Expert Opin Invest Drugs* **28**: pp. 399–409.

44 Shamshina JL, Barber PS, Rogers RD. (2013) Ionic liquids in drug delivery. *Expert Opin Drug Deliv* **10(1)**:1367–81.

Chapter 20

Cannabis and cannabinoid for pain

Amir Minerbi[1] **& Tali Sahar**[2,3]

[1] *Institute for Pain Medicine, Rambam Health Campus, Haifa, Israel*
[2] *Pain Relief Unit, Department of Anesthesia, Hadassah Medical Center, Jerusalem, Israel*
[3] *Department of Family Medicine, Hebrew University of Jerusalem, Jerusalem, Israel*

Introduction

A brief history of human cannabis use

Few treatment modalities for pain evoke as much emotion as does cannabis. Fewer are as ancient: humans have utilized cannabis as a source of fiber (ropes, fabrics and paper) and food, as well as for medicinal and ritual purposes throughout the millennia and over vast areas of the globe [1]. Medical use of cannabis declined through the first half of the twentieth century due to the introduction of new pharmaceutical agents and the adoption of restrictive and prohibition policies worldwide. Following the discovery of the active metabolites Δ^9-tetrahydrocannabinol (THC) and cannabidiol (CBD), as well as the cannabinoid receptors and the endocannabinoid system, interest in the potential therapeutic utility of cannabis has been increasing. This chapter will review the indications and evidence for the use of cannabinoids for pain in light of the complexity of their clinical use.

The endocannabinoid system

Endocannabinoid receptors

The human body hosts a vast and intricate innate cannabinoid system, comprising both receptors and ligands, as well as enzymes that synthesize and degrade the ligands. This system, known as the endocannabinoid system (ECS), forms a vast network throughout the body, with an important role in many aspects of human physiology. Acting as a modulatory, homoeostatic system, the ECS is involved in cognitive, behavioral, immunologic and metabolic functions [2, 3] in multiple organ systems. ECSs have been identified in various organisms, ranging from invertebrates to mammals, highlighting its putative evolutionary importance [4]. Two cannabinoid receptors have been identified: CB1 and CB2. Both are G-protein coupled receptors, found predominantly on cell membranes, which vary in their physiologic effects and their distribution on target organs.

Ligand binding to CB1 initiates an intracellular signaling cascade while also exerting a modulatory effect on membrane excitability. In the nervous system, CB1 is expressed preferentially on presynaptic terminals, where they modulate synaptic activity. Given their widespread expression, activation of CB1 receptors affects multiple physiologic processes, including memory, appetite, analgesia, anxiety, convulsions, cell proliferation and more.

CB2 is abundantly expressed by immune cells, and to a lesser degree in peripheral tissues and in the central nervous system (CNS), where it is thought to play a role in nociception and addiction. The physiologic effects of CB2 are less well understood.

In addition to the highly selective cannabinoid receptors CB1 and CB2, other receptors show affinity

Clinical Pain Management: A Practical Guide, Second Edition. Edited by Mary E. Lynch, Kenneth D. Craig, and Philip W. Peng.

for endocannabinoid ligands. These include the transient receptor potential cation channel subfamily V member 1 (TRPV1), considered by some as the third cannabinoid receptor CB3.

Endocannabinoid ligands

The two most-studied endocannabinoid ligands are N-arachidonoyl-ethanolamine (AEA, also known as anandamide) and 2-arachidonoylglycerol (2-AG). Other less-well studied CB1-interacting peptides have recently been reported. While both AEA and 2-AG are produced on demand, they differ in their synthesis, transport and degradation. They also differ in their affinity for cannabinoid receptors: AEA shows high affinity for CB1, of which it is a partial agonist, and negligible effect on CB2. In contrast, 2-AG is a full agonist of both CB1 and CB2, showing moderate-low affinity for both. Endocannabinoids also differ in their degradation pathways. While AEA is hydrolyzed by fatty acid amide hydrolase (FAAH), 2-AG is degraded by monoacylglycerol lipase (MAGL) [3].

The vast distribution of the endocannabinoid system and its role in multiple physiologic systems makes it an attractive target for therapeutic interventions, while also explaining the abundance of side effects associated with its manipulation.

Plant-derived cannabinoids and pharmaceutical cannabinoids

The taxonomy of cannabis is controversial. Decades of interbreeding of the two species (*Cannabis indica* and *Cannabis sativa*) – have led to intermixing such that they can no longer be considered distinct species or strains [5–7]. Thus, the common attribution of stimulating effects to *Cannabis sativa* and sedative effects to *Cannabis indica* is no longer accurate [8]. Cannabis plants produce hundreds of active metabolites, many of which may have biologic effects and are classified as cannabinoids, terpenoids and flavonoids. Plant-derived cannabinoids (phytocannabinoids) are lipophilic molecules, which act on endogenous cannabinoid receptors [9]. The two major cannabinoids, THC and CBD, play an essential role in the beneficial and adverse effects of cannabis. Minor cannabinoids and terpenoids may interact in a synergistic way to modulate the clinical effects of cannabis. This phenomenon, termed the "entourage effect" [10], may explain some of the differential response to various cannabis cultivars. The entourage effect may also account for the differences in the clinical effects of phytocannabinoids compared to synthetic cannabinoids. Pharmaceutical cannabinoids in clinical use include THC either alone or in combination with CBD, and may be synthetic or plant-derived [11] (Tables 20.1 and 20.2).

Increasing interest in cannabis for medical use

Interest in cannabis for medical purposes, and specifically for pain, has increased considerably in recent years, a trend that can be attributed to several factors: 1. Growing science demonstrating the endocannabinoid system and potential for therapeutic effects in human health; 2. The high prevalence of chronic pain and the difficulty of many patients to achieve adequate pain relief [12]; 3. The prevalence of comorbid symptoms associated with chronic pain, including impaired sleep, mood and overall quality of life, all of which could be influenced by cannabis; 4. Favorable media coverage of cannabis for medical use, overestimating its beneficial effects while downplaying possible adverse effects [13]; 5. Economic interests in cannabis, driven by a vast global market, both legal and illegal, estimated at hundreds of billions of dollars [14]. This shift in public opinion has facilitated the legalization of cannabis for medical use, generally followed by decriminalization and subsequent recreational legalization, which has been the pattern in many jurisdictions worldwide.

The complexity of cannabinoids as a medication

Evidence for the efficacy of cannabis and cannabinoids for pain is a constant source of confusion and frustration [15]. Cannabis is widely perceived by the lay public as an effective analgesic, however, well-designed studies supporting this opinion are scarce, indicating a marginal effect on pain at best [16]. Nevertheless, some patients seem to derive considerable analgesic benefits. How can these discrepancies be settled? Unlike other pharmaceutical agents,

Table 20.1 Characteristics of commonly available cannabinoid preparations classified by their route of delivery[40,43,63,68]. (min – minutes; hrs – hours; THC - Δ^9-tetrahydrocannabinol; CBD – cannabidiol)

Route of delivery	Oral	Inhaled	Trans-mucosal
Absorption	Enteral absorption followed by 1st & 2nd pass liver metabolism accounts for 20-30% absorption and high inter-individual variation.	Direct absorption to systemic circulation at rates of 10-60%	Direct absorption over mucous membranes
Onset of action	60-180 min; unpredictable	5-10 min	15-45 min
Duration of action	6-8 hrs	2-4 hrs	6-8 hrs
Factors affecting the absorbed dose	Dietary consumption of fats and alcohol	Type of vaporizer Technique and duration of inhalation	
Advantages	Simple, odorless	Rapid onset of action	Convenient
Disadvantages	Gastrointestinal side effect Unpredictable absorption	Requires dexterity May contain toxins (vaporizing<smoking) Exposure to combustion bi-products (smoking) Respiratory symptoms Concerns of vaping-associated lung disease	Requires dexterity

Table 20.2 Cannabinoid agents currently available in many countries

Agent	Source	On label indications	Dose supplied	Start dose	Maximum dose
Nabilone (Cesamet)	Synthetic analog of THC	Chemotherapy induced nausea and vomiting	0.5 mg, 1 mg	0.5 mg once or twice daily	6 mg/day
Dronabinol (Marinol)	Synthetic THC	Chemotherapy induced nausea and vomiting Anorexia in AIDS	2.5 mg, 5 mg, 10 mg capsules	2.5 mg once or twice daily	20 mg/day
Nabiximols (Sativex)	Extract of cannabis as oromucosal spray with THC and CBD	Neuropathic pain in MS Adjunctive analgesic in cancer pain	Each spray contains 2.7 mg THC, 2.5 mg CBD	1 spray once or twice daily	12 sprays/day
Epidiolex Cannabidiol	Extract of CBD from cannabis plant	Anticonvulsant Lennox- Gastaut or Dravet syndrome	100mg/ml	2.5 mg/kg twice daily	10 mg/kg twice daily
Medical cannabis programs in several nations	Cannabis plant	Non-specific, patient choice but most commonly used for pain in most surveys	Multiple strains and preparations for smoked, oral and topical use	Start low and go slow, watch for side effects	Product dependent

cannabis cannot be considered as a single medication. Cannabis hosts hundreds of molecules, with concentrations varying between strains, areas of cultivation, seasonality and route of administration [17].

Furthermore, while most studies focus on THC and CBD composition, evidence is mounting that other metabolites may be as important. An interesting lesson can be learned from studies conducted on the anti-tumor effect of cannabis extracts on cancer cells, which differs considerably depending on the composition of active metabolites in these extracts [18]. It thus appears that certain *combinations* of active components are needed for the anti-tumor effect to be achieved, an effect that is independent of the concentration of THC or CBD in the extract. Extrapolating these observations to the field of pain medicine, one should consider the myriad possible combinations of cannabis-derived active ingredients in a therapeutic preparation interacting with variables pertaining to the patients and their disease. This may explain why meta-analyses on the use of cannabis struggle to demonstrate significant benefits. The complexity of the problem (involving multiple ligands, receptors and target organs) may call for a reductionist approach investigating the effects of *combinations* of active ingredients on various symptoms.

Indications for cannabinoids in the management of pain

Cannabis is widely used to treat chronic pain either by clinicians' prescriptions or through self-treatment. Despite its wide public acceptance as an analgesic agent, evidence supporting the use of cannabis and cannabinoids for pain remains limited. Available studies are often assessed as poor quality due to small subject numbers, short follow-up time and heterogenous pain conditions. Furthermore, meta-analyses often include various cannabinoid treatments. In a recent systematic review, published by the IASP Presidential Task Force on Cannabis and Cannabinoid Analgesia, the authors conclude that "the evidence neither supports nor refutes claims of efficacy and safety for cannabinoids, cannabis, or cannabis-based medicines in the management of pain." [16]. The number needed to treat of cannabinoids for chronic pain has been estimated at 24 [19]. However, there seems to be a difference in the efficacy of cannabinoids in various pain conditions [20, 21].

Neuropathic pain - Several studies have explored the efficacy and safety of cannabinoids in patients with neuropathic pain. In a recent meta-analysis, including 1750 patients participating in 16 randomized controlled studies, cannabinoids were marginally superior to placebo, with 30% or higher pain relief achieved in 21% of patients treated with cannabinoids compared with 17% of placebo-treated patients [11]. The number needed to treat was estimated at 20. Adverse effects were more common among individuals treated with cannabinoids (number needed to harm = 3), probably accounting for the higher withdrawal rate. Other meta-analyses reached similar results [21]. In conclusion, limited evidence supports the use of herbal cannabis and nabiximols (but not dronabinol or nabilone) as a third-line treatment for neuropathic pain [16, 22].

Musculoskeletal pain - Few clinical trials on cannabinoids for musculoskeletal pain have been published. Nabilone was not associated with significant pain reduction in patients with low back pain [23] and no clinical trials of herbal cannabis in low back pain or arthritis are available. While some observational studies suggest perceived benefit among patients with low back pain and arthritis [24, 25], several systematic reviews of the use of cannabinoids in rheumatic diseases have concluded that the evidence for efficacy is lacking [15, 24, 26].

Nociplastic pain –As patients with fibromyalgia and other nociplastic pain disorders often experience symptoms in multiple body systems, many show interest in cannabinoids. Few clinical trials have explored the efficacy of cannabinoids in fibromyalgia. A Cochrane review was published in 2016, including two studies comparing nabilone (a synthetic THC) with amitriptyline for 4–6 weeks [27]. These studies provided low-quality evidence suggesting a slightly greater reduction in pain in the nabilone treated participants but at the cost of a higher frequency of adverse events. Several observational studies have indicated that cannabis use might be associated with lower pain intensity and improved sleep in fibromyalgia [28–30]. As individuals with fibromyalgia are often hypersensitive to the side effects of medications, they may also be more prone to developing adverse effects when using cannabinoids [30].

Cancer pain - Cannabis is often prescribed for oncological symptom management, although its effects on pain are not established. Recent meta-analyses demonstrated no added value for cannabinoids in pain reduction among patients with advanced cancer both for cannabinoids used alone and for cannabinoids added to opioids [16, 31, 32]. The addition of cannabinoids did increase the risk of adverse events, most notably somnolence and dizziness. The effects of cannabinoids on tumors are beyond the scope of this chapter. However, one should bear in mind that cannabinoids have been shown to possess anti-tumor effects (in-vitro and in-vivo)[18], but also to compromise the efficacy of certain anti-cancer treatments [33].

Headaches – Evidence for the clinical efficacy and safety of cannabinoids in primary headaches is lacking. In the absence of randomized controlled trials, current evidence relies on observational reports, case series and anecdotal reports [9]. In one retrospective study, patients reported a 50% reduction in their pain in 50% of the cases when using cannabis, but typically with the need for increasing doses over time [34]. To conclude, there is inadequate evidence on efficacy of cannabis in the management of headache. Moreover, headache is a common side effect of cannabinoids [16, 35].

Acute pain - Several systematic reviews have concluded that cannabinoids were not superior to placebo in acute pain [20, 21, 36].

Accompanying symptoms – individuals affected by chronic pain experience an increased prevalence of comorbid symptoms, including sleep problems, affective disorders, post-traumatic stress disorder (PTSD) and overall compromised quality of life. Cannabis and cannabinoids have been proposed to offer a beneficial effect on sleep, anxiety, PTSD and well-being in some patients [19, 28, 37].

In conclusion, when a strict evidence-based approach is taken, cannabinoids can be recommended as a third-line treatment for patients with neuropathic pain. There is currently no tangible evidence to support their use in other pain indications.

Maximizing the safety and efficacy of cannabinoids

Proper patient selection is a key to safe and efficient use of cannabinoids [20, 38], along with the intelligent choice of appropriate cannabinoid preparations, open and accurate communication[40] and gradual titration of low doses of cannabinoids ("start low, go slow and stay low") [39–42].

Patient selection

Cannabinoids may be considered for most chronic pain conditions as a part of a comprehensive treatment plan. They should not be an immediate first choice or an isolated treatment modality. Patients should be informed regarding the evidence supporting cannabinoids for the treatment of their illness [38, 43]. Common side effects should be explained, including gastrointestinal, cognitive, affective, motor and balance symptoms and serious adverse events should be mentioned, including psychotic episodes, myocardial infarctions, ischemic strokes and falls. The effect of cannabis on driving should be discussed and patients should be warned not to drive within several hours following the administration of THC-containing preparations. Preset goals for outcome should be established prior to initiation of a trial of cannabis.

Contraindications - Compared to other pain medications, cannabis is considered relatively safe and life-threatening adverse events of cannabinoids are rare [20,44]. Absolute contraindications are few and include acute psychosis and unstable psychiatric disorders, hypersensitivity, pregnancy (or planned pregnancy) and breastfeeding. Relative contraindications include severe liver diseases, severe cardiovascular or respiratory disease and first-degree family history of serious mental disorders [45].

Pregnancy & breastfeeding – Cannabis is not safe to use in pregnancy. THC crosses the placenta [46] and is found in high concentrations in breast milk [47]. As the ECS plays an essential role in fetal neurodevelopment, gestational exposure to cannabinoids may impair the proper development of fetal neuronal circuitry [48, 49]. Cannabinoids in pregnancy have been associated with adverse fetal and maternal outcomes, including low birth weight, more need for neonatal intensive unit care and also stillbirth, but not neonatal death [50]. Furthermore recent study suggests that offspring exposed to cannabis during pregnancy have a greater risk of psychopathology during middle childhood [51]. Therefore it is strongly advised that cannabis in any form be avoided when a pregnancy is planned, during pregnancy and while breast feeding [52, 53].

Choice of preparation

The availability of cannabis for medical use and cannabis-based medications varies globally. When considering the different available preparations [54], clinicians should first choose between pharmaceutical cannabinoids and herbal cannabis (Tables 20.1 and 20.2). The advantage of pharmaceutical preparations lies in their well-defined chemical content, which allows for a more reproducible clinical effect.

In contrast, herbal cannabis is often preferred by patients and can be administered by inhalation (smoking or vaping) or by ingestion. Oral preparations are generally associated with lower peak concentration and longer duration of activity at the cost of higher prevalence of gastrointestinal symptoms [40]. Inhaled administration is associated with less gastrointestinal side effects and may be considered in patients with anorexia or breakthrough pain episodes. Evidence to direct the choice of THC and CBD composition in the preparation is scant. Still, as a rule of thumb, lower THC concentrations are preferred in individuals with mental health or cardiovascular risk factors and older or fragile patients [55]. Herbal cannabis preparations should be obtained from a regulated source and patients should be strongly discouraged from turning to the illegal market. Chemical content of products that are not regulated are unknown and there is risk of contamination with pesticides, bacteria and fungi, as well as additive synthetic products to boost the psychoactive effect. Labelling of artisanal CBD products is often inaccurate [56].

Dosing and titration – As with other medications acting on the central nervous system, cannabinoids should be started with a low dose and gradually uptitrated [40]. It has been demonstrated that even very low doses of THC (1.25 to 10 mg) administered acutely to healthy young individuals may induce psychotic effects, negative mood symptoms and other psychiatric symptoms [57]. Initiating treatment with high doses of cannabinoids may expose patients to side effects without providing symptomatic benefits [55]. Furthermore, a growing body of evidence suggests that the analgesic effects of cannabinoids may exhibit an inverted U-shaped dose-effect, whereby in the low-doses produce analgesia while higher doses lead to a decreased analgesic effect or even to hyperalgesia [58–62].

Oil extracts are typically started with one drop or a fraction of a milliliter at bedtime, increased after a few days to twice- and then three times-daily. High CBD and low THC preparations are often preferred as a first step, although evidence is lacking. THC concentration and the overall dose may then be gradually increased as needed and tolerated. Administration with food will enhance gastrointestinal absorption of lipophilic cannabinoids.

Inhaled preparations (smoked or vaporized) are started at 0.25-0.5 grams per day divided into 3-5 doses and increased as needed, typically to 1-2 gr/day. It is recommended to begin with 2.5 mg THC/dose and to increase as needed to 15 mg/day [55]. In sensitive or fragile patients, including older individuals and patients with fibromyalgia, a slower titration of 'micro-doses' is recommended to avoid side effects and treatment discontinuation. Vaporizing should be preferred over smoking and mixing cannabis with tobacco should be discouraged [63].

Follow-up and reassessment –Regular follow up visits are recommended after treatment initiation for evaluation of the clinical efficacy and potential side effects. The presence of significant side effects should prompt consideration of dose reduction, changing THC and CBD concentration, choosing a different route of administration or discontinuating cannabinoid treatment. Follow-up should be provided by qualified clinicians independent of medical cannabis companies.

Side effects and drug-drug interactions of cannabinoids

While cannabinoids are considered safe and are rarely associated with life-threatening events [64], their use is frequently associated with side effects [65]. Because long-term follow-up studies are scant, reported side effects are primarily obtained from short-term studies [16]. Side effects depend both on the dose and the route of administration (Table 20.3). They may be classified based on affected systems, of which the most common side effects involve the central nervous system and gastrointestinal system (mostly with enteral administration). Cannabis use is associated with psychosis, sleep problems, anxiety, cognitive failures, respiratory events, cardiovascular and gastrointestinal events. Cannabis was also noted to be a risk factor for motor vehicle accidents, suicidal behaviour and partner and child violence [66]. Gradual titration, starting with low doses, may minimize the risk of adverse effects. Minor side effects can typically be treated by dose adjustment, alteration of CBD/THC composition and by choosing a different route of administration. In light of the inverted U-shape dose effect, decreasing the administered dose may minimize side effects without compromising the analgesic effect.

Table 20.3 Side effects associated with cannabinoid use classified by affected physiologic systems (CV – cardiovascular; THC - Δ⁹-tetrahydrocannabinol; CBD – cannabidiol; LH – luteinising hormone; FSH – follicle stimulating hormone; GH – growth hormone)

System	Common side effects	Serious side effects	Special considerations
Neurological and cognitive [16, 21, 39, 65, 70–76]	**Impaired alertness**: drowsiness, fatigue, lethargy, somnolence, disorientation **Imbalance**: dizziness, vertigo **Impaired cognition**: confusion, impaired attention, lack of concentration, mental clouding, impaired memory **Slurred speech** **Sensory impairments**: blurred vision and diplopia, impaired hearing and tinnitus **Pain**: headache, hyperalgesia	Impaired psychomotor skills leading to susceptibility to motor-vehicle and work-related accidents	Increased risk among: • drivers • young or older individuals • individuals with fibromyalgia or other hypersensitization syndromes • individuals receiving polypharmacy
Psychological [21, 45, 65, 70, 73–80]	Restlessness, anxiety, nervousness, hyperactivity Depression and dysphoria Euphoria Nightmares Disinterest	Dissociation Hallucinations Paranoia Psychosis	Increased risk among individuals: • younger than 25 years • with strong family history of serious psychiatric disorders
Cardiovascular [39, 65, 71–74, 78, 81–83]	Tachycardia, palpitations Hypertension / hypotension	Myocardial infarction Ischemic stroke	Increased risk with: • CV risk factors • ↑ THC
Gastrointestinal and metabolism [21, 39, 65, 72, 75, 76, 78]	Nausea, vomiting Loss of / increased appetite or thirst; Anorexia Abdominal discomfort or pain Altered taste, dry mouth Constipation / diarrhea Dyspepsia and epigastric symptoms	Cannabinoid hyperemesis syndrome Liver injury	Increased risk with: • oral administration • ↑ doses / ↑ THC • drastic weight change • oncological patients • older individuals
Respiratory [84, 86]	Cough and hoarseness Chronic lung disease (when smoked with tobacco)	Dyspnea	Smoking and mixing cannabis and tobacco should be avoided
Miscellaneous [85, 87]	Immune suppression (with ↑ doses) Depression of LH/FSH/GH/prolactin secretion	May interfere with immunotherapy (especially CBD)	
Side effects related to cannabis breeding [85]	Infections and infestations: aspergillosis, allergies Withdrawal and overdose symptoms due to change in cultivars	Heavy metals toxicity	

Serious side effects are rarely encountered but may necessitate discontinuation of treatment. Long term side effects related to use of medical cannabinoids are unknown, although there is now considerable evidence for harms associated with recreational cannabis use [66].

Drug-drug interactions of cannabinoids

Cannabinoids may interact with other medications taken by patients in two ways: First, they may augment or counteract other medicines' intended effect (pharmacodynamic interactions). For example, combining cannabinoids with sedative medications can increase their sedative effects. Similar interactions have been described with other pharmaceutical classes, including glucose-lowering medications, muscle relaxants, sympathomimetics and others [42]. Particular attention should be given to alcohol consumption as concomitant use may seriously increase both drugs' side effects. Second, cannabinoids act as substrates, inhibitors or inducers of various CYP-450 isoforms [67], whereby they may exert important effects on the pharmacokinetics of other medications [68]. A theoretical reduction in serum levels of the anticoagulants clopidogrel and warfarin is a concern. To date, information on drug-drug interaction is theoretical without any specific study in patients. Thus, prior to the prescription of cannabinoids, it is advisable to query the available databases [67, 69] for possible drug-drug interaction. Tapering off coadministered medications [38, 40, 41] and proper follow up may reduce the incidence of unwanted interactions [42].

Conclusions

Cannabis and cannabinoids pose a unique dilemma to the clinician: on the one hand, there is increasing public interest fueled by anecdotal positive personal experience and media coverage. On the other hand, there is a striking lack of high-quality evidence to support the use of cannabis and cannabinoids for pain. The puzzled clinician may also be deterred by the risk for adverse effects, particularly those pertaining to mental health and the cardiovascular system. Nevertheless, in clinical practice, there are some patients who derive considerable benefit from cannabis or cannabinoids. Adding to the conundrum is the large variability in the composition of herbal-cannabis preparations with variable routes of delivery.

Cannabinoids have the potential to become a powerful therapeutic tool for pain and its accompanying symptoms. As research in the field advances, it is realistic to expect a growing variety of pharmaceutical-grade medications backed by solid evidence on efficacy and safety and better insights into exogenous cannabinoids' interactions with the endocannabinoid system and the multiple body systems it modulates. In the meanwhile, cannabis and cannabinoids should not be abandoned but preferably used with caution. A practical approach should include proper patient selection, choice of preparation, cautious dosing and titration, patient education, follow-up and reassessment. Treating patients with cannabinoids remains more an art form than a science and a careful approach, aiming to avoid harm, is advisable.

References

1 Pisanti S, Bifulco M. (2019) Medical cannabis: a plurimillennial history of an evergreen. *J. Cell. Physiol* **234(6)**:8342–51.

2 Joshi N, Onaivi ES. (2019) Endocannabinoid system components: overview and tissue distribution. *Adv. Exp. Med. Biol* **1162**:1–12.

3 Zou S, Kumar U. (2018) Cannabinoid receptors and the endocannabinoid system: signaling and function in the central nervous system. *Int. J. Mol. Sci* **19(3)**:833.

4 Elphick MR, Egertová M. (2001) The neurobiology and evolution of cannabinoid signalling. *Philos. Trans. R. Soc. Lond. B. Biol. Sci* **356(1407)**:381–408.

5 McPartland JM, Small E. (2020) A classification of endangered high-THC cannabis (cannabis sativa subsp. indica) domesticates and their wild relatives. *PhytoKeys* **144**:81–112.

6 McPartland JM. (2018) Cannabis systematics at the levels of family, genus, and species. *Cannabis Cannabinoid Res* **3(1)**:203–12.

7 Reimann-Philipp U, Speck M, Orser C *et al.* (2020) Cannabis chemovar nomenclature misrepresents chemical and genetic diversity; survey of variations in chemical profiles and genetic markers in Nevada medical cannabis samples. *Cannabis Cannabinoid Res* **5(3)**: 215–230.

8 Stith SS, Vigil JM, Brockelman F, Keeling K, Hall B. (2018) Patient-reported symptom relief following medical cannabis consumption. *Front. Pharmacol* **9**:916.

9 Baron EP. (2018) Medicinal properties of cannabinoids, terpenes, and flavonoids in cannabis, and benefits in migraine, headache, and pain: an update on current evidence and cannabis science. *Headache* **58(7)**:1139–86.

10 Ben-Shabat S, Fride E, Sheskin T *et al.* (1998) An entourage effect: inactive endogenous fatty acid glycerol esters enhance 2-arachidonoyl-glycerol cannabinoid activity. *Eur. J. Pharmacol* **353(1)**: 23–31.

11 Mücke M, Phillips T, Radbruch L, Petzke, F, Häuser W. (2018) Cannabis-based medicines for chronic neuropathic pain in adults. *Cochrane Database Syst. Rev* **3(3)**:CD012182.
12 Minerbi A, Vulfsons S. (2013) Pain medicine in crisis-a possible model toward a solution: empowering community medicine to treat chronic pain. *Rambam Maimonides Med. J* **4(4)**:e0027.
13 Lewis N, Sznitman SR. (2019) Engagement with medical cannabis information from online and mass media sources: Is it related to medical cannabis attitudes and support for legalization? *Int. J. Drug Policy* **73**:219–27.
14 Global Cannabis Report: 2019 Industry Outlook. New Front Data. https://newfrontierdata.com/product/global-cannabis-2019/.
15 Sarzi-Puttini P, Ablin J, Trabelsi A, Fitzcharles, M-A, Marotto D, Häuser W. (2019) Cannabinoids in the treatment of rheumatic diseases: pros and cons. *Autoimmun. Rev* **18(12)**:102409.
16 Moore RA, Fisher E, Finn DP *et al.* (2020) Cannabinoids, cannabis, and cannabis-based medicines for pain management: an overview of systematic reviews. *Pain* **18(12)**:102409.
17 McPartland JM, Russo EB. (2001) Cannabis and cannabis extracts. *J. Cannabis Ther* **1(3–4)**:103–32.
18 Baram L, Peled E, Berman P *et al.* (2019) The heterogeneity and complexity of cannabis extracts as antitumor agents. *Oncotarget* **10(41)**:4091–106.
19 Stockings E, Campbell G, Hall WD *et al.* (2018) Cannabis and cannabinoids for the treatment of people with chronic noncancer pain conditions: a systematic review and meta-analysis of controlled and observational studies. *Pain***159(10)**:1932–54.
20 National Academies of Sciences, Engineering, and Medicine, Health and Medicine Division, Board on Population Health and Public Health Practice, Committee on the Health Effets of Marijuana: An Evidence Review and Research Agenda. (2017) *The Health Effects of Cannabis and Cannabinoids: The Current State of Evidence and Recommendations for Research.* National Academies Press (US), Washington, D.C.
21 Aviram J, Samuelly-Leichtag G. (2017) Efficacy of cannabis-based medicines for pain management: a systematic review and meta-analysis of randomized controlled trials. *Pain Physician* **20(6)**:E755–96.
22 Häuser W, Petzke F, Fitzcharles MA. (2018) Efficacy, tolerability and safety of cannabis-based medicines for chronic pain management - an overview of systematic reviews. *Eur. J. Pain* **22(3)**:455–70.
23 Pinsger M, Schimetta W, Volc D, Hiermann E, Riederer F, Pölz W. (2006) Nutzen einer Add-On-Therapie mit dem synthetischen Cannabinomimetikum Nabilone bei Patienten mit chronischen Schmerzzuständen – eine randomisierte kontrollierte Studie. *Wien. Klin. Wochenschr* **118(11–12)**:327–35.
24 Perrot S, Trouvin A-P. (2019) Cannabis for musculoskeletal pain and arthritis: evidence is needed. *Joint Bone Spine* **86(1)**:1–3.
25 Madden K, van der Hoek N, Chona S *et al.* (2018) Cannabinoids in the management of musculoskeletal pain: a critical review of the evidence. *JBJS Rev* **6(5)**:e7.
26 Johal H, Vannabouathong C, Chang Y, Zhu M, Bhandari M. (2020) Medical cannabis for orthopaedic patients with chronic musculoskeletal pain: does evidence support its use? *Ther. Adv. Musculoskelet. Dis* **12**:1759720X20937968.
27 Walitt B, Klose P, Fitzcharles M-A, Phillips T, Häuser W. (2016) Cannabinoids for fibromyalgia. *Cochrane Database Syst. Rev* **7(7)**:CD011694.
28 Fiz J, Durán M, Capellà D, Carbonell J, Farré M. Cannabis use in patients with fibromyalgia: effect on symptoms relief and health-related quality of life. *PloS One* **6(4)**:e18440.
29 Habib G, Artul S. (2018) Medical cannabis for the treatment of fibromyalgia. *J. Clin. Rheumatol. Pract. Rep. Rheum. Musculoskelet. Dis*, **24(5)**:255–8.
30 Sagi I, Bar-Lev Schleider L, Abu-Shakra M, Novack V. (2019) Safety and efficacy of medical cannabis in fibromyalgia. *J. Clin. Med* **8(6)**:807.
31 Boland EG, Bennett MI, Allgar V, Boland JW. (2020) Cannabinoids for adult cancer-related pain: systematic review and meta-analysis. *BMJ Support. Palliat. Care* **10(1)**:14–24.
32 Mücke M, Weier M, Carter C *et al.* (2018) Systematic review and meta-analysis of cannabinoids in palliative medicine. *J. Cachexia Sarcopenia Muscle* **9(2)**:220–34.
33 Taha T, Meiri D, Talhamy S, Wollner M, Peer A, Bar-Sela G. (2019) Cannabis impacts tumor response rate to nivolumab in patients with advanced malignancies. *The Oncologist* **24(4)**:549–54.
34 Cuttler C, Spradlin A, Cleveland MJ, Craft RM. (2020) Short- and long-term effects of cannabis

on headache and migraine. *J. Pain* **21(5–6)**: 722–30.

35 Aviram J, Samuelly-Leichtag G. (2017) Efficacy of cannabis-based medicines for pain management: a systematic review and meta-analysis of randomized controlled trials. *Pain Physician* **20(6)**:E75 5–E796.

36 Allan GM, Finley CR, Ton J et al. (2018) Systematic review of systematic reviews for medical cannabinoids: pain, nausea and vomiting, spasticity, and harms. *Can. Fam. Physician* **64(2)**:e78–e94.

37 Black N, Stockings E, Campbell G, Tran LT, Zagic D, Hall WD, Farrell M, Degenhardt L. (2019) Cannabinoids for the treatment of mental disorders and symptoms of mental disorders: a systematic review and meta-analysis. *Lancet Psychiatry* **6(12)**:995–1010.

38 Allan GM, Ramji J, Perry D *et al.* (2018) Simplified guideline for prescribing medical cannabinoids in primary care. *Can. Fam. Physician* **64(2)**:111–20.

39 Kalant H, Porath AJ. (2016) Clearing the smoke on cannabis: medical use of cannabis and cannabinoids – an update. Canadian Centre on Substance Use and Addiction. Available at: https://www.ccsa.ca/clearing-smoke-cannabis-medical-use-cannabis-and-cannabinoids-update Accessed Nov 2, 2019.

40 MacCallum CA, Russo EB. (2018) Practical considerations in medical cannabis administration and dosing. *Eur. J. Intern. Med* **49**: 12–19.

41 Leeat B. (2017) A unique protocol - medical cannabis treatment for oncological patients. *Israeli J. Oncol. Nurs* **29**:13–8.

42 Lucas CJ, Galettis P, Schneider J. (2018) The pharmacokinetics and the pharmacodynamics of cannabinoids. *Br. J. Clin. Pharmacol* **84(11)**:2477–82.

43 Clark A, Lynch M, Ware M, Beaulieu P, McGilveray I, Gourlay D. (2005) Guidelines for the use of cannabinoid compounds in chronic pain. *Pain Res. Manag* **10** Suppl A:44A–6A.

44 Ablin J, Ste-Marie PA, Schäfer M, Häuser W, Fitzcharles M-A. (2016) Medical use of cannabis products: lessons to be learned from Israel and Canada. *Schmerz* **30(1)**:3–13.

45 Moore TH, Zammit S, Lingford-Hughes A *et al.* (2007) Cannabis use and risk of psychotic or affective mental health outcomes: a systematic review. *The Lancet* **370(9584)**:319–28.

46 Bailey JR, Cunny HC, Paule MG, Slikker W. (1987) Fetal disposition of delta 9-tetrahydrocannabinol (THC) during late pregnancy in the rhesus monkey. *Toxicol. Appl. Pharmacol* **90(2)**:315–21.

47 Garry A, Rigourd V, Amirouche A, Fauroux V, Aubry S, Serreau R. (2009) Cannabis and breastfeeding. *J. Toxicol* **2009**:596149.

48 Tortoriello G, Morris CV, Alpar A, *et al.* (2014) Miswiring the brain: Δ9-tetrahydrocannabinol disrupts cortical development by inducing an SCG10 Neurodegeneration /stathmin-2 degradation pathway. *EMBO J* **33(7)**:668–85.

49 Basavarajappa BS, Nixon RA, Arancio O. (2009) Endocannabinoid system: emerging role from neurodevelopment to neurodegeneration. *Mini Rev. Med. Chem* **9(4)**:448–62.

50 Gunn JKL, Rosales CB, Center KE et al. (2016) Prenatal exposure to cannabis and maternal and child health outcomes: a systematic review and meta-analysis. *BMJ Open* **6(4)**:e009986.

51 Paul SE, Hatoum AS, Fine JD, *et al.* (2021) Associations between prenatal cannabis exposure and childhood outcomes: results from the ABCD study. *JAMA Psychiatry* **78(1)**:64–76.

52 Food and Drug Administration. (2019) What you should know about using cannabis, including CBD, when pregnant or breastfeeding. Available at: https://www.fda.gov/consumers/consumer-updates/what-you-should-know-about-using-cannabis-including-cbd-when-pregnant-or-breastfeeding. Accessed Nov 8, 2020.

53 Office of the Surgeon General, U.S. Department of Health and Human Services. (2019) A.S. for H. (ASH) Surgeon General's Advisory: marijuana use and the developing brain Available at: https://www.hhs.gov/surgeongeneral/reports-and-publications/addiction-and-substance-misuse/advisory-on-marijuana-use-and-developing-brain/index.html. Accessed Nov 14, 2019.

54 Lewis MM, Yang Y, Wasilewski E, Clarke HA, Kotra LP. (2017) Chemical profiling of medical cannabis extracts. *ACS Omega* **2(9)**:6091–103.

55 MacCallum CA, Russo EB. (2018) Practical considerations in medical cannabis administration and dosing. *Med Eur. J. Intern* **49**:12–19.

56 Bonn-Miller MO, Loflin MJE, Thomas BF, Marcu JP, Hyke T, Vandrey R. (2017) Labeling accuracy of cannabidiol extracts sold online. *JAMA* **318(17)**:1708–9.

57 Hindley G, Beck K, Borgan F *et al*. (2020) Psychiatric symptoms caused by cannabis constituents: a systematic review and meta-analysis. *Lancet Psychiatry* **7(4)**:344–53.

58 Mechoulam R, Parker LA. (2013) The endocannabinoid system and the brain. *Annu. Rev. Psychol* **64**:21–47.

59 Sulcova E, Mechoulam R, Fride E. (1998) Biphasic effects of anandamide. *Pharmacol. Biochem. Behav* **59(2)**:347–52.

60 Wallace M, Schulteis G, Atkinson JH *et al*. (2007) Dose-dependent effects of smoked cannabis on capsaicin-induced pain and hyperalgesia in healthy volunteers. *Anesthesiology* **107(5)**:785–96.

61 Wallace MS, Marcotte TD, Atkinson JH, Padovano HT, Bonn-Miller MA. (2020) Secondary analysis from a randomized trial on the effect of plasma tetrahydrocannabinol levels on pain reduction in painful diabetic peripheral neuropathy. *J. Pain* **21(11–12)**:1178–86.

62 Beaulieu P. (2006) Effects of nabilone, a synthetic cannabinoid, on postoperative pain. *Can. J. Anesth* **53(8)**:769–75.

63 Gieringer D, St. Laurent J, Goodrich S. (2004) Cannabis vaporizer combines efficient delivery of THC with effective suppression of pyrolytic compounds. *J. Cannabis Ther* **4(1)**:7–27.

64 Calabria B, Degenhardt L, Hall W, Lynskey M. (2010) Does cannabis use increase the risk of death? Systematic review of epidemiological evidence on adverse effects of cannabis use. *Drug Alcohol* Rev **29(3)**:318–30.

65 Deshpande A, Mailis-Gagnon A, Zoheiry N, Lakha SF. (2015) Efficacy and adverse effects of medical marijuana for chronic noncancer pain. *Can. Fam. Physician* **61(8)**:e372–81.

66 Campeny E, López-Pelayo H, Nutt D, *et al*. (2020) The blind men and the elephant: systematic review of systematic reviews of cannabis use related health harms. *Eur. Neuropsychopharmacol. J. Eur. Coll. Neuropsychopharmacol* **33**:1–35.

67 Stout SM, Cimino NM. (2014) Exogenous cannabinoids as substrates, inhibitors, and inducers of human drug metabolizing enzymes: a systematic review. *Drug Metab. Rev* **46(1)**:86–95.

68 Kocis PT, Vrana KE. (2020) Delta-9-tetrahydrocannabinol and cannabidiol drug-drug interactions. *Med. Cannabis Cannabinoids* **3**:61–73.

69 U.S. Food and Drug Administration. (2020) Drug Development and Drug Interactions: Table of Substrates, Inhibitors and Inducers. Available at: https://www.fda.gov/drugs/drug-interactions-labeling/drug-development-and-drug-interactions-table-substrates-inhibitors-and-inducers. Accessed Nov 20, 2020.

70 Brown JD, Winterstein AG. (2019) Potential adverse drug events and drug–drug interactions with medical and consumer cannabidiol (CBD) *Use. J. Clin. Med* **8(7)**:989.

71 Haroutounian S, Ratz Y, Ginosar Y *et al*. (2016) The effect of medicinal cannabis on pain and quality-of-life outcomes in chronic pain: a prospective open-label study. *Clin. J. Pain* **32(12)**:1036–43.

72 Lynch ME, Campbell F. (2011) Cannabinoids for treatment of chronic non-cancer pain; a systematic review of randomized trials. *Br. J. Clin. Pharmacol* **72(5)**:735–44.

73 van de Donk T, Niesters M, Kowal MA, Olofsen E, Dahan A, van Velzen M. (2019) An experimental randomized study on the analgesic effects of pharmaceutical-grade cannabis in chronic pain patients with fibromyalgia. *Pain* **160(4)**:860.

74 Walitt B, Klose P, Fitzcharles M, Phillips T, Häuser W. (2016) Cannabinoids for fibromyalgia. *Cochrane Database Syst.* Rev **7(7)**:CD011694.

75 Wang T, Collet J-P, Shapiro S, Ware, MA. (2008) Adverse effects of medical cannabinoids: a systematic review. *CMAJ* **178(13)**:1669–78.

76 Whiting PF, Wolff RF, Deshpande S, *et al*. (2015) Cannabinoids for medical use: a systematic review and meta-analysis. *JAMA* 313(24): 2456–73.

77 Dannon PN, Lowengrub K, Amiaz R, Grunhaus L, Kotler M. (2004) Comorbid cannabis use and panic disorder: short term and long term follow-up study. *Hum. Psychopharmacol* 19(2):97–101.

78 Lynch ME, Ware MA. (2015) Cannabinoids for the treatment of chronic non-cancer pain: an updated systematic review of randomized controlled trials. *J. Neuroimmune Pharmacol. Off. J. Soc. NeuroImmune Pharmacol* 10(2):293–301.

79 Volkow ND, Baler RD, Compton WM, Weiss SRB. (2014) Adverse health effects of marijuana use. *N Engl J Med* **370(23)**:2219–27.

80 Fischer B, Russell C, Sabioni P et al. (2017) Lower-risk cannabis use guidelines: a comprehensive update of evidence and recommendations. *Am. J. Public Health* **107(8)**:e1–12.

81 Minerbi A, Häuser W, Fitzcharles M.-A. (2019) Medical cannabis for older patients. *Drugs Aging* **36(1)**:39–51.

82 Patel RS, Manocha P, Patel J, Patel R, Tankersley WE. (2020) Cannabis use is an independent predictor for acute myocardial infarction related hospitalization in younger population. *J. Adolesc. Health Off. Publ. Soc. Adolesc. Med* **66(1)**:79–85.

83 Goyal H, Awad HH, Ghali JK. (2017) Role of cannabis in cardiovascular disorders. *J. Thorac. Dis* **9(7)**: 2079–92.

84 Owen KP, Sutter ME, Albertson TE. (2014) Marijuana: respiratory tract effects. *Clin. Rev. Allergy Immunol* **46(1)**:65–81.

85 Jackson B, Cleto E, Jeimy S. (2020) An emerging allergen: cannabis sativa allergy in a climate of recent legalization. *Allergy Asthma Clin. Immunol* 16:53.

86 Moore BA, Augustson EM, Moser RP, Budney AJ. (2005) Respiratory effects of marijuana and tobacco use in a U.S. sample. *J. Gen. Intern. Med* 20(1):33–7.

87 Alexander SPH, Kendall D.A. (2007) The complications of promiscuity: endocannabinoid action and metabolism. *Br. J. Pharmacol.* 2007, **152(5)**:602–23.

Chapter 21

Combined pharmacotherapy for chronic pain management

Ian Gilron[1], Troels Staehelin Jensen[2,3], & Anthony H. Dickenson[4]

[1]*Departments of Anesthesiology & Perioperative Medicine and Biomedical & Molecular Sciences, Queen's University, Kingston, Ontario, Canada*
[2]*Danish Pain Research Center, Aarhus University, Aarhus, Denmark*
[3]*Department of Neurology, Aarhus University Hospital, Aarhus, Denmark*
[4]*Department of Neuroscience, Physiology and Pharmacology, Division of Biosciences, University College, London, United Kingdom*

Introduction

Chronic pain affects 20-30% of the population in developed countries, [1, 2] imposes an adverse financial impact greater than that of cancer, diabetes and cardiovascular disease, [3] and contributes substantially to the global burden of disease [4]. Pharmacotherapy with a variety of drug classes continues to be an important component of multimodal, multidisciplinary chronic pain management [5, 6]. However, individual drugs often have limited utility due to incomplete analgesic efficacy and/or dose-limiting adverse effects [7]. In addressing these limitations, it has been hypothesized that combining two (or more) different analgesic drugs could provide additional benefit by: 1) increasing efficacy through concurrent targeting of multiple analgesic sites and/or mechanisms; and/or 2) reducing adverse effects – particularly if additive analgesic effects can facilitate dose reduction of each drug in the combination [8], In other therapeutic areas, rational combination therapy has long been used in various conditions such as asthma [9], cancer [10] and hypertension [11], but only more recently so for pain management. Although combining two or more analgesic drugs continues to be a common practice in clinical pain management [12, 13], the evidence base supporting this practice is somewhat limited and only starting to emerge [14-16] and experts have recommended further research on the safety and efficacy of combination drug therapy for chronic pain [5, 17]. In this chapter, we review preclinical, clinical and other information regarding the rationale, practice and future directions of combination pharmacotherapy for chronic noncancer pain with the exclusion of headache, which is discussed elsewhere [18].

Current status of drug therapy for chronic pain

Various different drug classes have been recommended for the treatment of chronic noncancer pain – as first- or second-line therapy depending on pain condition – including acetaminophen, nonsteroidal anti-inflammatory drugs, antidepressant drugs, anticonvulsant drugs and tramadol (Table 21.1). Strong opioids have been recommended as third-line therapy for neuropathic pain [5] and low back pain [19] only, but are otherwise not recommended for fibromyalgia or osteoarthritis;

Clinical Pain Management: A Practical Guide, Second Edition. Edited by Mary E. Lynch, Kenneth D. Craig, and Philip W. Peng.

Table 21.1 Recommendations for pharmacological treatment of chronic noncancer pain

Pain Condition	First-line or Second-line Recommendation	Weaker recommendation	Not recommended
Neuropathic pain[5]	1st line: – tricyclic antidepressants – SNRI antidepressants – gabapentin/pregabalin	2nd line: – tramadol* 3rd line: – strong opioids*	– cannabinoids – valproate – levetiracetam – mexiletine
Osteoarthritis of the hand, hip or knee[6]	Strong recommendation: – oral NSAIDs	Conditional recommendation: – acetaminophen – tramadol* – duloxetine	– chondroitin – glucosamine – 'non-tramadol' opioids
Fibromyalgia*[49]		Weak recommendation: – amitriptyline – duloxetine – milnacipran – tramadol – pregabalin – cyclobenzaprine	- opioids
Low back pain[19]	1st line: – oral NSAIDs 2nd line: – tramadol – duloxetine	– opioids (only if 1st/2nd line treatments failed)*	

SNRI – serotonin-norepinephrine reuptake inhibitor; NSAID – nonsteroidal anti-inflammatory drug

* Despite weak recommendations *for* tramadol or strong opioids shown in these previously published guidelines, some experts have more recently advocated against tramadol and strong opioids for general use in chronic noncancer pain.

separate guidelines for opioids in chronic pain have also been disseminated [20, 21]. Chronic pain conditions often feature sensory hyperexcitability that manifests as hyperalgesia (increased response to noxious stimuli) and allodynia (pain produced by normally non-noxious stimuli) [22]. This sensory hyperexcitability may be reduced by antidepressants, anticonvulsants and opioids [23] through actions on calcium channels, sodium channels and uptake mechanisms for monoamines or G-protein coupled membrane receptors expressed in neurons that are widespread throughout the nervous system such as peripheral, spinal, brainstem, limbic and cortical structures. In addition to potential analgesic and antihyperalgesic effects, adverse effects of most of these drugs may be experienced and include sedation, dizziness and memory or cognitive problems. Therefore, additive or synergistic analgesic interactions of two different drugs administered in combination could result in fewer adverse effects if the analgesic interaction allows for optimal pain relief at lower drug doses that are associated with fewer side effects.

Clinical rationale for analgesic combinations

As one of several treatment modalities for chronic pain, drug therapy is often ineffective in a substantial proportion of patients and only partially effective in another patient subgroup. Identifying specific drug combinations that provide better combined effectiveness versus monotherapy could increase the overall effectiveness of drug therapy for chronic pain. Since multiple, concurrent neural mechanisms of pain generation and transmission are often involved in chronic pain, combining two or more different drug classes to concurrently target these underlying mechanisms provides a rational approach to improve the effectiveness of drug therapy. In a clinical setting where a patient reports only partial benefit in response to a single analgesic drug, prescribers often then pursue "add-on" polypharmacy (e.g. see [25]) with the intention of attaining additional pain relief.

In principle, adding a second analgesic – "drug B" – to an only partially effective first treatment – "drug A" – could provide: A) better analgesia by adding a second drug with complementary actions, or a treatment that in some other way potentiates "drug A"; B) fewer side effects with "drug B" that directly antagonizes adverse effects of "drug A" [e.g. opioid plus central nervous system (CNS) stimulant] or with an "A+B" combination that provides maximal analgesia at lower drug doses such that overall side effects are reduced; or C) treatment of other pain-related symptoms (e.g. sleep disturbance, depression, anxiety), such as the nighttime addition of a sedating antidepressant drug to a nonsteroidal anti-inflammatory. Also, since multiple different pain mechanisms may be important within an individual patient (e.g., inflammatory and neuropathic sources of low back pain), another rationale for combination therapy could include the concurrent targeting of multiple pain mechanisms, e.g. both an anti-inflammatory and an anti-neuropathic treatment.

However, despite the observation that polypharmacy for chronic pain is a common practice, evidence shows that – for some combinations and in some clinical conditions – combination therapy does not always confer added benefit and in some cases may simply increase adverse effects. For example, in one trial of participants with lumbar radiculopathy, monotherapy with nortriptyline or morphine failed to demonstrate efficacy and combining the two provided no added benefit [26]. In another trial, ketamine, but not calcitonin, demonstrated efficacy for phantom limb pain but their combination was no better than ketamine monotherapy [27]. In a trial of participants suffering from postherpetic neuralgia, combining the phenothiazine, fluphenazine, to amitriptyline provided no added analgesia compared to amitriptyline alone and, furthermore, sedation was increased during combination therapy [28]. Thus, these are examples pointing to the need for expanded research on combination pharmacotherapy, so as to guide rational, evidence-based identification of specific analgesic combinations that safely provide improved outcomes versus monotherapy. Recent research efforts have sought to identify predictors of a favorable treatment response to combination treatment. For example, one recent genetic study identified a polymorphism (rs1045642) of the drug efflux pump ABCB1 transporter that predicted a positive analgesic response to the combination of morphine and nortriptyline, but not to either monotherapy [29]. Also, clinical algorithms have been used to predict responses to treatment in patients with low back pain using tapentadol alone and in combination with pregabalin [30]. These types of approaches are badly needed as pain control moves towards using sensory phenotypes and other potential predictors.

Optimizing the potential benefits of combination pharmacotherapy

Providing the optimal balance between beneficial and adverse drug effects is central to optimizing outcomes with combination pharmacotherapy. Table 21.2 lists several considerations for optimal combination pharmacotherapy in chronic pain. Emphasizing the combination of analgesic agents that have the best possible efficacy and safety is perhaps the first, and most intuitive, principle of optimal combination therapy. Ensuring the best possible understanding of potential pharmacokinetic (e.g., understanding time courses of individual drug levels and actions) and pharmacodynamics interactions between the combined drugs is also critical to optimize the selection and implementation of specific drug combinations [31].

Safety issues

Avoiding and preventing adverse drug interactions is likely the first and foremost safety consideration for combination pharmacotherapy [32]. One example relevant to chronic pain comes from case reports and/or in vitro studies indicating that combining two or more serotonin reuptake inhibiting antidepressant drugs (e.g. serotonin-specific reuptake inhibitors, serotonin-norepinephrine reuptake inhibitors, tricyclic antidepressants, tramadol) may increase the risk of developing serotonin syndrome

Table 21.2 Considerations for optimal combination pharmacotherapy in chronic pain†

Characteristics of each agent in the combination:
- *maximal efficacy*, *minimal toxicity* and *minimal adverse interactions* with other commonly used medications
- *minimal adverse drug interactions* with other component(s) of the combination
- *minimal overlap of adverse effects* for each component of the combination§
- different pharmacological mechanism*
- different site of action*

† N.B. These are general considerations to be applied to a generic treatment combination. However, other unique considerations may arise for specific combinations and certain pain conditions. Adapted from: Gilron I, Jensen TS, Dickenson AH. (2013) Combination pharmacotherapy for management of chronic pain: from bench to bedside. *Lancet Neurol* **12(11)**:1084-95.

§ Optimal combinations include treatments with differing adverse effect profiles (e.g. NSAID+SNRI antidepressant). However, many available effective treatments for some conditions such as neuropathic pain have similar side effect profiles (e.g. central nervous system depression). Despite this, some of these treatments have still been shown to provide added benefit in combination without substantial overlap of side effects.

* Theoretically, combining treatments with different pharmacological mechanisms and/or sites of action could be expected to provide maximal synergy. However, it should be noted that some examples have been described where treatments with common mechanisms and/or sites of action can provide added benefit.

(a potentially life-threatening adverse drug reaction associated with changes in mental status, autonomic hyperactivity and neuromuscular dysfunction) [33, 34]. Another example of a possible safety concern is related to combining drugs that share the adverse effect of electrocardiographic QT prolongation, which has been reported with tricyclic antidepressants, SNRI antidepressants and methadone such that combining agents with these effects can increase the risk of torsades de pointes – a lethal cardiac arrhythmia [34]. Yet other potential interactions [34] come from reports of increased risk of gastrointestinal bleeding when non-steroidal anti-inflammatory drugs are co-administered with antidepressants (e.g. amitriptyline, venlafaxine).

Identifying combinations with an optimal therapeutic profile

Combining two drugs with complementary analgesic mechanisms, and also with different side effect profiles, may provide an optimal therapeutic profile compared to monotherapy. For example, treatment of postoperative pain with NSAIDs (which are associated with a low incidence of sedation, nausea and vomiting) often result in less pain, sedation and nausea/vomiting when combined with opioids, partly due to analgesia-related reductions in patient-administered opioid doses [35]. However, commonly used treatments for some conditions (such as neuropathic pain), such as antidepressants, anticonvulsants and opiods, cause CNS depressant effects [5]. As such, the benefits of combining such CNS depressants may be more difficult to appreciate in this setting given the possibility that adverse effects may also be additive. However, previous studies have indicated that some combinations can provide overall benefit superior to that of monotherapy. Three trials by Gilron *et. al.* evaluated combinations of gabapentin plus morphine [36], nortriptyline plus gabapentin [37] and morphine plus nortriptyline [38] in participants with peripheral neuropathic pain. Using a simultaneous double-dummy, multiple period crossover design, doses of each single-agent and the combination were titrated over several weeks, to each patient's individual maximal tolerated dose (MTD) and then continued at MTD for a final week. In these trials, CNS side effects common to both agents and expected to be additive (e.g. sedation), were not significantly more frequent during combination therapy [36-38] – likely because the trial protocol stopped the individualized flexible dose titration upon encountering disabling side effects. Although these CNS side effects were not significantly more frequent during combination treatment, it is important to note that MTD drug doses were significantly lower during combination versus monotherapy – likely due to some overlap of CNS side effects [36-38]. However, even at lower MTD doses, pain intensity was significantly lower during combination versus either monotherapy (e.g. see Figure 21.1). Since the overlap of CNS side effects may explain lower MTD drug doses during combination therapy, it is remains unclear that, even at lower drug doses, pain intensity was decreased during

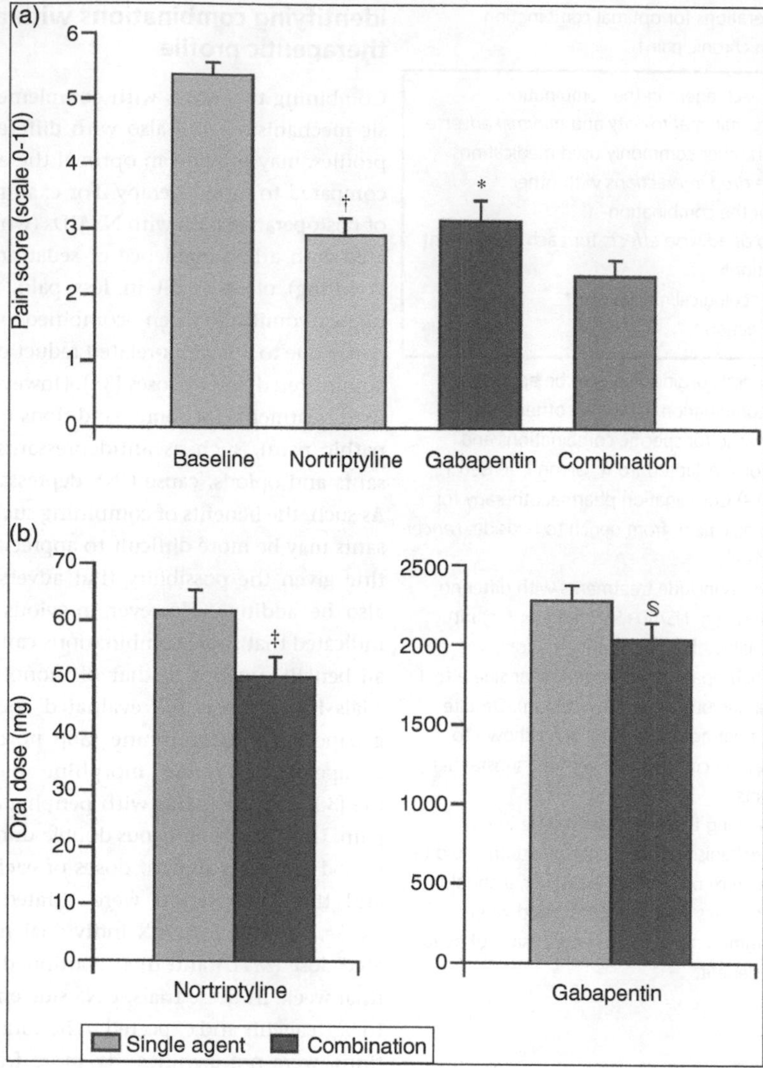

Figure 21.1 Randomized controlled trial of a nortriptyline-gabapentin combination in neuropathic pain In this double-blind, double-dummy, crossover trial, 56 patients with neuropathic pain were enrolled and randomized in a 1:1:1 ratio with a balanced Latin square design to receive one of three sequences of daily oral gabapentin, nortriptyline and a combination of both. During each 6-week treatment period, drug doses were titrated towards maximum tolerated dose. The primary outcome was mean daily pain at maximum tolerated dose. Forty-seven patients completed at least two treatment periods and 45 completed the entire trial. Mean daily pain (0–10; numerical rating scale) was 5.4 (95% CI 5.0 to 5.8) at baseline. At the maximum tolerated dose, pain was 3.2 (2.5 to 3.8) for gabapentin, 2.9 (2.4 to 3.4) for nortriptyline and 2.3 (1.8 to 2.8) for combination treatment (Panel A). Pain with combination treatment was significantly lower than with gabapentin***** (–0.9, 95% CI –1.4 to –0.3, p = 0.001) or nortriptyline**†** alone (–0.6, 95% CI –1.1 to –0.1, p = 0.02). At maximum tolerated dose, the most common adverse event was dry mouth, which was significantly less frequent in patients on gabapentin than on nortriptyline (p<0.0001) or combination treatment (p < 0.0001). *Mean maximum tolerated dose of gabapentin (Panel B) was 2433 mg (SE 106) as monotherapy versus 2180 mg (108) in combination (p = 0.0009). For nortriptyline (Panel B), maximum tolerated dose was 61.6 mg (3.6) as monotherapy versus 50.1 mg (3.5) in combination (p = 0.0006). (*Adapted from*: Gilron I, Bailey JM, Tu D, Holden RR, Jackson AC, Houlden RL. (2009) Nortriptyline and gabapentin, alone and in combination for neuropathic pain: a double-blind, randomised controlled crossover trial. *Lancet* **374(9697)**:1252-61.)

combination therapy whereas CNS SE frequencies were not higher (i.e., there was more additivity for analgesia than for side effects). One possible explanation for this discrepancy between additive analgesia versus additive side effects in these trials is that analgesic mechanisms of gabapentin, morphine and nortriptyline are peripheral, spinal and supraspinal whereas sedative and other CNS depression mechanisms of these drugs are predominantly supraspinal. As such, even if the two treatments being combined are CNS depressants, a superior therapeutic profile could be attained with such combinations. These treatment outcome patterns, however, have not been observed in all combination trials and may therefore depend on the specific drug combination studied, their sites of action and/or the details of the dose-titration protocol. For example, another antidepressant plus anticonvulsant neuropathic pain combination trial (involving imipramine plus pregabalin) also reported significantly lower pain intensity during combination treatment, however, side effects and trial withdrawals were higher during combination treatment [39]. In contrast to the other three trials mentioned above, the higher adverse effect frequency noted with this combination could be related to the specific drugs used (e.g. imipramine is associated with more frequent side effects than is nortriptyline) and also to the use of a forced dose titration in this trial versus the flexible titration to MTD used in the three trials mentioned above. Also, a large (N=804), multicenter trial using a double-blind, two-stage parallel design to compare an oral pregabalin-duloxetine combination (300 mg/day + 60 mg/day respectively) to high-dose monotherapy (600 mg/day pregabalin or 120 mg/day duloxetine) in painful diabetic neuropathy patients failing to respond to lower dose monotherapy (300 mg/day pregabalin or 60 mg/day duloxetine). The primary analysis of this trial was negative (i.e., no significant difference between combination and high-dose monotherapy for the primary pain outcome), however, the primary and all secondary outcome measures exhibited trends favoring combination therapy and side effects were generally similar in both groups [40]. The overall lack of any significant superiority of combination therapy versus monotherapy in this trial could be, in part, related to the trial design where participants experiencing as low as 30% pain reduction with low dose pregabalin or duloxetine treatment were considered treatment successes and withdrawn from the trial [40].

Combination pharmacotherapy for different chronic pain conditions – current status

As mentioned above, treatment pattern studies in various pain conditions suggest that approximately half of patients with chronic pain concurrently receive two or more different analgesic drugs [1213 41]. Commonly used analgesic drug combinations include: fixed-dose formulations of acetaminophen combined either with opioids (e.g. codeine) or tramadol, NSAIDs plus opioids, muscle relaxants plus opioids, antidepressants plus anticonvulsants, antidepressants plus opioids and anticonvulsants plus opioids. Despite these observed prescribing patterns, the evidence base supporting these combinations is relatively limited.

In the field of inflammatory arthritis, a Cochrane review of combination pharmacotherapy identified 23 eligible studies [16]. Combinations of an NSAID with an antipyretic analgesic (acetaminophen or benorylate) were compared only to NSAID alone in 12 studies; combinations of two different co-administered NSAIDs were compared to one NSAID alone in 5 studies; and various other combinations were evaluated in 6 other studies. Included RCTs, all published before 1994, were identified to be at high risk of bias leading to the conclusion that there is insufficient evidence to support combination therapy for inflammatory arthritis [16]. Most studies, included in this review notably compared two-drug combinations to *only one* of the monotherapies leaving in question the relative contribution of the other agent. For osteoarthritis, there have been no systematic reviews of combination trials and relatively few formal combination pharmacotherapy trials. These include studies of acetaminophen plus NSAID [42] whereas other fixed dose combination formulations (e.g. acetaminophen-opioid or acetaminophen-tramadol) were not compared to each respective combination component. This lack of evidence is reflected in the 2019 American College of Rheumatology treatment recommendations for hand, hip and knee OA where no specific recommendations are made for, or against, combination therapy except for one unreferenced comment stating "*. . .Evidence suggests that duloxetine has efficacy in the* *treatment of OA when used alone or in combination with NSAIDs."* [6].

In neuropathic pain, 21 RCTs were included in a Cochrane Collaboration systematic review published in 2012 [14]. Several additional trials [e.g. see 38, 39, 43] have since been published and an update to this review is currently underway. Based on the 2012 review, combinations of gabapentin or pregabalin with an opioid were evaluated in four RCTs (n=578); fluphenazine combined with a tricyclic antidepressant was evaluated in three RCTs (n=90); combinations of an opioid with a tricyclic antidepressant were evaluated in two RCTs (n=77); a combination of gabapentin and nortriptyline was evaluated in one RCT (n=56) and several other combinations were evaluated in 11 other RCTs. The review concluded that there are multiple, good-quality studies demonstrating superior efficacy of some two-drug combinations, versus monotherapy, but that the number of available studies for any one specific combination currently preclude the recommendation of any specific drug combination(s) for neuropathic pain [14].

In fibromyalgia, a 2018 Cochrane Collaboration systematic review identified 14 trials (1,289 participants) of drug combinations that were eligible for inclusion [15]. Among these trials, three (306 participants) evaluated an NSAID-benzodiazepine combination; two (89 participants) evaluated a double-antidepressant combination of amitriptyline plus fluoxetine; two (92 participants) evaluated the combination of amitriptyline with a different agent; two (164 participants) evaluated a melatonin-antidepressant combination; one (58 participants) evaluated a triple combination of the muscle relaxant, carisoprodol, paracetamol (acetaminophen) and caffeine; one (315 participants) evaluated a tramadol plus paracetamol (acetaminophen) combination; one (24 participants) evaluated a malic acid plus magnesium combination; one (200 participants) evaluated the combination of a monoamine oxidase inhibitor with 5-hydroxytryptophan; and one (41 participants) evaluated the combination of pregabalin with duloxetine [15]. Similar to other clinical pain conditions, several methodological limitations of combination trials were highlighted in this review (Table 21.3) that may guide future improvements for combination pharmacotherapy. Firstly, only about half of the studies compared the drug combination to *each* monotherapy (Table 21.3). The problem with such an 'incomplete' study design is that any differences between a combination of drugs 'A + B' versus only drug 'A' alone could be due strictly to differences in efficacy between drugs 'A' and 'B' and, thus, additional comparison of 'A + B' also with 'B' alone is necessary for the comprehensive evaluation of the combination.

Relevant to chronic low back pain – likely the most common chronic pain condition – it is notable that a relevant systematic review [44] identified only four eligible trials. Two of these compared a fixed dose tramadol-acetaminophen combination to placebo only. In addition to the small number of trials identified, it is also problematic here that studies of lumbar radiculopathy were mixed with those of largely non-neuropathic back pain. One trial of a morphine-nortriptyline combination has been discussed above [26] and another trial (n=36) suggested that a combination of pregabalin plus celecoxib was superior to either drug alone [45].

Clinical implementation of combination pharmacotherapy

At the time of writing, there is not yet enough confirmatory evidence to warrant a strong recommendation for any specific drug combination for any specific pain condition. However, there are at least two positive trials reporting superior pain reduction with combination therapy over monotherapy for: 1) an opioid+gabapentinoid combination in neuropathic pain [14, 25, 36]; and 2) a gabapentinoid+antidepressant combination for neuropathic pain [37, 39]. In the setting of patient care, it is helpful to distinguish between simultaneous combination therapy versus sequential combination therapy (i.e., in an "add-on" fashion) [46]. In the interest of improving patient safety by minimizing polypharmacy [47], a guiding principle is to first assess response to a single drug ('drug A'). If drug A is well tolerated and pain relief is good, this monotherapy could be continued and regularly re-evaluated. If drug A either produces intolerable adverse effects or inadequate relief, it should be abandoned with consideration for switching to another treatment ('drug B'). If, however, drug A is well tolerated with only partial pain relief, then consideration could be given to continuing drug A and initiating drug B in an "add-on" fashion. When drugs A and B are both CNS depressants (e.g. antidepressants, anticonvulsants or opioids), the dose of drug A is often titrated

Table 21.3 Methodology of fibromyalgia combination trials.

		Trial comparisons			
First author, year	**Combination Studied**	**Placebo-controlled**	**Combination vs. only 1 component**	**Combination vs. both components**	**Combination vs. other**
Albertoni Giraldes 2016		+	+		
Bennett 2003		+			
de Zanette 2014				+	
Gilron 2016		+		+	
Goldenberg 1986		+		+	
Goldenberg 1996		+		+	
Hussain 2011				+	
Kravitz 1994		+		+	
Nicolodi 1996				+	+*
Pridgen 2017		+			+
Quijada-Carrera 1996		+		+	
Russell 1991		+		+	
Russell 1995		+			
Vaeroy 1989		+			
Vlainich 2010			+		
Zucker 2006			+		

* Nicolodi 1996 compared a monoamine oxidase inhibitor, 5-hydroxytryptophan, their combination and amitriptyline.
(Adapted from: Thorpe J, Shum B, Moore RA, Wiffen PJ, Gilron I. Combination pharmacotherapy for the treatment of fibromyalgia in adults. Cochrane Database Syst Rev. 2018 Feb 19;2(2):CD010585.)

to the patient's maximal tolerated dose in order to maximize relief. In this situation, the dose of drug A is often near the limits of tolerability and the amount of "add-on" dose titration of drug B may be limited if the side effects of drug A are further compounded by the addition of drug B. Therefore, sequential combination therapy may not allow the titration of sufficiently efficacious doses of drug B due to overlapping side effects. If instead, both drugs A and B are started simultaneously at low doses and similarly titrated to maximal tolerated dose, this may allow for a more balanced dose ratio. Thus, the application of trial data to clinical practice should be done in the context of how the drugs were combined in the relevant trial (i.e. simultaneously versus sequentially).

Conclusions

In light of ongoing challenges to developing more effective pain treatments, combination pharmacotherapy remains an important (and understudied) treatment strategy. Continued improvement in the development and implementation of combination treatment strategies will be enhanced by preclinical strategies to predict optimal drug combinations, including methods to concurrently evaluate interactions between analgesic and adverse effects relevant to patient care. As reviewed in this chapter and also from considerations relevant to other therapeutic areas [48], optimal trials must evaluate *all* components of the combination on their own in order to best demonstrate value added in the combination. Also, given the need to understand pharmacokinetic and pharmacodynamics interactions between components of an analgesic combination, attention is also needed to define the optimal dose ratio between components although this may further complicate clinical study design. For combinations of drugs with similar side effect profiles that require gradual dose titration towards a maximal tolerated dose: a sequential method of "add-on" combination therapy will likely result in an unbalanced ratio which includes preferentially higher doses of the first drug titrated; alternatively, a method of simultaneous combination will likely result in a more evenly balanced dose ratio. Lastly, academic research funding agencies should recognize that analgesic combinations have not been, and may continue not to be, a research priority for the pharmaceutical industry. This may be due to the greater cost and complexity of combination trials but also due to the "head-to-head" element of combination trial designs whereby proprietary single agents "compete" with one another. Thus, creative strategies must be promoted to encourage drug developers, but also other research funding agencies, to support this important aspect of pain management research.

Widespread use of combination pharmacotherapy in pain management reflects the current limitations of various available pharmacotherapies (as single agents) and, furthermore, emphasizes the need for combination-specific research to distinguish between beneficial versus useless or even harmful drug combinations. Evidence showing that some, but not all, combinations provide more benefit versus monotherapy supports the value of continued research in this area with potential to improve clinical outcomes. Well integrated "bench-to-bedside" combination research programs with input from academia, industry and government regulators is expected to identify new, badly needed, treatment strategies to improve the management of chronic pain.

Acknowledgments

Work related to this chapter was supported, in part, by funding from the Canadian Institutes of Health Research (CIHR) and the Physicians' Service Incorporated (PSI) Foundation to IG. AHD is part of the Wellcome Trust funded London Pain Consortium. TSJ and AHD are part of the EU-IMI consortium: EUROPain. The authors thank Dr. Shafaq Sikandar for invaluable assistance related to this review.

References

1 Verhaak PFM, Kerssens JJ, Dekker J, Sorbi MJ, Bensing JM. (1998) Prevalence of chronic benign pain disorder among adults: a review of the literature. *Pain* **77(3)**:231–9.

2 Mills SEE, Nicolson KP, Smith BH. (2019) Chronic pain: a review of its epidemiology and associated factors in population-based studies. *Br J Anaesth* 123(2):e273–83.

3 Gaskin DJ, Richard P. (2012) The economic costs of pain in the United States. *J Pain* **13(8)**:715–24.

4 Rice ASC, Smith BH, Blyth FM. (2016) Pain and the global burden of disease. *Pain* **157(4)**:791–6.

5 Finnerup NB, Attal N, Haroutounian S *et al.* (2015) Pharmacotherapy for neuropathic pain in adults: a systematic review and meta-analysis. *Lancet Neurol* **14(2)**:162–73.

6 Kolasinski SL, Neogi T, Hochberg MC *et al.* (2020) 2019 American College of Rheumatology/Arthritis Foundation guideline for the management of osteoarthritis of the hand, hip, and knee. *Arthritis Care Res* (Hoboken) **72(2)**:149–62.

7 Gilron I, Jensen TS, Dickenson AH. (2013) Combination pharmacotherapy for management of chronic pain: from bench to bedside. *Lancet Neurol* **12(11)**:1084–95.

8 Gilron I, Max MB. (2005) Combination pharmacotherapy for neuropathic pain: current evidence and future directions. *Expert Rev Neurother* **5(6)**:823–30.

9 Juniper EF, Jenkins C, Price MJ, James MH. (2002) Impact of inhaled salmeterol/fluticasone propionate combination product versus budesonide on the health-related quality of life of patients with asthma. *Am J Respir Med* **1(6)**:435–40.

10 Lilenbaum RC, Langenberg P, Dickersin K. (1998) Single agent versus combination chemotherapy in patients with advanced nonsmall cell lung carcinoma: a meta-analysis of response, toxicity, and survival. *Cancer* **82(1)**:116–26.

11 Law MR, Wald NJ, Morris JK, Jordan RE. (2003) Value of low dose combination treatment with blood pressure lowering drugs: analysis of 354 randomised trials. *BMJ* **326(**7404**)**:1427.

12 Berger A, Sadosky A, Dukes E, Edelsberg J, Oster G. (2012) Clinical characteristics and patterns of healthcare utilization in patients with painful neuropathic disorders in UK general practice: a retrospective cohort study. *BMC Neurol* **12**:8.

13 Gore M, Tai KS, Sadosky A, Leslie D, Stacey BR. (2011) Clinical comorbidities, treatment patterns, and direct medical costs of patients with osteoarthritis in usual care: a retrospective claims database analysis. *J Med Econ* **14(4)**:497–507.

14 Chaparro LE, Wiffen PJ, Moore RA, Gilron I. (2012) Combination pharmacotherapy for the treatment of neuropathic pain in adults. *Cochrane Database Syst Rev* **2012(7)**:CD008943.

15 Thorpe J, Shum B, Moore RA, Wiffen PJ, Gilron I. (2018) Combination pharmacotherapy for the treatment of fibromyalgia in adults. *Cochrane Database Syst Rev* **2(2)**:CD010585.

16 Ramiro S, Radner H, van der Heijde D *et al.* (2011) Combination therapy for pain management in inflammatory arthritis (rheumatoid arthritis, ankylosing spondylitis, psoriatic arthritis, other spondyloarthritis). *Cochrane Database Syst Rev* **(10)**:CD008886.

17 Attal N, Cruccu G, Baron R, *et. al.* (2010) EFNS guidelines on the pharmacological treatment of neuropathic pain: 2010 revision. *Eur J Neurol* **17(**9**)**:1113–e88.

18 Straube A, Aicher B, Fiebich BL, Haag G. (2011) Combined analgesics in (headache) pain therapy: shotgun approach or precise multi-target therapeutics? *BMC Neurol* **11**:43.

19 Qaseem A, Wilt TJ, McLean RM *et al.* (2017) Noninvasive treatments for acute, subacute, and chronic low back pain: a clinical practice guideline from the American College of Physicians. *Ann Intern Med* **166(**7**)**:514–30.

20 Busse JW, Craigie S, Juurlink DN *et al.* (2007) Guideline for opioid therapy and chronic noncancer pain. *CMAJ* **189(**18**)**:E659–66.

21 Dowell D, Haegerich TM, Chou R. (2016) CDC Guideline for prescribing opioids for chronic pain--United States, 2016. *JAMA* **315(**15**)**:1624–45.

22 Jensen TS, Baron R. (2003) Translation of symptoms and signs into mechanisms in neuropathic pain. *Pain* **102(**1-2**)**:1–8.

23 Finnerup NB, Jensen TS. (2006) Mechanisms of disease: mechanism-based classification of neuropathic pain – a critical analysis. *Nat Clin Pract Neurol* **2(2)**:107–15.

24 Hoffman EM, Watson JC, St Sauver J, Staff NP, Klein CJ. (2017) Association of long-term opioid therapy with functional status, adverse outcomes, and mortality among patients with polyneuropathy. *JAMA Neurol* **74(**7**)**:773–79.

25 Hanna M, O'Brien C, Wilson MC. (2008) Prolonged-release oxycodone enhances the effects of existing gabapentin therapy in painful diabetic neuropathy patients. *Eur J Pain* **12(**6**)**:804–13.

26 Khoromi S, Cui L, Nackers L, Max MB. (2007) Morphine, nortriptyline and their combination vs. placebo in patients with chronic lumbar root pain. *Pain* **130(**1-2**)**:66–75.

27 Eichenberger U, Neff F, Sveticic G *et al.* (2008) Chronic phantom limb pain: the effects of calcitonin, ketamine, and their combination on pain and sensory thresholds. *Anesth Analg* **106(**4**)**:1265–73.

28 Graff-Radford SB, Shaw LR, Naliboff BN. (2000) Amitriptyline and fluphenazine in the treatment of postherpetic neuralgia. *Clin J Pain* **16(**3**)**: 188–92.

29 Benavides R, Vsevolozhskaya O, Cattaneo S *et al.* (2020) A functional polymorphism in the ATP-Binding Cassette B1 transporter predicts pharmacologic response to combination of nortriptyline and morphine in neuropathic pain patients. *Pain* **161(**3**)**:619–29.

30 Otto JC, Forstenpointner J, Sachau J *et al.* (2019) A novel algorithm to identify predictors of treatment response: tapentadol monotherapy or tapentadol/pregabalin combination therapy in chronic low back pain? *Front Neurol* **10**:979.

31 Spilker B. (1991) Combination medicine trials. In: B Spilker, ed. *Guide to Clinical Trials*. Raven Press, New York.

32 Virani A, Mailis A, Shapiro LE, Shear NH. (1997) Drug interactions in human neuropathic pain pharmacotherapy. *Pain* **73(**1**)**:3–13.

33 Boyer EW, Shannon M. (2005) The serotonin syndrome. *N Engl J Med* **352(**11**)**:1112–20.

34 Haanpää ML, Gourlay GK, Kent JL *et al.* (2010) Treatment considerations for patients with neuropathic pain and other medical comorbidities. *Mayo Clin Proc* **85(**3 Suppl**)**:S15–25.

35 Elia N, Lysakowski C, Tramèr MR. (2005) Does multimodal analgesia with acetaminophen, nonsteroidal antiinflammatory drugs, or selective cyclooxygenase-2 inhibitors and patient-controlled analgesia morphine offer advantages over morphine alone? Meta-analyses of randomized trials. *Anesthesiology* **103(**6**)**:1296–304.

36 Gilron I, Bailey JM, Tu D, Holden RR, Weaver DF, Houlden RL. (2005) Morphine, gabapentin, or their combination for neuropathic pain. *N Engl J Med* **352(**13**)**:1324–34.

37 Gilron I, Bailey JM, Tu D, Holden RR, Jackson AC, Houlden RL. (2009) Nortriptyline and gabapentin, alone and in combination for neuropathic pain: a double-blind, randomised controlled crossover trial. *Lancet* **374(**9697**)**: 1252–61.

38 Gilron I, Tu D, Holden RR, Jackson AC, DuMerton-Shore D. (2015) Combination of morphine with nortriptyline for neuropathic pain. *Pain* **156(**8**)**:1440–8.

39 Holbech JV, Bach FW, Finnerup NB, Brøsen K, Jensen TS, Sindrup SH. (2015) Imipramine and pregabalin combination for painful polyneuropathy: a randomized controlled trial. *Pain* **156(**5**)**: 958–66.

40 Tesfaye S, Wilhelm S, Lledo A *et al*. (2013) Duloxetine and pregabalin: high-dose monotherapy or their combination? The "COMBO-DN study"--a multinational, randomized, double-blind, parallel-group study in patients with diabetic peripheral neuropathic pain. *Pain* **154(**12**)**: 2616–25.

41 Gore M, Sadosky A, Stacey BR, Tai KS, Leslie D. (2012) The burden of chronic low back pain: clinical comorbidities, treatment patterns, and health care costs in usual care settings. *Spine* (Phila Pa 1976) **37(**11**)**:E668–77.

42 Buescher JS, Meadows S, Saseen J. (2004) Clinical inquiries. Does acetaminophen and NSAID combined relieve osteoarthritis pain better than either alone? *J Fam Pract* **53(**6**)**:501–3.

43 Baron R, Martin-Mola E, Müller M, Dubois C, Falke D, Steigerwald I. (2015) Effectiveness and safety of tapentadol prolonged release (PR) versus a combination of tapentadol PR and pregabalin for the management of severe, chronic low back pain with a neuropathic component: a randomized, double-blind, phase 3b study. *Pain Pract* **15(**5**)**:455–70.

44 Romanò CL, Romanò D, Lacerenza M. (2012) Antineuropathic and antinociceptive drugs combination in patients with chronic low back pain: a systematic review. *Pain Res Treat* **2012**:154781.

45 Romanò CL, Romanò D, Bonora C, Mineo G. (2009) Pregabalin, celecoxib, and their combination for treatment of chronic low-back pain. *J Orthop Traumatol* **10(**4**)**:185–91.

46 Raja SN, Haythornthwaite JA. (2005) Combination therapy for neuropathic pain--which drugs, which combination, which patients? *N Engl J Med* **352(**13**)**:1373–5.

47 Jyrkkä J, Enlund H, Korhonen MJ, Sulkava R, Hartikainen S. (2009) Patterns of drug use and factors associated with polypharmacy and excessive polypharmacy in elderly persons: results of the Kuopio 75+ study: a cross-sectional analysis. *Drugs Aging* **26(**6**)**:493–503.

48 Podolsky SH, Greene JA. (2011) Combination drugs--hype, harm, and hope. *N Engl J Med* **365(**6**)**:488–91.

49 Macfarlane GJ, Kronisch C, Atzeni F *et al*. (2017) EULAR recommendations for management of fibromyalgia. *Ann Rheum Dis* **76(**12**)**:e54.

Part 5

Interventional

Chapter 22

Diagnostic and therapeutic blocks

Agnes Stogicza[1] & Philip W. Peng[2]

[1] *Department of Anesthesiology and Pain Medicine, Saint Magdolna Private Hospital, Budapest, Hungary*

[2] *Professor, Department of Anesthesiology and Pain Medicine, University Health Network and Sinai Health System, University of Toronto, Toronto, Canada*

Patients with chronic pain can present with two patterns: generalized/diffuse (e.g. fibromyalgia) or localized/regional (e.g. meralgia paresthetica). In the latter case, interventional techniques including nerve blocks can be considered for pain relief or employed as a diagnostic tool to assist in the evaluation of the source of pain or prognosticate the treatment strategies.

Diagnostic block

There are two main roles of a diagnostic block in pain management. The first is to locate the source of the pain. Even though the pain is restricted to a region such as the lower back, the pain generators can be from the facet joints, disc, ligaments, osseous or myofascial components. Using facet joint related pain as an example, the literature suggests that it cannot be reliably diagnosed with clinical assessment or radiologic imaging [1]. By interrupting the nociceptive input from the facet joint, the clinician can determine whether the facet joints are the source of the pain. Another example is the situation when a patient has multiple disc herniations and the clinical assessment is inconclusive of the symptomatic level. A selective nerve root block provides valuable information for determining the symptomatic level [2]. Another role of the diagnostic block is to prognosticate regarding treatment response. A positive diagnostic block increases the likelihood of a positive outcome from a more definitive procedure as in facet joint disease [3].

There are a few basic requirements in considering a diagnostic block. The suspected pain generator should be confined to a region allowing an interventional procedure to interrupt the pain signals. The block can be in form of a nerve block, local infiltration or joint injection. The local anesthetic used for the interruption of the pain signal should be precisely administered to the target. The patient should be cognitively intact to interpret the pain response and document the pain scores over a period of time in a diary.

Based on the pain response following the diagnostic block, the clinician will evaluate the source of pain and plan the management accordingly. When assessing a diagnostic test, a 2x2 table is typically used based on the test response and the presence of disease [4] and from there, the sensitivity, specificity and positive/negative predictive value can be estimated (Figure 22.1). In interpreting the response to a diagnostic test, a similar 2x2 table can help the clinician to understand the complexity of the evaluation (Figure 22.1).

Typically, the clinician dichotomizes response as a positive or negative responder (response A and B in Figure 22.2. A positive response (A) confirms the source of pain is the target of the block. A positive

Clinical Pain Management: A Practical Guide, Second Edition. Edited by Mary E. Lynch, Kenneth D. Craig, and Philip W. Peng.

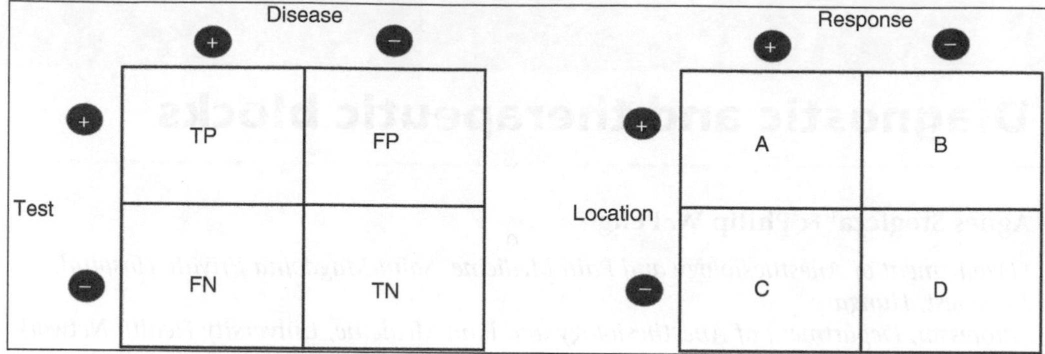

Figure 22.1 Conventional 2x2 table showing the true and false positive, true and false negative result (TP, FP, TN, and FN respectively) Image courtesy of Dr. Philip Peng.

response can, however, be influenced by higher center as a result of expectation or non-specific treatment effect [5]. Thus, the concept of controlled block is proposed (1 block with local anesthetic and another one with placebo). More commonly, comparative local anesthetic blocks can be done in which case two local anesthetic agents with different durations of action are used [6]. Some investigators may inaccurately use a positive response (A) to placebo to conclude that the complaint of pain is the result of 'malingering', hypervigilance or somatization of symptoms when in reality it is simply a placebo response [7]. A negative response (B) generally suggests that the source of the pain is not from the structure targeted by the block. An alternative interpretation is that the target structure is simply a non-responder to the local anesthetic block discouraging further treatment. This can be explained by the influence of higher centers (depression, anxiety or pain catastrophizing) or the effect of central sensitization [8]. When interpreting the response to the diagnostic block, clinicians make an assumption that the diagnostic block accurately interrupts the pain pathway. This is not always the case (response C and D). In some cases even with the use of image-guidance one may not be able to block the pain generator and a misguided block can lead to a false negative result [9]. To complicate the interpretation further, a misguided diagnostic block can lead to a positive response from the expectant or non-specific treatment effect or due to the spilling local anesthetic outside the target [10]. Overall, the clinician who performs the diagnostic block should be aware of these limitations.

Therapeutic intervention/block

The term therapeutic block typically refers to the insertion of a needle into the target site or nerves followed by the administration of local anesthetic with or without steroid. However, over the last few decades, there are additional percutaneous interventions available (Table 22.1).

In terms of nerve management, the nerve entrapment can be managed by hydrodissection [11] or minimally invasive ultrasound-guided decompression [12]. Different types of neural ablation (chemical, thermal and cryotherapy) techniques [13] as well as different types of neuromodulation (pulsed radiofrequency treatment, peripheral nerve and spinal cord stimulation) have been described.

Injection around the tendon aims at disease around the tendon but it is of minimal value to the intrinsic disease of the tendon such as tendinopathy or calcific tendinitis. Fenestration is a potential treatment for tendinosis or tendinopathy with or without administration of biologic agents (autologous blood or platelet rich plasma) that stimulates the growth [14]. In patients with calcific tendinitis, the calcium crystals can be managed with fenestration and barbotage [15].

In general, interventional procedures can be broadly classified as targeting three anatomic categories: peripheral nerve, neuraxial and musculoskeletal structures. Two examples in each category will be used to exemplify the application of interventional procedure in pain management.

Table 22.1 Spectrum of percutaneous interventional procedures. Reproduced with permission from Philip Peng Educational Series.

Nerve management	MSK management	Types of injectate
Perineural injection	Tendon	Local anesthetics
Nerve release/ hydro-dissection	• Fenestration	Adjuvants (e.g. steroids)
Chemical ablation (alcohol, phenol)	• Barbotage	Hyaluronic acid
Thermal (radiofrequency/RF) ablation	Cyst	Botulinum toxin
Cryoablation	• aspiration	Dextrose
Nerve decompression	• cyst neck fenestration	Platelet rich plasma
Neuromodulation		Biologic agents
• Pulsed RF		
• Peripheral nerve stimulation		
• Spinal cord stimulation		

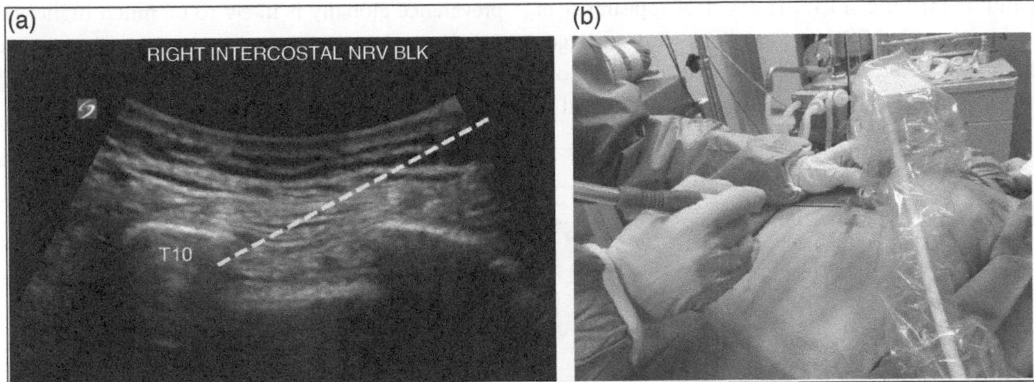

Figure 22.2 Identification and diagnostic injection of the intercostal nerve (a) is followed by cryoablation (b) Images courtesy of Agnes R. Stogicza, MD (a) and Eleni Episkopu, MD (b).

Peripheral nerve intervention

Pathologic states (injury or entrapment) of the peripheral nerves can cause persistent pain. These nerves can be the targets for interventional pain management. The prerequisites for performing procedures on these nerves are the ability to precisely identify their location and understand their functions (motor and sensory). Smaller nerve intervention has attracted significant interest in recent years. When the area of pain can be linked to an individual and identifiable nerve, one can perform a diagnostic injection to confirm the hypothesis. If that injection leads to an appropriate response, a definitive treatment can be offered.

Interventional treatment for intercostal neuralgia has been well investigated. Persistent pain after thoracotomy is common, affecting about 67% of thoracotomy patients [16]. Thoracic postherpetic neuralgia affects about 47% of herpes zoster patients older than 60 [17]. Intercostal neuralgia may also develop after rib fractures.

Typically, a diagnostic injection is performed under ultrasound guidance with 1-2ml of local anesthetic administered to the intercostal nerves in the painful region (Figure 22.2). If this leads to an appropriate response (sensory block in the area of nerve distribution with analgesia duration concordant with the duration of local anesthetic), definitive treatment can follow. Cryoablation is the most commonly studied ablation modality for intercostal neuralgia (Figure 22.2), resulting in 6-9 months of pain relief in most cases [18–24]. It causes Wallerian degeneration of the axon. As the connective tissue around the nerve such as epineurium remains intact, the nerve can regenerate in the same pathway. The procedure can be repeated if the pain recurs. Another less commonly used type of ablation is radiofrequency ablation [25, 26].

A classic example of small nerve intervention is the treatment for meralgia paresthetica, of which the reported incidence is 4.3 cases per 10,000 patient years in the general population [27]. This condition refers to the entrapment of the lateral femoral cutaneous nerve (LFCN) under the inguinal ligament, causing numbness and painful burning sensation on the lateral aspect of the thigh. The LFCN is a pure sensory nerve, readily identifiable by ultrasound in the fat-filled grove between the sartorius and tensor fascia-lata. Easy access and the lack of a motor component make it an excellent target for both diagnostic and therapeutic blocks. The typical appearance of the entrapped LFCN is swollen and enlarged (Figure 22.3). Following a successful diagnostic block with 1-2 mL of local anesthetic and steroid a sustained effect can be provided with cryoablation (Figure 22.3) or pulsed radiofrequency.

In theory, any peripheral nerve can be a target for interventions [28–32], as long as they are carefully evaluated as the source of pain with a very precise and specific (low volume) local anesthetic injection and the clinician and patient understand the risk and benefit of the definitive treatment modalities (Table 22.2).

Spinal intervention

Low back pain is very common, with an annual point prevalence of 13%. These data arise from high income populations, which suggests that the true prevalence globally is likely to be much higher [33, 34]. The source of pain contributing to the low back pain can be multifactorial. Two of them can be the targets for intervention and are discussed below.

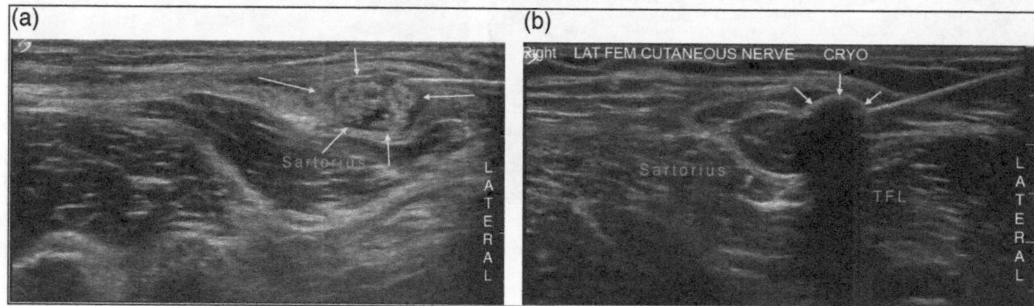

Figure 22.3 Identification and diagnostic injection of the lateral femoral cutaneous nerve (a) is followed by cryoablation (b). Arrows point at the nerve (a) and the ice-ball (b). Image courtesy of Agnes R. Stogicza, MD.

Table 22.2 Main characteristics of the various approaches to the definitive minimally invasive treatments of nerves. RFA = radiofrequency ablation, CRYO = cryoablation, PRF = Pulsed.

	RFA	CRYO	PRF
Myelinated nerves	Irreversible lesion	Reversible	Reversible
Motor loss	Yes	Yes	No
Sensory loss	Yes	Yes	No
Neuroma formation, potential for increased pain	Yes	No	No
Targets in non-cancer pain	Small, non-myelinated nerves only	All nerves	All nerves
Cancer pain	All nerves	All nerves	All nerves
Placement	Easy	Harder	Easy
Denervation certainty	✓	✓✓	×
Pain relief	✓✓	✓✓	✓
How long it lasts?	6M+	6M	?

Diagnostic and therapeutic intervention for the zygapophyseal joints (facets) of the lumbar spine have been studied extensively. The estimated prevalence of facet pain in patients with low back pain is 31% [35]. The typical presentation involves pain with prolonged rest, extension and rotation and often associated with spasm in the paravertebral musculature. The targets for diagnostic injection are the medial branches of the dorsal rami of the exiting nerve roots. Each facet joint receives dual innervation from the symptomatic level and the level above. For instance, the L4-5 facet joint receives innervation from L3 and L4 medial branches. The diagnostic block is typically performed with 0.3-0.5mL local anesthetic at each level. If the patient reports concordant response, that is, decreased pain appropriate to the duration of the local anesthetic, then radiofrequency ablation may follow. The latter involves the placement of the specialized needle to the same target resulting in ablation of the nerve with heat (typically 78-82°C). According to the American Society of Interventional Pain Physician's recent publication, the level of evidence is Level II with moderate strength of recommendation for lumbar radiofrequency ablation. Evidence included 11 relevant randomized controlled trials (RCTs) with 2 negative studies and 4 studies with long-term improvement [36].

Discogenic pain is common among younger populations with an estimated prevalence of 26–42 % in patients with back pain. Patients typically present with an excruciating pain on sitting although standing may also provoke pain. Pain is usually relieved somewhat with laying down and light activity. Annular tear of the disc is shown as a high intensity zone in the T2 weighted magnetic resonance imaging (MRI) (Figure 22.4) [37]. These imaging and clinical findings are correlated with the diagnostic injection of the disc (provocative discography), which is performed with the insertion of a needle into the intervertebral disc followed by injection of contrast under fluoroscopy. From there, the clinician observes concordant pain (reproducing the patient's usual pain) on injection and patterns of the contrast spread. The contrast patterns are graded using a Dallas discogram score, the most commonly used grading system based upon the radial spread of the contrast towards the annulus [38]. Once the problematic disc is identified, therapeutic injection can follow. Although there are a number of

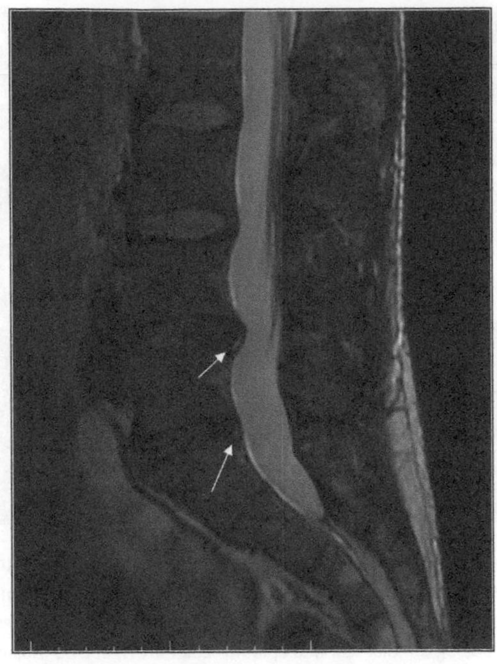

Figure 22.4 T2 weighted MRI image of the lumbar spine. Arrows point at the high intensity zones. Image courtesy of Agnes R Stogicza, MD.

interventions proposed in the past, the most promising is the use of biologic treatments in the form of platelet rich plasma (PRP) and bone marrow concentrate (BMC). After the contrast is injected into the disc with the annular tear or disrupted disc anatomy (Figure 22.5), 1-2 cc of PRP or BMC is administered. There are 13 trials (2 level I and 11 level IV) investigating the analgesic efficacy and functional improvement of PRP and BMC intradiscal administration based on a recent review. With the exception of one level IV study, all trials found significant improvement [39].

Musculoskeletal intervention

Musculoskeletal pain is a major cause of disability. In a recent global burden of disability study, musculoskeletal conditions were ranked the highest contributor to global disability, accounting for 16% of all years lived with disability [40] is Osteoarthritis of joints is a common cause of musculoskeletal pain with hip and knee joints most commonly affected. Osteoarthritis of hip and knee were ranked as the 11th highest contributor to global disability [41].

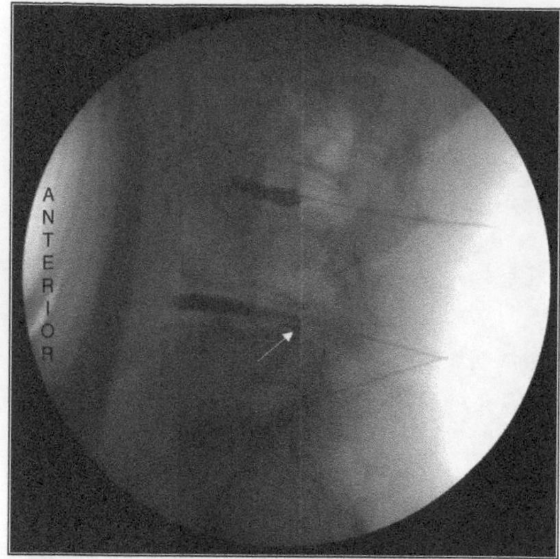

Figure 22.5 Fluoroscopy image of the lumbar spine, with needles placed in the L3-4, L4-5 and L5-S1 discs. Discogram demonstrates good central filling of the L3-4 disc (Dallas Grade 0), annular tear and epidural leak (arrow) at L4-5 (Dallas Grade 3) and annular filling, but no rupture (Dallas Grade 2) at L5-S1 disc. Image courtesy of Agnes R. Stogicza, MD.

When conservative therapy fails to control the pain, interventional therapy plays an important role. It can be in form of joint injection or denervation which can be exemplified in knee osteoarthritis.

Knee joint injection is indicated in patient with moderate to severe knee osteoarthritis not responding to conservative therapy. Traditionally, knee injection is performed with landmark guided technique. However, ultrasound improves the accuracy of knee intra-articular (IA) injection [42]. The accuracy of landmark guided injection is approximately 79% compared with 95% from ultrasound guidance based on the pooled data [43]. The commonly used agents for IA knee injection are steroid, viscosupplement and platelet rich plasma [44]. In general, the duration of IA steroid is short (<3 weeks) but repeated injection can lead to acceleration of cartilage loss. Both viscosupplement and platelet rich plasma result in longer duration of effect but in general are not very effective in advanced osteoarthritis (Table 22.3).

An emerging technique for the management of pain from knee osteoarthritis is radiofrequency (RF) ablation. The indication for RF ablation is the same as for total knee arthroplasty. Since the first randomized controlled trial of RF ablation of knee was published with promising results in 2011 [45], there has been a growing interest in this technique with 13 randomized trials published in the subsequent 8 years [46]. Unlike knee intra-articular injection, the targets are the articular branches to the anterior capsule; superomedial, superolateral and inferomedial genicular nerves (Figure 22.6). With the use of either fluoroscopy or ultrasound, the radiofrequency needle is inserted into those targets followed by ablation of those nerves [47]. The literature supports significant analgesic efficacy and functional improvement for 6 to 12 months [46]. During this period, patients can resume rehabilitation to strengthen the lower limb, if the knee pain returns, the RF ablation can be repeated.

Conclusion

Interventional procedures are non-surgical minimally invasive techniques that are commonly considered in the pain management. It should be considered as part of the armamentarium in a multidisciplinary approach to the management of pain. These procedures serve both diagnostic and therapeutic purposes. The target is not necessary a nerve but any discrete source of pain including joints. The therapeutic intervention is not necessary injection but includes a diversified array of options as presented in this chapter.

Table 22.3 Comparison of various injectate for knee. Reproduced with permission from Philip Peng Educational Series.

	Steroid	Viscosupplement	Platelet rich plasma
Mechanism	Anti-inflammatory	Supplementation of synovial fluid	Restore joint hemostasis
Duration	<3 weeks	<3 months	<12 months
Comments	Accelerate cartilage loss	Less effect for end stage OA	Less effect for end stage OA

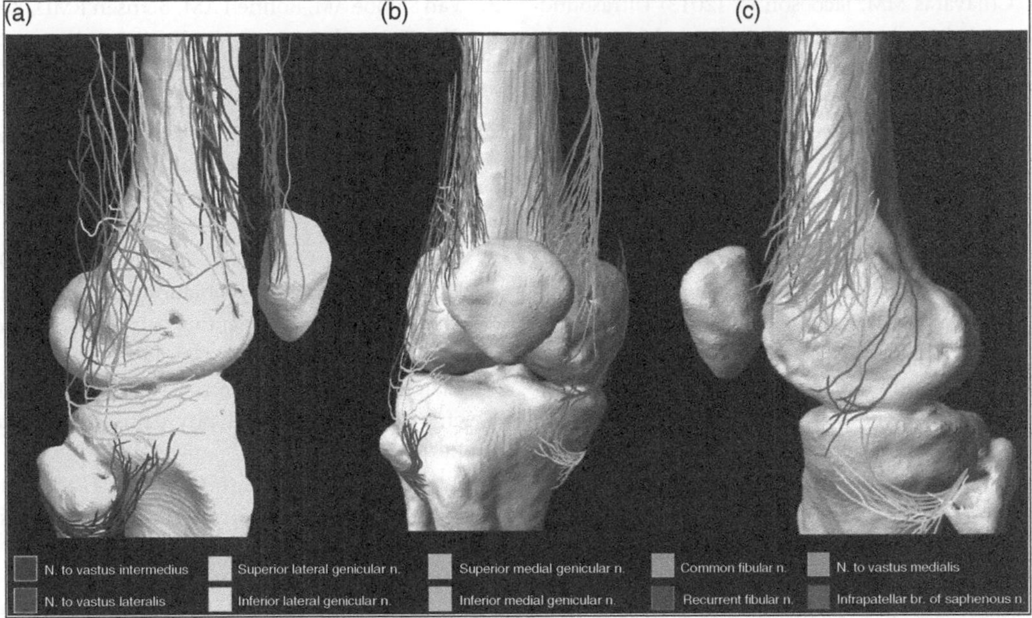

Figure 22.6 Articular branches of the anterior capsule of knee (A–C). Image courtesy of Dr. Philip Peng (Color Plate 7).

References

1 Perolat R, Kastler A, Nicot B *et al.* (2018) Facet joint syndrome: from diagnosis to interventional management. *Insights Imaging* **9(5)**:773–89.

2 Yeom JS, Lee JW, Park KW *et al.* (2008) Value of diagnostic lumbar selective nerve root block: A prospective controlled study. *Am J Neuroradiol* **29(5)**:1017–23.

3 Cohen SP, Doshi TL, Constantinescu OC *et al.* (2018) Effectiveness of lumbar facet joint blocks and predictive value before radiofrequency denervation. *Anesthesiology* **129(3)**:517–35.

4 Lalkhen AG, McCluskey A. (2008) Clinical tests: sensitivity and specificity. *Contin Educ Anaesthesia, Crit Care Pain* **8(6)**:221–3.

5 Ballentyne JC. (2011) Nonspecific treatment effects in pain medicine. *Pain Clin Updat* **XIX(2)**:1–8.

6 Barnsley L, Lord S, Bogduk N. (1993) Comparative local anaesthetic blocks in the diagnosis of cervical zygapophysial joint pain. *Pain* **55(1)**:99–106.

7 Bogduk N. (2004) Diagnostic blocks: a truth serum for malingering. *Clin J Pain* 20:409–14

8 Peng PWH. (2016) Descending mechanisms. Clinical perspective. In: Peng PWH, Casasola de L, eds. *Basic Science of Pain: an Illustrated and Clinical Orientated Guide.* IBook Apple INC, Cupertino. pp. 107–15.

9 Narouze S, Peng PWH. (2010) Ultrasound-guided interventional procedures in pain medicine: a review of anatomy, sonoanatomy, and procedures: Part II: Axial structures. *Reg Anesth Pain Med* **35(4)**:386–96.

10 Hogan Q, Abram S. (1998) Diagnostic and prognostic neural blockade. In: Cousins MJ, Bridenbaugh P, eds. *Neural Blockade in Clinical Anesthesia and Management of Pain.* Lippincott-Raven Publishers, Hagertown. pp. 837–974.

11 Chang K-V, Wu W-T, Özçakar L. (2020) Ultrasound imaging and guidance in peripheral nerve entrapment: hydrodissection highlighted. *Pain Manag* **10(2)**:97–106.

12 Petrover D, Richette P. (2018) Treatment of carpal tunnel syndrome : from ultrasonography to ultrasound guided carpal tunnel release. *Jt Bone Spine* **85(5)**:545–52.

13 Spinner D. (2019) General Principles of musculoskeletal scanning and intervention. In: Peng PWH, ed. *Ultrasound for Interventional Pain Management - An Illustrated Procedure Guide.* Springer, Cham. pp. 207–12.

14 Chiavaras MM, Jacobson JA. (2013) Ultrasound-guided tendon fenestration. *Semin Musculoskelet Radiol* **17(1)**:85–90.

15 Peng PWH, Cheng P. (2015) Calcific tendinitis. In: Peng PWH, ed. *Regional Nerve Blocks in Anesthesia and Pain Management*, 6th edn. Springer Germany, Heidelberg. pp. 313–20.

16 Karmakar MK, Ho AMH. (2004) Postthoracotomy pain syndrome. *Thorac Surg Clin* **14(3)**:345–52.

17 Calandria L. (2011) Cryoanalgesia for post-herpetic neuralgia: a new treatment. *Int J Dermatol* **50(6)**:746–50.

18 Yasin J, Thimmappa N, Kaifi JT *et al.* (2020) CT-guided cryoablation for post-thoracotomy pain syndrome: A retrospective analysis. *Diagnostic Interv Radiol* **26(1)**:53–7.

19 Yang MK, Cho CH, Kim YC. (2004) The effects of cryoanalgesia combined with thoracic epidural analgesia in patients undergoing thoracotomy. *Anaesthesia* **59(11)**:1073–7.

20 Sepsas E, Misthos P, Anagnostopulu M, Toparlaki O, Voyagis G, Kakaris S. (2013) The role of intercostal cryoanalgesia in post-thoracotomy analgesia. *Interact Cardiovasc Thorac Surg* **16(6)**: 814–8.

21 Vossler JD, Zhao FZ. (2019) Intercostal nerve cryoablation for control of traumatic rib fracture pain: A case report. *Trauma Case Reports* **23**: 100229.

22 Koethe Y, Mannes AJ, Wood BJ. (2014) Image-guided nerve cryoablation for post-thoracotomy pain syndrome. *Cardiovasc Intervent Radiol* **37(3)**:. 843–6.

23 Mustola ST, Lempinen J, Saimanen E, Vilkko P. (2011) Efficacy of thoracic epidural analgesia with or without intercostal nerve cryoanalgesia for postthoracotomy pain. *Ann Thorac Surg* **91(3)**:869–73.

24 Gabriel RA, Finneran JJ, Swisher MW *et al.* (2020) Ultrasound-guided percutaneous intercostal cryoanalgesia for multiple weeks of analgesia following mastectomy: A case series. Korean *J Anesthesiol* **73(2)**:163–8.

25 Abd-Elsayed A, Lee S, Jackson M. (2018) Radiofrequency ablation for treating resistant intercostal neuralgia. *Ochsner J* **18(1)**:91–3.

26 Engel AJ. (2012) Utility of intercostal nerve conventional thermal radiofrequency ablations in the injured worker after blunt trauma. *Pain Physician* **15(5)**:E711–8.

27 Van Slobbe AM, Bohnen AM, Bernsen RMD, Koes BW, Bierma-Zeinstra SMA. (2004) Incidence rates and determinants in meralgia paresthetica in general practice. *J Neurol* **251(3)**:294–7.

28 Stogicza A, Trescot A, Rabago D. (2019) New technique for cryoneuroablation of the proximal greater occipital nerve. *Pain Pract* **19(6)**:594–601.

29 Campos NA, Chiles JH, Plunkett AR. (2009) Ultrasound-guided cryoablation of genitofemoral nerve for chronic inguinal pain. *Pain Physician* **12(6)**:997–1000.

30 Callesen T, Bech K, Thorup J *et al.* Cryoanalgesia: effect on postherniorrhaphy pain. *Anesth Analg* **87(4)**:896–9.

31 Byas-Smith MG, Gulati A. (2006) Ultrasound-guided intercostal nerve cryoablation. *Anesth Analg* **103(4)**:1033–5.

32 Moesker AA, Karl HW, Trescot AM. (2014) Treatment of phantom limb pain by cryoneurolysis of the amputated nerve. *Pain Pract* **14(1)**:52–6.

33 Shmagel A, Foley R, Ibrahim H. (2016) Epidemiology of chronic low back pain in US adults: National Health and Nutrition Examination Survey 2009–2010. *Arthritis Care Res* **68(11)**:1688–94.

34 Smith E, Hoy DG, Cross M *et al.* (2014) The global burden of other musculoskeletal disorders: estimates from the Global Burden of Disease 2010 study. *Ann Rheum Dis.*73(**8**):1462–9.

35 Manchikanti L, Boswell M V, Singh V *et al.* (2004) Prevalence of facet joint pain in chronic spinal pain of cervical, thoracic, and lumbar regions thoracic, and lumbar regions. *BMC Musculoskelet Disord* **5**:15.

36 Manchikanti L, Kaye AD, Soin A *et al.* (2020) Comprehensive evidence based guidelines for facet joint interventions in the management of chronic spinal pain: American Society of Interventional Pain Physicians (ASIPP). *Guidelines Facet Joint Interventions 2020 Guidelines. Pain Physician* **23**:S1–127.

37 Aprill C, Bogduk N. (1992) High-intensity zone: a diagnostic sign of painful lumbar disc on magnetic resonance imaging. *Br J Radiol* **65**:361–9.

38 Sachs BL, Vanharanta H, Spivey MA *et al.* (1987) Dallas discogram description. A new classification of CT/discography in low back disorders. *Spine* (Phila Pa 1976) **12(3)**:287–94.

39 Desai MJ, Mansfield JT, Robinson DM, Miller BC, Borg-Stein J. (2020) Regenerative medicine for axial and radicular spine-related pain: a narrative review. *Pain Pract* **20(4)**:437–53.

40 James SL, Abate D, Abate KH *et al*. (2018) Global, regional, and national incidence, prevalence, and years lived with disability for 354 Diseases and Injuries for 195 countries and territories, 1990-2017: a systematic analysis for the Global Burden of Disease Study 2017. *Lancet* **392(10159)**:1789–858.

41 Cross M, Smith E, Hoy D *et al*. (2014) The global burden of hip and knee osteoarthritis: Estimates from the Global Burden of Disease 2010 study. *Ann Rheum Dis* **73(7)**:1323–30.

42 Peng PWH, Shankar H. (2014) Ultrasound-guided interventional procedures in pain medicine: a review of anatomy, sonoanatomy, and procedures. Part V: Knee joint. *Reg Anesth Pain Med* **39(5)**:368–80.

43 Berkoff DJ, Miller LE, Block JE. (2012) Clinical utility of ultrasound guidance for intra-articular knee injections: A review. *Clin Interv Aging* **7**:89–95.

44 Nouer FT, Peng PWH. (2019) Ultrasound-guided knee interventions. In: Peng PWH, ed. *Ultrasound for Interventional Pain Management - An Illustrated Procedure Guide*. Springer, Cham. pp. 283–300.

45 Choi WJ, Hwang SJ, Song JG *et al*. (2011) Radiofrequency treatment relieves chronic knee osteoarthritis pain: a double-blind randomized controlled trial. *Pain* **152(3)**:481–7.

46 Ajrawat P, Radomski L, Bhatia A, Peng P, Nath N, Gandhi R. (2019) Radiofrequency procedures for the treatment of symptomatic knee osteoarthritis: a systematic review. *Pain Med* 21(**2**);333–48.

47 Tran J, Peng PWH, Lam K, Baig E, Agur AMR, Gofeld M. (2018) Anatomical study of the innervation of anterior knee joint capsule: implication for image-guided intervention. *Reg Anesth Pain Med* 43(**4**):407–14.

Chapter 23

Neuromodulation therapy

Vishal P. Varshney[1,2], Jonathan M. Hagedorn[3], & Timothy R. Deer[4]

[1] *Department of Anesthesia, Providence Healthcare, Vancouver, British Columbia, Canada*
[2] *Department of Anesthesiology, Pharmacology and Therapeutics, Faculty of Medicine, University of British Columbia, Vancouver, British Columbia, Canada*
[3] *Department of Anesthesiology and Perioperative Medicine, Division of Pain Medicine, Mayo Clinic, Rochester, Minnesota, USA*
[4] *The Spine and Nerve Center of the Virginias, Charleston, West, Virginia, USA*

Introduction

Neuromodulation is defined by the International Neuromodulation Society as "the alteration of nerve activity through targeted delivery of a stimulus, such as electrical stimulation or chemical agents, to specific neurological sites in the body" [1]. It involves utilizing implantable devices to modulate abnormal neural pathways with either pharmacologic or electrical stimuli. Neuromodulation therapies can be directed to various anatomical locations along the central and peripheral nervous system. This explains the many forms of neuromodulation therapies that exist today, which include deep brain stimulation, spinal cord stimulation, dorsal root ganglion stimulation, peripheral nerve stimulation and intrathecal drug delivery systems. These therapies have been used to achieve clinical benefit in many disease conditions such as spasticity, epilepsy, peripheral vascular disease, urinary and fecal incontinence and chronic pain [2]. While the applications of neuromodulation are broad, this chapter aims to focus on its application to chronic pain conditions.

The history of neuromodulation dates back thousands of years, when ancient Egyptians used the electrical discharge of torpedo fish to treat gout, arthritis and epilepsy [3]. Its applicability with implantable devices began in the early 1960s, first with deep brain stimulation, then with spinal cord stimulation by N. Shealy in 1967 [4]. Over the last few decades, and particularly in the last 5–10 years, the growth in neuromodulation research has been exponential, with significant progress made into our understanding of how neuromodulation works, what anatomical locations are more clinically effective to target and how we can deliver electrical signals, among other areas. Because of this, neuromodulation has emerged as an increasingly valuable and clinically effective chronic pain therapy.

Deep Brain Stimulation

Deep brain stimulation (DBS) offers direct stimulation of cortical regions of the brain responsible for pain perception (Figure 23.1). It has been used to manage neuropathic pain resistant to pharmacotherapy for more than 60 years [5]. In patients with centrally mediated pain syndromes, such as post-stroke pain or neuropathic pain post-spinal cord injury, thalamic or anterior cingulate cortex (ACC) stimulation has demonstrated limited, but favorable responses [6, 7]. DBS is also indicated in the management of atypical facial pain that has not responded

Clinical Pain Management: A Practical Guide, Second Edition. Edited by Mary E. Lynch, Kenneth D. Craig, and Philip W. Peng.

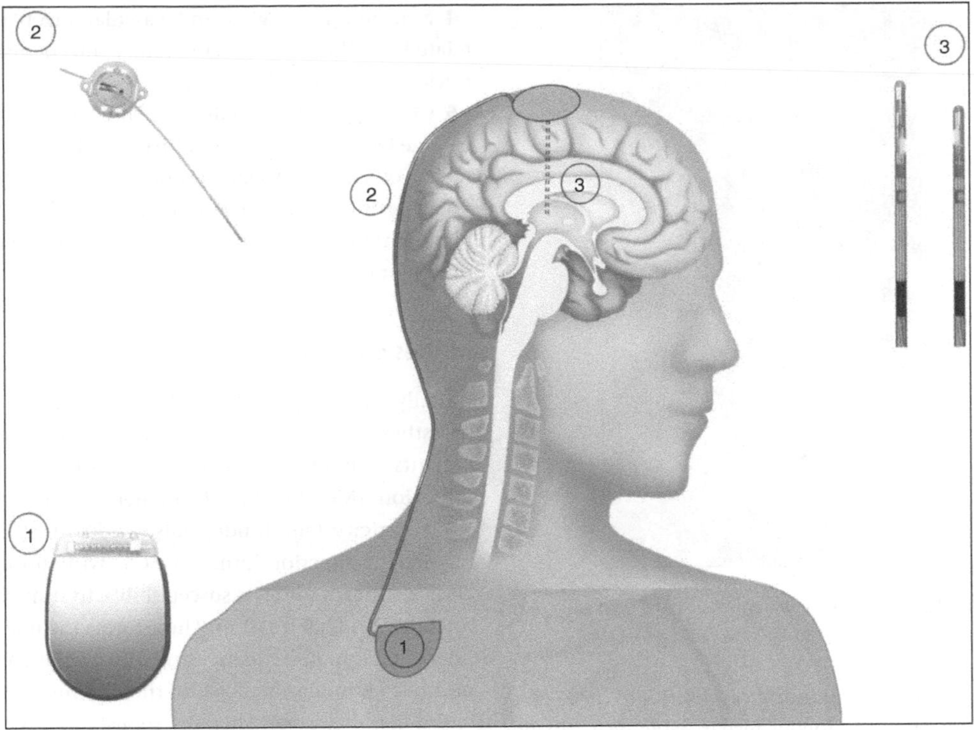

Figure 23.1 Schematic diagram of a deep brain stimulator system. 1. Implantable pulse generator. 2. Extension cable and burr hole lead. 3. Electrode.

to spinal cord stimulation or peripheral nerve stimulation [6]. Because of limited evidence, this therapy has been used in only end of therapy situations.

Boccard et al. reported a cohort study of 24 patients with refractory neuropathic pain who underwent bilateral ACC DBS [7]. Patient-reported outcome measures were collected before and after surgery, including the Numerical Rating Scale (NRS), Short-Form 36 quality of life (SF-36), McGill Pain Questionnaire (MPQ) and the EuroQol 5-domain quality of life (EQ-5D) questionnaire. Six months after surgery, the mean NRS score decreased from 8.00 to 4.27 ($p = 0.004$). There was a significant improvement in the MPQ (mean, –36%; $p = 0.021$) and the EQ-5D score significantly decreased (mean, –21%; $p = 0.036$). The physical functioning domain of SF-36 was significantly improved (mean, +54.2%; $p=0.01$). These findings were sustained at 1 year follow-up, as NRS score decreased by 43% ($P < 0.01$), EQ-5D was significantly reduced (mean, –30.8; $P = 0.05$) and significant improvements were also observed for different domains of the SF-36. Patients were followed up to 42 months after implant and efficacy was noted to be sustained, with some patients reporting an NRS score as low as 3. Long-term stimulation was, however, associated with an increased risk of seizures/epilepsy and this may be related to the pattern of stimulation, which is being investigated by the study authors.

Spinal Cord Stimulation

History

The first spinal cord stimulator was inserted in 1967 by N. Shealy, where he performed a thoracic laminectomy to implant a Vitallium electrode measuring 3 by 4 mm, sutured to dura [4]. In the late 1970's, implantable pulse generators (IPGs) came to market with technology adapted from space satellite power and telemetry systems [8]. This has formed the foundation of what we currently use today, with percutaneous leads developed that allow for superior

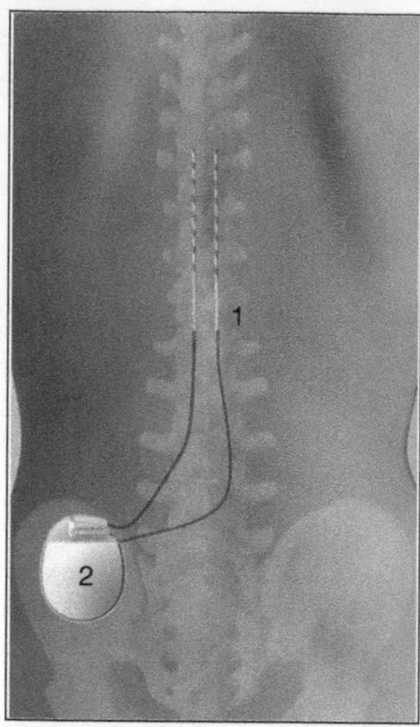

Figure 23.2 Schematic diagram of a spinal cord stimulator system. 1. Electrode. 2, Implantable pulse generator.

steering and programming capabilities (8 or 16 contacts) and transcutaneous rechargeable IPGs capable of lasting 5–10 years resulting in reduced morbidity, less frequent IPG replacement and cost savings [9] (Figure 23.2).

Review of Mechanisms of Actions

The underlying mechanism of how spinal cord stimulation (SCS) works to treat chronic pain has evolved over the last few decades, with Wall and Melzack's gate control theory thought to be the most accepted proposed mechanism [10]. Gate control theory asserts that stimulation of nonpainful afferent signals "closes the gate" to transmission of painful afferent signals, thereby preventing pain sensations from reaching the brain. Multiple other mechanisms have been elucidated, including:

1 Supraspinal activation of the descending antinociception system (DAS), modulating post-synaptic nociceptive projection neurons and the dorsal horn of the spinal cord [11, 12]

2 Substantia gelatinosa-mediated presynaptic inhibition of nociceptive signals

3 Activation of interneuron networks in the laminae I-III of the dorsal horn, which modulate nociceptive signaling and balance excitatory and inhibitory neurotransmitter release [13, 14]

4 Neuroimmune, glial and vascular mechanisms related to the neuroinflammatory mechanism of nociception [15]

5 Changes in the medial thalamic pathways to change the suffering aspect of pain (DeRidder's 2010 review of his burst theory, [16]).

6 Differing modes of stimulation are thought to preferentially target one or many of these mechanisms for optimal clinical efficacy.

Modes of Stimulation

Initially, the only form of SCS available was paresthesia-based, or tonic, stimulation, where patients would feel paresthesias covering their painful regions. Modification of parameters used to delivery electricity (amplitude, pulse width, frequency) has led to superior forms of SCS, with improved clinical efficacy and less susceptibility to stimulation tolerance and habituation. These forms include nonlinear burst, high-frequency and differential targeted multiplex stimulation. Each of these forms of stimulation has been validated in robust clinical trials (Table 23.1).

Indications

Most chronic neuropathic pain conditions have demonstrated response to SCS, such as failed back surgery syndrome, complex regional pain syndrome and chronic peripheral neuropathies [2, 9]. Additional indications include refractory angina, diabetic neuralgia, post-herpetic neuralgia and visceral or peripheral ischemic pain. Contraindications include active infections, immunosuppression and inability to withhold anticoagulation. Patients with a history of unmanaged psychological and mental health conditions tend to have poorer outcomes and expert mental health assessment is recommended prior to proceeding with trial or device implantation.

Technique

SCS is typically performed in two phases – a trial phase and a permanent implant phase. Recent evidence has questioned the utility of the trial phase [20]. In the trial period, a percutaneous cylindrical lead or a paddle lead facilitated by laminectomy is inserted under fluoroscopic guidance to the

Table 23.1 Evidence for novel modes of SCS in recent trials. NPRS: numerical pain rating scale

Form of stimulation studied/study name	Study design	Pain presentation studied	Primary outcome	Results
Non-linear burst (SUNBURST, 2017) [17]	Multicenter. randomized, controlled, crossover noninferiority trial	Chronic intractable pain of the trunk and/or limbs	Establish non- inferiority of pain intensity after three months of burst stimulation compared to three months of tonic stimulation	Burst stimulation is noninferior to tonic stimulation ($p < 0.001$), and superior to tonic stimulation ($p < 0.017$)
High frequency (SENZA, 2015) [18]	Multicenter, randomized, pragmatic, parallel-arm, noninferiority trial	Chronic, intractable pain of the trunk and/ or limbs	50% or greater back pain reduction with no stimulation-related neurological deficit	High-frequency stimulation is superior to tonic stimulation in reducing back and leg pain (79% vs. 51.3%; $p < 0.001$)
Differential targeted multiplex (DTM, 2020) [19]	Prospective, multicenter, feasibility study	Chronic intractable back pain with or without leg pain	Change in low back pain relative to a baseline score after a trial period of 3 to 5 days	In DTM group, mean low back NPRS score was 2.4. Difference between mean low back NPRS scores for standard and DTM programming was significant ($p < 0.0001$)

level of the spinal cord corresponding to the patient's pain area. Trial durations are approximately 5–10 days. A positive trial typically demonstrates at least 50% improvement from baseline pain to proceed to the permanent implant phase. In this phase, either the percutaneous or surgical paddle lead are internalized and attached to an IPG that can be nonrechargeable or rechargeable. The IPG can be inserted subcutaneously in the posterior flank, buttock or anterior abdominal wall region.

Complications

The 2014 Neuromodulation Appropriateness Consensus Committee established that SCS has a low risk of major complications, but minor complications are more common [21]. These typically include electrode fracture or lead migration, which are rectified by either replacing or repositioning the lead. The occurrence rate of lead fracture is estimated to be 5.9–9.1% and lead migration is up to 13.6%. Other complications of SCS include battery/IPG failure (1.7%), biological complications like infection (3.4–10%), epidural hematoma (0.3%) or pain localized to the incision, electrode or IPG site.

Cost-Effectiveness

Although associated with a high upfront cost, SCS has demonstrated cost-effectiveness overall when compared to conventional medical management (CMM) alone [22–24]. In a variety of disease conditions reviewed, SCS was found to have a significant benefit in incremental cost-effectiveness ratio (ICER) per quality-adjusted life years when compared to CMM, which is a generic measure of health benefit that allows the cost-effectiveness of pain treatments to be compared with other treatments in non-pain therapy areas as well [22]. Hoelscher et al. also studied cost-effectiveness analyses, which found that efficacy of SCS fell within usual third-party "willingness-to-pay" thresholds of US$50 000–US$100 000 quality-adjusted life-years gained and that initial costs can be recovered within 2–3 years [25].

DRG Stimulation

Given the difficulty of covering focal pain with traditional SCS, updated stimulation methods and targets were sought and dorsal root ganglion (DRG) stimulation was developed. The idea of targeting the DRG for chronic pain was first considered in 1949, but it wasn't until 2009 that Deer et al. performed the feasibility study for DRG stimulation in humans [26, 27]. More recently, Deer et al. reported the results from a randomized controlled trial comparing DRG stimulation to SCS for the treatment of CRPS Type I and II in the lower extremities [28]. In the prospective, randomized, controlled, multicenter study, an evaluation of the safety and efficacy of DRG stimulation compared to traditional SCS in subjects with CRPS type I and II at three and 12 months was performed. If the patient had a successful trial period with a given device (greater than 50% pain relief), they were implanted with the trialed device. Over the course of 12 months, implanted subjects were followed with the primary endpoint being the difference in success rate (great than 50% reduction in VAS from preimplant levels) between DRG stimulation and SCS at three months. At three months, 59 DRG and 52 SCS patients were available and 81.2% of DRG stimulation patients achieved success and 55.7% of SCS reaching the same result. This established superiority with DRG stimulation as compared to traditional SCS for this patient population ($p < 0.0004$). At 12 months, 55 DRG and 50 SCS patients completed the visit and a successful outcome was achieved in 74.2% for DRG stimulation versus 53.0% with SCS. Again, this showed superiority of DRG stimulation over SCS ($p < 0.0004$). In addition, DRG stimulation patients experienced less paresthesia in non-painful regions [28].

The mechanism of action for DRG stimulation is theorized to be different than traditional SCS. Traditional SCS is dependent on changes in GABA within the dorsal horn of the spinal cord, while DRG stimulation produces its pain relieving effects without GABA changes [29]. Additional work has shown DRG stimulation reduces the number of action potentials reaching the dorsal horn through augmentation of the DRG T-junction, in addition to cytokine and ionic changes, decreased hyperexcitability of neurons, activation of central nervous system centers and changes in gene expression within the DRG and spinal cord [30–32].

Dorsal root ganglion stimulation is currently approved by the Food and Drug Administration for chronic intractable pain of the lower extremities in adults with complex regional pain syndrome types I and II (causalgia). It is labeled in the United States for device implantation placed at or below the T10 vertebral level. In addition to CRPS Types I and II, there have been a number of manuscripts highlighting DRG stimulation for other focal pain conditions, including pelvic pain, discogenic low back pain, phantom limb pain and post-hernia pain [33, 34].

Peripheral Nerve Stimulation

Given on-going technological advances and debate regarding optimal neurostimulation targets, peripheral nerve stimulation (PNS) has emerged as an effective adjunct for both acute and chronic pain conditions. Recent evidence points to PNS being effective in neuropathic pain of the extremities, back pain due to failed back surgery syndrome and post-amputation pain. In 2016, Deer et al. performed a prospective, randomized, double-blind multicenter study to assess the safety and efficacy of PNS in the treatment of neuropathic pain of the extremities and trunk. Ninety-four patients were implanted and randomized to either the treatment arm (N=45) or control arm (N=49). The treatment arm had a 27.2% mean pain reduction compared to 2.3% reduction in the control arm ($p < 0.0001$) [35]. In 2019, Eldabe et al. conducted a multicenter randomized controlled trial (RCT) comparing the effectiveness of PNS with optimized medical management (OMM) versus OMM alone for patients with back pain related to failed back surgery syndrome. The primary endpoint was at least 50% pain improvement compared to baseline at nine months post-implant. Seventy-four patients completed the nine month follow-up visit. At nine months, 33.9% of patients in the PNS+OMM arm compared to 1.7% of patients in the OMM alone arm had at least a 50% decrease in their low back pain [36]. Recently, Gilmore et al. reported the 12 month results on the use of a 60-day PNS implant for chronic pain following amputation. The study included 28 traumatic lower extremity amputation patients with residual limb and/or phantom limb pain who were randomized to receive either eight weeks of PNS or four weeks of placebo followed by crossover to four weeks of PNS. Responder was defined as at least 50% decrease in pain. At 12 months, the eight week PNS group had a responder rate of 67% compared to the crossover group which had a responder rate of 15% [37].

There are currently both temporary and permanent PNS devices available for use. The technique for each involves placement of a thin electrical wire in proximity to the specific nerve in question. This is typically performed with local anesthesia at the insertion site under the guidance of an ultrasound. A monopolar needle is inserted and guided to within 0.5 to 1.0 cm from the target nerve. Stimulation testing is performed with this needle and an appropriate response is paresthesia in the expected nerve distribution without muscle contraction or uncomfortable superficial sensations. When an appropriate response is felt, an introducer needle is pre-loaded with the PNS lead and this is guided to the tested location. The needle is withdrawn over the lead, leaving the PNS lead in place. Depending on the system, the externalized lead can be attached to an external battery and attached to the skin or tunneled underneath the skin with an overlying receiver.

Intrathecal Drug Delivery Systems

Intrathecal (IT) analgesia was first described over 100 years ago by August Bier, but it wasn't until the 1990s that a battery powered implantable pump was released. Since then, intrathecal drug delivery systems (IDDS) have proven to be cost-effective, efficacious and associated with high patient satisfaction for a variety of conditions [38–42]. In a study from 2013, it was theorized that the IDDS financial break-even point for noncancer pain occurs around 27 months post-implantation and, on a per patient basis over a lifetime, that IDDS led to savings of $3,111 per year compared to conventional pain therapies [38]. Similarly, in an earlier study looking at patients with failed back surgery syndrome, the break-even point was found to be around 28 months and after that time period IDDS became increasingly cost effective [39]. In studies involving cancer pain patients, similar results were reported. Stearns et al. concluded that patients with IDDS had lower healthcare utilization over the first year post-implantation compared with conventional medical management, which amounted to $3,195 lower per patient when IDDS was utilized [40]. More recently, Stearns et al. showed more substantial savings of $15,142 at two months ($p = 0.0097$) and $63,498 at 12 months ($p = 0.03$) compared to conventional medical management after implantation of IDDS for cancer pain [41].

Indications for IDDS include axial neck or back pain, failed back surgery syndrome, abdominal and pelvic pain, trunk pain, extremity pain, complex regional pain syndrome, cancer pain and those patients who are finding relief with systemic opioids but have intolerable side effects. However, the decision to pursue IT therapy varies based on a number of patient specific factors, including diagnosis (malignant versus non-malignant pain), pain characteristics (neuropathic versus nociceptive versus mixed), distribution of pain (localized versus widespread), patient factors and response to other therapies. Typically, IDDS is considered in patients who have been unable to find appropriate pain relief with less invasive options. Randomized clinical trials show IT therapy is effective for malignant and non-malignant pain with both opioids and non-opioid medications over significant periods of time [43–45]. Contraindications to IDDS therapy include widespread pain without a definite cause, active systemic infection, poorly controlled diabetes, active coagulopathy, immune dysfunction, spinal anatomy that doesn't allow safe device placement and presence of an uncontrolled psychiatric disorder. All of these conditions should be treated prior to IT trialing and certainly before IDDS implantation.

There are three FDA approved medications labeled for IT use: ziconotide, morphine and baclofen. Ziconotide is an IT non-opioid FDA-approved medication for chronic pain. It is considered first-line for diffuse and localized neuropathic and nociceptive pain of cancer and noncancer etiologies [46]. Its mechanism of action involves a selective N-type calcium channel block, which limits release of nociceptive neurotransmitters, including Substance P, glutamate and CGRP [47]. The side effect profile is primarily neurologic, including sedation, nausea, vision changes and memory loss. Psychiatric side effects regarding mood, anxiety and psychosis have also been described. Advantages include a lack of tolerance and no withdrawal when discontinued abruptly. The single-shot IT bolus trialing dose is 1–5 mcg. For continuous infusion, the recommended starting rate is 0.5–1.2 mcg/day. The maximum concentration is 100 mcg/mL and the maximum daily dose is 19.2 mcg [46].

Morphine is the only opioid approved and labeled by the FDA for IT use and is considered first-line for both neuropathic and nociceptive pain conditions, whether used as a single agent or combined with bupivacaine [48]. Its analgesic mechanism of action is based on activation of mu, kappa and delta receptors within the substantia gelatinosa and rexed lamina II in the dorsal horn of the spinal cord. The single-shot IT bolus trialing dose is 0.1 – 0.5 mg. For continuous infusion, the maximum recommended concentration is 20 mg/mL, with a starting rate of 0.1–0.5 mg/day and a maximum daily dose of 15 mg [48]. Other commonly utilized opioid medications include hydromorphone, fentanyl and sufentanil. These three synthetic opioids are not FDA-approved, but remain commonly used in the spectrum of IDDS infusion options. Hydromorphone and fentanyl are both considered first line for varying painful conditions. Additionally, these synthetic opioids have greater lipophilicity and one would expect less travel of the medication within the IT space.

Local anesthetics are commonly used in clinical practice, typically in combination with an opioid. In particularly, bupivacaine is an amide local anesthetic that is considered first-line for diffuse and localized cancer and noncancer related pain. Bupivacaine is the only local anesthetic currently recommended in consensus guidelines [48]. Its mechanism of action relies on its ability to block sodium channels, thus inhibiting sodium influx and neuronal depolarization. Side effects include hypotension, paresthesias and motor block and urinary retention at higher dosages. The single-shot trialing IT bolus dose is 0.5–2.5 mg. For continuous infusion, the maximum concentration is 30 mg/mL, with a starting rate of 0.01–4 mg/day and a maximum daily dose of 15 – 20 mg [48].

Like other treatments, complications are unavoidable. These can be categorized into procedural, equipment related and pharmacological [49, 50]. Procedural complications include delayed wound healing, surgical site infections, surgical site seroma or hematoma, epidural hematoma and spinal headache. With appropriate surgical preparation and intraoperative technique, these risks can be mitigated. However, even with meticulous surgical preparation and handling, these complications are unplanned and unavoidable. Equipment related complications include catheter or pump issues. Catheter-related complications include catheter kinking, migration, occlusion or fracture.

Pump-related complications include motor stall and pump flipping/rotation. Pharmacological complications can include medication side effects, such as nausea, vomiting, pruritis or motor block with higher dosages, but also more sinister complications such as catheter tip granuloma which may decrease IT infusion amounts and potentially lead to spinal cord compression.

Conclusion

In appropriate patients, neuromodulation therapies are highly efficacious and cost-effective. Thankfully, the clinical evidence continues to expand and guide therapeutic decision making. We are hopeful that future researchers will be able to develop additional electroceuticals and intrathecal agents with novel targets and mechanisms of action. In this future landscape, clinical results will continue to improve, devices will become smaller and more usable and the overall neuromodulation experience will evolve in a patient-centric manner.

References

1 International Neuromodulation Society. (2021) Neuromodulation Defined. Neuromodulation, or neuromodulatory effect. Available at: https://www.neuromodulation.com/neuromodulation-defined. Accessed December 17, 2020.

2 Deer TR, Mekhail N, Provenzano D *et al.* (2014) The appropriate use of neurostimulation of the spinal cord and peripheral nervous system for the treatment of chronic pain and ischemic diseases: The neuromodulation appropriateness consensus committee. *Neuromodulation* **17(6)**:515–50.

3 Deer TR, Hagedorn JM, Jameson JB, Mekhail N. A new horizon in neuromodulation. *Pain Med* 22(**4**):1012–14.

4 Shealy CN, Mortimer JT, Reswick JB. (1967) Electrical inhibition of pain by stimulation of the dorsal columns: preliminary clinical report. *Anesth Analg* **46(4)**:489–91.

5 Pereira EAC, Aziz TZ. (2014) Neuropathic pain and deep brain stimulation *Neurotherapeutics* **11(3)**:496–507.

6 Farrell S, Green A, Aziz T. The current state of deep brain stimulation for chronic pain and its context in other forms of neuromodulation. *Brain Sci* **8(8)**:158.

7 Boccard SGJ, Prangnell SJ, Pycroft L *et al.* (2017) Long-term results of deep brain stimulation of the anterior cingulate cortex for neuropathic pain. *World Neurosurg* **106**:625–37.

8 Kirk J. (2001) *Machines in Our Hearts: The Cardiac Pacemaker, the Implantable Defibrillator, and American Health Care.* Johns Hopkins University Press, Baltimore.

9 Hong A, Varshney V, Hare GMT, David Mazer C. (2020) Spinal cord stimulation: a nonopioid alternative for chronic pain management. *CMAJ* **192(42)**:E1264–7.

10 Melzack R, Wall P. (1965) Pain mechanisms: a new theory. *Science* **150(3699)**:971–9.

11 Ahmed S, Yearwood T, De Ridder D, Vanneste S. (2018) Burst and high frequency stimulation: underlying mechanism of action. *Expert Rev Med Devices* **15(1)**:61–70.

12 Chakravarthy K, Fishman MA, Zuidema X, Hunter CW, Levy R. (2019) Mechanism of action in burst spinal cord stimulation: review and recent advances. *Pain Med* **20(1)**:S13–22.

13 Jensen MP, Brownstone RM. (2019) Mechanisms of spinal cord stimulation for the treatment of pain: still in the dark after 50 years. *Eur J Pain* **23(4)**:652–9.

14 Caylor J, Reddy R, Yin S *et al.* (2019) Spinal cord stimulation in chronic pain: evidence and theory for mechanisms of action. *Bioelectron Med* **5(1)**:1–41.

15 Sdrulla AD, Guan Y, Raja SN. (2018) Spinal cord stimulation: clinical efficacy and potential mechanisms. *Pain Pract* **18(8)**:1048–67.

16 De Ridder D, Vanneste S, Plazier M *et al.* (2010) Burst spinal cord stimulation: toward paresthesia-free pain suppression. *Neurosurgery* **66(5)**: 986–990.

17 Deer T, Slavin K V., Amirdelfan K *et al.* (2018) Success Using Neuromodulation with BURST (SUNBURST) study: results from a prospective, randomized controlled trial using a novel burst waveform. *Neuromodulation* **21(1)**:56–66.

18 Kapural L, Yu C, Doust MW, Gliner BE *et al.* (2015) Novel 10-kHz high-frequency therapy (HF10 Therapy) is superior to traditional low-frequency spinal cord stimulation for the

treatment of chronic back and leg pain. *Anesthesiology* **123(4)**:851–60.

19 Fishman MA, Calodney A, Kim P *et al.* (2020) Prospective, multicenter feasibility study to evaluate differential target multiplexed spinal cord stimulation programming in subjects with chronic intractable back pain with or without leg pain. *Pain Pract* **20(7)**:761–8.

20 Eldabe S, Duarte R V., Gulve A *et al.* (2020) Does a screening trial for spinal cord stimulation in patients with chronic pain of neuropathic origin have clinical utility and cost-effectiveness (TRIAL-STIM)? A randomised controlled trial. *Pain* **161(12)**:2820–9.

21 Deer TR, Mekhail N, Provenzano D *et al.* (2014) The appropriate use of neurostimulation: avoidance and treatment of complications of neurostimulation therapies for the treatment of chronic pain. *Neuromodulation* **17(6)**:571–98.

22 Kumar K, Rizvi S. (2013) Cost-effectiveness of spinal cord stimulation therapy in management of chronic pain. *Pain Med* **14**:1631–49.

23 Ontario Health Quality. (2019) 10-kHz high-frequency spinal cord stimulation for adults with chronic noncancer pain: a health technology assessment. *Ont Health Technol Assess Ser* **20(6)**:1–109.

24 Zucco F, Ciampichini R, Lavano A *et al.* (2015) Cost-effectiveness and cost-utility analysis of spinal cord stimulation in patients with failed back surgery syndrome: results from the PRECISE study. *Neuromodulation Technol Neural Interface* **18(4)**:266–76.

25 Hoelscher C, Riley J, Wu C, Sharan A. (2017) Cost-effectiveness data regarding spinal cord stimulation for low back pain. *Spine (Phila PA 1976)* **42 Suppl 14**:S72-9.

26 Soresi AL. (1949) Control of "intractable pain" by spinal ganglia block. *Am J Surg* **77(1)**:72–8.

27 Deer TR, Grigsby E, Weiner RL, Wilcosky B, Kramer JM. (2013) A prospective study of dorsal root ganglion stimulation for the relief of chronic pain. *Neuromodulation* **16(1)**:67–72.

28 Deer TR, Levy RM, Kramer J *et al.* (2017) Dorsal root ganglion stimulation yielded higher treatment success rate for complex regional pain syndrome and causalgia at 3 and 12 months: A randomized comparative trial. Pain. 2017;158(**4**):669–81.

29 Koetsier E, Franken G, Debets J *et al.* (2020) Mechanism of dorsal root ganglion stimulation for pain relief in painful diabetic polyneuropathy is not dependent on GABA release in the dorsal horn of the spinal cord. *CNS Neurosci Ther* **26(1)**:136–43.

30 Groom JE, Foreman RD, Chandler MJ, Barron KW. (1997) Cutaneous vasodilation during dorsal column stimulation is mediated by dorsal roots and CGRP. *Am J Physiol - Hear Circ Physiol* **272(2 Pt 2)**:H950–7.

31 Yi GS, Wang J, Wei X Le, Tsang KM, Chan WL, Deng B. (2014) Neuronal spike initiation modulated by extracellular electric fields. *PLoS One* **9(5)**:97481.

32 Koopmeiners AS, Mueller S, Kramer J, Hogan QH. (2013) Effect of electrical field stimulation on dorsal root ganglion neuronal function. *Neuromodulation Technol Neural Interface* **16(4)**:304–11.32.

33 Hunter CW, Yang A. (2019) Dorsal root ganglion stimulation for chronic pelvic pain: a case series and technical report on a novel lead configuration. *Neuromodulation Technol Neural Interface* **22(1)**:87–95.

34 Morgalla MH, Bolat A, Fortunato M, Lepski G, Chander BS. (2017) Dorsal root ganglion stimulation used for the treatment of chronic neuropathic pain in the groin: a single-center study with long-term prospective results in 34 cases. *Neuromodulation Technol Neural Interface* **20(8)**:753–60.

35 Deer T, Pope J, Benyamin R *et al.* (2016) Prospective, multicenter, randomized, double-blinded, partial crossover study to assess the safety and efficacy of the novel neuromodulation system in the treatment of patients with chronic pain of peripheral nerve origin. *Neuromodulation Technol Neural Interface* **19(1)**:91–100.

36 Eldabe SS, Taylor RS, Goossens S *et al.* (2019) A randomized controlled trial of subcutaneous nerve stimulation for back pain due to failed back surgery syndrome: the SubQStim study. *Neuromodulation Technol Neural Interface* **22(5)**:519–28.

37 Gilmore C, Ilfeld B, Rosenow J *et al.* (2019) Percutaneous peripheral nerve stimulation for the treatment of chronic neuropathic postamputation pain: a multicenter, randomized,

placebo-controlled trial. *Reg Anesth Pain Med* **44(6)**:637–45.

38 Guillemette S, Witzke S, Leier J, Hinnenthal J, Prager JP. (2013) Medical cost impact of intrathecal drug delivery for noncancer pain. *Pain Med 14(***4***)*:504–15.

39 Kumar K, Hunter G, Demeria DD. (2002_ Treatment of chronic pain by using intrathecal drug therapy compared with conventional pain therapies: a cost-effectiveness analysis. *J Neurosurg* **97(4)**:803–10.

40 Stearns LJ, Hinnenthal JA, Hammond K, Berryman E, Janjan NA. (2016) Health services utilization and payments in patients with cancer pain: a comparison of intrathecal drug delivery vs. conventional medical management. *Neuromodulation Technol Neural Interface* **19(2)**:196–205.

41 Stearns LJ, Narang S, Albright RE *et al.* (2019) Assessment of health care utilization and cost of targeted drug delivery and conventional medical management vs conventional medical management alone for patients with cancer-related pain. *JAMA Netw Open* **2(4)**:e191549.

42 Schultz DM, Orhurhu V, Khan F, Hagedorn JM, Abd-Elsayed A. (2020) Patient satisfaction following intrathecal targeted drug delivery for benign chronic pain: results of a single-center survey study. *Neuromodulation Technol Neural Interface* **23(7)**:1009–17.

43 Smith TJ, Staats PS, Deer T *et al.* (2002) Randomized clinical trial of an implantable drug delivery system compared with comprehensive medical management for refractory cancer pain: impact on pain, drug-related toxicity, and survival. *J Clin Oncol* **20(19)**:4040–9.

44 Wallace MS, Charapata SG, Fisher R *et al.* (2006) Intrathecal ziconotide in the treatment of chronic nonmalignant pain: a randomized, double-blind, placebo-controlled clinical trial. *Neuromodulation* **9(2)**:75–86.

45 Bolash R, Udeh B, Saweris Y *et al.* (2015) Longevity and cost of mplantable intrathecal drug delivery systems for chronic pain management: a retrospective analysis of 365 patients. *Neuromodulation Technol Neural Interface* **18(2)**:150–6.

46 Deer T, Rauck RL, Kim P *et al.* (2017) Effectiveness and safety of intrathecal ziconotide: interim analysis of the Patient Registry of Intrathecal Ziconotide Management. *Pain Pract* **18(2)**:230–9.

47 Deer T, Hagedorn JM. (2020) How has ziconotide impacted non-cancer pain management? *Expert Opin Pharmacother* **21(5)**:507–11.

48 Deer TR, Pope JE, Hayek SM *et al.* (2016) The Polyanalgesic Consensus Conference (PACC): recommendations on intrathecal drug infusion systems best practices and guidelines. *Neuromodulation* **20**:96–132.

49 Goel V, Yang Y, Kanwar S, Banik RK *et al.* (2020) Adverse events and complications associated with intrathecal drug delivery systems: insights from the Manufacturer and User Facility Device Experience (MAUDE) database. *Neuromodulation Technol Neural Interface* Online ahead of print.

50 Delhaas EM, Huygen FJPM. (2020) Complications associated with intrathecal drug delivery systems. *BJA Education*20(**2**):51–7.

Chapter 24

Neurosurgical management of pain

Marshall T. Holland[1], **Ashwin Viswanathan**[2], **& Kim J. Burchiel**[3]

[1] *Department of Neurosurgery, Heersink School of Medicine, The University of Alabama at Birmingham, Birmingham, AL*

[2] *Department of Neurosurgery, Baylor College of Medicine, Houston, Texas, USA*

[3] *Department of Neurosurgical Surgery, Oregon Health and Science University, Portland, USA*

Introduction

Pain is the most common reason for patients to seek the care of a neurosurgeon. Neurosurgical interventions for the management of pain can broadly be categorized as anatomic, neuromodulatory and neuroablative. Anatomic procedures for the treatment of pain seek to correct structural abnormalities leading to pain, as in the case of spondylolysis with spondylolisthesis or in entrapment neuropathies. Neuromodulatory procedures include both drug infusion therapies and neurostimulation procedures such as peripheral nerve stimulation, spinal cord stimulation, motor cortex stimulation and deep brain stimulation. In contrast, neuroablative procedures seek to interrupt the pathways of pain transmission and may be directed towards the peripheral nerve, root entry zone, spinal cord or brain. To the degree that evidence to support the particular procedure can be classified, it will be listed according to contemporary standards. In general, Class I evidence derives from randomized controlled trials, Class II from well-constructed prospective cohort trials, or in some cases high-quality meta-analysis and Class III evidence pertains to case series, case reports or expert opinion.

Anatomic

Most patients who consult neurosurgeons do so to understand the etiology of, and to relieve, a pain problem. In the subset of patients in whom an anatomic etiology for the pain can be identified, neurosurgical intervention may prove an effective intervention.

Spinal Disorders

The most common pain problems neurosurgeons address are related to the spine. A full discussion of indications and surgical strategies for spinal surgery are beyond the scope of this chapter. In general, radicular pain is tractable to neurosurgical intervention, while axial pain in the absence of a structural abnormality is more difficult to treat and outcome from surgery uncertain. Indications for spinal surgery include the relatively straight-forward removal of a herniated disk producing a clear radicular syndrome, to stabilization of spondylolisthesis associated with spondylolysis. Our understanding of the indications for spinal fusion in the setting of degenerative disease of the cervical and lumbar spine are still developing; recent reviews seek to clarify patient selection and outcomes [1, 2].

Clinical Pain Management: A Practical Guide, Second Edition. Edited by Mary E. Lynch, Kenneth D. Craig, and Philip W. Peng.

Trigeminal Neuralgia

In selected cases of trigeminal neuralgia (TN) surgery is indicated (for clinical presentation see Chapter 32) [3]. Before considering surgical therapy for patients with TN, patients must have undergone an adequate trial of one or more oral medications such as carbamazepine, oxcarbazepine or a gabapentinoid and have become either intolerant of, or refractory to, the medications. Microvascular decompression is a surgical option that can lead to long-term pain relief. This surgical therapy addresses what is thought to an anatomic correlate of TN – arterial compression of the root entry zone (REZ) of the trigeminal nerve. High resolution magnetic resonance imaging aimed at delineating the arterial and neural anatomy can demonstrate compression at the REZ. Microvascular decompression (MVD) is associated with a 0.2% mortality and < 5% morbidity, which includes hearing loss in 1%, cerebrospinal fluid leakage in 2–3% and rare (<1%) cranial nerve deficits. Use of microvascular decompression for TN is supported by Class III evidence, but no Class I–II studies have been completed.

Additionally, it is important to note there is evidence for a group of patients, often younger onset and skewed female, with a clear diagnosis of classic trigeminal neuralgia without vascular compression [4]. In these patient's, microvascular decompression with internal neurolysis offers favorable outcomes (85% pain free and 96 % with satisfactory pain relief) with comparable morbidity to TN patients undergoing MVD [5].

Entrapment Neuropathies

A number of peripheral nerve compression syndromes exist that can be improved through surgical decompression. The most common entrapment neuropathy is compression of the median nerve by the transverse carpal ligament at the wrist (carpal tunnel syndrome). Patients may present with diffuse aching of the arm and forearm, associated with numbness and weakness of the hands. Symptoms are typically worse at night. Physical examination may reveal weakness of thumb abduction or opposition and provocative tests such as tapping the median nerve over wrist may induce paresthesias. In a Cochrane review it was found that surgery for carpal tunnel syndrome relieved symptoms significantly better than splinting. The authors concluded that further research is needed in order to determine whether this applies to people with mild symptoms and whether surgical treatment is better than steroid injections [6].

Neuromodulatory

Deep Brain Stimulation

The mechanism of pain relief from deep brain stimulation (DBS) is hypothesized to involve activation of descending inhibitory pain pathways. Multiple targets for neurostimulation have been proposed: the thalamic ventralis caudalis (Vc) nucleus, the ventral striatum/anterior limb of the internal capsule and the periaqueductal gray/periventricular gray matter. DBS should only be considered for patients in whom all other treatment modalities have not shown adequate improvement. Symptoms should have been present for more than 6 months and the patient should have been evaluated by a multidisciplinary pain center first [7].

A frame-based or frameless stereotactic system may be used to place DBS electrodes. Following implantation, patients undergo an externalized trial period of 3–7 days. During this time, patients maintain a pain diary and various stimulation parameters are used. If a patient has a successful stimulation trial, they undergo implantation of the generator. If the trial is unsuccessful, the electrodes are then removed. Surgical complications associated with DBS include infection (5%), stroke (3%), asymptomatic intracerebral bleeding (4%) and other hardware related complications (7%).

Only case series and case reports (Class III) support the use of DBS for chronic pain. Chronic pain conditions that have been treated with DBS include failed back syndrome, cancer pain, anesthesia dolorosa, stroke pain, thalamic syndromes and others. Published series report better long-term outcomes for nociceptive pain than for neuropathic pain [8]. Given the lack of substantiating evidence and recent unsuccessful randomized study, DBS for chronic pain remains an off label, non-FDA approved procedure [9].

Motor cortex stimulation

Motor cortex stimulation (MCS) was introduced as a treatment modality for central deafferentation pain in the early 1990s. Investigators noted that stimulation of the motor cortex led to inhibition of thalamic hyperactivity associated with deafferentation. Epidural electrodes for MCS may be placed through either burr holes or craniotomy. The surgical target can be adjusted based upon the location of the pain. Placement of the epidural electrodes is typically followed by a 5 to 10 day trial period. Patients who have a successful trial are then implanted with a generator [10].

Case series evidence (Class III) indicates that MCS *may* provide benefit for patients with neuropathic pain. In contrast, there is no evidence to support the use of MCS in patients with nociceptive pain. MCS has been applied to various neuropathic pain syndromes including facial pain, central pain secondary to stroke and peripheral deafferentation pain including phantom limb pain. Overall, approximately 40–70% of appropriately selected patients may have a successful trial period of MCS, warranting implantation of a generator. Patients with TN pain form a subgroup of patients in whom generally positive results have been reported. Despite these promising initial results, MCS is still a treatment modality in development. Particularly, as long term studies with extending follow up have failed to demonstrated significant improvement in pain, this intervention is rarely covered by insurance [11, 12].

Spinal cord stimulation

Spinal cord stimulation (SCS) was first used as treatment modality for cancer pain in the 1960s. The surgical technique evolved from subdural electrode placement, to intradural placement to epidural placement today. A more detailed discussion of SCS is presented in Chapter 24.

Other Neuromodulatory Interventions

As with SCS, intrathecal opiates have significantly expanded the treatment options available to the pain management physician. This therapy is discussed further in Chapter 20. Intracerebroventricular opioids have been shown to be an effective intervention in patients with malignant pain unresponsive to other therapies. This route of administration may be particularly useful in patients with malignancy involving the head and neck or in whom respiratory depression may be a risk with high spinal administration. The surgical technique involves implantation of a ventricular catheter into the lateral ventricle for delivery of opiates near target receptors around the aqueductal wall of the midbrain [13]. Side effects from intraventricular administration of opioids can include somnolence, nausea and respiratory depression.

Neuroablation

The increased use of SCS and intrathecal drug delivery has led to a decrease in the use of neuroablative procedures to manage pain. A systematic review identified that destructive techniques for the treatment of pain have had a long and important history with 146 studies examining the use of neuroablative procedures in non-cancer pain [14]. This review found the majority of studies constituted Class III evidence with the majority of Level I and II studies focused on radiofrequency rhizotomies (Table 24.1). Further research is needed, but in the meantime this review identifies that there is a wealth of experience to date and for the appropriately selected patient

Table 24.1 Number of studies by class of evidence assessing ablative procedures for non-malignant pain.

Procedure	Class I	Class II	Class III
Cingulotomy	0	0	13
Cordotomy	0	0	11
DREZ lesioning	0	0	26
Ganglionectomy	2	0	15
Mesencephalotomy	0	0	9
Myelotomy	0	0	3
Rhizotomy for:			
trigeminal neuralgia	0	2	18
lumbar facet syndrome	4	1	9
discogenic back pain	1	0	0
cervical pain	4	1	4
cluster headache	0	0	3
Thalamotomy	0	0	12

DREZ, dorsal root entry zone.

Table 24.2 Ablative procedures, appropriate clinical application and pitfall application.

Ablative procedure	Clinical application	Pitfall application
Neurectomy	Stump or traumatic neuroma; Meralgia paresthetica; Post-herniorrhaphy pain	Phantom limb pain; Post-herpetic neuralgia
Dorsal rhizotomy and dorsal root ganglionectomy	Chest wall pain; Post-thoracotomy syndrome; Occipital neuralgia	Lumbar radiculopathy; Low back pain; Post-herpetic neuralgia
Sympathectomy	Causalgia*; Reflex sympathetic dystrophy*;Abdominal cancer pain	Non-sympathetically mediated pain
Trigeminal system procedures: radiofrequency balloon compression glycerol rhizolysis	Classic trigeminal neuralgia; Facial pain due to multiple sclerosis	Neuropathic trigeminal pain
DREZ	Nerve root avulsion (brachial plexus injury); Local segmental pain after spinal cord injury; Localized cancer pain	Post-herpetic neuralgia; Facial pain
Cordotomy	Unilateral cancer pain below C5; Paroxysmal neuropathic pain after traumatic spinal cord injury	Caution with midline and central pain
Myelotomy	Pelvic and sacral cancer pain; Midline cancer pain	
Mesencephalotomy (Trigeminal Tractotomy)	Head and neck cancer pain; Central, post stroke pain	Facial pain
Thalamotomy	Cancer pain; Central pain	Deafferentation pain
Cingulotomy	Diffuse cancer pain; Failed back syndrome; Best in patients with depressive symptoms	

DREZ, dorsal root entry zone. * Based on limited evidence.

with pain unresponsive to other interventions, neuroablative procedures can serve as an invaluable therapy (Table 24.2).

Neuroablative lesions can be created mechanically by surgical scalpel, chemically, thermally by radiofrequency lesioning and through radiation therapy. Figures 24.1 and 24.2 illustrate spinal and cerebral neuroablative and neuromodulatory procedures, respectively.

Peripheral nervous system

Neurectomy

Neurectomy is the surgical sectioning of a nerve [15, 16]. Application is limited because it involves sacrifice of a nerve, which may carry motor and sensory fibers. In the long-term, intact sensory neurons, which are adjacent to the denervated area, can sprout axons, leading to a smaller region of denervation and denervation hypersensitivity. Local anesthetic blockade should always be performed diagnostically and to demonstrate the expected postoperative deficit that may be incurred from sectioning the nerve. Indications are listed in Table 24.2.

Dorsal rhizotomy and dorsal root ganglionectomy

Dorsal rhizotomy involves sectioning the dorsal nerve root. Evidence suggesting that up to one-third of axons in the ventral nerve root are derived from the dorsal root ganglion, led surgeons to consider resection of the dorsal root ganglion as an alternative procedure. Both rhizotomy and ganglionectomy lead to the loss of proprioception and, consequently, the procedure is not appropriate for extremity pain. Despite these drawbacks, long-term pain relief can be achieved when treating chest wall pain, post-thoracotomy syndrome and occipital neuralgia through sectioning of the C2 ganglion [17]. Application of rhizotomy and ganglionectomy to lumbar radiculopathy, lower back pain and

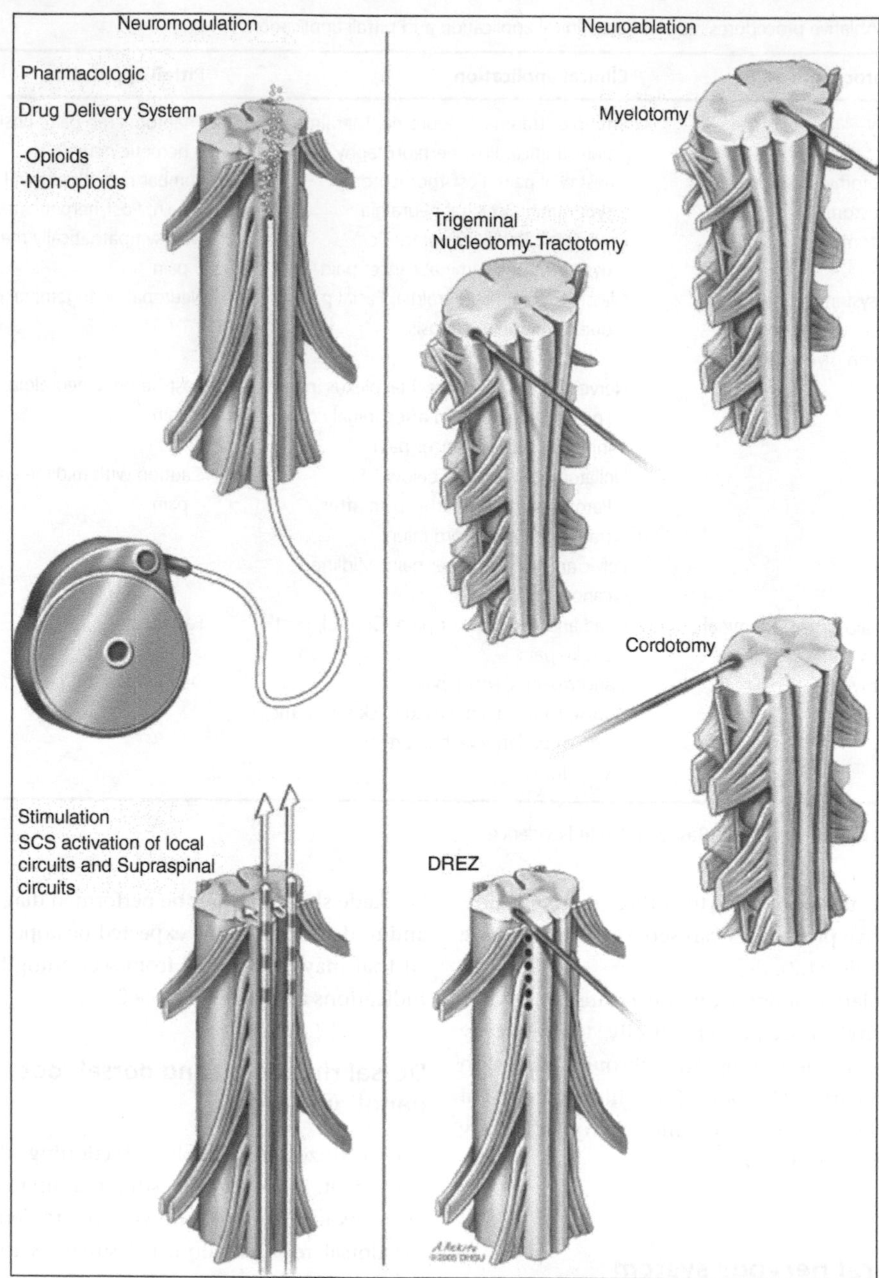

Figure 24.1 Diagrammatic representation of spinal neuromodulation and neuroablation procedures. Reproduced with permission from Raslan AM, McCartney S, Burchiel KJ. (2007) Management of chronic severe pain: spinal neuromodulatory and neuroablative approaches. In: Sakas DE, Simpson B, Krames ES, eds. *Acta Neurochir Suppl*, Springer-Verlag, New York. pp. 33–41.

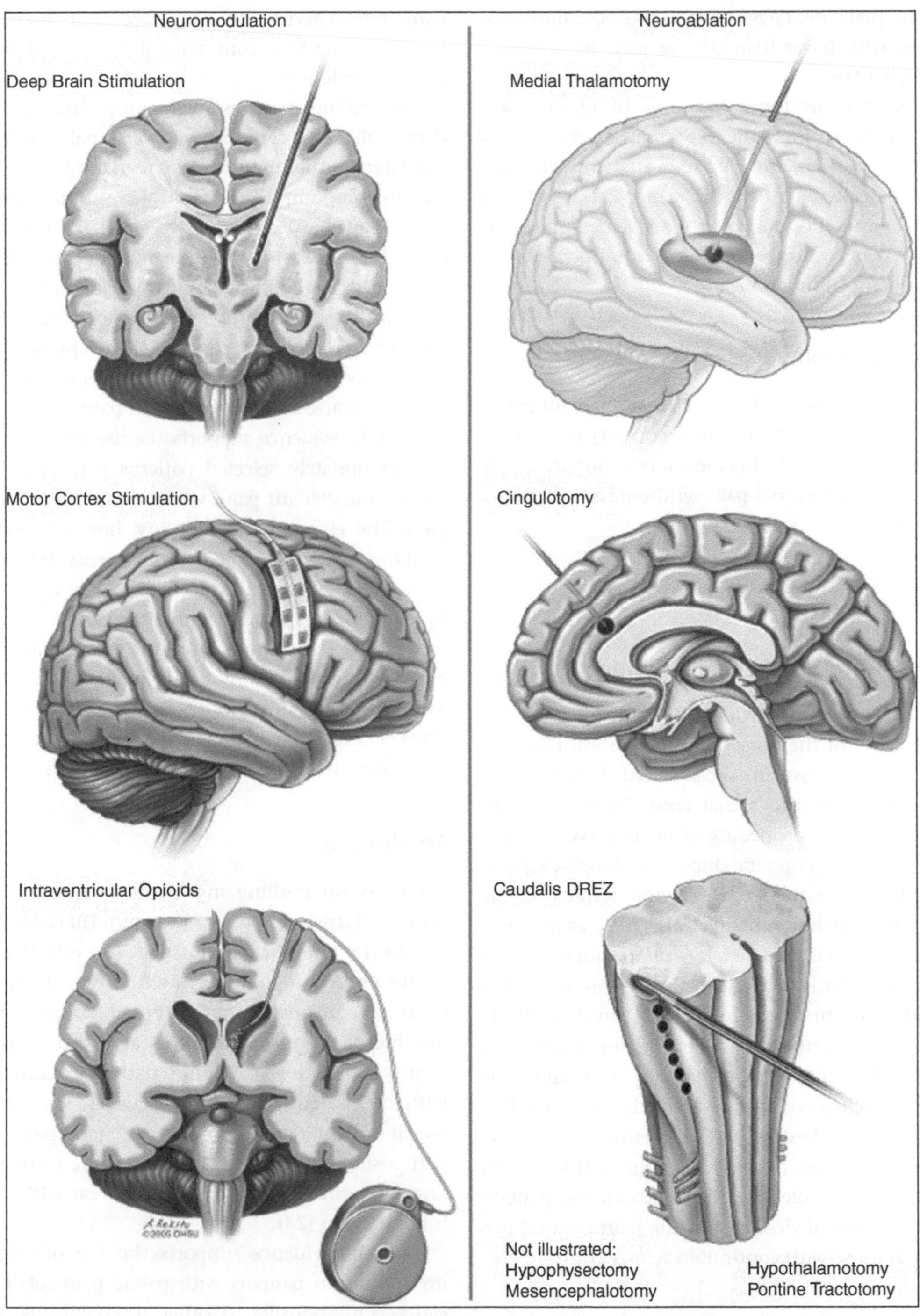

Figure 24.2 Diagrammatic representation of cerebral neuromodulation and neuroablation procedures. Reproduced with permission from Raslan AM, McCartney S, Burchiel KJ. (2007) Management of chronic severe pain: cerebral neuromodulatory and neuroablative approaches. In: Sakas DE, Simpson B, Krames ES, eds. *Acta Neurochir Suppl*. Springer-Verlag, New York. pp.17–26.

post-herpetic neuralgia have shown disappointing results, with fewer than 30% of patients obtaining pain relief [18].

As with neurectomy, sprouting of adjacent sensory axons can limit the long-term effectiveness of this procedure. In the long-term, patients may also develop deafferentation pain, which can lead to significant disability. Rhizotomy and ganglionectomy lead to denervation, which further limits the future use of neurostimulation.

Sympathectomy

Reviews have identified that treating neuropathic pain by sympathectomy is based on very limited evidence [14, 19-21]. Sympathetically maintained pain and complex regional pain syndrome are presented in Chapter 37.

Spinal Cord

Dorsal Root Entry Zone Lesioning

The dorsal root entry zone (DREZ) includes the central portion of the dorsal or sensory root, Lissauer's tract and the most superficial Rexed laminae of the dorsal horn of the spinal cord. These areas are involved in the processing of nociceptive information. Altered peripheral input to these areas can result in hyperactivity of this region, leading to pain syndromes. By lesioning the DREZ, the area of hyperactivity can be eliminated, leading to pain relief [22].

In a systematic review, a total of 26 case series were included. All studies reported more than 50% relief in pain in a majority of patients and the results were durable. Patients with brachial plexus avulsion and traumatic spinal cord injury tended to have the best response [14]. Results of DREZ lesioning for post-herpetic neuralgia or for post-amputation pain have not been favorable. For these indications, patients with paroxysmal electric shooting pain respond better than those with continuous aching pain.

Cordotomy

Cordotomy targets the lateral spinothalamic tract located in the anterolateral quadrant of the spinal cord. As the spinothalamic tract carries information regarding pain and temperature sensation from the contralateral body, the goal of cordotomy is abolishing pain sensation contralateral to and below the level of the lesion.

Lancinating, paroxysmal, neuropathic and allodynic pain secondary to cancer or spinal cord injury and lateral rather than midline pain tend to respond well to cordotomy. Treatment of continuous neuropathic pain has been less successful. The treatment of midline pain may require bilateral cordotomy, which carries a higher risk of weakness, sexual dysfunction and respiratory depression. The highest level of analgesia that can be reliably produced by cordotomy is at the C5 dermatome, thus cordotomy is not indicated for head and neck pain.

Class III evidence supports the use of cordotomy for appropriately selected patients with malignant and non-malignant pain, with best results in cancer pain. The efficacy of cordotomy, however, reduces with time, with less than 50% of patients still having pain relief after 1 year. The level of analgesia produced by cordotomy also falls with increasing time from procedure. The introduction of the percutaneous approach for cordotomy has reduced the morbidity associated with this procedure. Potential complications of cordotomy include sleep apnea, post cordotomy dysesthesia and mirror-image pain [23].

Myelotomy

Commissural midline myelotomy seeks to interrupt the crossing fibers of the spinothalamic tract within the anterior commissure. The effectiveness of this procedure in patients with visceral pain led to the recognition of a visceral pain pathway at the midline of the dorsal columns also known as the post-synaptic dorsal column pathway. Compared with other neuroablative procedures, myelotomy has the advantages of providing bilateral pain relief with a single procedure and is effective in treating visceral pain, which is difficult to treat with other interventions [24].

Class III evidence supports the use of midline myelotomy in patients with pelvic pain related to cancer unresponsive to other interventions. Case series have demonstrated satisfactory pain relief in 60–80% of cancer patients who underwent myelotomy [25]. Potential surgical complications include bladder and bowel dysfunction, diminished proprioception and gait disturbances.

Brainstem

Brainstem lesioning is indicated in the treatment of pain involving the head, face and neck, carried by fibers of the trigeminal, glossopharyngeal, vagus, nervus intermedius and upper cervical nerves. Neuroablative procedures targeting the brainstem include mesencephalotomy, trigeminal tractotomy and caudalis DREZ.

Mesencephalotomy (Trigeminal Tractotomy)

When applied to face and head pain, mesencephalotomy targets the trigeminothalamic (trigeminal tractotomy) and reticulothalamic tracts contralateral to the patient's pain. If a patient has bilateral pain, a lesion placed contralateral to the more painful side can provide bilateral pain relief. Case series of mesencephalotomy for cancer pain report that 85% of patients having complete or good pain relief and 60% experience good results in the long-term. Mesencephalotomy for central post-stroke pain has not proven as efficacious with 60% of patients reporting acceptable pain relief but with poor long-term benefit. Other indications, including facial pain, have not shown promising results.

Potential complications associated with mesencephalotomy include changes in ocular motility, which are usually mild and asymptomatic. Use of a stereotactic approach to mesencephalotomy has reduced the incidence of dysesthesia to less than 15%; an open technique has been associated with a 50% or greater risk of postoperative dysesthesias [26].

Intracranial

The introduction of stereotaxis and the ability to target deep brain structures led to the development of several intracranial targets for pain management. Ablative procedures for the management of pain have been directed towards the thalamus, pulvinar, pituitary, cinglate gyrus and the precentral and postcentral gyrus [27]. However, the exact mechanisms through which these procedures relieve pain are not fully understood. The limited number of patients who have undergone these procedures and few published series make treatment recommendations difficult.

Thalamotomy

Because of the wide involvement of thalamic nuclei in pain processing, the thalamus has been a target of interest for both neuroablative and neurostimulative procedures for pain management. The main sensory nucleus, Vc nucleus, was the first target for neuroablation. However, targeting of the Vc nucleus was associated with the development of significant deafferentation pain. The medial thalamus including the centralis lateralis, centrum medianum and parafascicularis have become the more common target for thalamotomy. Medial thalamotomy is thought to influence pain transmission through the non-specific spinoreticulothalamic tract.

Outcome after thalamotomy is difficult to ascertain due to the lack of controlled studies. Although thalamotomy is thought to be more effective in the treatment of nociceptive, rather than neuropathic pain, it has been applied to a variety of pain syndromes including cancer pain, central and peripheral deafferentation pain, spinal cord injury pain and arthritis [28]. Medial thalamotomy has been demonstrated to provide good short-term pain relief in more than 50% of patients, but the long-term success rate is only 30%. Consequently, thalamotomy is most appropriate for the treatment of cancer pain in selected patients with a short life expectancy.

Cingulotomy

The goal of cingulotomy is to disrupt the anterior cingulate gyrus, usually bilaterally. Cingulotomy is thought to alter the patient's emotional reaction to pain through interruption of the Papez circuit of the limbic system. The major indication for cingulotomy is in the terminally ill cancer patient with widely metastatic disease, whose pain has not responded to other therapeutic modalities. Success rates of up to 68% have been reported, but efficacy decreases with time, reaching 50% by 6-month follow-up. Cingulotomy has also been applied to non-malignant chronic pain, with failed back syndrome being the dominant indication. In a series of 18 patients with a median follow-up of 6 years, 72% of patients reported useful pain relief, with 70% patients having improved social function and 25% of patients returning to work. Postoperative seizures can occur and should be managed medically with antiepileptic medicines [29].

Conclusions

Neurosurgical techniques for the management of pain include a wide array of interventions. Correction of an anatomic abnormality where clearly identified in spinal pain is reasonable to consider in appropriately selected patients. Neuromodulation is a promising field and is discussed in more detail in Chapter 20. For some procedures, including DBS and MCS, the indications are still being developed and long term outcomes have not been the most encouraging. Further studies are necessary to determine the most appropriate candidates for these therapies. With regards to neuroablative techniques, there is a long history with significant clinical experience but most support for ablative procedures in chronic non-cancer pain is based on Class III evidence. Again, further research is needed. In the meantime, this chapter provides guidance into situations where an ablative procedure may be considered.

Acknowledgment

We thank Shirley McCartney, PhD, for editorial assistance.

References

1 Mummaneni PV, Kaiser MG, Matz PG, *et al.* (2009) Cervical surgical techniques for the treatment of cervical spondylotic myelopathy. *J Neurosurg Spine* **11(2)**:130–41.

2 Gibson JN, Waddell G. (2005) Surgery for degenerative lumbar spondylosis: updated Cochrane Review. *Spine (Phila Pa 1976)* **30(20)**:2312–20.

3 Miller JP, Acar F, Burchiel KJ. (2009) Classification of trigeminal neuralgia: clinical, therapeutic, and prognostic implications in a series of 144 patients undergoing microvascular decompression. *J Neurosurg* **111(6)**:1231–4.

4 Magown P, Ko AL, Burchiel KJ. (2019) The spectrum of trigeminal neuralgia without neurovascular compression. *Neurosurgery* **85(3)**:E553–E9.

5 Ko AL, Ozpinar A, Lee A, Raslan AM, McCartney S, Burchiel KJ. (2015) Long-term efficacy and safety of internal neurolysis for trigeminal neuralgia without neurovascular compression. *J Neurosurg* **122(5)**:1048–57.

6 Verdugo RJ, Salinas RA, Castillo JL, Cea JG. (2008) Surgical versus non-surgical treatment for carpal tunnel syndrome. *Cochrane Database Syst Rev* 2008(4):CD001552.

7 Raslan AM, McCartney S, Burchiel KJ. (2007) Management of chronic severe pain: cerebral neuromodulatory and neuroablative approaches. *Acta Neurochir Suppl* 97(Pt 2):17–26.

8 Whitworth L, Fernandez, J., and Feler, C. (2005) Deep brain stimulation for chronic pain. In: Fisher W, Burchiel K, eds. Seminars in *Neurosurgery: Pain Management for the Neurosurgeon: Part 2/3.*Thieme Medical Publishers, New York. pp 183–93.

9 Lempka SF, Malone DA, Jr., Hu B *et al.* (2017) Randomized clinical trial of deep brain stimulation for poststroke pain. *Ann Neurol* **81(5)**:653–63.

10 Fontaine D, Hamani C, Lozano A. (2009) Efficacy and safety of motor cortex stimulation for chronic neuropathic pain: critical review of the literature. *J Neurosurg* **110(2)**:251–6.

11 Raslan AM, Nasseri M, Bahgat D, Abdu E, Burchiel KJ. (2011) Motor cortex stimulation for trigeminal neuropathic or deafferentation pain: an institutional case series experience. *Stereotact Funct Neurosurg* **89(2)**:83–8.

12 Sachs AJ, Babu H, Su YF, Miller KJ, Henderson JM. (2014) Lack of efficacy of motor cortex stimulation for the treatment of neuropathic pain in 14 patients. *Neuromodulation* **17(4)**:303–10; discussion 310-1.

13 Lazorthes YR, Sallerin BA, Verdie JC. (1995) Intracerebroventricular administration of morphine for control of irreducible cancer pain. *Neurosurgery* **37(3)**:422–8; discussion 428-9.

14 Cetas JS, Saedi T, Burchiel KJ. (2008) Destructive procedures for the treatment of nonmalignant pain: a structured literature review. *J Neurosurg* **109(3)**:389–404.

15 Burchiel KJ, Johans TJ, Ochoa J. (1993) The surgical treatment of painful traumatic neuromas. *J Neurosurg* **78(5)**:714–9.

16 Williams PH, Trzil KP. (1991) Management of meralgia paresthetica. *J Neurosurg* **74(1)**:76–80.

17 Acar F, Miller J, Golshani KJ, Israel ZH, McCartney S, Burchiel KJ. (2008) Pain relief after cervical ganglionectomy (C2 and C3) for the treatment of medically intractable occipital neuralgia. *Stereotact Funct Neurosurg* **86(2)**:106–12.

18 North RB, Kidd DH, Campbell JN, Long DM. (1991) Dorsal root ganglionectomy for failed back surgery syndrome: a 5-year follow-up study. *J Neurosurg* **74(2)**:236–42.
19 Mailis A, Furlan A. (2003) Sympathectomy for neuropathic pain. *Cochrane Database Syst Rev* 2003(2):CD002918.
20 Sweet W, ed. (1990) *Sympathectomy for Pain.* 3rd edn. W.B. Saunders, Philadelphia.
21 Furlan AD, Mailis A, Papagapiou M. (2000) Are we paying a high price for surgical sympathectomy? A systematic literature review of late complications. *J Pain* **1(4)**:245–57.
22 Sindou MP, Blondet E, Emery E, Mertens P. (2005) Microsurgical lesioning in the dorsal root entry zone for pain due to brachial plexus avulsion: a prospective series of 55 patients. *J Neurosurg* **102(6)**:1018–28.
23 Kanpolat Y, Ugur HC, Ayten M, Elhan AH. (2009) Computed tomography-guided percutaneous cordotomy for intractable pain in malignancy. *Neurosurgery* **64(3 Suppl)**:ons187–93; discussion ons193-4.
24 Nauta HJ, Soukup VM, Fabian RH, *et al.* (2000) Punctate midline myelotomy for the relief of visceral cancer pain. *J Neurosurg* **92(2 Suppl)**:125–30.
25 Nauta HJ, Westlund, K, Willis W, eds. (2002) *Midline Myelotomy*. Thieme Medical Publishers, New York.
26 Shieff C, Nashold BS, Jr. (199) Stereotactic mesencephalotomy. *Neurosurg Clin N Am* **1(4)**:825–39.
27 Raslan AM, McCartney S, Burchiel KJ. (2007) Management of chronic severe pain: spinal neuromodulatory and neuroablative approaches. *Acta Neurochir Suppl* **97(Pt 1)**:33–41.
28 Gybels J, Kupers R, Nuttin B. (1993) Therapeutic stereotactic procedures on the thalamus for pain. *Acta Neurochir (Wien)* **124(1)**:19–22.
29 Wilkinson HA, Davidson KM, Davidson RI. (1999) Bilateral anterior cingulotomy for chronic noncancer pain. *Neurosurgery* **45(5)**:1129–34; discussion 1134-6.

Part 6

Psychological

Chapter 25

Pain self-management: theory and process for clinicians

Michael McGillion[1], Sandra M. LeFort[2], Karen Webber[2], Jennifer N. Stinson[3,4,5], & Chitra Lalloo[3]

[1]*School of Nursing, McMaster University, Hamilton, Ontario, Canada*
[2]*Faculty of Nursing, Memorial University of Newfoundland, St. John's, Newfoundland and Labrador, Canada*
[3]*Child Health Evaluation Sciences, The Hospital for Sick Children, Toronto, Ontario, Canada*
[4]*Department of Anesthesia and Pain Medicine, The Hospital for Sick Children, Toronto, Ontario, Canada*
[5]*Lawrence S. Bloomberg, Faculty of Nursing, University of Toronto, Ontario, Canada*

Introduction

Chronic non-cancer pain remains an important public health problem that seriously affects people's everyday lives including their family, social and working lives. Chronic pain, defined as pain lasting 6 months or longer, affects 19% of Europeans and 20% (1 in 5) of Canadians [1–4]. Among Canadians afflicted, approximately 67% report that their chronic pain is moderate to severe and half of these individuals have endured chronic pain for over ten years [3]. The burden of chronic pain on individuals includes functional limitations and high rates of depression, sleep problems, loneliness, low self-esteem as well as significant job change or job loss [3–7]. The economic burden of the problem is monumental. The total annualized costs of chronic pain in the United States and Canada—including direct health care costs and lost productivity—are estimated at $560 billion and between $38 to $40 billion, respectively [5, 6].

Because prevalence rates are so high, access to appropriate care continues to be a major problem. Choinière et al. found that the median wait time for multidisciplinary pain care for adults (2017 – 2018) is approximately 5.5 months and some people wait up to 4 years for their first appointment [8]. While the onus is on primary care providers (most of whom are generalists) to fill the gap in care, most have inadequate training in the effective prevention management of chronic pain [9].

One approach to improving patient care at the primary care level is self-management education [10]. Traditional patient education provides information and teaches technical skills about how to manage the condition itself. By contrast, self-management education is broader in scope, emphasizing problem solving, action planning for behavior change, contingency planning when desired goals are not reached and confidence building to enable people to deal better with everyday problems that result from chronic conditions [11]. In other words, self-management education helps people with a chronic condition better manage their lives. Cumulative evidence from studies conducted in multiple countries support that low-cost community-based and digital self-management programs, as adjuncts to usual care, are effective in improving health outcomes and quality of life for individuals with a variety of

Clinical Pain Management: A Practical Guide, Second Edition. Edited by Mary E. Lynch, Kenneth D. Craig, and Philip W. Peng.

chronic health conditions including chronic pain [12–32]. This chapter provides an overview of key self-management principles, successful program models, critical process elements and their impact on patient outcomes and practical tips for program start-up.

What is self-management?

Active self-managers are people who are willing to learn about and take responsibility for the daily management of their chronic condition and its consequences. The goal of self-management is to maintain a wellness focus in the foreground, even in the midst of a chronic health problem, to improve overall quality of life. The daily tasks that need self-management are threefold:

1 Taking care of one's overall health (e.g. healthy eating, being physically active, relaxing and reducing stress, connecting with like-minded others, learning about one's condition, treatments and medications);

2 Planning and problem solving to carry on with normal activities and roles in life as best as possible (e.g. maintaining healthy social relationships and staying involved in home, social and work activities); and

3 Managing the emotional changes that are inherent in the chronic illness experience such as anger, fear, frustration, depression, etc. [37].

To manage these tasks successfully, people need a set of core self-management skills: problem-solving skills; decision-making skills; how to find, evaluate and utilize appropriate resources; how to work effectively in partnership with healthcare providers; and how to take action to change behavior [36]. Like other chronic conditions, managing chronic pain on a daily basis requires the acquisition and use of these core self-management skills. But many people with pain have not had the opportunity to learn these skills in a constructive and supportive environment; rather, they have been told that they will have to "learn to live with the pain." This is where pain self-management education programs can help at the primary care level. These programs have been developed to provide patients with the skills to live an active and meaningful life even with a complex and difficult problem such as chronic pain.

Background: Stanford self-management program model

The Chronic Pain Self-Management Program (CPSMP) [12, 13] and the Chronic Angina Self-Management Program (CASMP) [14] are pain-focused self-management programs that were derived from the Stanford University Patient Education Research Center model of self-management. These programs are now administered centrally at the Self Management Resource Center (SMRC) based in Palo Alto, California. By all accounts, the self-management programs developed by Dr. Kate Lorig and colleagues have been the most rigorously developed and evaluated over the last 35 years with over 80 research publications from this research group [34]. The first such program was the Arthritis Self-Management Program (ASMP) which was designed with "bits and -pieces taken from theory, accepted practice and good intentions" [35, p. 356]. However, over time, it evolved to become a program grounded in Albert Bandura's concept of self-efficacy, defined as "the exercise of human agency through people's beliefs in their capabilities to produce desired effects by their actions" [36, p. 3]. This is also referred to as a sense of control. The ASMP program design was fully revised to incorporate the four confidence-building strategies known to enhance self-efficacy, including mastery, modeling, reinterpretation of symptoms and social persuasion [35]. All the current evidence-based SMRC self-management programs including the CPSMP and the CASMP incorporate these important confidence-enhancing strategies.

Content, process and strategies to enhance self-efficacy

Self-management education is, by definition, problem-based and is designed to address the common problems and difficulties that arise for a given chronic health problem [33]. Using the CPSMP as an example, the program content, delivered to groups of participants over 2.5 hours per week for 6 weeks, includes the following topics: self-management- tasks; differences between acute and chronic pain; the role of the brain and pain; balancing activity and rest; exercise and physical activity; relaxation and stress management; depression; nutrition; evaluating non-traditional treatments; problem solving; decision making; communication skills with family, friends and healthcare providers; medications and medication responsibilities; fatigue and sleep; and action planning and goal setting to change behavior [37].

As part of the program,, participants are introduced to the idea of a "self-management toolbox" and that, like a carpenter's toolbox, different tools work best for different types of problems (Figure 25.1). Hence, over the 6 weeks of the program, participants practice these different techniques and begin to use problem-solving and decision-making skills about which types of tools work best for them given their day-to-day circumstances. They begin to understand that there is no "magic bullet" that will take the pain away, but that working at managing their overall health and their pain and other symptoms by using these tools can improve their enjoyment of life.

Self-management programs are structured to maximize active involvement of group participants. They are not the passive receivers of information. Therefore, the critical process components of the program are also standardized and include the following components:

1 *Mini-lectures*: provide an opportunity for brief information sharing about all topics.

2 *Self-reflection*: provides an opportunity to share feelings as participants discuss how chronic pain affects their lives and what kinds of difficult emotions are associated with their chronic pain.

3 *Brainstorming*: allows group members to discuss the benefits of exercise, good nutrition, symptoms of depression, etc.

4 *Setting weekly action plans*: allows participants to learn the process of setting achievable short-term goals each week.

5 *Feedback*: reporting report back to the group each week about allows participants to share how they did with their action plan and receive feedback from the group.

6 *Group problem solving*: allows opportunities to problem solve a variety of common problems.

7 *Support*: provides a way to receive mid-week support from a peer in the group by telephone e-mail or text.

The confidence-building strategies are embedded in the processes of the program. Opportunities for skills mastery or taking action are provided at every session of the 6-week program and participants are encouraged to try new techniques each week at home. In this model of self-management, action planning is the key element to skills mastery [33, 35]. Modeling is a key strategy to enhance self-efficacy and is accomplished in a number of ways including the use of appropriate resource materials, the use of peer leaders (not always healthcare professionals) as facilitators for the program and program participants acting as models for each other. It is powerful for people with chronic pain to see others like themselves problem solve and achieve desired goals; they begin

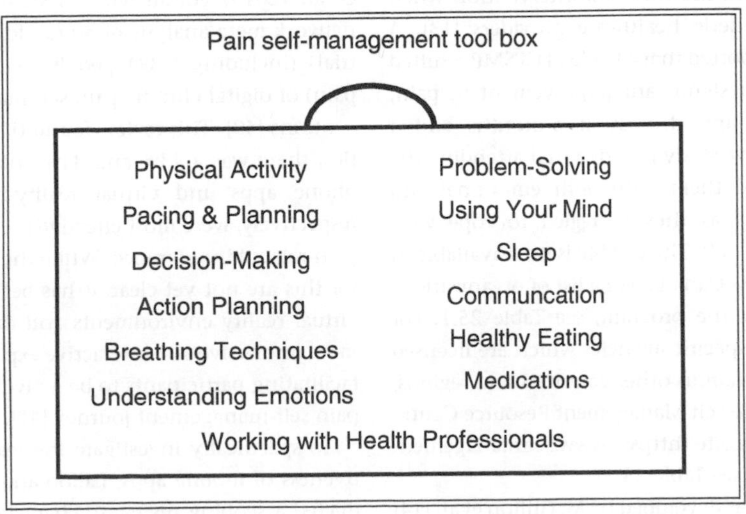

Figure 25.1 Self-management toolbox.

to see that, "if they can do it, I can do it." The reinterpretation of physiologic symptoms as having multiple causes rather than just one cause (i.e. their pain) helps participants realize that many of the tools in their toolbox might be useful. Finally, social persuasion, by being involved in a group that provides gentle support and encouragement to change behaviors, can be a powerful tool to enhance confidence.

Effectiveness of pain self-management programs: main findings

Community-based programs

The CPSMP [12] was adapted from Dr. Lorig's ASMP and later the Chronic Diseases Self-Management Program (CDSMP) in order to make it more directly applicable to people with chronic non-cancer pain. Specific modifications were made with regard to content but all process elements to enhance self-efficacy remained the same. In a first randomized controlled trial (n = 110), LeFort et al. [12] found that the CPSMP significantly improved pain outcomes, dependency on others, aspects of role functioning, sense of vitality and life-satisfaction and self-efficacy and resourcefulness to self-manage pain at 3 months. Subsequently, a multisite effectiveness trial (n = 279) found that the positive effects of the CPSMP on aspects of mental health and resourcefulness were retained up to 12 months post-intervention when delivered by generic healthcare providers [13]. A Danish study reported that a lay-lead CPSMP resulted in a modest but significant improvement in pain, pain cognition and distress at 5-months and a Danish qualitative study reported that attending the CPSMP provided them with both emotional and practical support as they struggled to cope with chronic pain [38, 39]. The CPSMP is now available in 49 agencies across Canada. For a list of organizations licensed to offer the program, see Table 25.1. For information on specific agencies which are licensed to offer the program in other countries and regions, please contact the Self Management Resource Centre through their website (https://www.selfmanagementresource.com/) (see Table 25.1).

The CASMP was developed by McGillion et al. [14] at the University of Toronto. Like the CPSMP, adaptations were made from the CDSMP to address issues specific to living with persistent cardiac pain arising from chronic stable angina (CSA) including fear and anxiety management, chest pain symptom monitoring, decision making about seeking emergency medical assistance, correct use of antianginal medications, heart healthy diet and communicating with life partners and healthcare professionals about cardiac pain [14]. In a randomized controlled trial (RCT) (n = 130), McGillion et al. [14] found that the CASMP was effective for improving angina pain, self-efficacy, physical functioning and general health status.

Digital programs

In addition to community-based models, recent years have seen advancements made in digital pain self-management programs [19, 20, 43]. In adults, an array of digital programs have been developed using multiple modalities including automated, interactive voice response support through telephone; internet and virtual reality-based programs; videoconferencing platforms, as well as mobile phone applications (apps) [39]. While this proliferation of modalities has led to increased options for chronic pain self-management, a challenge has been a lack of clear understanding of which modalities are most effective for end users and, hence, show promise for continued investment, clinical application and continued research. To inform this issue, Slattery et al. (2019) conducted a systematic review and network meta-analysis of 30 randomized controlled trials (including 5,394 people living with chronic pain) of digital chronic pain self-management interventions [40]. This review found that across modalities, there was a 43% and 34% chance that mobile phone apps and virtual reality-based programs, respectively, were most effective for the reduction of pain-related interference. While the possible reasons for this are not yet clear, it has been proposed that virtual reality environments and mobile apps offer more immersive and interactive experiences, thereby facilitating participants to be active in their chronic pain self-management journey [40].

To specifically investigate the features and effectiveness of mobile apps, Lalloo and colleagues conducted a scoping review to characterize the field of publicly available smartphone apps for pain

Table 25.1 Key resources.

US	Self Management Resource Center (SMRC), Palo Alto, CA. www.selfmanagementresource.com
Canadian Centers offering CPSMP	
British Columbia	Available through Self-Management BC, a Ministry of Health, Patients as Partners initiative administered by the University of Victoria. The CPSMP is offered throughout the province.www.selfmanagementbc.ca/chronicpainselfmanagement
Alberta	Available through Alberta Health Services as *Better Choices, Better Health – Chronic Pain* www.albertahealthserivces.ca/services/bcbh.aspx
Saskatchewan	Available through the Saskatoon Health Region as *Living Well with Chronic Pain* Program. www.saskatoonhealthregion.ca/locations_services/Services/cdm/Pages/Programs/Chronic-Pain.aspx
Manitoba	Available through the Wellness Institute and health authorities across the provinces as *Getting Better Together – Chronic Pain*. http:/sogh.mb.ca/wellness
Ontario	Available through many regions of Ontario through Family Health Teams, local health authorities and other health care organizations under a variety of names. www.selfmanagementtc.ca/about-us/self-management-programs-in-ontario
Quebec	Available through Association Quebecoise de la Douleur Chronique as *My Toolbox*. www.douleurchronique.org
Nova Scotia	Available through the Nova Scotia Health Authority, Primary Care Division. www.nshealth.ca/programs-and-services
Other Countries where CPSM is offered	
	Argentina / Peru
	Australia / Portugal
	Bermuda / Republic of Korea
	Chile / South Africa
	China / Japan
	France / Spain
	Hong Kong / Taiwan
	Ireland / United Kingdom
	Italy / United States (all States)
	Netherlands / Peurto Rico
	New Zealand / Virgin Islands

self-management [22]. A total of 279 apps were identified and characterized based on the App Store description. Pain self-care skill support was the most commonly reported self-management function (77.4%). Apps also offered pain education (45.9%), self-monitoring (19%), social support (3.6%) and goal setting (0.72%). No apps were comprehensive in terms of pain self-management, with the majority (58.5%) including only a single self-management function. Critically, only 8.2% of apps included a health care professional in app development and none provided a theoretical rationale for pain self-management content. The employ of multiple pain self-management modalities and functions within apps is an evolving area for study [22, 40].

Similar to adult populations, the use of digital interventions has evolved over time in pediatric and adolescent populations, progressing from internet-based programs to mobile apps. Stinson et al. [41] developed an Internet-based self-management program for adolescents living with juvenile idiopathic arthritis (JIA) entitled Teens Taking Charge: Managing Arthritis Online. This is a 12-week program consisting of web modules dedicated to cognitive behavioral coping skills, stress management and other self-management topics, as well as disease-specific education. Trained non-healthcare professionals provided brief monthly telephone support to help participants tailor online information to their needs and review weekly assignments. A recent RCT (n = 333) was conducted to evaluate effectiveness of the intervention in adolescents with JIA [21]. Significant overall reductions in pain intensity ($p = 0.02$) and pain interference ($p = 0.007$) were observed for intervention group participants compared to those in the education control group. There was a significant overall improvement in health-related quality of life (HRQL) related to problems with pain ($p = 0.02$) and problems with daily activities ($p = 0.01$). There was also a significant improvement in the intervention group over time ($p = 0.008$) for HRQL related to treatment problems [21]. These effects were sustained for up to 12 months following program completion [21]. The Teens Taking Charge: Managing Arthritis Online program is publicly available at no cost: https://teens.aboutkidshealth.ca/jiateenhub

To help address the aforementioned theoretical and design-related gaps in apps for pain self-management, Stinson and Lalloo developed a self-management app for adolescents and young adults living with a painful condition called iCanCope (http://icancope.ca) [23]. iCanCope applies cognitive behavioral therapy principles to help youth learn and practice pain self-management skills with the aim of improving function. Specifically, it is designed to empower youth with personalized daily symptom tracking (pain, pain interference, mood, physical activity, sleep, energy), goal setting, library of pain coping strategies, peer-based social support and pain education. Since development of the original app, disease-specific iterations of iCanCope have been developed and are under evaluation for youth with chronic pain, juvenile idiopathic arthritis and sickle cell disease [24–29]. Adaptations are also under development for post-operative pain and neurofibromatosis. A pilot study is also underway to integrate Apple's Researchkit technology for the purpose of remote electronic consent, the first such implementation in a Canadian pediatric settling [31].

User-level engagement data [24, 32] from ongoing trials indicate that youth with chronic pain demonstrate moderate-to-high adherence with the daily symptom tracking feature of the iCanCope app [34]. The program also has emerging evidence of positive clinical impact. A recently published pilot RCT (N=60) in adolescents with juvenile idiopathic arthritis reported preliminary reductions in pain intensity after two months of use [26]. Upon completion of the ongoing RCTs, the iCanCope app will be publicly released (iOS and Android) with the aim of increasing the accessibility and availability of pain self-management support for young people living with painful conditions.

Getting started: conducting a needs assessment

Whether community-based in person or delivered in digital formats, a critical first step in launching a pain self-management program is conducting a comprehensive needs assessment. Many patient education programs in the past have fallen short because their content has been driven by the input of clinicians alone [42]. This is problematic because clinicians often have particular beliefs about priorities for patient pain-related education that differ from those of patients. Moreover, aside from potential discrepancies between clinicians' and patients' views, there may be other stakeholder viewpoints to consider that will have implications for program success (e.g. family, institutional administrators, non-governmental agencies) [43, 44]. The following are a list of key questions that can assist in deciding which key stakeholder representatives to involve in a needs assessment:

1 Who should give input into development of the program and why?

2 Who will deliver it and who will support its ongoing implementation?

3 Where will it take place?

4 How will it be advertised and who will pay for this?

5 What are the cost and resource implications for day-to-day program delivery?

6 Are there public policies, guidelines or practice standards that should be considered in the approach?

In addition to learning needs, it is also critically important to examine the salient pain-related beliefs of those involved. Understanding these beliefs can have major implications for optimizing program adherence and benefits. Maladaptive or incorrect pain-related beliefs are common and have been increasingly recognized as key factors in treatment and education program failure [45, 46]. Inclusion of questions about pain-related beliefs will help to ensure that common underlying assumptions are targeted and related cognitions associated with the particular pain problem that the program will be designed to address.

Focus groups

A convenient way of collecting needs assessment data is to run focus groups. Focus groups involve hosting a group of participants to have a focused discussion and share ideas. Cumulative evidence has demonstrated that the ideal number of participants in order to foster productive discussion is between 8 and 12 [46, 47]. For depth and clarity, participants should also be from similar cohorts, so it is usually best practice to hold separate groups for patients and other stakeholder representatives (e.g. family members, clinicians, administrators) [42].

Like the discussion on pain-related beliefs, the steps involved in executing focus groups are best explained by example; we will refer to the development of the CASMP program. McGillion et al. [49] held four focus groups to identify CSA patients' pain self-management learning needs; two groups involved patients and two involved clinicians and administrator stakeholders. Each group lasted approximately 1.5 hours and utilized a semi-structured interview format. Questions were developed for each group to generate thinking and discussion about: (a) key angina-related beliefs; (b) the day-to-day problems that patients with CSA face; and (c) the corresponding self-management learning needs. Each participant was asked to provide input and the discussion format remained as open as possible. All of the discussions were audio taped and transcribed; an assistant also made note of key discussion points. The data were then coded for major themes via content analysis [49].

There are a couple of caveats worth mentioning. It is important to remember that clinicians inevitably have preconceived ideas of the learning priorities for patients and so having an impartial third party conduct the process, when possible, is ideal. Also, focus groups typically generate quite a lot of data and thematic content analyses of these data require some methodological expertise. If this is an unfamiliar practice, it is a good idea to consult with a methods expert to plan an organized and comprehensive approach. There are several ways to conduct a needs assessment and the use of focus groups is an example of one method we have found helpful. Choice of method ultimately depends on individual preferences, institutional program goals, depth and breadth of information required and suitability to the particular patient population.

Conclusions and resources

This chapter provides background and an overview of the concept of self-management, key strategies for enhancing self-efficacy to self-manage pain and practical suggestions for getting started. Considerable progress has been made in the field of pain self-management but work remains to be done. While much of our work has been focused on adaptations of the group-based model developed by Lorig and colleagues, alternative approaches, such as individual pain self-management training, require attention. Digital pain self-management is also a major area of focus. For those interested in developing in person or digital programs, we suggest that processes similar to those we have reviewed (assessment of beliefs, identification of key learning priorities, program development and testing) could be followed.

We conclude this chapter by referring those wishing to incorporate pain self-management into their practices to helpful websites and a list of agencies currently offering the CPSMP in Canada (Table 25.1).

References

1 Breivik H, Eisenberg E, O'Brien T, OPENMinds. (2011) The individual and societal burden of chronic pain in Europe: the case for strategic prioritisation and action to improve knowledge and availability of appropriate care. *BMC Public Health* **13**:1229.

2 Schopflocher D, Taenzer P, and Jovey, R. (2011) The prevalence of chronic pain in Canada. *Pain Res Manag* **16**:445–50.

3 Reitsma ML, Tranmer JE, Buchanan DM *et al.* (2011). The prevalence of chronic pain and pain-related interference in the Canadian population from 1994 to 2008. *Chronic Diseases and Injuries in Canada* **31(4)**:157–64.

4 Steingrimsdottir OA, Landmark T, Macfarlane GI *et al.* (2017) Defining chronic pain in epidemiological studies: a systematic review and meta-analysis. *Pain* **158**:2092–107.

5 Gaskin DJ, Richard P. (2012) The economic costs of pain in the United States. *J Pain* **13**:715–24.

6 Wilson MG, Lavis JN, amd Ellen ME. (2015) Supporting chronic pain management across provincial and territorial health systems in Canada: findings from two stakeholder dialogues. *Pain Res Manag* **20**:269–79.

7 Campbell F, Hudspith M, Choinière M. (2020) Working Together to Better Understand, Prevent, and Manage Chronic Pain: What We Heard. A

Report by the Canadian Pain Task Force, **October 2020**. Available at: https://www.canada.ca/content/dam/hc-sc/documents/corporate/about-health-canada/public-engagement/external-advisory-bodies/canadian-pain-task-force/report-2020-rapport/report-2020.pdf
8 Choinière M, Peng P, Gilron I *et al.* (2020) Accessing care in multidisciplinary pain treatment facilities continues to be a challenge in Canada. *Reg Anesth Pain Med* **45**:943–8.
9 Thompson K, Johnson MI, Milligan J *et al.* (2018). Twenty-five years of pain education research-what have we learned? Findings from a comprehensive scoping review of research into pre-registration pain education for health professionals. *Pain* **159**:2146–58.
10 Smith BH, Elliott, AM. (2005) Active self-management of chronic pain in the community. *Pain* **113**:249–50.
11 Bodenheimer T, Lorig K, Holman H *et al.* (2002) Patient self-management of chronic disease in primary care. *JAMA* **288**:2469–75.
12 LeFort SM, Gray-Donald K, Rowat KM *et al.* (1998) Randomized controlled trial of a community-based psychoeducation program for the self-management of chronic pain. *Pain* **74**:297–306.
13 LeFort S, Watt-Watson J, Webber K. (2003) Results of a randomized trial of the chronic pain self-management program in three Canadian provinces. *Pain Res Manag* **8(Suppl B)**:73.
14 McGillion M, Watt-Watson J, Stevens B *et al.* (2008) Randomized controlled trial of a psychoeducation program for the self-management of chronic cardiac pain. *J Pain Symptom Manag* **36**:126–40.
15 Newman S, Steed L, Mulligan K. (2004) Self-management interventions for chronic illness. *Lancet* **364**:1523–37.
16 King-Vanvlack C, Di Rienzo G, Kinlin M *et al.* (2007) Education and exercise program for chronic pain patients. *Pract Pain Manag* **7**:17–27.
17 Harris MF, Williams AM, Dennis SM *et al.* (2008) Chronic disease self-management: implementation with and within Australian general practice. *Med J Aust* **189**:S17–20.
18 Mann E, LeFort S, Vandenkerkhof E. (2013) Self-management interventions for chronic pain. *Pain Manag Nsg* **3**:211–22.
19 Heapy AA, Higgins DM, Cervone D *et al.* (2015) A systematic review of technology-assisted self-management interventions for chronic pain: looking across treatment modalities. *Clin J Pain* **31**:470–92.
20 Gogovor, A Visca R, Auger C. (2017) Informing the development of an Internet-based chronic pain self-management program. *Int J Med Inform* **97**:109–19.
21 Stinson JN, Lalloo C, Hundert AS *et al.* (2020) Teens Taking Charge: a randomized controlled trial of a web-based self-management program with telephone support for adolescents with juvenile idiopathic arthritis. *J Med Internet Res* **22(7)**:e16234.
22 Lalloo C, Jibb LA, Rivera J, Agarwal A, Stinson JN. (2015) "There's a pain app for that": review of patient-targeted smartphone applications for pain management. *Clin J Pain* **31(6)**:557–63.
23 Stinson JN, Lalloo C, Harris L *et al.* (2014) iCanCope with Pain™: user-centred design of a web- and mobile-based self-management program for youth with chronic pain based on identified health care needs. *Pain Res Manag* **19(5)**:257–65.
24 Stinson J, White M, Isaac L *et al.* (2013) Understanding the information and service needs of young adults with chronic pain: perspectives of young adults and their providers. *Clin J Pain* **29(7)**:600–12.
25 Lalloo C, Hundert A, Harris L *et al.* (2019) Capturing daily disease experiences of adolescents with chronic pain: mHealth-mediated symptom tracking. *JMIR Mhealth Uhealth* **7(1)**:e11838.
26 Lalloo C, Harris LR, Hundert AS *et al.* (2021) The iCanCope pain self-management application for adolescents with juvenile idiopathic arthritis: a pilot randomized controlled trial. *Rheumatology (Oxford)* 60(**1**):196–206.
27 Lalloo C, Pham Q, Cafazzo J, Stephenson E, Stinson J. (2020) A ResearchKit app to deliver paediatric electronic consent: protocol of an observational study in adolescents with arthritis. *Contemp Clin Trials Commun* **17**:100525.
28 Kulandaivelu Y, Lalloo C, Ward R *et al.* (2018) Exploring the needs of adolescents with sickle cell disease to inform a digital self-management and transitional care program: qualitative study. *JMIR Pediatr Parent* **1(2)**:e11058.

29 Palermo TM, Zempsky WT, Dampier CD *et al.* (2018) iCanCope with sickle cell pain: design of a randomized controlled trial of a smartphone and web-based pain self-management program for youth with sickle cell disease. *Contemp Clin Trials* **74**:88–96.

30 Birnie KA, Campbell F, Nguyen C *et al.* (2019) iCanCope PostOp: user-centered design of a smartphone-based app for self-management of postoperative pain in children and adolescents. *JMIR Form Res* **3(2)**:e12028.

31 Lalloo C, Pham Q, Cafazzo J, Stephenson E, Stinson J. (2020) A ResearchKit app to deliver paediatric electronic consent: Protocol of an observational study in adolescents with arthritis. *Contemp Clin Trials Commun* **17**:100525.

32 Pham Q, Graham G, Lalloo C *et al.* (2018). An analytics platform to evaluate effective engagement with pediatric mobile health apps: design, development, and formative evaluation. *JMIR Mhealth Uhealth* **6(12)**:e11447.

33 Lorig KR, Holman H. (2003) Self-management education: history, definition, outcomes, and mechanisms. *Ann Behav Med* **26**:1

34 Bibliography. (2021) Self-Management Resource Center. Available at: www.selfmanagementresource.com/resources/bibliography. Accessed December 18, 2020.

35 Lorig KR, Gonzalez V. (1992) The integration of theory with practice: a 12-year case study. *Health Educ Q* **19**:355–368.

36 Bandura A. (2000) *Self-Efficacy: The Exercise of Control*. W.H. Freeman, New York.

37 LeFort SM. (2015) *Chronic Pain Self-Management Program Leader's Manual*. Stanford, Palo Alto, CA.

38 Mehlsen M, Heegaard L, Frostholm L. (2015) A prospective evaluation of the Chronic Pain Self-Management Programme in a Danish population of chronic pain patients. *Patient Educ Couns* **98**:677–80.

39 Andersen LN, Kohberg M, Herborg LG *et al.* (2014) "Here we're all in the same boat" – a qualitative study of group based rehabilitation for sick-listed citizens with chronic pain. *Scand J Psych* **55**:333–42.

40 Slattery BW, Haugh S, O'Connor L et al. (2019) An evaluation of the effectiveness of the modalities used to deliver electronic health interventions for chronic pain: systematic review with network meta-analysis. *J Med Internet Res* **21**:e11086.

41 Stinson JN, McGrath PJ, Hodnett E *et al.* (2009) Feasibility testing of an online self-management program for adolescents with juvenile idiopathic arthritis (JIA): a pilot randomized controlled trial. *Arthritis Rheum* **60**:S87.

42 Lorig K. (2000) How do I know what patients want and need? Needs assessment. In: Lorig K and associates, eds. *Patient Education: A Practical Approach*, 3rd edn. Sage, London. pp. 1–20.

43 McGillion M, LeFort SM, Stinson J. (2008) Chronic pain self-management. In: Rashiq S, Schopflocher D, Taenzer P *et al. Chronic Pain: A Health Policy Perspective.* Wiley-Blackwell, Weinheim. pp. 167–181.

44 Horvath AO, Greenberg LS. (1989) Development and validation of the working alliance inventory. *J Couns Psychol* **36**:223–33.

45 DeGrood DE, Tait RC. (2001) Assessment of pain beliefs and pain coping. In: Turk DC, Melzack R, eds. *Handbook of Pain Assessment*, 2nd edn. Guilford Press, New York. pp. 320–345.

46 Watt-Watson J. (1992) Misbeliefs about pain. In: Watt-Watson J, Donovan M, eds. *Pain Management: Nursing Perspective*. Mosby, St. Louis. pp. 36–58.

47 Madriz E. (2000) Focus groups in feminist research. In: Denzin KN, Lincoln YS, eds. *Handbook of Qualitative Research*, 2nd edn. Sage, London. pp. 835–50.

48 Morgan DL. (1997) *Focus Groups as Qualitative Research*, 2nd edn. Sage, Thousand Oaks.

49 McGillion M, Watt-Watson J, Kim J *et al.* (2004) Learning by heart: a focused groups study to determine the psychoeducational needs of chronic angina patients. *Can J Cardiovasc Nurs* **14**:12–22.

Chapter 26

Psychological interventions: a focus on cognitive-behavioral therapy

Melissa A. Day[1,2] & Beverly E. Thorn[3]

[1] *School of Psychology, The University of Queensland, Brisbane, Queensland, Australia*
[2] *Department of Rehabilitation Medicine, University of Washington, Seattle, Washington, USA*
[3] *Department of Psychology, The University of Alabama, Tuscaloosa, Alabama, USA*

Introduction

Psychosocial interventions have demonstrated efficacy in the management of chronic pain across a variety of pain types, settings and modes of delivery. The current "gold standard" psychosocial approach is Cognitive-Behavioral Therapy (CBT) which has been shown to significantly reduce pain intensity, pain interference, disability and distress, as well as improve self-efficacy and quality of life [1–3]. Moreover, research is now showing that CBT engenders measurable neurological functional and structural changes that are associated with pain outcome improvement [4, 5].

Arguably important to the delivery of any pain treatment (psychosocial or otherwise), is the provision of psychoeducation around the rationale for that treatment in order to gain patient buy-in [6, 7]. Hence, an understanding of how pain is processed in the brain and how this is influenced by a complex interconnection between regions involved in not just the somatosensory aspect, but also areas associated with cognitions, emotions, motivations and behaviors is an important component of therapy.

We will therefore start this chapter by describing the therapeutic rationale for CBT with a focus on a simplified version of the "Gate Control Theory". We will then provide an overview of those psychosocial factors that influence the processing of pain in the brain. Mapping on to this we will describe the techniques that CBT uses to target risk factors for poor pain coping and to enhance self-efficacy and adaptive behaviors. We will provide an overview of the body of research supporting the efficacy of CBT, as well as touch upon some needed future directions.

How pain is processed in the brain: An overview and therapeutic rationale

With the advent of modern brain imaging techniques, it is now widely understood that pain is primarily the end result of supraspinal cortical processes which are influenced by a complex range of biopsychosocial factors [8]. This understanding was first described by Melzack and Wall in their revolutionary Gate Control Theory [9, 10], a theory that sparked the subsequent plethora of research testing the proposed brain mechanisms in pain and that is now known as the Neuromatrix model [11].

What has consistently emerged from the body of research testing and advancing this theory – using electroencephalography (EEG), magnetic resonance

Clinical Pain Management: A Practical Guide, Second Edition. Edited by Mary E. Lynch, Kenneth D. Craig, and Philip W. Peng.

imaging (MRI) and functional MRI (fMRI) – is that a set of neural networks are reliably activated in response to pain and that these networks select, filter and modulate pain signals. Specifically, the majority of nociceptive pathways terminate in the thalamus, with thalamic nuclei responsible for then relaying sensory information to a highly distributed network including regions associated with pain processing (e.g. the primary and secondary somatosensory cortices, insula) and cognitive-emotional demands (e.g. prefrontal cortex, anterior cingulate cortex, amygdala). Importantly, this functional network is not just the passive recipient of pain signals from the periphery, rather this network is actively involved in regulating and modulating the sensory perception of pain [12–16]. That is, this network can either "turn up the volume on pain" (i.e., leading to increased perceived pain intensity) or it can "turn down the volume on pain" (i.e., leading to decreased pain intensity), depending on a range of biopsychosocial factors.

Providing a simplified psychoeducational overview of this model, without jargon, and engaging patients in a collaborative discussion is an excellent way to provide a rationale for targeting psychosocial factors in treatment, which have the capacity to directly influence the processing of pain in the brain. The following points are important to emphasize: (1) Pain is not a sensation in and of itself, the brain – and many filters in the brain – determine the perception of pain; (2) Pain signals coming from the spinal cord are filtered through brain sites involving memory, emotion and thought processes; and (3) The brain activity in the filtering sites can enhance or diminish incoming pain signals (See [17] for additional details).

What "turns up the volume on pain" versus "what turns down the volume on pain"?

A vast body of research has consistently shown that chronic pain is influenced by a range of biopsychosocial factors including behaviors (at the individual and broader social level), emotions and cognitions. Research has reliably identified factors within each of these domains that are adaptive versus maladaptive and have the capacity to influence function, even in the presence of on-going pain. In this section, we provide an overview of the most robust predictors of pain outcomes within each of these domains. Although the field has been predominantly focused on examining "unhelpful" and/or maladaptive aspects of pain, here we also note those factors associated with adaptive function that are important to emphasize and harness in treatment. Then, in the subsequent section, we describe how these factors are targeted by CBT techniques to improve pain management.

Behavioral and wider social factors. Fordyce [18] was one of the first to describe how behavioral factors contribute to the experience of chronic pain. Fordyce proposed that observable pain behaviors, such as limping, grimacing, resting and medication consumption (e.g. opioids) contribute to worse pain outcomes over time. For example, these behaviors may reinforce being a "pain patient" and they interfere with engagement in well behaviors, such as appropriately paced activity (as opposed to resting which contributes to muscular deconditioning). Although discussion of the current so-called opioid epidemic is beyond the scope of this chapter, it is worth noting that the long-term use of opioids for chronic pain is associated with significant side-effects including analgesic tolerance, physical dependence, opioid-induced hyperalgesia and risk of misuse, addiction and diversion and other negative impacts on function (e.g. sedation), with only modest effects on pain intensity [19–29]. Hence, while in the short term such medications might "turn down the volume on pain" it is also important to discuss with patients the ways in which, when taken long-term, these medications can increase pain and disability and "turn up the volume on pain".

Another major behavioral factor to address is avoidance, which has repeatedly been associated with heightened pain, more disability and lower return to work rates [30, 31]. The functional opposite of avoidance is engagement in paced activity as well as engagement in meaningful activities (or those that provide a sense of mastery). Recent literature reviews have demonstrated that appropriately paced engagement in valued activities despite the pain is associated with multiple positive pain-related outcomes, including less pain intensity, depression, pain-related anxiety, lower levels of physical and psychosocial disability and improved globally rated daily activity and overall emotional wellbeing [32–34].

Fordyce [18] was also a pioneer in emphasizing that pain does not occur in isolation, but rather it occurs within a social context. Demographically, women, racial and ethnic minorities, the elderly and those with low socioeconomic status have higher pain prevalence, more pain-associated disability and greater levels of treatment disparities than their demographic counterparts [19]. Further, pain and disability affect work, family, leisure, healthcare and other environments. Vocational concerns (job stress, job dissatisfaction, vocational uncertainty and downward socioeconomic drift) and family concerns all feed into the complexities of pain and related disability. These in turn influence the behaviors, emotions and thoughts of the individual, as well as their pain. What has also been shown in the literature though is that social support – in the form of social, informational, behavioral and/or tangible sources – is associated with better pain-related outcomes [35]. This adaptive role of social support can be built upon and harnessed in treatment via consideration of mode of delivery and whether group delivery, couples or family therapy modalities might be appropriate [35]. Within group-delivered treatments, we have found that a common theme qualitatively reported by many participants is that the support provided by the group and the sense of "not being alone" was highly valued by individuals living with chronic pain [36].

Emotional factors. In the context of persistent pain, emotional concomitants naturally arise and for a proportion of people, emotional symptoms reach clinical levels. Rates of co-morbid depression are estimated to affect up to 50% of people [37–39], and rates of anxiety disorders (most commonly Post-Traumatic Stress Disorder, Panic Disorder and Generalized Anxiety Disorder) affect up to an estimated 57% of people [40–42].However, these are likely underestimates as psychological co-morbidities typically go undiagnosed and undertreated.[43] Co-morbid depression and anxiety are important to assess and treat in the context of chronic pain though, as these conditions are associated with an array of worse pain outcomes [44, 45], including interference with treatment and premature drop-out [43, 46, 47]. Furthermore, symptoms of anxiety and fear might be a particularly common response when the source of pain is undiagnosed. In this context, the Fear Avoidance Model of pain [48, 49] proposes that widespread fear of increased pain or of injury or re-injury, is subsequently related to behavioral avoidance and significantly contributes to disability among individuals with chronic pain. In support for this model, research has shown that fear-related factors more accurately predict functional limitations than even pain severity, pain duration or other biomedical factors [30, 50].

The potential buffering role of resilience and positive affect/emotion has been a topic of increasing investigation over the past decade. Research supports the role that positive emotions play in fostering recovery from pain flare-ups [51]. Further, subjective happiness and humor have been linked to improved pain thresholds, reduced pain intensity and the release of endorphins, as well as better general health in chronic pain [52–56]. Thus, appropriate use of positive themes and humor in therapy – which has at various times been recognized as a feature of cognitive therapy – might not only contribute to facilitating therapeutic bonds, but also might improve pain outcomes [56, 57].

Cognitive factors. Given the important contribution of negative thoughts to distress and unhelpful behavior, psychosocial interventions often focus on cognitive content or habits of processing. Negative thoughts about pain have been organized into descriptive categories such as threat and harm appraisals (e.g. "pain is life-threatening"), automatic thoughts (e.g. "I can't cope with this pain") acquired beliefs about pain (e.g. "pain should be treated with rest and medication") and deep beliefs about oneself (e.g. "I am a failure").[7] Generally, though, research often focuses on negative thoughts about pain in relation to pain catastrophizing [58]. Across various theoretical models (including the Fear Avoidance Model noted above [48] as well as the Communal Coping Model [58]) pain catastrophizing is theorized as the antecedent to engendering fear and maladaptive pain behaviors, including avoidance. An extensive body of research has consistently shown pain catastrophizing predicts a range of poor outcomes, including pain intensity, disability, poorer social functioning, longer recovery times following surgery, greater healthcare utilization and worse mood (e.g. depression and anxiety), even when important covariates such as disease severity, pain intensity, anxiety and neuroticism are controlled [59–66].

The other cognitive variable that repeatedly emerges as critical to bolster in pain management programs is self-efficacy [67]. This is the belief that one can manage pain and initiate strategies to achieve personal goals despite continuing pain [69]. Self-efficacy represents an example of a positive appraisal that has been shown to be important in pain. Other cognitive process variables are also emerging as protective in the context of chronic pain. Two such cognitive processes are mindfulness and pain acceptance, both of which have been shown to predict an array of positive outcomes including lower pain intensity, negative affect, pain catastrophizing, fear of pain, pain hypervigilance and disability [69, 70]. Although CBT does not theoretically target the cognitive process variables of mindfulness or pain acceptance, research suggests CBT does result in improvements in mindfulness and acceptance and that these processes might be important to the positive outcome gains achieved in CBT [71].

Cognitive-Behavioral Therapy for chronic pain management

Psychological pain treatments have developed considerably over the past 50 years, as have treatment targets. The operant approach was the first systematically applied psychological treatment for pain and focused on overt behavior [18]; the respondent and stress management approaches which followed tended to emphasize muscle tension [72]. Family, couples and system therapies addressed interpersonal processes and conflict [35, 73]; and, more recently, mindfulness-based stress reduction [74, 75] and mindfulness-based cognitive therapy [6], as well as acceptance and commitment therapy [76, 77] have been successfully applied for improving a range of pain-related outcomes. To date however, of the psychological approaches that have been shown to be helpful for chronic pain, CBT has accumulated the most high quality evidence to support its efficacy.

The CBT approach for chronic pain management took hold in the 1980's following the early behavioral work [78–80]. Since this time, CBT has accumulated empirical support across various types of pain, settings, populations and modes of delivery with respect to its efficacy and cost-effectiveness, with these benefits maintained at short- and long-term follow-up [3, 81–88]. Most of the research to date has established the efficacy of CBT within adult populations with chronic back pain, headache, orofacial pain or arthritis related pain, with a smaller number of trials completed within other pain conditions [1, 88]. Further, more recent research by Seminowicz and colleagues[4] has demonstrated the positive outcomes associated with CBT extend beyond self-report indicators, with increased gray matter volume in several areas of the brain related to pain processing found following an 11-week CBT treatment. Based on the wealth of high quality, well-controlled trials supporting the use of CBT for chronic pain, it is currently considered the gold standard psychological treatment approach [1–3, 88]. Ideally, CBT is delivered within an interdisciplinary context in which the multifaceted nature of chronic pain is targeted by a team of professionals from various disciplines (e.g. pain medicine, psychology, physiotherapy and occupational therapy, and others). Given that access to the ideal interdisciplinary delivery approach is limited, it is important to note that research does also support CBT as a stand-alone therapy [88].

Although the precise techniques included within CBT protocols vary, there are general theoretical principles that are consistent across researchers and practitioners. For example, the idea that cognitions and emotions influence pain coping is an overarching principle. Within clinical practice (i.e., where adherence to a specific manual, as in clinical trials, is not required), tailoring of CBT content is often made on the basis of treatment goals and to map on to a careful psychological assessment (Chapter 11). Both patient objectives and the interests of referral sources can be diverse and poorly specified, however, and patient goals may diverge or conflict with those specified by the referrer or by treatment staff. In the sections that follow, attention is directed to common targets of CBT techniques in relation to the behaviors, emotions and cognitions described in the earlier sections that have been shown to predict pain-related outcomes. Although we have grouped the techniques in relation to these domains, it is most probable that such techniques may have multiple effects (i.e., changing cognitions will likely have effects on also changing emotions and vice versa, for example).

1 Psychoeducation about pain, how the brain processes pain and how biopsychosocial factors influence pain perception is critical information to convey. As we described above, we have found that it is clinically most useful to provide this psychoeducation in session 1 to provide a rationale for psychological treatments, to convey understanding that the patient's pain is real (i.e., not just "in their head") and that CBT is effective for real pain.

2 A variety of behavioral techniques may be used to address maladaptive avoidance behaviors and to increase engagement in appropriately paced, valued activities. This includes quota based behavioral activation plans and goal-directed paced physical activity, as well as activity scheduling (i.e., pleasant activities and activities that provide a sense of mastery). These techniques are initially based around goal setting by the patient with assistance from the therapist, to identify appropriate short and long-term goals, skills deficits and methods for achieving these goals. Pacing and activity scheduling start from a modest baseline and build the patient's capacity for activity (by small increments over time), with non-pain contingent, programmed breaks or changes of activity interspersed. The aim is to achieve more "up time" (i.e., engagement in activity) and more reliably, within the limits of pain, rather than to make one-time heroic efforts to achieve goals despite pain, often unsuccessfully. Finally, assertive communication skills training is also often included as a behavioral technique and may be particularly useful when relationship factors are contributing to pain, pain behaviors and coping.

3 The emotional concomitants of pain are indirectly targeted through both behavioral and cognitive techniques. Expressive writing is one way in which emotional responses to pain and stress can be effectively acknowledged (as opposed to avoided) and processed [7]. Expressive writing is considered an emotional disclosure technique and has been shown to be beneficial in dealing with unresolved stressful or traumatic experiences, both of which often accompany chronic pain [7]. Relaxation strategies (including one or more types of relaxation techniques such as biofeedback, autogenic relaxation, progressive or passive muscle relaxation, meditation and/or self-hypnosis) are another way to decrease stress and negative emotional states and engender a sense of calm and positive affect [89]. Alternatively, other work by Vlaeyen and colleagues has emphasized the use of graded exposure techniques to address fear of pain specifically [90, 91]. Occasionally, stress inoculation training is also included.

4 Cognitive therapy is the cornerstone of CBT and various cognitive techniques are used to address not only maladaptive cognitions but also to bolster adaptive cognitions, particularly self-efficacy. This includes cognitive restructuring strategies, as well as problem solving and coping self-statements. These techniques address patients' elicited concerns and emotional difficulties, teach them to identify catastrophizing and other unhelpful habits of thinking (e.g. pain fortune telling, overgeneralization etc.) and provide them with a means to challenge and change their thoughts. This is not readily accomplished through didactic instruction alone, but typically requires substantial Socratic dialogue with the patient and personal practice.

Across each of these behavioral, emotional and cognitive CBT techniques, the importance of between-session skills practice (i.e., homework) is emphasized. CBT provides "tools for the toolkit" for patients to self-manage their pain, however as with any skill, these techniques take practice to learn. Thus, acquisition of skills for self-management of pain is encouraged not only through direct instruction during sessions, but through rehearsal, behavioral experiments and thought records, as well as other take home activities. Within this context, attention to motivational enhancement is increasingly recognized as critical and many programs integrate motivational interviewing principles for this purpose [92]. Relatedly, generalization, relapse prevention and maintenance plans are similarly emphasized. Skills are practiced in different settings and barriers to change are anticipated and the patient is prepared to address them. Essentially, patients are encouraged to anticipate setbacks/lapses/relapses and plan for successful management.

Taken together, there are a wide range of techniques that are subsumed under the "CBT umbrella". Due to this, it is not known which specific treatment components account for the demonstrated treatment efficacy [88]. Research is beginning to examine ways to match specific sub-sets of these techniques to patient's presenting cognitive-behavioral patterns.

For example, one study by van Koulil and colleagues [93] classified individuals with fibromyalgia into two groups at baseline and mapped treatment on to these profiles: (1) a pain-avoidance group (i.e., who avoided activities due to fear of pain) that received techniques targeted towards increasing daily activities, reducing pain and avoidance behaviors and increasing physical condition; and (2) a pain-persistence group (i.e., individuals who persisted in activities despite pain), which was trained in techniques targeted towards regulating daily activity, increasing activity pacing, restructuring pain-persistence cognitions and increasing physical condition. Compared to a wait list, the tailored treatments resulted in significantly greater improvements on pain outcomes, with large effect sizes found. However, given a "mis-matched" condition was not included, the benefit of such tailoring is not fully known. Other research examining an individually tailored CBT protocol compared to a standard CBT protocol found no significant differences in outcomes [94].

As described earlier, other treatments such as mindfulness-based stress reduction [74, 75], mindfulness-based cognitive therapy [6], and acceptance and commitment therapy [76, 77] have a building research base supporting their efficacy across chronic pain conditions. Future research is needed to identify those patient profiles that might be best matched to one of these alternative evidence-based treatments, as opposed to simply various combinations of CBT techniques [95]. Advancing such precision medicine with the development of patient-treatment matching algorithms has the potential to substantially boost effect sizes [95]. Moreover, identifying the critical mediators that underlie treatment gains will inform streamlining treatment protocols, including those based on CBT as well as acceptance and mindfulness principles.

Conclusions

The pain experience is a perception mediated by the brain and involves not only sensory input but neural filters that increase or decrease the "volume" of pain experienced by an individual. Since the brain is responsible for thoughts, emotions, memories and sensory phenomena, it stands to reason that one important aspect of treating pain would involve psychosocial treatments. These treatments do not negate or ignore biologic factors that contribute to pain, but include other important aspects of the overall perception and adjustment to pain. When provided, psychological interventions make an important contribution to interdisciplinary treatment.

References

1 Ehde DM, Dillworth TM, Turner JA. (2014) Cognitive behavioural therapy for indiviudals with chronic pain: efficacy, innovations and directions for research. *Am Psychol* **69(2)**: 153–66.

2 Day MA, Thorn, B.E., Burns, J. (2012) The continuing evolution of biopsychosocial interventions for chronic pain. *Journal of Cognitive Psychotherapy: An International Quarterly* **26(2)**:114–29.

3 Williams AC, Eccleston C, Morley S. (2012) Psychological therapies for the management of chronic pain (excluding headache) in adults. *Cochrane Database of Syst. Rev* 11(**11**):CD007407.

4 Seminowicz D, Shpaner M, Keaser ML *et al.* (2013) Cognitive-behavioral therapy increases prefrontal cortex gray matter in patients with chronic pain. *J Pain* **14(12)**:1573–84.

5 Shpaner M, Kelly C, Lieberman G *et al.* (2014)_ Unlearning chronic pain: A randomized controlled trial to investigate changes in intrinsic brain connectivity following cognitive behavioral therapy. *NeuroImage: Clinical* **5**:365–76.

6 Day MA. (2017) *Mindfulness-Based Cognitive Therapy for Chronic Pain: A Clinical Manual and Guide*. Wiley, Chichester.

7 Thorn BE. (2017) *Cognitive Therapy for Chronic Pain: A Step-by-Step Guide*, 2nd edn. The Guilford Press, New York.

8 Jensen MP. (2010) A Neuropsychological model of pain: research and clinical implications. *Journal of Pain* **11**:2–12.

9 Melzack R, Wall PD. (1965) Pain mechanisms: a new theory. *Science* **150(3699)**:971–9.

10 Melzack R, Wall PD. (1982) *The Challenge of Pain*. Basic Books, New York.

11 Melzack R. (1999) From the gate to the neuromatrix. *Pain* **Suppl 6**:S121–126.

12 Seminowicz DA, Moayedi M. (2017) The dorsolateral prefrontal cortex in acute and chronic pain. *J Pain* **18(9)**:1027–35.

13 Duerden EG, Albanese MC. (2013) Localization of pain-related brain activation: a meta-analysis of neuroimaging data. *Hum Brain Mapp* **34**:109–49.

14 Bornhovd K, Quante M, Glauche V, Bromm B, Weiller C, Buchel C. (2002) Painful stimuli evoke different stimulus-response functions in the amygdala, prefrontal, insula and somatosensory cortex: a single-trial fMRI study. *Brain* **125**:1326–36.

15 Moayedi M, Salomons TV. (2016) Brain imaging in experimental pain. In: Battaglia A, ed. *An Introduction to Pain and Nervous System Disorders*. John Wiley & Sons Ltd, London. pp. 225–48.

16 Garland EL. (2012) Pain processing in the human nervous system: a selective review of nociceptive and biobehavioral pathways. *Primary Care* **39(3)**:561–71.

17 Thorn BE. (2020) Ronald Melzack Award Lecture: Putting the brain to work in cognitive behavioral therapy for chronic pain. *Pain* **161**:S27–S35.

18 Fordyce WE. (1976) *Behavioral Methods for Chronic Pain and Illness*. Mosby, St. Louis.

19 Institute of Medicine. (2011) *Relieving Pain in America: A Blueprint for Transforming Prevention, Care, Education, and Research*. The National Academics Press, Washington, D.C.

20 National Institutes of Health (2011). National Pain Strategy: A comprehensive population health-level strategy for pain. https://www.iprcc.nih.gov/national-pain-strategy-overview/national-pain-strategy-report. Accessed October 11, 2021.

21 Volkow ND, McLellan AT. (2016) Opioid abuse in chronic pain: misconceptions and mitigation strategies. *New Engl J Med* **374(13)**:1253–63.

22 Deyo RA, Von Korff M, Duhrkoop D. (2015) Opioids for low back pain. *BMJ* **350**:G6380.

23 Cooper TE, Chen J, Wiffen PJ, *et al.* (2017) Morphine for chronic neuropathic pain in adults. *Cochrane Database Syst Rev* **5(5)**:CD011669.

24 Gaskell H, Derry S, Stannard C, Moore RA. (2016) Oxycodone for neuropathic pain in adults. *Cochrane Database Syst Rev* **7(7)**:CD010692.

25 Krebs EE, Gravely A, Nugent S *et al.* (2018) Effect of opioid vs nonopioid medications on pain-related function in patients with chronic back pain or hip or knee osteoarthritis pain. *JAMA* **319(9)**:872–82.

26 Noble M, Treadwell JR, Tregear SJ *et al.* (2010) Long-term opioid management for chronic noncancer pain. *Cochrane Database of Syst Rev***20 10(1)**:CD006605.

27 Trescot AM, Glaser, S.E., Hansen, H., Benyamin, R., Patel, S., Manchikanti, L. (2008) Effectiveness of opioids in the treatment of chronic non-cancer pain. *Pain Physician* **11(2)**:S181–200.

28 Dowell D, Haegerich TM, Chou R. (2016) CDC guideline for prescribing opioids for chronic pain—United States, 2016. *JAMA* **315(15)**:1624–45.

29 Davis MP, Behm B, Balachandran D. (2017) Looking both ways before crossing the street: assessing the benefits and risk of opioids in treating patients at risk of sleep-disordered breathing for pain and dyspnea. *J Opioid Manag* **13(3)**:183–96.

30 Vlaeyen JWS, Kole-Snijders A, Rotteveel A, Ruesink R, Heuts P. (1995) The role of fear of movement/(re)injury in pain disability. *J Occup Rehabil* **5**:235–52.

31 Vlaeyen JW, Kole-Snijders AM, Boeren RG, van Eek H. (1995) Fear of movement/(re)injury in chronic low back pain and its relation to behavioral performance. *Pain.* **62**:363–72.

32 Thompson M, McCracken LM. (2011) Acceptance and related processes in adjustment to chronic pain. *Curr Pain Headache Rep* **15(2)**:144–51.

33 McCracken LM, Vowles KE. (2006) Acceptance of chronic pain. *Curr Pain Headache Rep* **10(2)**:90–4.

34 McCracken LM, Samuel VM. (2007) The role of avoidance, pacing, and other activity patterns in chronic pain. *Pain* **130**:119–25.

35 Keefe FJ, Somers TJ. (2010) Psychological approaches to understanding and treating arthritis pain. *Nat Rev Rheumatol* **6(4)**:210–6.

36 Day MA, Thorn BE, Kapoor S. (2011) A qualitative analysis of a randomized controlled trial comparing a cognitive-behavioral treatment with education. *J Pain* 12(**9**):941–52.

37 Banks SM, Kerns RD. (1996) Explaining high rates of depression in chronic pain: A diathesis-stress framework. *Psychological Bulletin* **119**:95–110.

38 Dersh J, Gatchel RJ, Mayer TG, Polatin PB, (2006) Temple OW. Prevalence of psychiatric disorders in patients in patients with chronic disabling occupational spinal disorders. *Spine* **31**:1156–62.

39 Romano J, Turner JA. (1985) Chronic pain and depression: Does the evidence support a relationship? *Psychological Bulletin* **97**:18–34.

40 Siqveland J, Hussain A, Lindstrøm JC, Ruud T, Hauff E. (2017) Prevalence of posttraumatic stress disorder in persons with chronic pain: a meta-analysis. *Front Psychiatry* **8**:164.

41 Wolfe F, Smythe HA, Yunus MB *et al.* (1990) The American College of Rheumatology 1990 criteria for the classification of fibromyalgia: Report of the Multicenter Criteria Committee. *Arthritis Rheum* **33**:160–172.

42 Asmundson G, Katz J. (2009) Understanding the co-occurrence of anxiety disorders and chronic pain: state-of-the-art. *Depress Anxiety* **26(20)** :888–901.

43 Shmuely Y, Baumgarten M, Rovner B, Berlin J. (2001) Predictors of improvement in health-related quality of life among elderly patients with depression. *Int Pyschogeriatr* **13**:63–73.

44 Gore M, Sadosky A, Stacey B, Tai K, Leslie D. (2012) The burden of chronic low back pain. *Spine* **37(11)**:E668–77.

45 O'Brien EM, Waxenberg LB, Atchison JW *et al.* (2010) Negative mood mediates the effect of poor sleep on pain among chronic pain patients. *Clinical J Pain* **26(4)**:310–9.

46 Day MA, Ward LC, Ehde DM *et al.* (2019) A pilot randomized controlled trial comparing mindfulness meditation, cognitive therapy, and mindfulness-based cognitive therapy for chronic low back pain. *Pain Medicine* **20(11)**:2134–48.

47 Rolfson O, Dahlberg LE, Nilsson JA, Malchau H, Garellick G. (2009) Variables determining outcome in total hip replacement surgery. *J Bone Joint Surg Br* **91**:157–161.

48 Vlaeyen JWS, Linton SJ. (2000) Fear-avoidance and its consequences in chronic musculoskeletal pain: a state of the art review. *Pain* **85**:317–32.

49 Vlaeyen JWS, Linton SJ. (2012) Fear-avoidance model of chronic musculoskeletal pain: 12 years on. *Pain* **153(6)**:1144–7.

50 Crombez G, Vlaeyen JWS, Heuts P. (1999) Pain related fear is more disabling that pain itself: evidence on the role of pain-related fear in chronic back pain disability. *Pain* **80**:329–39.

51 Zautra AJ, Smith B, Affleck G, Tennen H. (2001) Examinations of chronic pain and affect relationships: applications of a dynamic model of affect. *J Consult Clin Psychol* **69**:786–795.

52 Mahony DL, Burroughs DL, Hieatt AC. (2001) The effects of laughter on discomfort thresholds: does expectation become reality? *J Gen Psychol* **128(2)**:217–26.

53 Tse M, Lo A, Cheng T, Chan E, Chan A, Chung H. (2010) Humor therapy: relieving chronic pain and enhancing happiness for older adults. *J Aging Res* **2010**:343574.

54 Haig RA. (1988) *The Anatomy of Humor*. Charles C. Thomas Publishing Ltd, Springfield.

55 Takeyachi Y, Konno S, Otani K *et al.* (2003) Correlation of low back pain with functional status, general health perception, social participation, subjective happiness and patient satisfaction. *Spine* **28(13)**:1461–7.

56 Gelkopf M, Kreitler S. (1996) Is humor only fun, an alternative cure, or magic? The cognitive therapeutic potential of humor. *Journal of Cognitive Psychotherapy* 10(**4**):235–54.

57 Dionigi A, Canestrari C. (2018) The use of humour by therapists and clients in cognitive therapy. *European Journal of Humour Research* **6(3)**:50–67.

58 Sullivan MJ, Thorn B, Haythornthwaite JA *et al.* (2001) Theoretical perspectives on the relation between catastrophizing and pain. *Clinical Journal of Pain* **17(1)**:52–64.

59 Geisser ME, Robinson ME, Keefe FJ, Weiner ML. (1994) Catastrophizing, depression and the sensory, affective and evaluative aspects of chronic pain. *Pain* **59(1)**:79–83.

60 Sullivan MJ, Rodgers WM, Kirsch I. (2001) Catastrophizing, depression and expectancies for pain and emotional distress. *Pain* **91(1-2)**: 147–54.

61 Day MA, Thorn BE. (2010) The relationship of demographic and psychosocial variables to pain-related outcomes in a rural chronic pain population. *Pain* **151(2)**:467–74.

62 Flor H, Behle DJ, Birbaumer N. (1993) Assessment of pain-related cognitions in chronic pain patients. *Behav Res Ther* **31(1)**:63–73.

63 Keefe FJ, Rumble ME, Scipio CD, Giordano LA, Perri LM. (2004) Psychological aspects of persistent pain: current state of the science. *J Pain* **5(4)**:195–211.

64 Sullivan MJL, Thorn B, Haythornthwaite JA *et al.* (2001) Theoretical perspectives on the relation between catastrophizing and pain. *Clin J Pain* **17(1)**:52–64.

65 Edwards RR, Cahalan C, Mensing G, Smith M, Haythornthwaite JA. (2011) Pain, catastrophizing, and depression in the rheumatic diseases. *Nat Rev Rheumatol* **7(4)**:216–24.

66 Drahovzal D, Stewart S, Sullivan M. (2006) Tendency to catastrophize somatic sensations: pain catastrophizing and anxiety sensitivity in predicting headache. *Cognitive Behaviour Therapy* **35(4)**:226–35.

67 Rudy TE, Lieber SJ, Boston JR, Gourley LM, Baysal E. (2003) Psychosocial predictors of physical performance in disabled individuals with chronic pain. *Clin J Pain* 19:18–30.

68 Turner JA, Holtzman S, Mancl L. (2007) Mediators, moderators, and predictors of therapeutic change in cognitive-behavioral therapy for chronic pain. *Pain* **127**:276–86.

69 Schutze R, Rees C, Preece M, Schutze M. (2010) Low mindfulness predicts pain catastrophizing in a fear-avoidance model of chronic pain. *Pain* **148**:120–7.

70 McCracken LM, Eccleston C. (2003) Coping or acceptance: what to do about chronic pain? *Pain* **105**:197–204.

71 Turner JA, Anderson ML, Balderson BH, Cook AJ, Sherman KJ, Cherkin DC. (2016) Mindfulness-based stress reduction and cognitive-behavioral therapy for chronic low back pain: similar effects on mindfulness, catastrophizing, self-efficacy, and acceptance in a randomized controlled trial. *Pain* **157(11)**:2434–44.

72 Linton SJ. (1982) A critical review of behavioural treatments for chronic benign pain other than headache. *Br J Clin Psychol* **21**:321–37.

73 Kerns RD, Payne A. (1996) Treating families of chronic pain patients. In: Gatchel RJ, Turk D, eds. *Psychological Approaches to Pain Management*. Guilford Press, New York. pp. 283–304.

74 Kabat-Zinn J. (2013) *Full Catastrophe Living (Revised Edition): Using the Wisdom of Your Body and Mind to Face Stress, Pain, and Illness*. Bantam Books, New York.

75 Kabat-Zinn J. (2003) Mindfulness-based interventions in context: past, present, and future. *Clinical Psychology: Science and Practice* **10**:144–56.

76 Vowles KE, McCracken LM. (2008) Acceptance and values-based action in chronic pain: a study of treatment effectiveness and process. *Journal of Consulting and Clinical Psychology* **76(3)**:397–407.

77 McCracken LM, Vowles KE. (2014) Acceptance and commitment therapy and mindfulness for chronic pain: model, process and progress. *American Psychologist* **69(2)**:178–87.

78 Holzman AD, Turk DC, Kerns RD. (1986) The cognitive-behavioral approach to the management of chronic pain. In: Holzman AD, Turk DC, eds. *Pain Management: A Handbook of Psychological Treatment Approaches*. Pergamon Press, New York. pp. 31–50.

79 Kerns RD, Turk DC, Holzman AD, Rudy TE. (1986) Comparison of cognitive-behavioral and behavioral approaches to the outpatient treatment of chronic pain. *Clin J Pain* **1**:195–203.

80 Turner JA, Clancy S. (1988) Comparison of operant behavioral and cognitive-behavioral group treatment for chronic low back pain. *Journal of Consulting and Clinical Psychology* **56**:261–6.

81 Bruns D, Mueller K, Warren PA. (2012) Biopsychosocial law, health care reform, and the control of medical inflation in Colorado. *Rehabilitation Psychology* **57(2)**:81–97.

82 Eccleston C, Palermo TM, Williams AC, Lewandowski A, Morley S. (2009) Psychological therapies for the management of chronic and recurrent pain in children and adolescents. *Cochrane Database of Syst Rev.* **2009(2)**:CD003968.

83 Morley S, Williams A. (2015) New developments in the psychological management of chronic pain. *The Can J Psychiatry* **60(4)**:168–75.

84 Schweikert B, Jacobi E, Seitz R *et al.* (2006) Effectiveness and cost-effectiveness of adding a cognitive behavioral treatment to the rehabilitation of chronic low back pain. *J Rheumatol* **33(12)**:2519–26.

85 Lami MJ, Martinez MP, Sanchez AI. (2013) Systematic review of psychological treatment in fibromyalgia. *Curr Pain Headache Rep* 17(**7**):345.

86 Eccleston C, Hearn L, Williams AC. (2015) Psychological therapies for the management of chronic neuropathic pain in adults. *Cochrane Database of Syst Rev* 2015(**10**):CD011259.

87 Fisher E, Heathcote LC, Palermo TM, De C Williams AC, Lau J, Eccleston C. (2014) Systematic review and meta-analysis of psychological therapies for children with chronic pain. *J Pediatr Psychol* **39(8)**:763–82.

88 Day MA, Thorn BE. In press. Group therapy for chronic pain. In: Rathmell J, ed. *Bonica's Management of Pain*, 5th edn, Wolters Kluwer, Baltimore.

89 Day MA, Eyer, J, Thorn, BE. (2013) Therapeutic relaxation. In: Hofmann SG, ed. *The Wiley Handbook of Cognitive Behavioral Therapy: A Complete Reference Guide. Volume 1: CBT General Strategies*. Vol 1. Wiley-Blackwell, Hoboken. pp. 157–80.

90 Vlaeyen JW, de Jong J, Geilen M, Heuts PH, van Breukelen G. (2002) The treatment of fear of movement/(re)injury in chronic low back pain: further evidence on the effectiveness of exposure in vivo. *Clin J Pain* **18(4)**:251–61.

91 Leeuw M, Goossens ME, Linton SJ, Crombez G, Boersma K, Vlaeyen JW. (2007) The fear-avoidance model of musculoskeletal pain: current state of scientific evidence. *Journal of Behavioral Medicine*. **30**:77–94.

92 Miller WR, Rollnick S. (2012) *Motivational Interviewing: Helping People Change*, 3rd ed. Guilford Press, New York.

93 Van Koulil S, van Lankveld W, Kraaimaat, FW *et al.* (2016) Tailored cognitive–behavioral therapy and exercise training for high-risk patients with fibromyalgia. *Arthritis Care Res* **62**:1377–85.

94 Kerns RD, Burns JW, Shulman M et al. (2014) Can we improve cognitive-behavioral therapy for chronic back pain treatment engagement and adherence? A controlled trial of tailored versus standard therapy. *Health Psychology* **33(9)**: 938–47.

95 Day MA, Ehde DM, Jensen MP. (2015) Psychosocial pain management moderation: the limit, activate and enhance model. *J Pain* **16(10)**:947–60.

Chapter 27

Pain catastrophizing and fear of movement: detection and intervention

Catherine Paré & Michael J.L. Sullivan

Department of Psychology, McGill University, Montréal, Québec, Canada

Over the past two decades, considerable research has accumulated indicating that medical status variables cannot fully account for presenting symptoms of pain and disability in individuals with chronic pain conditions [1]. Biopsychosocial models have been put forward suggesting that a complete understanding of pain experience and pain-related outcomes will require consideration of physical, psychological and social factors [2]. Catastrophic thinking and fear of movement are two psychological variables that have been shown to be significant determinants of pain and disability associated with persistent pain conditions. This chapter will briefly review what is currently known about the impact of pain catastrophizing and fear of movement on pain outcomes. The chapter will describe assessment techniques and intervention approaches for individuals who present with high levels of pain catastrophizing and fear of movement.

Pain catastrophizing

Pain catastrophizing has emerged as one of the most robust and powerful predictors of pain-related outcomes [3, 4]. Pain catastrophizing has been defined as "an exaggerated negative mental set brought to bear during actual or anticipated pain" [5]. The term pain catastrophizing is used to describe a particular response to pain symptoms that includes elements of rumination (i.e. excessive focus on pain sensations), magnification (i.e. exaggerating the threat value of pain sensations) and helplessness (i.e. perceiving oneself as unable to cope with pain symptoms). To date, several hundred studies have been published showing a relation between pain catastrophizing and adverse pain outcomes [3, 6].

Investigations have revealed a relation between pain catastrophizing and adverse pain outcomes in patients with a wide range of acute and persistent pain conditions [4]. High levels of pain catastrophizing have been associated with increased pain and pain behavior, increased use of healthcare services, poor surgical outcomes, longer hospital stays, increased use of analgesic medication, opioid misuse and higher rates of occupational disability [7, 8]. In samples of patients with chronic pain, pain catastrophizing has been associated with heightened disability, predicting the risk of chronicity and the severity of disability better than illness-related variables or pain itself [9]. Numerous investigations have revealed that pain catastrophizing is associated with a number of markers of pathological pain processing, including temporal summation of pain [10], sensitivity to movement-evoked pain [11], neuroendocrine responses [12], conditioned pain modulation [13] and widespread pain [14].

Clinical Pain Management: A Practical Guide, Second Edition. Edited by Mary E. Lynch, Kenneth D. Craig, and Philip W. Peng.

Pain catastrophizing has been shown to be associated with poor response to numerous pain management interventions. For example, high scores on pain catastrophizing have been associated with less pain reduction following joint injection [15], radiofrequency neurotomy [16] and multidisciplinary rehabilitation [17]. Pain catastrophizing has been shown to predict poor response to physical therapy [18], analgesic medication [19, 20], opioids [21] and surgical interventions [22, 23]. Our group has recently shown that high post-treatment scores on a measure of pain catastrophizing predict failure to maintain gains made in the rehabilitation of whiplash injury [24].

In the past decade, an increasing amount of research has been dedicated to understanding the relationship between pain catastrophizing and mental health and the consequent impact on pain-related outcomes. Pain catastrophizing has been associated with increased symptoms of depression, anxiety and PTSD [25, 26, 27]. One recent study revealed that clinically significant mental health difficulties mediated the relationship between pain catastrophizing levels and occupational disability [26]. Recently, pain catastrophizing has been proposed to play a role in the underlying mechanisms of problematic recovery from pain or mental health difficulties [28, 29].

Fear of movement associated with pain

Fear of pain, or kinesiophobia, has been defined as a "highly specific negative emotional reaction to pain eliciting stimuli involving a high degree of mobilization for escape/avoidance behavior" [30]. It can also be aroused by impending pain and encompasses present- and future-directed cognitions about pain [31, 32]. Fear of movement is a type of pain-related fear characterized by avoidance of activity associated with pain or premature termination (i.e., escape) of activity causing pain [33]. Escape refers to behaviors that are enacted with the goal of terminating pain experience. Avoidance behavior refers to behavior that postpones or prevents pain experience. Once learned, avoidance behaviors can be self-perpetuating. Self-perpetuation of avoidance behavior occurs when individuals develop the expectation that future activities will be associated with pain. Extreme avoidance of movement can contribute to significant disability. Although the role of fear of movement has been extensively studied in individuals with low back pain, only recently have investigators examined pain-related fears in patients with other types of pain conditions such as arthritis and whiplash injury [34].

The combined negative impact of pain catastrophizing and fear of movement has primarily been interpreted using the Fear-Avoidance Model of Pain [33]. According to the Fear-Avoidance Model, individuals will differ in the degree to which they interpret their pain symptoms in a 'catastrophic' or 'alarmist' manner. The model predicts that catastrophic thinking following the onset of pain will contribute to heightened fears of movement. In turn, fear is expected to lead to avoidance of activity that might be associated with pain [33]. Prolonged inactivity is expected to contribute to depression and disability. The model is recursive such that increased pain symptoms, distress and disability become the input for further catastrophic or alarmist thinking [33]. Since its inception in 2000, the same authors have provided an updated version of the model [35] (Figure 27.1). This updated version has moved away from detailing specific processes that arise following pain, such as pain catastrophizing, and shifted towards a conditioning-based explanation of an individual's response to pain [35]. Research findings have been consistent in showing that high levels of fear-avoidance beliefs are associated with more pronounced pain-related disability [34].

It has been suggested that assessment of catastrophizing and fear of movement should be part of the routine evaluation of patients with pain conditions. There has also been a call for the development of interventions that are designed to specifically target catastrophizing and fear of movement [9].

Assessment of catastrophizing

Several instruments have been developed to assess pain catastrophizing. Considerable research on catastrophizing has used the Coping Strategies Questionnaire (CSQ) [36]. The CSQ is a 48-item self-report measure consisting of seven coping subscales, including a 6-item catastrophizing subscale. Respondents are asked to rate the frequency with which they use the different strategies described by scale items. The catastrophizing subscale of the CSQ contains items reflecting pessimism and helplessness in relation to coping with pain. Two shortened versions of the CSQ have been developed to improve upon the clinical utility of the questionnaire [37, 38].

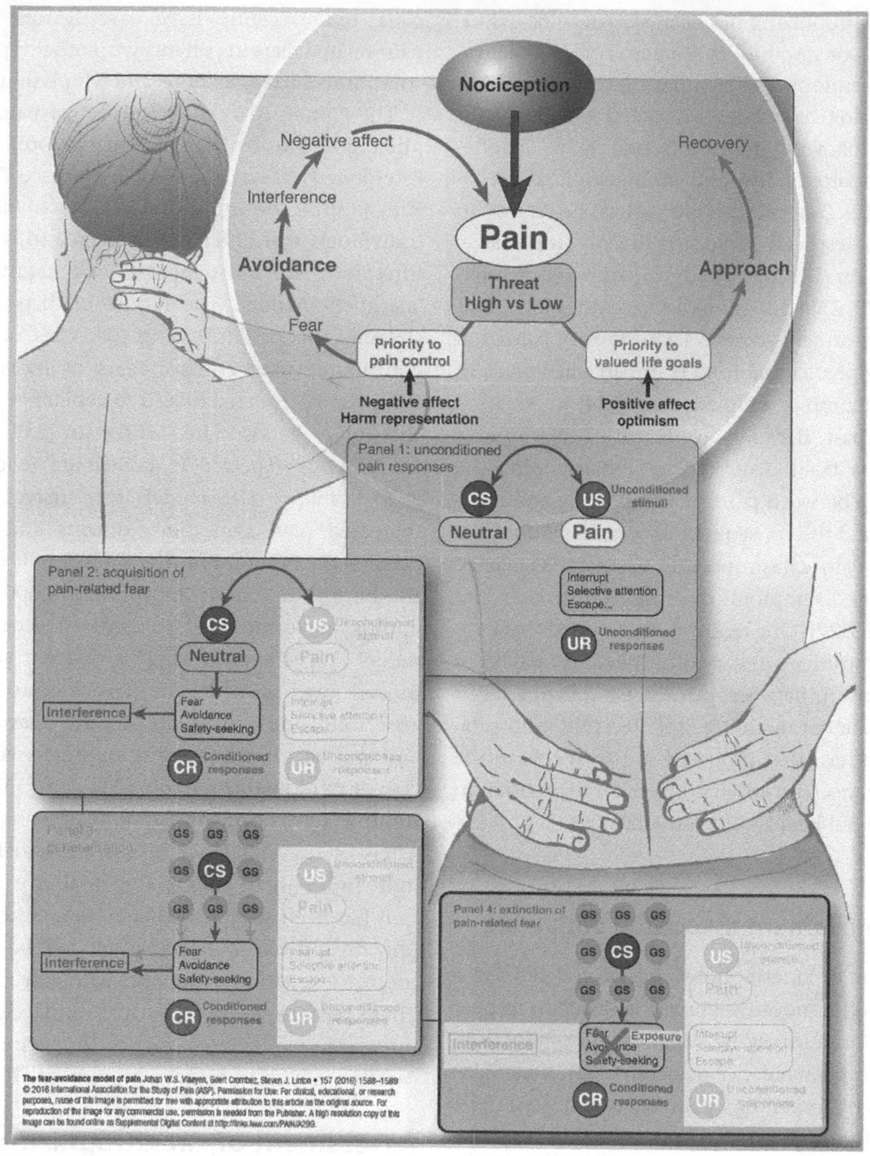

Figure 27.1 The fear-avoidance model of pain (Color Plate 8). *Source:* Vlaeyen et al. 2016. Reproduced with permission of Wolters Kluwer Health, Inc.

The Pain Catastrophizing Scale (PCS) is currently the most widely used measure of pain catastrophizing [4, 39]. The PCS is a self-report questionnaire that assesses three dimensions of catastrophizing: rumination ("I can't stop thinking about how much it hurts"), magnification ("I worry that something serious may happen") and helplessness ("It's awful and I feel that it overwhelms me"). The PCS consists of 13 items describing different thoughts and feelings that individuals may experience when they are in pain [39]. On this measure, respondents are asked to rate the frequency with which they experience different catastrophic thoughts and feelings when they are in pain on a 5-point scale with the end-points (0) not at all and (4) all the time. The reliability and validity of the PCS has been well established [40]. The PCS yields a total score and subscale scores for rumination, magnification and helplessness. Individuals who obtain scores above 20 are considered to fall within the risk range [41].

The PCS has been translated into over 27 languages. Adaptations of the PCS have been developed for different populations such as the PCS-child [42], PCS-significant other [43] and PCS-parent [44]. Recently, the PCS was adapted for daily use [45]. Shorter versions of the PCS have recently been developed and can be useful under conditions where assessment burden might need to be taken into consideration [46].

Treatments aimed at reducing catastrophizing

Findings linking pain catastrophizing to problematic recovery outcomes over the past two decades have provided the impetus for the development of interventions designed to reduce pain catastrophizing [47, 48, 49, 50, 51]. The content and structure of these interventions has varied widely, ranging from information-based web applications to psychosocial interventions delivered by trained professionals [47, 48, 52, 53, 54, 55]. Interventions targeting pain catastrophizing have generally ranged in duration from 4-10 weeks [49, 50, 54]. Techniques used to target catastrophizing include a host of cognitive behavioral techniques, such as education, thought monitoring, reappraisal, guided disclosure, validation, goal setting, emotional problem solving and activity scheduling [50, 56, 57]. Research has been consistent in showing that reductions in pain catastrophizing predict improvements in pain-related outcomes, suggesting that the success of pain or disability management interventions are at least partially dependent on reducing pain catastrophizing [47, 58, 59, 60].

A recent review by Schutze et al. (2018) highlighted that most interventions used to reduce pain catastrophizing have yielded only modest outcomes [61]. Mental health comorbidity might be a factor relevant to the modest impact of treatments aimed at reducing pain catastrophizing [52, 61, 62, 63, 64]. If high scores on measures of pain catastrophizing reflect a high probability of mental health comorbidity, it is likely that many psychoeducational or web-based interventions targeting pain catastrophizing might not be sufficient to yield meaningful improvement in clinical outcomes.

Assessment of fear of movement

Several scales have been developed to assess pain-related fears including the Tampa Scale for Kinesiophobia (TSK) [65], the Fear-Avoidance Beliefs Questionnaire (FAB-Q) [66], the Fear of Pain Questionnaire III (FPQ-III) [32] and the Pain and Anxiety Symptom Scale (PASS) [67]. The FAB-Q is most relevant for individuals who might have specific fears of work-related activities. The FPQ-III assesses the degree to which individuals are fearful of different pain-inducing situations (e.g. dental pain, surgery) but is not specific to activity or movement. The item-content of the PASS addresses anxiety-related symptoms (e.g, sweating, agitation, dread, fear) that might be associated with pain.

The TSK [65] is the most widely used measure of fear of movement. Respondents are asked to make ratings of their degree of agreement with each of the 17 statements. Four items of the TSK (items 4, 8, 12 and 16) are reversed such that higher scores represent less, as opposed to more, fear of movement. Respondents' ratings are summed to yield a total score where higher values reflect greater fear of movement. The item content of the TSK is most relevant for individuals who are suffering from pain due to musculoskeletal injury or from pain that is exacerbated by activity (e.g. arthritis). The TSK has been shown to have satisfactory validity and reliability for evaluating fear of movement and to be associated with various indices of disability [68]. The TSK has been shortened by some researchers to produce 11-, 13- and 14-item versions [69]. Although widely used, reviews of the literature have called into question the construct validity and responsiveness of most measures of fear of pain [70].

Treatments aimed at reducing fear of movement

Clinical interventions that have been shown to reduce levels of fear of movement include: 1) education, reassurance and activity encouragement; 2) graded exposure to feared activities; 3) activity monitoring, progressive goal setting and graded activity; 20) cognitive behavioral therapy (CBT) techniques and 5) acceptance and commitment therapy (ACT) [36, 69]. Each of these interventions can be effective when delivered independently in primary care settings or when combined within a multidisciplinary treatment program. Clinical trials that have evaluated the efficacy of the latter have shown that these programs are associated with meaningful improvement in measures of fear of movement, pain intensity, activity interference, psychosocial risk factors and work disability [49, 71, 72].

Interventions that use education, reassurance and activity encouragement aim to provide patients with information and advice about how to reduce their levels of fear-related disability [73]. Educational interventions are usually the precursor to encouraging the resumption of normal activities and typically inform patients about their pain condition, their expected recovery trajectory and the signs or symptoms that may indicate serious danger [74]. Regarding reassurance and activity encouragement, the key messages communicated are that pain is not a reliable signal of tissue damage, that the pain condition is not life threatening or permanently disabling and that it is safe and beneficial to engage in physical activity. Patients with elevated levels of fear will often require support in shifting their focus from the severity of their injury to prioritizing life goals, like returning to normal activity [71, 75]. It may therefore be helpful for clinicians to consider activity encouragement and reassurance as therapeutic strategies that permeate the recovery process rather than as discrete interventions. The mediums through which these interventions are implemented can vary significantly (e.g. one-on-one sessions, group classes, online forums), which makes them relatively easy to integrate into primary care and rehabilitation settings. Past research conducted with acute and sub-acute pain populations has shown that these interventions result in significant improvements in fear of movement, emotional functioning, pain intensity and self-report disability [71, 76].

Graded exposure to feared activities is a systematic, behavioral intervention that helps patients overcome their fears of specific movements by progressively engaging them in previously avoided activities [35]. Clinicians help patients to identify and rank feared activities in a hierarchy, from least to most feared. Next, patients are asked to rate their fear of performing their least feared activity on a scale of 0 (no fear) to 10 (extreme fear) and to communicate the negative physical consequences they expect to occur upon engaging in this behavior. Patients are then encouraged to perform the behavior and asked to rate their level of fear following exposure. Research suggests that as patients gain exposure to each activity, their level of fear for this specific movement declines [36]. As their fear dissipates, the next activity on the hierarchy is introduced and the procedure is repeated. This intervention is typically initiated in one-on-one clinical settings and complemented with, and ultimately progressed to, self-guided home exercises. While graded exposure is one of the most effective interventions for reducing the fear of specific movements, its effects do not seem to generalize to untargeted activities [77]. For this reason, this intervention is more likely to translate into improved disability levels when feared activities that hinder essential daily function are targeted (e.g. work-related activities).

It has been suggested that individuals' fears of movement and their ensuing avoidance of activity are fueled by over-predictions of harm or pain exacerbation [35]. If individuals can be encouraged to engage in activities that they fear will bring about pain (or symptom exacerbation), they are provided with an opportunity to correct their over-predictions [36]. In other words, experience can allow individuals to alter their exaggerated predictions of threat or harm associated with potentially pain-inducing activities and in turn, decrease the probability of avoidance behavior.

Activity monitoring, progressive goal setting and graded activity are therapeutic strategies that aim to provide patients with direction, structure and support to enable an increase in their levels of physical activity [49]. These interventions are initiated by establishing the patient's baseline activities level. Asking patients to record a week of daily activity logs can facilitate this step [50]. Once patients have identified and described their objectives, graded activity is used to progressively increase their activity participation. Daily activity quotas are established based on this information, which are updated at follow-up sessions. Care must be taken to start with activity quotas that have a high probability of success, to instill feelings of achievement and motivation for engaging in progressively higher quotas without increasing pain. These interventions have been associated with long-term improvements in fear of movement, pain intensity and activity limitations as well as a reduced number of work absenteeism days [72].

CBT techniques are a class of interventions that use a structured approach to modifying fear-related thoughts, feelings and activities [1]. Thought monitoring and thought restructuring are two CBT techniques that are commonly used in the treatment of fear of movement [1, 78]. Patients with elevated levels of fear commonly react to pain with thoughts that increase the threat value of the painful experience and with avoidant behavior that limits exposure to the pain-related activity [36]. The clinician works with the patient to alter his or her threat appraisals of pain eliciting situations. Exposure-based CBT protocols have also been used to focus on fear movements and activities for individuals suffering from chronic musculoskeletal pain [79]. Past research that has used CBT interventions to target fear of movement has shown that these treatments are associated with significant improvements in fear, activity interference and measures of work disability [1, 36].

ACT is based on concepts of mindfulness, acceptance and values-based action [80]. Although ACT addresses patients' cognitions, unlike CBT, the focus or objective is not on changing the content of the cognitions. Rather the focus is on changing the function of the cognitions [81]. The patient is encouraged to accept that pain is part of the present reality and to consciously choose to participate in valued activities in spite of ongoing symptoms [81]. A number of studies have supported the use of ACT as an intervention for reducing pain-related fear [71].

Summary

Research to date has highlighted the important role of catastrophizing and pain-related fear as significant determinants of pain severity and pain-related disability. Measurement instruments have been developed to assist clinicians in identifying pain patients at risk for problematic recovery or poor treatment response. There are also interventions that have been shown to reduce catastrophizing and pain-related fear. Because catastrophizing and pain-related fear are correlated, it is likely that intervention techniques designed to target catastrophizing will also have positive impacts on pain-related fear and vice versa. Disclosure techniques and cognitive behavioral approaches might impact preferentially on catastrophizing while activity mobilization and exposure techniques might impact preferentially on fear of movement. Although more research is needed to determine the most effective approaches to yield clinically meaningful reductions in catastrophizing and pain-related fear this chapter has presented the current evidence for best treatment options.

References

1 Gatchel RJ, Peng YB, Peters ML, Fuchs PN, Turk DC. (2007) The biopsychosocial approach to chronic pain: scientific advances and future directions. *Psychol Bull* **133(4)**:581–624.

2 Turk, DC, Monarch, ES. Biopsychosocial perspective on chronic pain (2018). In: Turk DC, Gatchel RJ, eds. *Psychological approaches to pain management: A practitioner's handbook*, 3rd Ed, pp. 1-586. New York: Guilford Press.

3 Leung L. (2012) Pain catastrophizing: an updated review. *Indian J Psychol Med* **34(3)**:204–17.

4 Quartana PJ, Campbell CM, Edwards RR. (2009) Pain catastrophizing: a critical review. *Expert Rev Neurotherapeutics* **29(5)**:745–58.

5 Sullivan MJL, Thorn B, Haythornthwaite JA *et al.* (2001) Theoretical perspectives on the relation between catastrophizing and pain. *Clin J Pain* **17(1)**:52–64.

6 Sullivan MJL, Adams H, Martel MO, Scott W, Wideman T. (2011) Catastrophizing and perceived injustice: risk factors for the transition to chronicity after whiplash injury. *Spine* **36(25 Suppl)**:S244–9.

7 Edwards RR, Dworkin RH, Sullivan MD, Turk DC, Wasan AD. (2016) The role of psychosocial processes in the development and maintenance of chronic pain. *J Pain* **17(9 Suppl)**:T70–92.

8 Neblett R. (2017) Pain catastrophizing: an historical perspective. *J Applied Biobehav Res* **22(1)**:e12086.

9 Sullivan MJL, Lynch ME, Clark AJ. (2005) Dimensions of catastrophic thinking associated with pain experience and disability in patients with neuropathic pain conditions. *Pain* **113(3)**:310–315.

10 Sullivan MJL, Lariviere C, Simmonds M. (2010) Activity-related summation of pain and functional disability in patients with whiplash injuries. *Pain* **151(2)**: 440–6.

11 Mankovsky-Arnold T, Wideman TH, Thibault P, Lariviere C, Rainville P, Sullivan MJL. (2017) Sensitivity to movement-evoked pain and multisite pain are associated with work-disability following whiplash injury: a cross-sectional study. *J Occ Rehab* **27**:413–21.

12 Edwards RR, Kronfli T, Haythornthwaite JA, Smith MT, McGuire L, Page GG. (2008) Association of catastrophizing with interleukin-6 responses to acute pain. *Pain* **140(1)**:135–44.

13 Nahman-Averbuch H, Nir RR, Sprecher E, Yarnitsky D. (2016) Psychological factors and conditioned pain modulation: A meta-analysis. *Clin J Pain* **32(6)**:541–54.

14 Julien N, Goffaux P, Arsenault P, Marchand S. (2005) Widespread pain in fibromyalgia is related to a deficit of endogenous pain inhibition. *Pain* **114(1-2)**:295–302.

15 Smith AD, Jull G, Schneider G, Frizzell B, Hooper RA, Sterling M. (2013) A comparison of physical and psychological features of responders and non-responders to cervical facet blocks in chronic whiplash. *BMC Musculoskelet Disord* **14**:313.

16 Smith AD, Jull GA, Schneider GM, Frizzell B, Hooper RA, Sterling MM. (2016) Low pain catastrophization and disability predict successful outcome to radiofrequency neurotomy in individuals with chronic whiplash. *Pain Pract* **16(3)**:311–9.

17 Scott W, Wideman TH, Sullivan MJL. (2014) Clinically meaningful scores on pain catastrophizing before and after multidisciplinary rehabilitation - a prospective study of individuals with subacute pain after whiplash injury. *Clin J Pain* **30(3)**:183–90.

18 Bergbom S, Boersma K, Overmeer T, Linton SJ. (2011) Relationship among pain catastrophizing, depressed mood, and outcomes across physical therapy treatments. *Physical Ther* **91(5)**:754–64.

19 Haythornthwaite JA, Clark MR, Pappagallo M, Raja SN. (2003) Pain coping strategies play a role in the persistence of pain in post-herpetic neuralgia. *Pain* **106(3)**:453–60.

20 Mankovsky T, Lynch M, Clark A, Sawynok J, Sullivan MJ. (2012) Pain catastrophizing predicts poor response to topical analgesics in patients with neuropathic pain. *Pain Res Manag* **17(1)**:10–4.

21 Martel MO, Wasan AD, Jamison RN, Edwards RR. (2013) Catastrophic thinking and increased risk for prescription opioid misuse in patients with chronic pain. *Drug Alcohol Depend* **132(1-2)**:335–41.

22 Pavlin DJ, Sullivan MJ, Freund PR, Roesen K. (2005)_ Catastrophizing: a risk factor for postsurgical pain. *Clin J Pain* **21(1)**:83–90.

23 Sullivan MJL, Tanzer M, Stanish W *et al.* (2009) Psychological determinants of problematic outcomes following total knee arthroplasty. *Pain* **143(1-2)**:123–9.

24 Moore E, Thibault P, Adams H, Sullivan MJL. (2016) Catastrophizing and pain-related fear predict failure to maintain treatment gains following participation in a pain rehabilitation program. *Pain Rep* **1(2)**:e567.

25 Borsbo B, Peolsson M, Gerdle B. (2009) The complex interplay between pain intensity, depression, anxiety and catastrophising with respect to quality of life and disability. *Disabil Rehabil* **31(19)**:1605–13.

26 Paré C, Thibault P, Cote P *et al.* (2019) The relationship between level of catastrophizing and mental health comorbidity in individuals with whiplash injuries. *Clin J Pain* **35(11)**:880–6.

27 Sullivan MJL, Simmonds M, Velly A. (2006) Pain, depression, disability and rehabilitation outcomes. Institut de recherche Robert-Sauvé en santé et en sécurité de travail.

28 Flink IL, Boersma K, Linton SJ. (2013) Pain catastrophizing as repetitive negative thinking: a development of the conceptualization. *Cogn Behav Ther* **42(3)**:215–23.

29 Gellatly R, Beck AT. (2016) Catastrophic thinking: A transdiagnostic process across psychiatric disorders. *Cogn Ther Res* **40(4)**:441–52.

30 McNeil DW, Au AR, Zvolensky MJ, Rettig McKee D, Klineberg IJ, Ho CK. (2001) Fear of pain in orofacial pain patients. *Pain* **89**:245–52.

31 Niederstrasser NG, Meulders A, Meulders M, Slepian PM, Vlaeyen JW, Sullivan MJ. (2015) Pain catastrophizing and fear of pain predict the experience of pain in body parts not targeted by a delayed-onset muscle soreness procedure. *J Pain* **16(11)**:1065–76.

32 Wideman TH, Asmundson GG, Smeets RJ *et al.* (2013) Rethinking the fear avoidance model: toward a multidimensional framework of pain-related disability. *Pain* **154(11)**:2262–5.

33 Vlaeyen JW, Linton SJ. (2000) Fear-avoidance and its consequences in chronic musculoskeletal pain: a state of the art. *Pain* **85(3)**:317–32.

34 Leeuw M, Goossens ME, Linton SJ, Crombez G, Boersma K, Vlaeyen JW. (2007) The fear-avoidance model of musculoskeletal pain: current state of scientific evidence. *J Behav Med* **30(1)**:77–94.

35 Vlaeyen JW, Crombez G, Linton SJ. (2016) The fear-avoidance model of pain. *Pain* **157(8)**:1588–9.

36 Rosenstiel A, Keefe F. (1983) The use of coping strategies in chronic low back pain patients: rela-

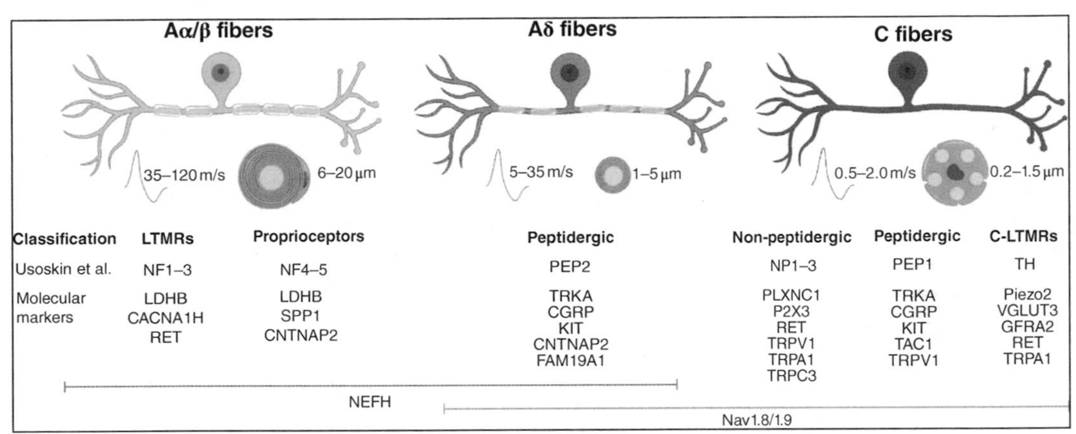

Plate 1 **Primary sensory neuron characteristics.** Primary sensory neurons are categorized based on their conduction velocity, degree of myelination and thickness of their axons and cell bodies. While the axons of Aα/β large-diameter and Aδ medium-diameter neurons are thickly and thinly myelinated, respectively, C fibres are unmyelinated and supported by Schwann cells organized in Remak bundles. Recent single cell RNA sequencing by Usoskin, Furlan [10] has revealed 11 sensory neuronal subtypes based on their molecular composition. Aα/β fibres are classified as low-threshold mechanoreceptors (LTMRs) and proprioceptors. Nociceptors (Aδ and C fibres) are further grouped by whether they produce neuropeptides (peptidergic), like calcitonin-gene related peptide (CGRP), or not (non-peptidergic). C-low threshold mechanoreceptors (C-LTMRs), a special class of C fibres, are involved in non-noxious, affective touch and are characterized by their expression of tyrosine hydroxylase. Myelinated fibres (Aα/β and Aδ) express the heavy neurofilament polypeptide (NEFH). Nociceptors (Aδ and C) are characterized by the presence of voltage-gated sodium channels 1.8 and 1.9 (Nav1.8/1.9). Other molecular markers are summarized.

Clinical Pain Management: A Practical Guide, Second Edition. Edited by Mary E. Lynch, Kenneth D. Craig, and Philip W. Peng.

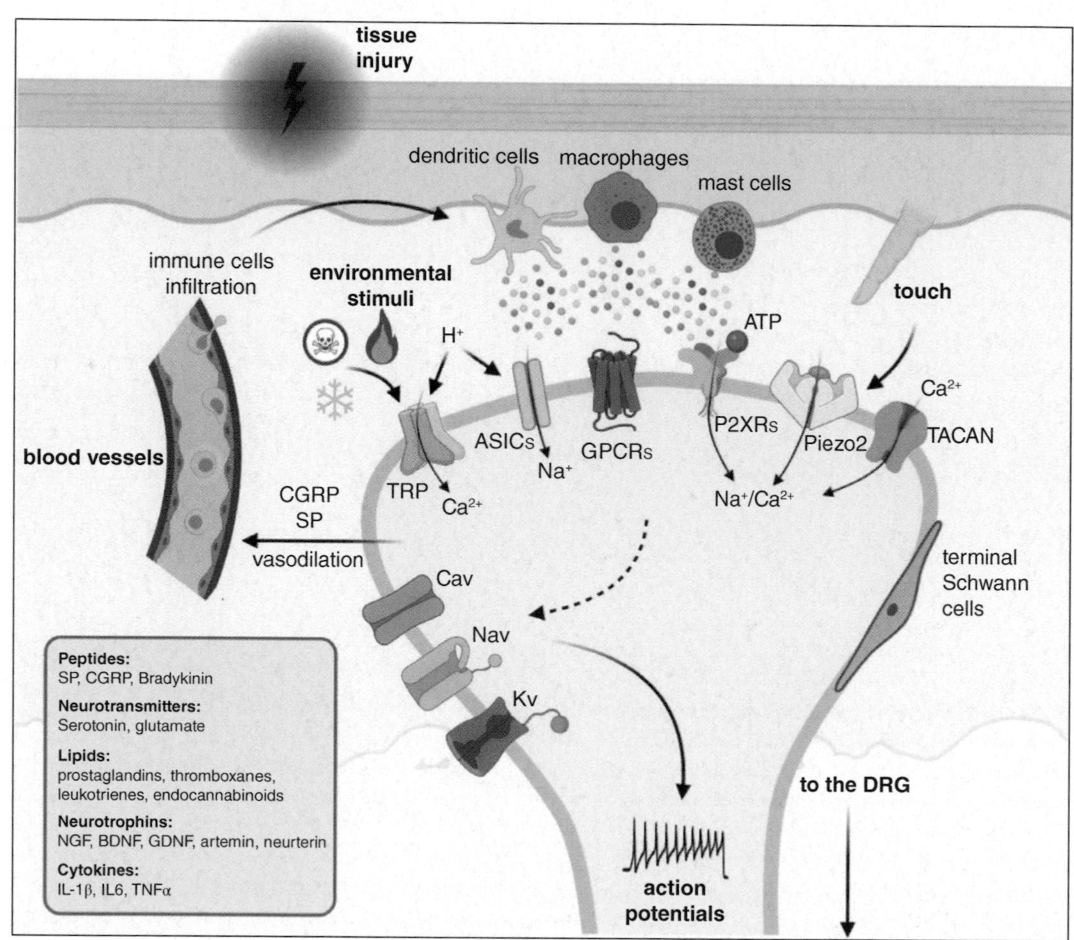

Plate 2 **Primary afferent terminals**. The sensory afferent terminal preferentially responds to a plethora of stimuli using a panoply of receptors and ion channels. Heat, cold and chemical toxins are encoded by Ca^{2+}-permeable transient receptor potential (TRP) channels such as TRPV1, TRPM8, and TRPA1. Low pH (pH<6) is also known to activate acid-sensing ion channels (ASICs). Purinergic receptors, particularly P2X receptors, respond to extracellular ATP usually released in response to an inflammatory insult. Recent characterization of pressure-sensitive receptors has identified Piezo2 and TACAN channels as selective mechanosensors important for the development of mechanical allodynia and hyperalgesia. More recently, a class of Schwann cells that transduce tactile nociception were discovered to ensheathe free nerve endings [86]. Tissue injury and inflammation causes the release of various factors that enhance the activity of nerve fibres and promote sensitization. These factors are summarized in the figure.

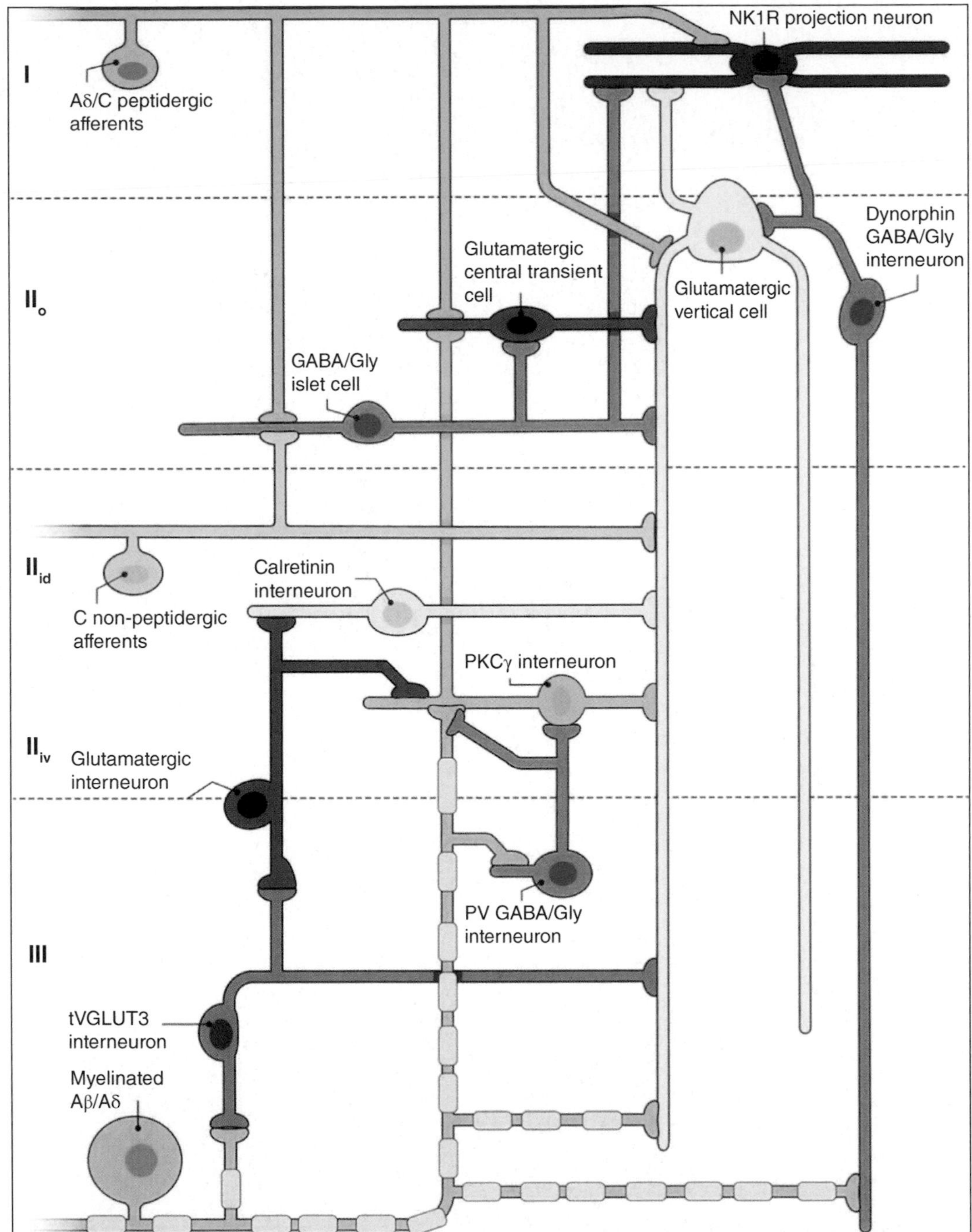

Plate 3 **Spinal dorsal horn circuitry.** The complex circuitry of the spinal cord allows for the integration of incoming noxious and non-noxious stimuli prior to relaying them forward to the brain. Nociceptive afferents terminate in lamina I and II while low-threshold mechanoreceptors (Aβ) terminate in deeper laminae. Local excitatory and inhibitory interneurons act as "gates", suppressing certain information while allowing other information to pass through. Spinal inhibitory circuits are impaired following neuropathy and inflammation, giving rise to hyperalgesia and allodynia. Peirs, Williams [59] recently described engagements of different microcircuits in the development of pain hypersensitivity following nerve injury and inflammation. Peirs, Williams [59] recently demonstrated that a loss of inhibitory tone following spared nerve injury allows Aβ fibres to activate PKCγ interneurons which ultimately lead to the activation of projection neurons. Inflammatory stimuli, such as carrageenan, instead engages calretinin interneurons that further transmit information to projection neurons. This figure is from Peirs and Seal [29] and was reprinted with permission from the American Association for the Advancement of Science.

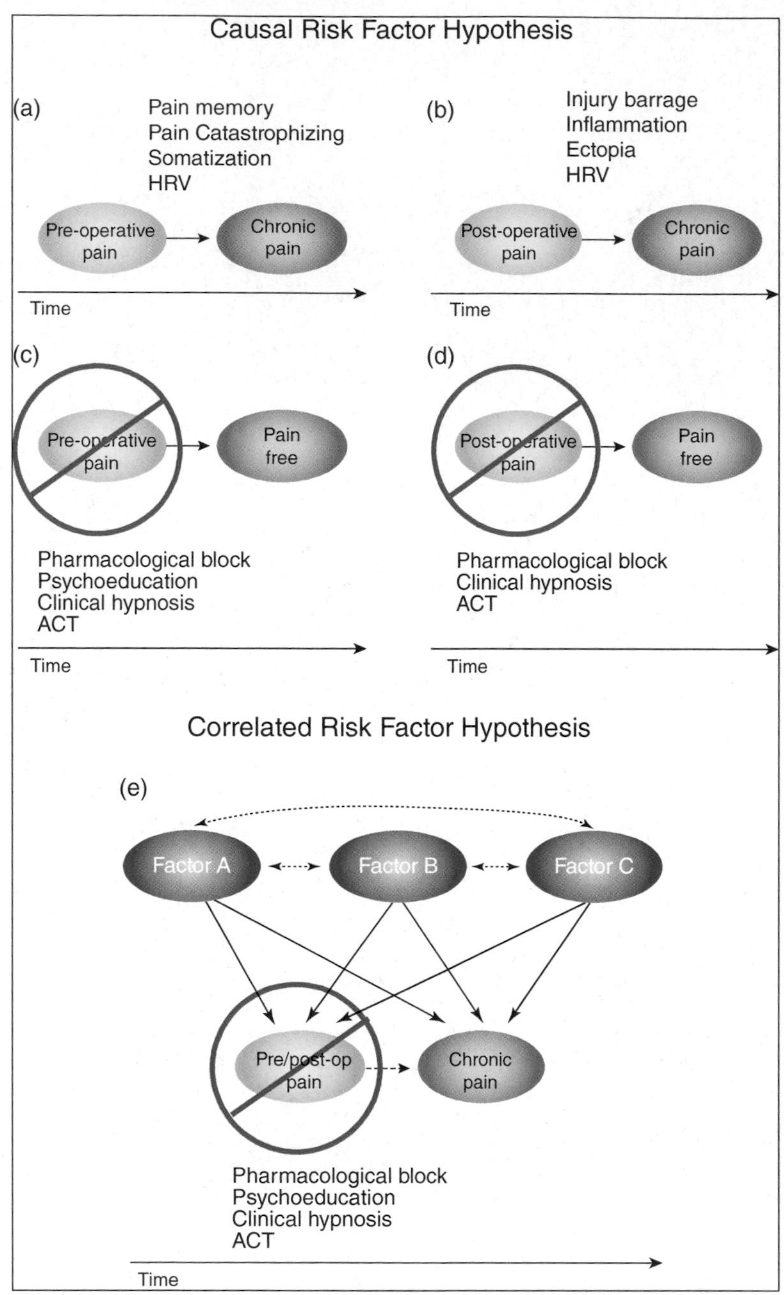

Plate 4 Figure depicting causal (top) and associative (bottom) hypotheses predicting the prevention and non-prevention of CPSP by pharmacologic blockade and/or psychological management at various times throughout the perioperative period. Top. Transition to chronicity (A, B) may be prevented by pharmacological blockade or psychological management of preoperative pain (C) and/or acute postoperative pain (D) assuming the former causes the latter. Bottom. Transition to chronicity will not be prevented if pains are merely correlated and caused by one or more higher-order, inter-related factors (E). HRV = heart rate variability; ACT = Acceptance and Commitment Therapy.

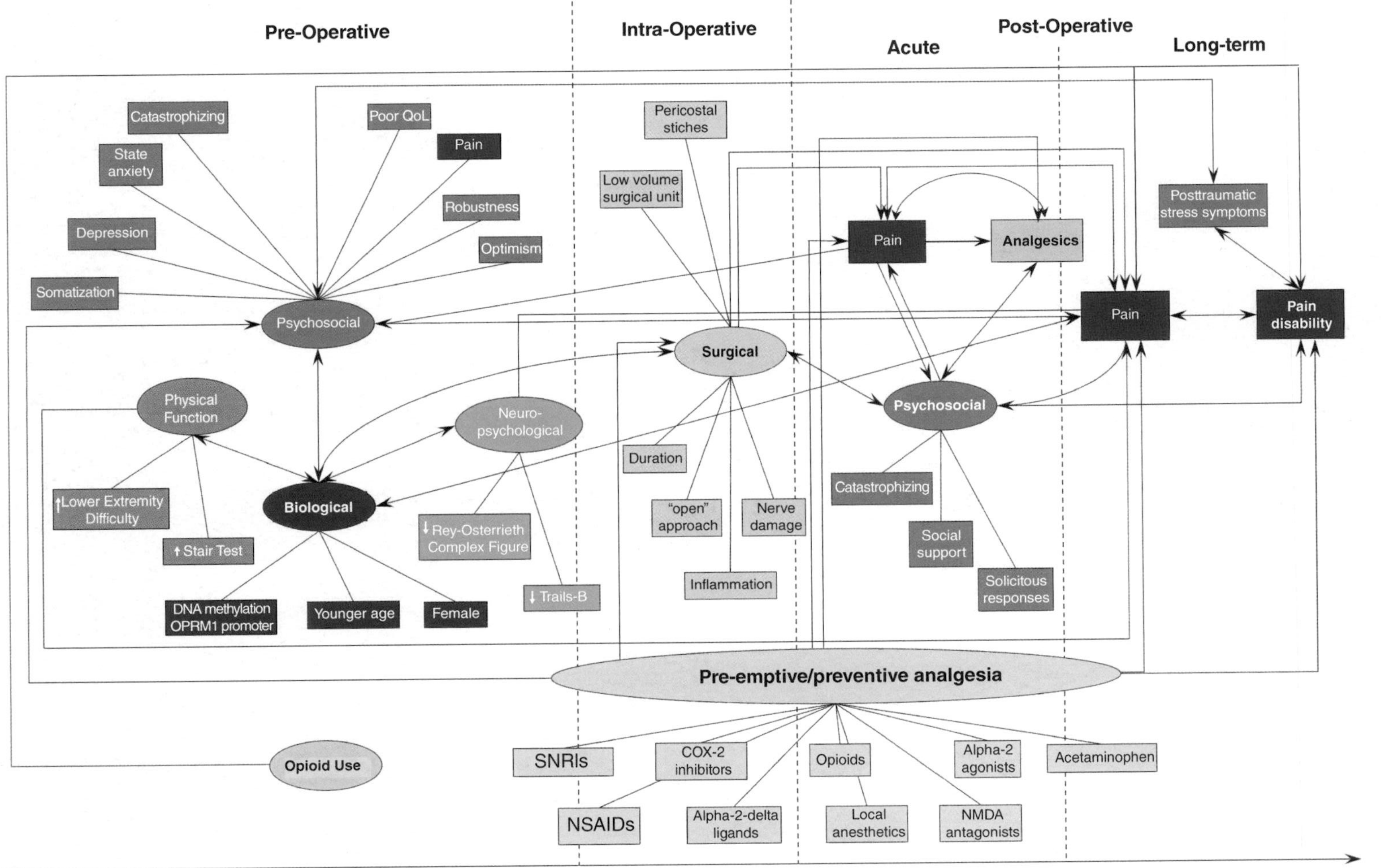

Plate 5 Schematic illustration of the processes involved in the development of CPSP and CPSP disability showing relationships (arrows) among pre-operative, intra-operative and post-operative factors. Lines with double arrows between variables show associative relationships reported in the literature. Lines with a single arrow show causal relationships based on randomized controlled trials of preventive analgesia.

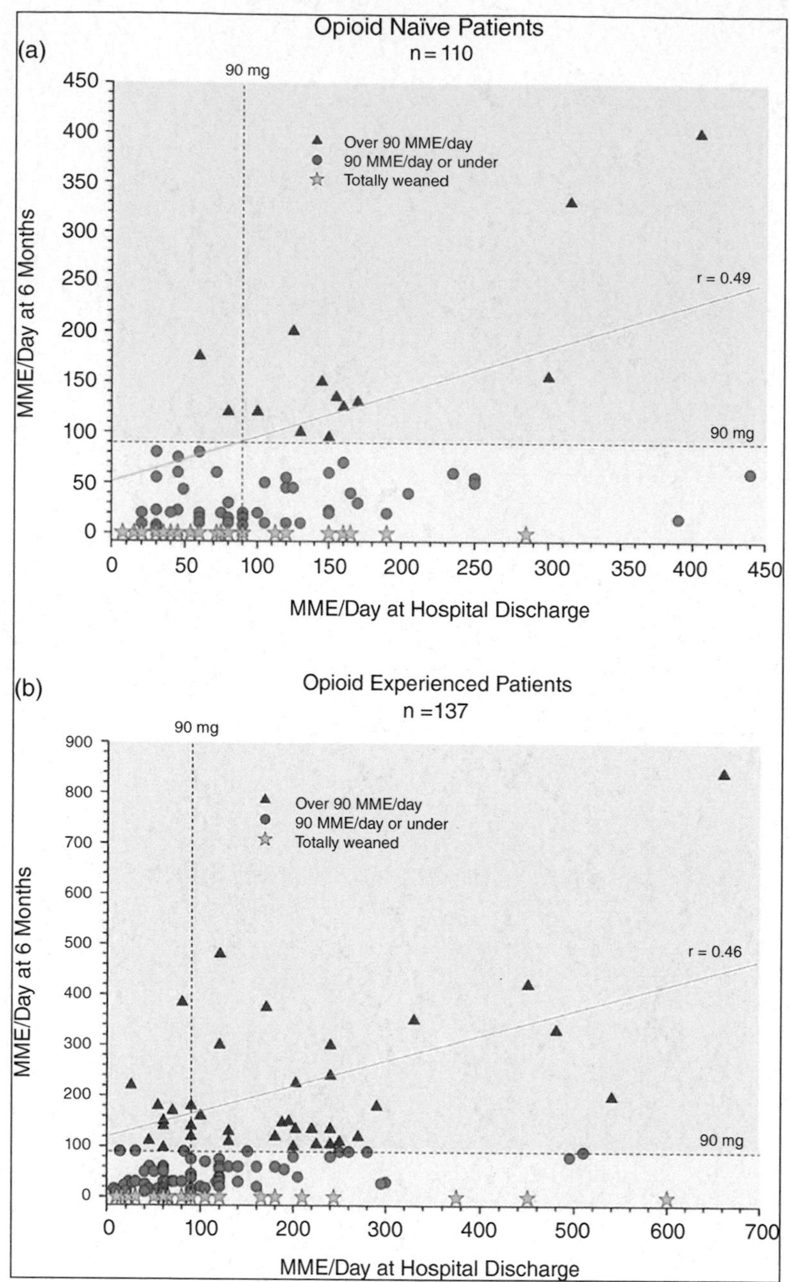

Plate 6 Mean daily opioid use in mg morphine equivalents (MME/day) at the end of Transitional Pain Service (TPS) treatment 6 months after surgery shown as a function of MME/day at hospital discharge prior to the first outpatient TPS visit among 110 patients who were not taking opioids before surgery (opioid-naïve) and 137 who were (opioid experienced). Also shown is the best-fitting straight line and correlation between MME/day at hospital discharge and at 6 months indicating that 21% and 24% of the latter dose can be predicted by the former for opioid-naïve and opioid experienced patients, respectively. The maximum dose of 90 MME/day recommended by the USA and Canadian opioid guideline is depicted by the dashed lines. Based on the maximum recommended dose, patients in the two lower quadrants (green shading) represent TPS treatment successes and those in the two upper quadrants (red shading) represent TPS treatment failures. Green circles represent patients who were under 90 MME/day at the end of TPS treatment 6 months after hospital discharge; cyan stars represent patients who were totally weaned (MME/day = 0) by 6 months; red triangles represent patients who were over 90 MME/day at 6 months. Adapted from Clarke et al. [18] with permission.

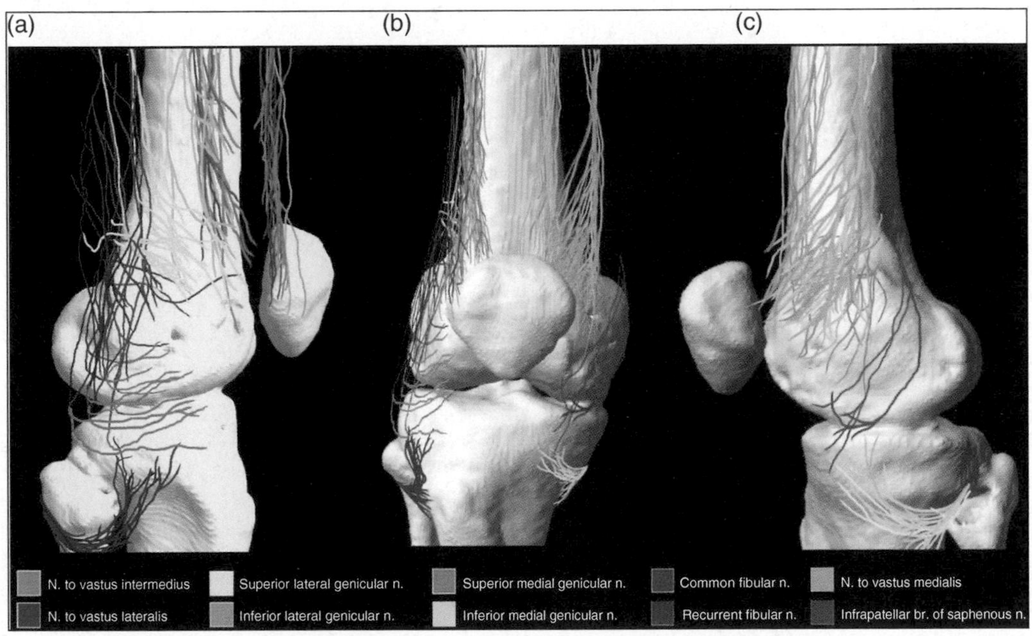

Plate 7 Articular branches of the anterior capsule of knee. Image courtesy of Dr. Philip Peng.

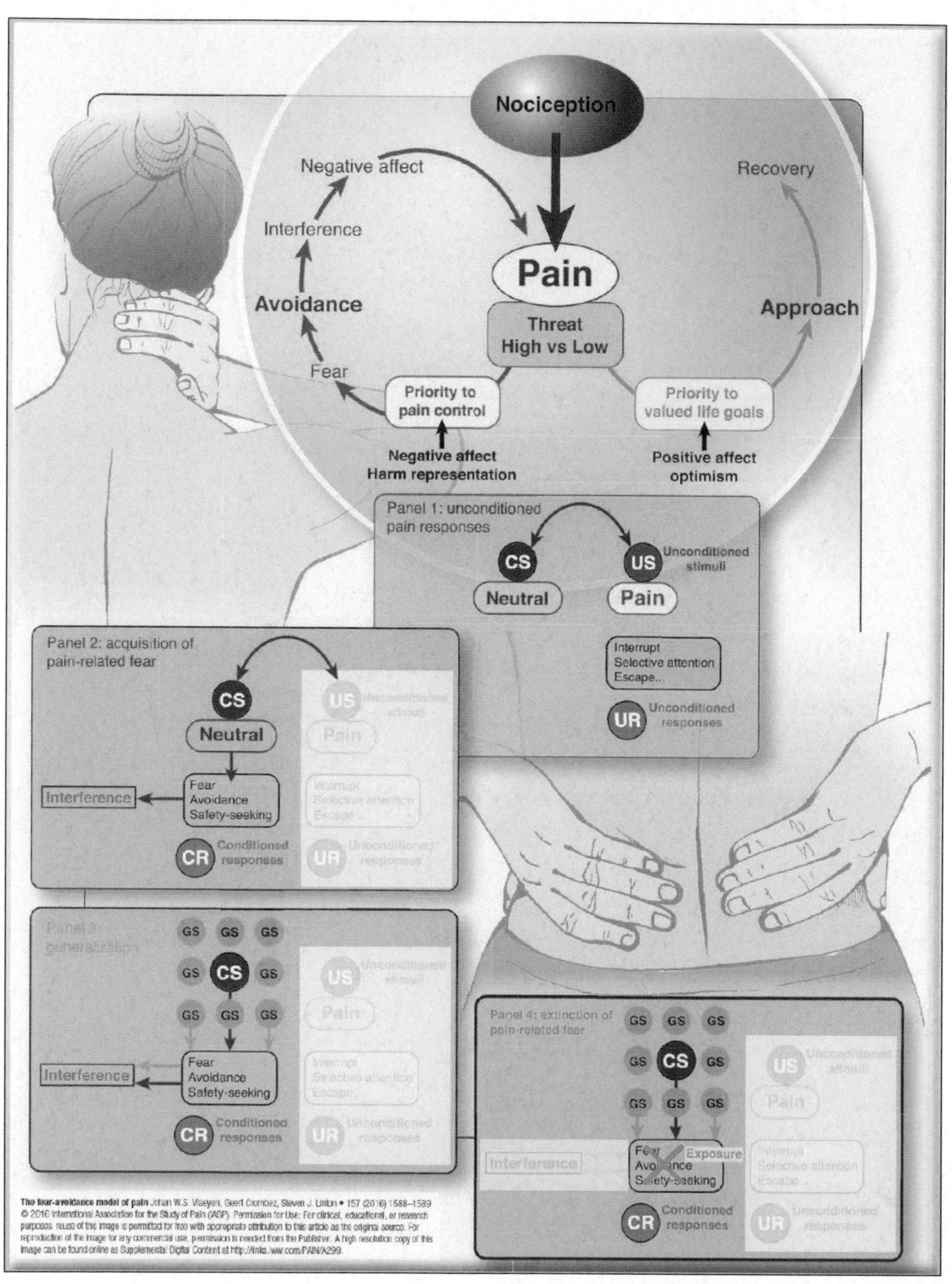

Plate 8 The fear-avoidance model of pain. Source: Vlaeyen et al. 2016.

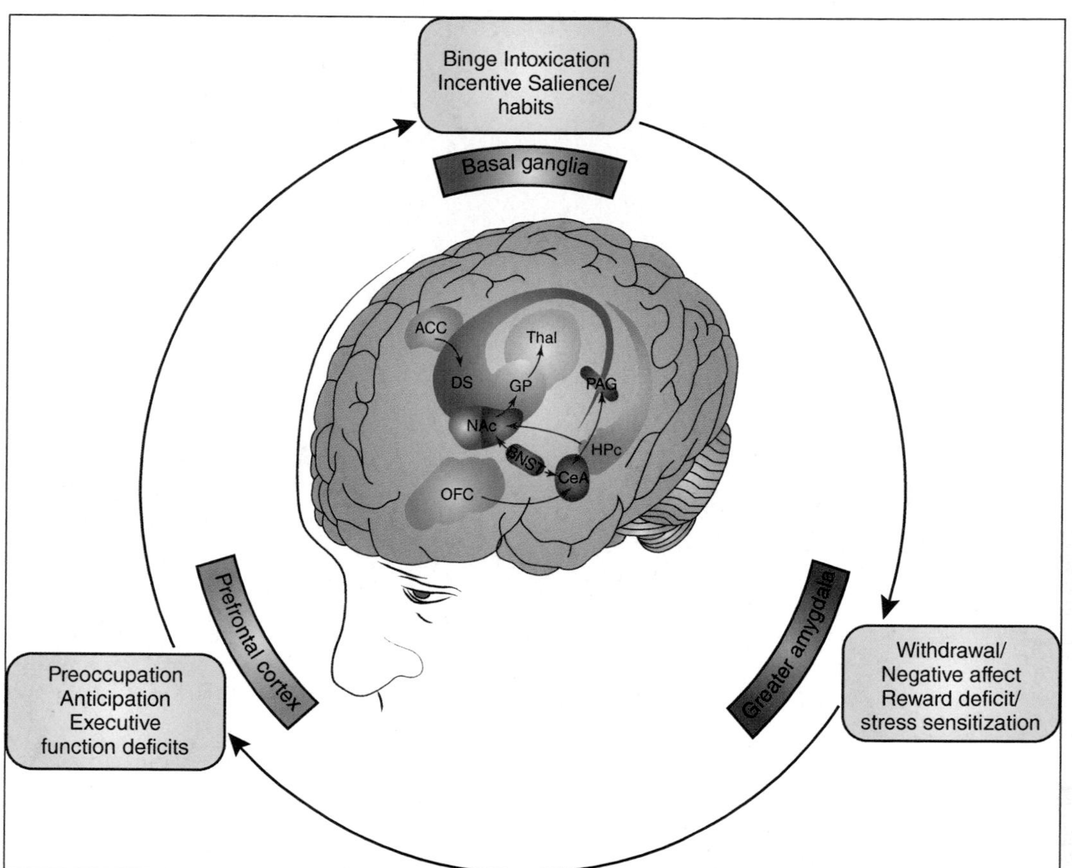

Plate 9 Stages of the addiction cycle. During intoxication, drug-induced activation of the brain's reward regions (in blue) is enhanced by conditioned cues in areas of increased sensitization (in green). During withdrawal, the activation of brain regions involved in emotions (in pink) results in negative mood and enhanced sensitivity to stress. During preoccupation, the decreased function of the prefrontal cortex leads to an inability to balance the strong desire for the drug with the will to abstain, which triggers relapse and reinitiates the cycle of addiction. The compromised neurocircuitry reflects the disruption of the dopamine and glutamate systems and the stress-control systems of the brain, which are affected by corticotropin-releasing factor and dynorphin. The behaviors during the three stages of addiction change as a person transitions from drug experimentation to addiction as a function of the progressive neuroadaptations that occur in the brain. ACC, anterior cingulate cortex; BNST, basal nucleus of the stria terminalis; CeA, central nucleus of the amygdala – change to Amyg on diagram (Amyg, central nucleaus of the amygdala); DS, dorsal striatum; GP, globus pallidus; HPC, hippocampus; NAC, nucleus accumbens; OFC, orbitofrontal cortex; PAG, periaqueductal gray; Thal, thalamus [Modified with permission from Koob and Volkow 105].

tionship to patient characteristics and current adjustment. *Pain* **17**:33–44.

37 Harland NJ, Georgieff K. (2003) Development of the coping strategies questionnaire 24, a clinically utilitarian version of the Coping Strategies Questionnaire. *Rehabil Psychol* **48(4)**:296–300.

38 Riley JL, Robinson ME. (1997) CSQ: Five factors of fiction? *Clin J Pain* **12(2)**:156–62.

39 Sullivan MJL, Bishop S, Pivik J. (1995) The pain catastrophizing scale: development and validation. *Psychol Assessm* **7**:524–32.

40 Wheeler CHB, Williams ACC, Morley SJ. (2019) Meta-analysis of the psychometric properties of the Pain Catastrophizing Scale and associations with participant characteristics. *Pain* **160(9)**:1946–53.

41 Scott W, Wideman TH, Sullivan MJL. (2014) Clinically meaningful scores on pain catastrophizing before and after multidisciplinary rehabilitation: a prospective study of individuals with subacute pain after whiplash injury. *Clin J Pain* **30(3)**:183–190.

42 Crombez G, Bijttebier P, Eccleston C, Mascagni T, Mertens G, Goubert L, Verstraeten K. (2003) The child version of the pain catastrophizing scale (PCS-C): a preliminary validation. *Pain* **104(3)**: 639–46.

43 Cano A, Leonard MT, Franz A. (2005) The significant other version of the Pain Catastrophizing Scale (PCS-S): preliminary validation. *Pain* **119(1-3)**:26–37.

44 Goubert L, Eccleston C, Vervoort T, Jordan A, Crombez G. (2006) Parental catastrophizing about their child's pain. The parent version of the Pain Catastrophizing Scale (PCS-P): a preliminary validation. *Pain* **123(3)**:254–63.

45 Darnall BD, Sturgeon JA, Cook KF et al. (2017) Development and validation of a Daily Pain Catastrophizing Scale. *J Pain* **18(9)**:1139–49.

46 Adams H, Thibault P, Ellis T, Moore E, Sullivan M. (2017) The relation between catastrophizing and occupational disability in individuals with major depression: concurrent and prospective associations. *J Occup Rehabil* **27(3)**:405–12.

47 Burns JW, Day MA, Thorn BE. (2012) Is reduction in pain catastrophizing a therapeutic mechanism specific to cognitive-behavioral therapy for chronic pain? *Transl Behav Med* **2(1)**:22–29.

48 Burns JW, Kubilus A, Bruehl S, Harden RN, Lofland K. (2003) Do changes in cognitive factors influence outcome following multidisciplinary treatment for chronic pain? A cross-lagged panel analysis. *J Consult Clin Psychol* **71(1)**:81–91.

49 Sullivan MJL, Adams H, Rhodenizer T, Stanish WD. (2006) A psychosocial risk factor--targeted intervention for the prevention of chronic pain and disability following whiplash injury. *Physical Ther* **86(1)**:8–18.

50 Sullivan MJL, Stanish WD. (2003) Psychologically-based occupational rehabilitation: the Pain-Disability Prevention Program. *Clin J Pain* **19(2)**:97–104.

51 Turner JA, Holtzman S, Mancl L. (2007) Mediators, moderators, and predictors of therapeutic change in cognitive-behavioral therapy for chronic pain. *Pain* **127(3)**:276–286.

52 Smeets RJ, Vlaeyen JW, Kester AD, Knottnerus JA. (2006) Reduction of pain catastrophizing mediates the outcome of both physical and cognitive-behavioral treatment in chronic low back pain. *J Pain* **7(4)**:261–71.

53 Spinhoven P, Ter Kuile M, Kole-Snijders AM, Hutten Mansfeld M, Den Ouden DJ, Vlaeyen JW. (2004) Catastrophizing and internal pain control as mediators of outcome in the multidisciplinary treatment of chronic low back pain. *Eur J Pain* **8(3)**:211–9.

54 Vowles KE, Gross RT, Sorrell JT. (2004) Predicting work status following interdisciplinary treatment for chronic pain. *Eur J Pain* **8(4)**:351–8.

55 Vowles KE, McCracken LM, Eccleston C. (2007) Processes of change in treatment for chronic pain: the contributions of pain, acceptance, and catastrophizing. *Euro J Pain* **11(7)**:779–87.

56 Brison RJ, Hartling L, Dostaler S *et al.* (2005) A randomized controlled trial of an educational intervention to prevent the chronic pain of whiplash associated disorders following rear-end motor vehicle collisions. *Spine* **30(16)**:1799–807.

57 Wideman TH, Sullivan MJL. (2011) Reducing catastrophic thinking associated with pain. *Pain Manag* **1**:249–56.

58 Flink IK, Boersma K, Linton SJ. (2014) Changes in catastrophizing and depressed mood during and after early cognitive behaviorally oriented interventions for pain. *Cogn Behav Ther* **43(4)**:332–41.

59 Gilliam WP, Craner JR, Morrison EJ, Sperry JA. (2017) The mediating effects of the different dimensions of pain catastrophizing on outcomes

in an interdisciplinary pain rehabilitation program. *Clin J Pain* **33(5)**:443–51.

60 Vowles KE, McCracken LM, Eccleston C. (2007) Processes of change in treatment for chronic pain: the contributions of pain, acceptance, and catastrophizing. *Eur J Pain* **11(7)**:779–87.

61 Schutze R, Rees C, Smith A, Slater H, Campbell JM, O'Sullivan P. (2018) How can we best reduce pain catastrophizing in adults with chronic noncancer pain? A systematic review and meta-analysis. *J Pain* **19(3)**:233–56.

62 Gardner-Nix J, Backman S, Barbati J, Grummitt J. (2008) Evaluating distance education of a mindfulness-based meditation programme for chronic pain management. *J Telemed Telecare* **14(2)**:88–92.

63 Turner JA, Anderson ML, Balderson BH, Cook AJ, Sherman KJ, Cherkin DC. (2016) Mindfulness-based stress reduction and cognitive behavioral therapy for chronic low back pain: similar effects on mindfulness, catastrophizing, self-efficacy, and acceptance in a randomized controlled trial. *Pain* **157(11)**:2434–44.

64 Williams AC, Eccleston C, Morley S. (2012) Psychological therapies for the management of chronic pain (excluding headache) in adults. *Cochrane Database Syst Rev* **11**:CD007407.

65 Kori S, Miller R, Todd D. (1990) Kinesiophobia: A new view of chronic pain behavior. *Pain Manag* **1990**:35–43.

66 Waddell G, Newton M, Henderson I, Somerville D, Main CJ. (1993) A Fear-Avoidance Beliefs Questionnaire (FABQ) and the role of fear-avoidance beliefs in chronic low back pain and disability. *Pain* **52**:157–68.

67 McCracken LM, Zayfert C, Gross RT. (1992) The Pain Anxiety Symptoms Scale: development and validation of a scale to measure fear of pain. *Pain* **50(1)**:67–73.

68 Roelofs J, Sluiter JK, Frings-Dresen MH *et al.* (2007) Fear of movement and (re)injury in chronic musculoskeletal pain: evidence for an invariant two-factor model of the Tampa Scale for Kinesiophobia across pain diagnoses and Dutch, Swedish, and Canadian samples. *Pain* **131(1-2)**:181–90.

69 Woby SR, Roach NK, Urmston M, Watson PJ. (2005) Psychometric properties of the TSK-11: a shortened version of the Tampa Scale for Kinesiophobia. *Pain* **117(1-2)**:137–44.

70 Lundberg M, Grimby-Ekman A, Verbunt J, Simmonds MJ. (2011) Pain-related fear: a critical review of the related measures. *Pain Res Treat* **2011**:494196.

71 Bailey KM, Carleton RN, Vlaeyen JW, Asmundson GJ. (2010) Treatments addressing pain-related fear and anxiety in patients with chronic musculoskeletal pain: a preliminary review. *Cogn Behav Ther* **39(1)**:46–63.

72 Staal JB, Hlobil H, Twisk JW, Smid T, Koke AJ, van Mechelen W. (2004) Graded activity for low back pain in occupational health care: a randomized, controlled trial. *Annals Intern Med* **140(2)**:77–84.

73 Waddell G. (2004) *The Back Pain Revolution*. Churchill Livingstone, Edinburgh.

74 de Jong JR, Vlaeyen JW, Onghena P, Goossens ME, Geilen M, Mulder H. (2005) Fear of movement/(re)injury in chronic low back pain: education or exposure in vivo as mediator to fear reduction? *Clin J Pain* **21(1)**:9–17.

75 Moseley GL, Vlaeyen JW. (2015) Beyond nociception: the imprecision hypothesis of chronic pain. *Pain* **156(1)**:35–8.

76 Asenlof P, Denison E, Lindberg P. (2005) Individually tailored treatment targeting activity, motor behavior, and cognition reduces pain-related disability: a randomized controlled trial in patients with musculoskeletal pain. *J Pain* **6(9)**:588–603.

77 Goubert L, Francken G, Crombez G, Vansteenwegen D, Lysens R. (2002) Exposure to physical movement in chronic back pain patients - no evidence for generalization across different movements. *Behav Res Ther* **40**:415–29.

78 Thorn B, Boothy J, Sullivan MJL. (2002) Targeted treatment of catastrophizing for the management of chronic pain. *Cogn Behav Prac* **9**:127–38.

79 Meulders A. (2020) Fear in the context of pain: lssons learned from 100 years of fear conditioning research. *Behav Res Ther* **131**:103635.

80 Hayes SC, Strosahl KD, Wilson KG. (1999) *Acceptance and Commitment Therapy: An Experiential Approach to Behavior Change*. Guilford Press, New York.

81 Vowles KE, McCracken LM. (2008) Acceptance and values-based action in chronic pain: a study of treatment effectiveness and process. *J Consult Clin Psychol* **76(3)**:397–407.

Part 7

Complementary Therapies

Chapter 28

Complementary and Integrative Approaches for Pain Relief

Inna Belfer, Wen Chen, Emmeline Edwards, David Shurtleff, & Helene Langevin

National Center for Complementary and Integrative Health (NCCIH), National Institutes of Health (NIH), Bethesda, Maryland, USA

Complementary health approaches include a broad range of practices, interventions, and natural products that are not typically part of conventional medical care (Table 28.1). The term *complementary* refers to the use of these approaches together with conventional therapies and is increasingly preferred to the term *alternative*, which denotes usage as a substitute for standard care [1].

The term *integrative health* care refers to conventional and complementary approaches used together in a coordinated way. Integrative health also emphasizes care of the whole person that aims to improve health in multiple interconnected domains: social, psychological, and physical, including multiple organs and systems (Figure 28.1) [1].

Painful conditions are the most common reasons why American adults use complementary health approaches [2]. About 40 million American adults experience severe pain in any given year [3], and they spend more than $14 billion out-of-pocket on complementary approaches to manage their pain [4]. The International Association for the Study of Pain recently revised its definition of pain to "...an unpleasant sensory and emotional experience associated with, or resembling that associated with, actual or potential tissue damage [5]." This new definition acknowledges that pain and nociception are different phenomena and that pain cannot be inferred solely from activity in sensory neurons. Many complementary and integrative health approaches are multimodal in nature and may contribute to pain relief by impacting several pain-processing structures simultaneously, and they address the cognitive, emotional, and physical complexities associated with pain.

Chronic pain management is often refractory to conventional medical approaches, and standard pharmacologic approaches have substantial drawbacks. Health care guidelines of the American College of Physicians and other professional organizations recognize the value of certain complementary approaches as adjuncts to pharmacologic management.[6][7] Research has shown that some complementary health modalities may reduce some pain conditions, including acupuncture, spinal manipulation, and yoga for chronic back pain and tai chi for fibromyalgia [8, 9, 10, 11, 12]

Categories of Complementary and Integrative Health Approaches Based on Primary Therapeutic Input

Although complementary approaches vary greatly, it is useful to classify them by their primary therapeutic input, which may be dietary (e.g. special diets,

Clinical Pain Management: A Practical Guide, Second Edition. Edited by Mary E. Lynch, Kenneth D. Craig, and Philip W. Peng.

Table 28.1 Glossary of Complementary Health Approaches Used for Managing Pain

Term	Definition
Acupuncture and acupressure	A family of procedures involving stimulation of defined anatomic points, a component of the major Asian medical traditions; most common application involves the insertion and manipulation of thin metallic needles
Ayurvedic medicine	The major East Indian traditional medicine system; treatment includes meditation, diet, exercise, herbs and elimination regimens (using emetics and diarrheals)
Biofeedback	The use of electronic devices to help people learn to consciously control body functions such as breathing and heart rate
Herbs	Herbal supplements—sometimes called botanicals—are a type of dietary supplement containing one or more herbs.
Hypnosis	The induction of an altered state of consciousness characterized by increased responsiveness to suggestion
Massage	Manual therapies that manipulate muscle and connective tissues to promote muscle relaxation, healing and sense of well-being
Meditation	A group of practices, largely based in Eastern spiritual traditions, intended to focus or control attention and obtain greater awareness of the present moment, or mindfulness
Mindfulness-based stress reduction	A type of meditation initially developed to help manage stress, but which has evolved to encompass the treatment of a variety of health-related conditions such as anxiety, depression and pain
Naturopathy	A clinical discipline that emphasizes a holistic approach to the patient, herbal medications, diet and exercise
Probiotics	Live microorganisms that are intended to have health benefits when consumed or applied to the body. They can be found in yogurt and other fermented foods, dietary supplements and beauty products.
Relaxation techniques	Relaxation techniques include a number of practices such as progressive relaxation, guided imagery, biofeedback, self-hypnosis and deep breathing exercises. The goal is similar in all: to produce the body's natural relaxation response, characterized by slower breathing, lower blood pressure and a feeling of increased well-being.
Spinal manipulation	A range of manual techniques, employed by chiropractors and osteopathic physicians, for adjustments of the spine to affect neuromuscular function and other health outcomes
Tai chi	A mind and body practice originating in China that involves slow, gentle movements and sometimes is described as "moving meditation"
Traditional Chinese medicine	A medical system that uses acupuncture, herbal mixtures, massage, exercise and diet
Yoga	An exercise practice, originally East Indian, that combines breathing exercises, physical postures and meditation

herbs), psychological (e.g. meditation), physical (e.g. massage, acupuncture) or the combination of psychological and physical (e.g. yoga).

Primary Dietary Input

Natural products, including plants and animal products, have been used for millennia for pain relief, and have been the source of many drugs (e.g. salicylates, opioids). Recent research to identify new sources of analgesics based on natural products also has yielded valuable tools for probing the molecular features of pain pathways. Coupled with human genetics, preclinical animal models, and clinical pharmacology, natural products have provided critical insights into the molecular basis of pain sensation and helped to validate new targets for pain relief.

Plant-Derived

Research has examined the effects of cannabis or cannabinoids on chronic pain, particularly neuropathic pain, and has found low- to moderate-quality evidence that these medicines produced better pain relief than placebos [13, 14]. Resiniferatoxin (RTX), produced by

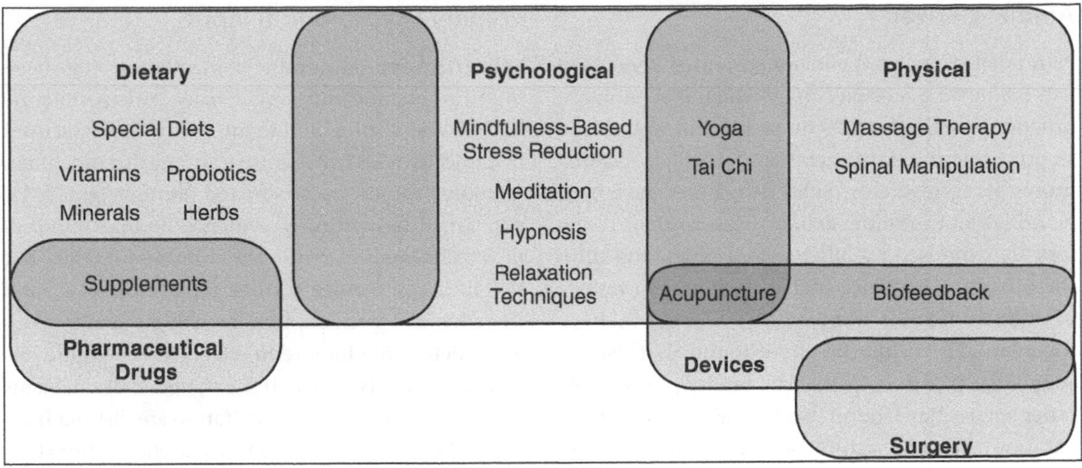

Figure 28.1 The integration of complementary and integrative health interventions with traditional drug-based and/or surgical pain management [1].

euphorbias, is effective as a long-duration, nonopioid single-administration treatment for bone cancer pain [15]. In recent laboratory studies, conolidine, derived from *Tabernaemontana divaricata*, is efficacious in pain assays and appears to have analgesic properties; however, its mechanism of action remains unknown [16]. There is some evidence that enteric-coated peppermint oil capsules may be modestly efficacious in reducing abdominal pain associated with irritable bowel syndrome (IBS) [17]. Devil's claw and white willow bark (taken orally) may be helpful for low-back pain over the short term [18]. Two compounds in kratom (*Mitragyna speciosa*) leaves, mitragynine and 7-hydroxymitragynine, interact with opioid receptors in the brain, decreasing pain when taken in high doses [19]; however, to date, there are no clinical trials to evaluate the health effects of kratom or to determine if kratom is an effective or safe treatment for any pain condition or for opioid addiction.

Challenges in the assessment of plant products include their complexity and variability, including possible instability of active components or the presence of impurities, conflicting or unreliable conclusions in the literature, and low statistical power of studies [20]. Further, there is a paucity of data on the safety of many products, including the safety of their use in a 21st century context (e.g. if taken with modern prescription drugs) [20, 21, 22] and their appropriate use in the context of traditional or indigenous practices.

Microbial-Derived

Botulinum toxin may relieve pain by blocking substance P and calcitonin gene-related peptide (CGRP) within the central nervous system, leading to reduction of central sensitization. It may also cause peripheral decreases of substance P, CGRP, glutamate, and TRPV receptor translocation, leading to a block of peripheral sensitization [23]. In addition, anthrax toxins are being studied as a molecular platform to target pain, and asymptomatic bacteriuria (ASB) strains of *E. coli* are being investigated for their analgesic properties [24]. There is some evidence that suggests some probiotics may improve abdominal pain from IBS; however, benefits have not been conclusively demonstrated, and not all probiotics have the same effects [25].

Marine-Based

Snail venoms have potentially valuable effects, including inhibition of pain without the potential for addiction, but they are peptides, and delivery to target sites is challenging [26]. The one marketed pain medicine derived from snail venom, ziconotide (Prialt), cannot cross the blood-brain barrier and therefore can only be administered intrathecally. For this reason, although ziconotide has advantages over morphine, it's only used when morphine is not a possibility [27].

Animal-Derived

Pain relief is one of the many purported benefits of fish oil, but the mechanism by which fish oil might produce beneficial effects for pain is not well understood. Omega-3 fatty acids and their specialized proresolving mediator (SPM) derivatives have both neuronal and immune actions because their receptors are expressed by different cell types, and thus, there is some evidence that they may help resolve both inflammation and pain [28]. Clinical trials on rheumatoid arthritis (RA) have found that fish oil supplements may help alleviate tender joints, while other studies have found that fish oil may reduce the daily nonsteroidal anti-inflammatory drug requirement of RA patients [29].

Vitamins

Laboratory studies have demonstrated that pretreatment and continuous treatment with nicotinamide riboside (NR), a vitamin B isoform, prevents the tactile hypersensitivity associated with paclitaxel-induced peripheral neuropathy, and behavioral testing has shown that animals treated with NR did not have an increase in pain behavior [30].

Riboflavin, also known as vitamin B_2, has been demonstrated as safe and effective prophylactic therapy for the prevention of migraines, especially in adults [31].

Primary Psychological and Physical Input

The evidence base for the effectiveness of mind and body practices is still relatively incomplete, but a few rigorous examples where there is promise of usefulness and safety include acupuncture and tai chi for pain associated with osteoarthritis (OA) of the knee [32, 33, 34, 35]; massage for neck pain [36]; tai chi for fibromyalgia [37]; relaxation techniques for headaches and migraine [38, 39]; and acupuncture, massage, yoga, and spinal manipulation for chronic back pain [7, 40]. New research is shedding light on the effects of meditation and acupuncture on central mechanisms of pain processing and perception and regulation of emotion and attention [41].

Primary Psychological Input

Mindfulness. Mindfulness meditation has been found to significantly reduce pain in experimental and clinical settings and to improve a wide spectrum of clinically relevant cognitive and health outcomes, including for low-back pain and fibromyalgia [7, 42, 43]. There is increasing evidence linking mindfulness techniques to improved immune function, but the findings require further replication [44], and there haven't been enough large, high-quality studies to determine long-term effects in rheumatic disease [45, 46]. It is unclear if the analgesic mechanisms supporting mindfulness meditation are distinct from or parallel to those engaged by placebo and/or slow, rhythmic breathing; however, there is emerging evidence suggesting that mindfulness meditation engages multiple unique neural mechanisms not mediated by endogenous opioids to reduce pain [47].

Hypnosis. A growing body of evidence suggests that hypnosis may be useful to manage some painful conditions [48, 49]. Findings from a few studies have demonstrated that training patients in the use of self-hypnosis significantly reduced their need for sedatives and analgesia when undergoing interventional radiological procedures [50].

Biofeedback. The efficacy of biofeedback has been evaluated in numerous studies for tension headaches, with positive results. Several studies have shown biofeedback decreased the frequency of both pediatric and adult migraines, with some showing an effect lasting over an average follow-up phase of 17 months [51, 52].

Placebo. Contextual factors, including patient–clinician interactions and the expectation of benefit, can contribute to improvements in pain. Although this phenomenon is called the "placebo effect," it can occur with any treatment, not just placebos, and may lead to enhanced outcomes [21, 53]. Understanding psychoneurobiological mechanisms underlying placebo analgesia may lead to shaping the clinician–patient relationship, reducing the use of analgesic drugs, and training the patient to become an active agent of the therapy [54].

Primary Physical Input

Acupuncture. For patients with low-back pain, acupuncture has been associated with lower pain intensity compared to usual care or simulated acupuncture [33]. Acupuncture can be a helpful and reasonable referral option for other chronic pain conditions [33], including fibromyalgia [55], headaches [33. 56], and OA [32, 57, 58]. Auricular acupuncture, either as a stand-alone therapy or as an adjunct technique, has shown potential benefits for acute pain relief [59].

Spinal manipulation. Spinal manipulation has been shown to produce modest, short-term effects on chronic low-back pain [6, 7]. Other studies have found that spinal manipulation is as effective as other interventions for reducing pain and improving function [60, 61].

Massage. There is low- to moderate-quality evidence that massage therapy is superior to nonactive therapies in reducing arthritis pain and improving functional outcomes [62]. Massage may provide short-term relief from low-back pain, but the evidence is not of high quality [11]. There is some evidence that massage has a positive effect on migraine, tension headaches, and neck pain [56, 63].

Psychological and Physical Input

Meditative Movements. There is evidence that yoga and tai chi may be beneficial for patients with fibromyalgia [37] or chronic low-back pain [6, 7[, and there is some evidence that yoga compared to nonexercise controls results in small to moderate improvements in back-related function at 3 and 6 months [64]. Some studies have demonstrated that tai chi produces beneficial effects similar to those of standard physical therapy in the treatment of knee OA [34, 58]. Regular yoga training may be helpful in reducing knee arthritis symptoms in patients with OA or RA [65].

Combined/Multimodal Input

Complementary health approaches are often used in combination, both in traditional health systems (e.g. traditional Chinese medicine) and in modern integrative practice [66]. The U.S. Veterans Health Administration uses a multimodal model of pain care that emphasizes nonpharmacologic methods, both conventional (e.g. physical therapy, cognitive behavioral therapy) and complementary (e.g. yoga, acupuncture), and may also include nutrition consultations [67].

Classic randomized controlled trial designs may not be well suited for research on multimodal complementary interventions [68, 69, 70]. Pragmatic comparative effectiveness designs with "usual care" comparators are widely used to study these types of interventions, and trials may need to take into account the individualization of interventions and the underlying theories of systems such as Ayurvedic medicine or naturopathy [71]. Pragmatic studies that compare multimodal treatments with usual care cannot determine which treatment components are responsible for benefits, but other kinds of translational studies can address this issue [72].

Therapeutic Output—Systems Impacted and Challenges of Mechanistic Research

As illustrated in Figure 28.2, complementary and integrative approaches whose therapeutic input is dietary, psychological, and/or physical may exert their effects, or therapeutic output, through a variety of mechanisms and impact multiple physiological systems. For example, peppermint oil may relieve pain associated with IBS by directly relaxing gastrointestinal smooth muscle [73], probiotics may have effects on the nervous system as well as the gut [74], and some components of traditional Chinese medicine [75] as well as omega-3 fatty acids and their derivatives have immune-mediated anti-inflammatory effects [28]. Interventions with psychological and/or physical therapeutic input such as meditation [76] and acupuncture [77] can have effects on the nervous system and may also target other body systems affected by the pain condition; for example, yoga may reduce low-back pain in part by increasing flexibility and core strength [78], and the stretching it involves may reduce connective tissue inflammation [79]. For all types of therapeutic input, psychosocial effects also may be important; for example, participation in an integrative group pain management program may provide tools to enable better self-management of pain [80].

While understanding the mechanisms of action of treatments is important for optimizing them, ensuring their safety, and identifying patients most likely to respond, pinpointing the mechanisms of

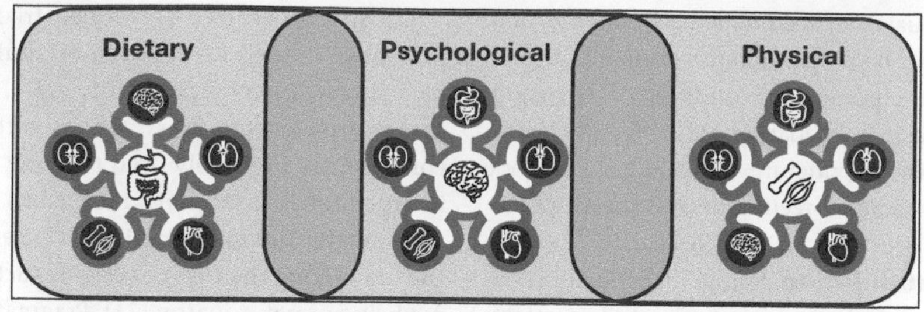

Figure 28.2 Complementary approaches that use dietary, psychological, and/or physical input may exert their therapeutic output through multiple mechanisms and may have effects on more than one physiological system.

complementary and integrative interventions is challenging because of their complex and multimodal nature [41, 80] and because their use often precedes scientific study [82, 83] Studies of complementary and integrative health approaches often require multidisciplinary expertise and use state-of-the-art techniques in areas such as neuroscience, immunology, pharmacognosy, proteomics, genetics and epigenomics. Further, there are limited preclinical pain models for complementary health interventions (e.g. no relevant model for meditative movements). Objective, validated measurement tools are essential, as are processes and procedures to ensure quality control, whether the intervention is mind- and body-based or a natural product.

Studying how mind and body approaches affect the nervous system is, in particular, scientifically challenging. This challenge is compounded by individual variability attributable to genetic, epigenetic and environmental factors. Nevertheless, recent advances in genomic science, neuroscience, stem cell research, systems biology and neuroimaging offer excellent resources and opportunities for neural mechanistic studies of complementary health approaches for pain.

Understanding biological signatures of complex natural products requires innovative approaches and tools beyond those traditionally used for analyzing a single molecule against a single mechanistic target. To move the field forward, there must be a renewed emphasis on multidisciplinary high-impact approaches to overcome conceptual, methodological and technological hurdles that hinder advances in natural products research. Regulatory challenges for studying natural products such as cannabis and kratom must also be addressed.

General Challenges with Integrating Complementary Approaches into Pain Medicine

Although patient self-report is the gold standard for assessing pain [84], the development of objective pain biomarkers to evaluate the efficacy of pain treatments may accelerate research and improve care [85]. For example, improved objective assessments such as imaging, biopsy and/or electrophysiological recordings of tissues involved in myofascial pain syndrome will be an important step toward incorporating soft tissues into the phenotyping of patients with "nonspecific" musculoskeletal pain [86]. Research is needed on complex chronic pain phenotypes, as there is increasing recognition that chronic pain conditions are heterogenous and that multiple pain conditions may overlap.[86] Recent research has linked specific genotypes to pain conditions. For example, a genome-wide association study identified a single nucleotide polymorphism associated with temporomandibular disorder in males [88], and research has identified blood gene expression markers for pain, which may allow for a precision medicine approach to treatment [89].

Primary prevention of pain can be considered the reduction of the functional impact/magnitude of acute pain, secondary prevention as the prevention of acute-to-chronic pain transition and tertiary prevention as decreasing the effect of chronic pain on overall health and quality of life [90]. Complementary health approaches may be helpful in secondary and tertiary prevention [90]. For example, studies have investigated acceptance and commitment therapy for prevention of postsurgical chronic pain [91]. Integrative health approaches may also have a role in health restoration efforts that may reduce the risk or severity of pain. Mind and body exercises and hands-on movement reeducation may correct faulty movement habits and offer opportunities to prevent or reverse tissue abnormalities and reduce pain [72, 92].

Implementation of complementary and integrative modalities for pain may be hindered by administrative barriers in health care settings, difficulties in providing access to services and limited insurance coverage. The Veterans Health Administration, a highly integrated health system, has successfully implemented multimodal integrative approaches; however, implementation of these approaches will be more challenging in private practice and community settings.[92] The national opioid crisis has provided an impetus for implementation of nonopioid pain management approaches; one component of the National Institutes of Health's major Helping to End Addiction Long-term (HEAL) Initiative specifically focuses on integrating nonopioid approaches into health care and includes research on acupuncture and mindfulness-based stress reduction [94].

Conclusions

Much pain research has been narrowly focused, reflecting the specific interests of the disciplines studying it, such as neuroscience and orthopedics. There is a need for cross-disciplinary research that can bridge between these disciplines and bring their knowledge together to enhance the treatment of pain. Research on integrative health practices can provide this bridge and encourage a "whole person" approach to pain.

Acknowledgments

The authors would like to thank Ms. Shawn Stout for contributing her writing and editorial expertise to the development of this chapter.

References

1 National Center for Complementary and Integrative Health. (2018) Complementary, Alternative, or Integrative Health: What's in a Name? Available at;https://www.nccih.nih.gov/health/complementary-alternative-or-integrative-health-whats-in-a-name. Accessed October 13, 2021.

2 Black LI, Clarke TC, Barnes PM, Stussman BJ, Nahin RL. (2015) Use of complementary health approaches among children aged 4–17 years in the United States: National Health Interview Survey, 2007–2012. National Health Statistics reports; no 78. National Center for Health Statistics, Hyattsville.

3 Nahin RL. (2015) Estimates of pain prevalence and severity in adults: United States, 2012. *J Pain* **16(8)**:769–80.

4 Nahin RL, Barnes PM, Stussman BJ. (2016) *Expenditures on complementary health approaches: United States, 2012*. National Health Statistics Reports. National Center for Health Statistics, Hyattsville.

5 International Association for the Study of Pain. (2020) *IASP announces revised definition of pain.* IASP, Washington, DC. Available at: https://www.iasp-pain.org/PublicationsNews/NewsDetail.aspx?ItemNumber=10475&navItemNumber=643. Accessed October 13, 2021.

6 Chou R, Deyo R, Friedly J, *et al.* (2017) Nonpharmacologic therapies for low back pain: a systematic review for an American College of Physicians clinical practice guideline. *Ann Intern Med* **166(7)**:493–505.

7 Qaseem A, Wilt TJ, McLean RM, Forceia MA. (2017) Clinical Guidelines Committee of the American College of Physicians. Noninvasive treatments for acute, subacute, and chronic low back pain: a clinical practice guideline from the American College of Physicians. *Ann Intern Med* **166(7)**:514–30.

8 Lee J-H, Choi T-Y, Lee MS, Lee H, Shin B-C, Lee H. (2013) Acupuncture for acute low back pain: a systematic review. *Clin J Pain* **29(2)**:172–85.

9 Hasegawa TM, Baptista AS, de Souza MC, Yoshizumi AM, Natour J. (2014) Acupuncture for acute non-specific low back pain: a randomised, controlled, double-blind, placebo trial. *Acupunct Med* **32(2)**:109–15.

10 Vas J, Aranda JM, Modesto M *et al.* (2012). Acupuncture in patients with acute low back pain: a multicentre randomised controlled clinical trial. *Pain* **153(9)**:1883–89.

11 Furlan AD, Imamura M, Dryden T, Irvin E. (2008) Massage for low-back pain. *Cochrane Database Syst Rev*. **(4)**:CD001929.

12 Williams K, Abildso C, Steinberg L *et al.* (2009) Evaluation of the effectiveness and efficacy of

Iyengar yoga therapy on chronic low back pain. *Spine (Phila Pa 1976)* **34(**19**)**:2066–76.
13 Stockings E, Campbell G, Hall WD *et al.* (2018) Cannabis and cannabinoids for the treatment of people with chronic noncancer pain conditions: a systematic review and meta-analysis of controlled and observational studies. *Pain* **159(**10**)**:1932–54.
14 Mücke M, Phillips T, Radbruch L, Petzke F, Häuser W. (2018) Cannabis-based medicines for chronic neuropathic pain in adults. *Cochrane Database Syst Rev* **3(**3**)**:CD012182.
15 Brown DC, Agnello K, Iadarola MJ. (2015) Intrathecal resiniferatoxin in a dog model: efficacy in bone cancer pain. *Pain* **156(**6**)**:1018–1024.
16 Tarselli MA, Raehal KM, Brasher AK *et al.* (2011) Synthesis of conolidine, a potent non-opioid analgesic for tonic and persistent pain. *Nat Chem* **3(**6**)**:449–53.
17 Ford AC, Moayyedi P, Chey WD *et al.* American College of Gastroenterology monograph on management of irritable bowel syndrome. *Am J Gastroenterol* **113(Suppl 2)**:1–18.
18 Oltean H, Robbins C, van Tulder MW, Berman BM, Bombardier C, Gagnier JJ. (2014) Herbal medicine for low-back *pain. Cochrane Database Syst Rev* **2014(**12**)**:CD004504.
19 Kruegel AC, Uprety R, Grinnell SG *et al.* (2019) 7-Hydroxymitragynine is an active metabolite of mitragynine and a key mediator of its analgesic effects. *ACS Cent Sc* **5(**6**)**:992–1001.
20 Sorkin BC, Kuszak AJ, Bloss G *et al.* (2020)Improving natural product research translation: from source to clinical trial. *FASEB J* **34(**1**)**:41–65.
21 Gaston TE, Mendrick DL, Paine MF, Roe AL, Yeung CK. (2020) "Natural" is not synonymous with "safe": toxicity of natural products alone and in combination with pharmaceutical agents. *Regul Toxicol Pharmacol* **113**:104642.
22 Rider CV, Walker NJ, Waidyanatha S. (2018) Getting to the root of the matter: challenges and recommendations for assessing the safety of botanical dietary supplements. *Clin Pharmacol Ther* **104(**3**)**:429–31.
23 Matak I, Tékus V, Bölcskei K, Lacković Z, Helyes Z. (2017) Involvement of substance P in the antinociceptive effect of botulinum toxin type A: evidence from knockout mice. *Neuroscience* **358**:137–45.
24 Rudick CN, Taylor AK, Yaggie RE, Schaeffer AJ, Klumpp DJ. (2014) Asymptomatic bacteriuria *Escherichia coli* are live biotherapeutics for UTI. *PLoS One* **9(**11**)**:e109321.
25 Ritchie ML, Romanuk TN. (2012) A meta-analysis of probiotic efficacy for gastrointestinal diseases. *PLoS One* **7(**4**)**:e34938.
26 Verdes A, Anand P, Gorson J *et al.* (2016)_ From mollusks to medicine: a venomics approach for the discovery and characterization of therapeutics from Terebridae peptide toxins. *Toxins (Basel)* **8(**4**)**:117.
27 McDowell GC, Saulino MF, Wallace M *et al.* (2020) Effectiveness and safety of intrathecal ziconotide: final results of the Patient Registry of Intrathecal Ziconotide Management (PRIZM). *Pain Med* 21(1):2925–38.
28 Zhang L, Terrando N, Xu Z-Z *et al.* (2018) Distinct analgesic actions of DHA and DHA-derived specialized pro-resolving mediators on post-operative pain after bone fracture in mice. *Front Pharmacol* **9**:412.
29 Galarraga B, Ho M, Youssef HM *et al.* Cod liver oil (n-3 fatty acids) as an non-steroidal anti-inflammatory drug sparing agent in rheumatoid arthritis. *Rheumatology (Oxford)* **47(**5**)**:665–9.
30 Hamity MV, White SR, Blum C, Gibson-Corley KN, Hammond DL. (2020) Nicotinamide riboside relieves paclitaxel-induced peripheral neuropathy and enhances suppression of tumor growth in tumor-bearing rats. *Pain* 161(10):2364–75.
31 Thompson DF, Saluja HS. (2017) Prophylaxis of migraine headaches with riboflavin: a systematic review. *J Clin Pharm Ther* **42(**4**)**:394–403.
32 Lin X, Huang K, Zhu G, Huang Z, Qin A, Fan S. (2016) The effects of acupuncture on chronic knee pain due to osteoarthritis: a meta-analysis. *J Bone Joint Surg Am* **98(**18**)**:1578–85.
33 Vickers AJ, Cronin AM, Maschino AC *et al.* (2012) Acupuncture for chronic pain: individual patient data meta-analysis. *Arch Intern Med* **172(**19**)**:1444–53.
34 Wang C, Schmid CH, Iversen MD *et al.* (2016) Comparative effectiveness of tai chi versus physical therapy for knee osteoarthritis: a randomized trial. *Ann Intern Med* **165(**2**)**:77–86.
35 Yan J-H, Gu WJ, Sun J, Zhang W-X, Li B-W, Pan L. (2013) Efficacy of tai chi on pain, stiffness and function in patients with osteoarthritis: a meta-analysis. *PLoS One* **8(**4**)**:e61672.

36 Patel KC, Gross A, Graham N *et al.* (2012) Massage for mechanical neck disorders. *Cochrane Database Syst Rev* **12;(9)**:CD004871.

37 Wang C, Schmid CH, Fielding RA *et al.*H(2018) Effect of tai chi versus aerobic exercise for fibromyalgia: comparative effectiveness randomized controlled trial. *BMJ* **360**:k851.

38 Cho S-J, Song T-J, Chu MK. (2017) Treatment update of chronic migraine. *Curr Pain Headache Rep* **21**(6):26.

39 Jong MC, Boers I, van Wietmarschen HA *et al.* (2019) Hypnotherapy or transcendental meditation versus progressive muscle relaxation exercises in the treatment of children with primary headaches: a multi-centre, pragmatic, randomised clinical study. *Eur J Pediatr* **178(2)**:147–54.

40 Skelly AC, Chou R, Dettori JR *et al.* (2018) Noninvasive nonpharmacological treatment for chronic pain: a systematic review. Comparative effectiveness review No. 209. AHRQ Publication No 18-EHC013-EF. Agency for Healthcare Research and Quality, Rockville.

41 Bushnell MC, Ceko M, Low LA. (2013) Cognitive and emotional control of pain and its disruption in chronic pain. *Nat Rev Neurosci* **14(7)**:502–11.

42 Macfarlane GJ, Kronisch C, Dean LE *et al.* (2017). EULAR revised recommendations for the management of fibromyalgia. *Ann Rheum Dis* **76(2)**:318–28.

43 Cherkin DC, Sherman KJ, Balderson BH *et al.* (2016) Effect of mindfulness-based stress reduction vs cognitive behavioral therapy or usual care on back pain and functional limitations in adults with chronic low back pain: a randomized clinical trial. *JAMA* **315(12)**:1240–9.

44 Black DS, Slavich GM. (2016) Mindfulness meditation and the immune system: a systematic review of randomized controlled trials. *Ann N Y Acad Sci* **1373**(1):13–24.

45 Chen L, Michalsen A. (2017) Management of chronic pain using complementary and integrative medicine. *BMJ* **357**:j1284.

46 Dissanayake RK, Bertouch JV. (2010) Psychosocial interventions as adjunct therapy for patients with rheumatoid arthritis: a systematic review. *Int J Rheum Dis* **13(4)**:324–34.

47 Wells RE, Collier J, Posey G (2020). Attention to breath sensations does not engage endogenous opioids to reduce pain. *Pain* **161**(8):1884–93.

48 Garland EL, Brintz CE, Hanley AW (2019) Mind-body therapies for opioid-treated pain: a systematic review and meta-analysis. *JAMA Intern Med* **180(1)**:91–105.

49 Thompson T, Terhune DB, Oram C *et al.* (2019) The effectiveness of hypnosis for pain relief: A systematic review and meta-analysis of 85 controlled experimental trials. *Neurosci Biobehav Rev* **99**:298–310.

50 Lang EV, Benotsch EG, Fick LJ *et al.* (2000) Adjunctive non-pharmacological analgesia for invasive medical procedures: a randomised trial. *Lancet* **355(**9214**)**:1486–90.

51 Nestoriuc Y, Martin A. (2007) Efficacy of biofeedback for migraine: a meta-analysis. *Pain* **128(**1–2**)**:111–127.

52 Stubberud A, Varkey E, McCrory DC, Pedersen SA, Linde M.B (2016) iofeedback as prophylaxis for pediatric migraine: a meta-analysis. *Pediatrics* **138(2)**:e20160675.

53 Colloca L, Jonas WB, Killen J, Miller FG, Shurtleff D. (2014) Reevaluating the placebo effect in medical practice. *Z Psychol* **222(3)**:124–7.

54 Colloca L, Klinger R, Flor H, Bingel U. (2013) Placebo analgesia: psychological and neurobiological mechanisms. *Pain* 154(4):511–14.

55 Deare JC, Zheng Z, Xue CC, Liu JP, Shang J, Scott SW, Littlejohn G. (2013) Acupuncture for treating fibromyalgia. *Cochrane Database Syst Rev* **2013(5)**:CD007070.

56 Millstine D, Chen CY, Bauer B. (2017) Complementary and integrative medicine in the management of headache. *BMJ* **357**:j1805.

57 Selfe TK, Taylor AG. (2008) Acupuncture and osteoarthritis of the knee: a review of randomized, controlled trials. *Fam Community Health* **31(3)**:247–54.

58 Kolasinski SL, Neogi T, Hochberg MC *et al.* (2020) 2019 American College of Rheumatology/ Arthritis Foundation guideline for the management of osteoarthritis of the hand, hip, and knee. *Arthritis Care Res (Hoboken)*. 72(2):149–62.

59 Jan AL, Aldridge ES, Rogers IR, Visser EJ, Bulsara MK, Niemtzow RC. (2017) Does ear acupuncture have a role for pain relief in the emergency setting? A systematic review and meta-analysis. *Med Acupunct* **29(5)**:276–89.

60 Rubinstein SM, van Middelkoop M, Assendelft WJJ, de Boer MR, van Tulder MW. (2011) Spinal

manipulative therapy for chronic low-back pain. *Cochrane Database Syst Rev* (2):CD008112.
61 Eklund A, Jensen I, Lohela-Karlsson M *et al.* (2018). The Nordic Maintenance Care Program: effectiveness of chiropractic maintenance care versus symptom-guided treatment for recurrent and persistent low back pain—a pragmatic randomized controlled trial. *PLoS One* **13(9)**:e0203029.
62 Nelson NL, Churilla JR. (2017) Massage therapy for pain and function in patients with arthritis: a systematic review of randomized controlled trials. *Am J Phys Med Rehabil* **96(9)**:665–72.
63 Sherman KJ, Cook AJ, Wellman RD *et al.* (2014) Five-week outcomes from a dosing trial of therapeutic massage for chronic neck pain. *Ann Fam Med* **12(2)**:112–20.
64 Wieland LS, Skoetz N, Pilkington K, Vempati R, D'Adamo CR, Berman BM. (2017) Yoga treatment for chronic non-specific low back pain. *Cochrane Database Syst Rev* **1(1)**:CD010671.
65 Wang Y, Lu S, Wang R *et al.* (2018) Integrative effect of yoga practice in patients with knee arthritis: a PRISMA-compliant meta-analysis. *Medicine (Baltimore).* **97(**31**)**:e11742.
66 National Center for Complementary and Integrative Health. (2013) Traditional Chinese medicine fact sheet..NCCIH, Bethesda. Available at:https://www.nccih.nih.gov/health/traditional-chinese-medicine-what-you-need-to-know. Accessed October 13, 2021.
67 Mattocks K, Rosen MI, Sellinger J *et al.* (2020) Pain care in the Department of Veterans Affairs: understanding how a cultural shift in pain care impacts provider decisions and collaboration. *Pain Medicine* 21(5):970–7.
68 Heron J. (1986) Critique of conventional research methodology. *Comp Med Res* 1:12–22.
69 Dossey L. (1995) How should alternative therapies be evaluated: an examination of fundamentals. *Altern Ther Health Med* **1(2)**:6–10, 79–85.
70 Carter B. (2003) Methodological issues and complementary therapies: researching intangibles? *Complement Ther Nurs Midwifery* **9(3)**:133–139.
71 Ijaz N, Rioux J, Elder C, Weeks J. (2019) Whole systems research methods in health care: a scoping review. *J Altern Complement Med* **25(**S1**)**:S21–51.
72 Langevin HM. (2020) Reconnecting the brain with the rest of the body in musculoskeletal pain research. *J Pain* 22(1):1–8.
73 Hills JM, Aaronson PI. (1991) The mechanism of action of peppermint oil on gastrointestinal smooth muscle. An analysis using patch clamp electrophysiology and isolated tissue pharmacology in rabbit and guinea pig. *Gastroenterology* **101(1)**:55–65.
74 Herndon CC, Wang Y-P, Lu C-L. (2020) Targeting the gut microbiota for the treatment of irritable bowel syndrome. *Kaohsiung J Med Sci* **36(3)**:160–70.
75 Wang M, Liu L, Zhang CS *et al.* (2020) Mechanism of traditional Chinese medicine in treating knee osteoarthritis. *J Pain Res* **13**:1421–9.
76 Zeidan F, Vago DR. (2016) Mindfulness meditation-based pain relief: a mechanistic account. *Ann N Y Acad Sci* **1373(1)**:114–27.
77 Napadow V, Beissner F, Lin Y, Chae Y, Harris RE. (2020) Editorial: Neural substrates of acupuncture: from peripheral to central nervous system mechanisms. *Front Neurosci* 13:1419.
78 Colgrove YM, Gravino-Dunn NS, Dinyer SC, Sis EA, Heier AC, Sharma NK. (2019) Physical and physiological effects of yoga for an underserved population with chronic low back pain. *Int J Yoga* **12(3)**:252–64.
79 Corey SM, Vizzard MA, Bouffard NA, Badger GJ, Langevin HM. (2012) Stretching of the back improves gait, mechanical sensitivity and connective tissue inflammation in a rodent model. *PLoS One* **7(1)**:e29831.
80 Bruns EB, Befus D, Wismer B *et al.* (2019) Vulnerable patients' psychosocial experiences in a group-based, integrative pain management program. *J Altern Complement Med* 25(7):719–26.
81 Colloca L, Raghuraman N, Wang Y et al. (2020). Virtual reality: physiological and behavioral mechanisms to increase individual pain tolerance limits. *Pain* 161(9):2010–21.
82 Musial F, Mist S, Warber S, Kreitzer MJ, Ritenbaugh C, Kessler C. (2019) Why and how should we integrate biomarkers into complex trials? A discussion on paradigms and clinical research strategies. *Complement Med Res* **26(5)**:343–52.
83 Bialosky JE, Beneciuk JM, Bishop MD *et al.* (2018) Unraveling the mechanisms of manual therapy: modeling an approach. *J Orthop Sports Phys Ther* **48(1)**:8–18.
84 Fillingim RB, Loeser JD, Baron R, Edwards RR. (2016) Assessment of chronic pain: domains, methods, and mechanisms. *J Pain* **17(**9 Suppl**)**:T10–20.

85 National Institutes of Health. NIH HEAL Initiative: Discovery and validation of biomarkers, endpoints, and signatures for pain conditions [internet]. NIH, Bethesda. Available at: https://heal.nih.gov/research/preclinical-translational/biomarkers. Accessed July 7, 2020.

86 National Center for Complementary and Integrative Health. Quantitative evaluations of myofascial tissues: potential impact on musculoskeletal pain research, project concept review. NCCIH, Bethesda, MD. Available at: https://www.nccih.nih.gov/grants/quantitative-evaluations-of-myofascial-tissues-potential-impact-on-musculoskeletal-pain-research. Accessed July 7, 2020.

87 Maixner W, Fillingim RB, Williams DA, Smith SB, Slade GD. (2016) Overlapping chronic pain conditions: implications for diagnosis and classification. *J Pain* **17(**9 Suppl**)**:T93–107.

88 Smith SB, Parisien M, Bair E *et al.* (2019) Genome-wide association reveals contribution of MRAS to painful temporomandibular disorder in males. *Pain* 160(3):579–91.

89 Niculescu AB, Le-Niculescu H, Levey DF *et al.* (2019) Towards precision medicine for pain: diagnostic biomarkers and repurposed drugs. *Mol Psychiatry* **24(**4**)**:501–22.

90 Gatchel RJ, Reuben DB, Dagenais S *et al.* (2018) Research agenda for the prevention of pain and its impact: Report of the work group on the prevention of acute and chronic pain of the Federal Pain Research Strategy. *J Pain* **19(**8**)**:837–51.

91 Dindo L, Zimmerman MB, Hadlandsmyth K *et al.* (2018) Acceptance and commitment therapy for prevention of chronic postsurgical pain and opioid use in at-risk veterans: a pilot randomized controlled study. *J Pain* 19(10):1211–21.

92 Cotton VA, Low LA, Villemure C, Bushnell MC. (2018) Unique autonomic responses to pain in yoga practitioners. *Psychosom Med* **80(**9**)**:791–8.

93 The National Academies of Sciences, Engineering, and Medicine. (2019) *The role of nonpharmacological approaches to pain management: proceedings of a workshop*. National Academies Press, Washington, D.C. Available at: https://www.nap.edu/catalog/25406/the-role-of-nonpharmacological-approaches-to-pain-management-proceedings-of. Accessed October 13, 2021.

94 National Institutes of Health. (2020) NIH HEAL Initiative: Pragmatic and implementation studies for the management of pain to reduce opioid prescribing (PRISM). Available at: https://heal.nih.gov/research/clinical-research/prism. Accessed October 13, 2021.

Part 8

Specific Clinical States

Chapter 29

Chronic low back pain

Eugene J. Carragee

Department of Orthopedic Surgery, Stanford University School of Medicine, Redwood City, California, USA

Introduction

Low back pain (LBP), either episodic or recurrent, is an extremely common symptom. However, only a very small proportion of persons having an episode of LBP seek medical attention. Back pain episodes, even when rising to clinical evaluation, are very rarely due to serious pathologic disease such as tumor, infection or fracture. In most instances the cause of LBP is unclear. In societies in which very heavy labor is a necessary component of subsistence living, LBP episodes resulting in an inability to perform heavy labor may threaten basic needs. However, in recent decades chronic LBP illness has become a major clinical and financial problem in industrialized societies. The treatment of non-specific LBP illness is recognized as a leading cause of "low-value care" in the United States [1]. This has been exacerbated specifically by the over-prescription, misuse and diversion of opioid medications in the United States, where LBP is the single most common reason for prescription of opioids [2]. To a great extent, non-specific LBP illness remains an enigmatic clinical entity. When there is neither serious systemic or local pathology, complex psychological, social or neurophysiological issues have been shown to often dominate the clinical picture.

Clinical evaluation

Most persons with LBP do not seek medical care. The majority of LBP episodes are benign and self- limited, although minor persistent pain or recurrences are common. In a prospective evaluation of 200 working adults, asymptomatic for LBP at baseline, followed over 5 years, nearly all subjects had at least one LBP episode during the study period [3]. In fact, there were 625 LBP episodes lasting greater than 48 hours reported: that is, middle-aged workers experience 1–2 LBP episodes per year. This is about as common as viral upper respiratory infections. Of these only 33 episodes (5%) were evaluated by a clinician. As in usual practice, the overwhelming majority of cases had no diagnosis made and no specific treatment prescribed. Only two subjects, of over 600 episodes of LBP, were found to have serious pathology on work up both had primary radicular symptoms with neurologic findings. [3]When an initial diagnostic assessment is performed in the acute period (days to several weeks of symptoms), the focus is usually on identifying or "ruling out" serious illness rather than definitively making a pathoanatomic diagnosis. This primary diagnostic evaluation usually involves a screening for "red flags" of serious disease by history and detecting systemic disease, spinal deformity and

Clinical Pain Management: A Practical Guide, Second Edition. Edited by Mary E. Lynch, Kenneth D. Craig, and Philip W. Peng.

Table 29.1 Red and yellow flags in the evaluation of low back pain.

Red flags	Yellow flags
Major trauma	Negative attitudes that back pain is harmful or potentially severely disabling
New onset age >55 years or bone disease resulting in bone fragility.	Fear-avoidance behavior, reduced activity levels, kinesophobia
Constitutional symptoms (fever, chills, weight loss), history of cancer, deep rheumatic or inflammatory disease.	An expectation that passive, rather than active, treatment will be beneficial
Recent infection, IV drug use, immune suppression,	A history of depression, anxiety, low morale and social withdrawal or isolation.
Severe pain with rest, night pain	Social, financial or compensation disincentives to recovery
Neurologic weakness or cauda equina symptoms/ signs (bowel, bladder symptoms, saddle sensory loss)	Substance abuse: tobacco, alcohol, opioid or sedative/ narcotic medication.

neurologic signs by history and examination (Table 29.1). In a large primary care setting (including primary care physical therapists), less than 1% of the 1200 patients newly referred for LBP evaluations had serious pathology [4]. Obviously, in other practices with more frequent, serious underlying diseases (such as cancer, major trauma exposure or immune suppression), this may be somewhat higher (3–4%).

It is important to clearly differentiate primary back and buttock pain from primary radicular pain (indicated by predominant leg pain, sensory changes, motor weakness or bowel and bladder disturbance) because the treatment will be very different. There is rarely any surgical or invasive intervention indicated for back pain syndromes early in the clinical course. Conversely, patients with primary neurological compression syndromes (e.g. radiculopathy from disc herniation or stenosis, neurogenic claudication symptoms and cauda equina symptoms) should be more closely evaluated and effective interventions might be indicated early on or even urgently. The treatment of neurological compression syndromes is beyond the scope of this chapter.

In the patient who does not recover good function in 4–8 weeks, a secondary diagnostic survey is indicated. This follow-on evaluation should re-examine both serious psychosocial and neurophysiological barriers to recovery ("yellow flags") and also definitely "rule out" those serious pathologic conditions considered initially (Table 29.1). Laboratory testing, erythrocyte sedimentation rate (ESR) or C-reactive protein (CRP) and imaging (most efficiently with a rapid sequence sagittal magnetic resonance scan of the lumbar spine) are extremely sensitive for inflammatory disease, infection, malignancy and insufficiency fracture [5]. These tests are so sensitive that these serious conditions are usually identified even in the early stages and very few serious pathologic findings will be missed.

Most commonly, however, only common degenerative changes are found on evaluation. Because the next phase of treatment is usually non-specific (analgesics, anti-inflammatory medication, conditioning, supportive measures and the expectant passage of time), an anatomic diagnosis of high precision is usually not pursued. It must be emphasized that a failure to report significant recovery by this time is unusual. The clinician must be concerned there are non-spinal issues (e.g. the illnesses is linked to a compensation dispute or is part of a widespread chronic pain illness or is complicated by major depression) that are contributing or predominating this patient's failure to return to usual activities.

In patients who report they are still having troubles that are highly bothersome after 3–6 months of illness, further anatomic evaluation may be considered. This tertiary diagnostic evaluation may be undertaken if the primary and secondary evaluations have revealed neither serious structural pathology nor significant confounding psychosocial or neurophysiological factors. This examination may include flexion and extension radiographs looking for instability, PET-computed tomography (CT) scan looking for occult pelvic, facet or pars fractures, gynecologic or vascular examination looking for visceral pathology (Table 29.2).

Diagnostic injections (discography, anesthetic facet or sacroiliac joint blockades) are highly

Table 29.2 Common pathologic findings and implications in patients with persistent low back pain and disability (no radicular symptoms).

Findings	Likelihood of causing symptoms	Course of action
Malignant primary or metastatic tumor	High	Specific to tumor, neurologic risk and spinal stability
Pyogenic or granulomatous osteomyelitis/discitis	High	Specific to infection, neurologic risk and spinal stability
Acute compression fracture	High	Specific to deformity, neurologic risk and spinal stability
Unstable isthmic or degenerative spondylolisthesis	High	Reassurance if neurologically normal and slip is small. Surgical evaluation if highly unstable, neurologic risk
Disc herniation without sciatica	Unclear. Suspect related if massive extruded herniation	Reassurance if small. Surgical evaluation if massive and causing severe stenosis
Scoliosis (>40°) or with rotatory listhesis	Moderate	Specific to deformity, neurologic risk and spinal stability
Reactive endplate changes (massive)	Moderate, associated with instability	Specific local treatment may be indicated (e.g. fusion or disc replacement)
Stable isthmic or degenerative spondylolisthesis	Moderate	Specific local treatment may be indicated (e.g. fusion)
Scoliosis (<15–40°)	Low	Reassurance, general measures
Schmorl's nodes (isolated)	Low	Reassurance in the absence of major kyphosis
Minor kyphosis	Very low	Reassurance, general measures
Scoliosis (<15%)	Extremely low	Reassurance, general measures
Disc degeneration	Extremely low	Reassurance, general measures
Annular fissure	Extremely low	Reassurance, general measures
Facet arthrosis without large cyst or deformity	Extremely low	Reassurance, general measures

controversial. There are no good validation studies to confirm the diagnostic accuracy of these studies nor is there evidence that these procedures improve symptoms. There is consensus among the American Pain Society Guidelines, American College of Occupational and Environmental Medicine Guidelines, Veterans Administration Guideline and European COST Guidelines that these diagnostics injections have weak or absent supporting evidence or are frankly not recommended. There is some evidence that the use of discography may result in worse outcomes in patients with psychological distress or compensation issues. Clinicians utilizing these tests should discuss their risks and limitations frankly with patients. More recent data on the use of discography has shown that the disc puncture and injection, even with small gauge needles and low-pressure injections, appear to cause accelerated disc degeneration. Extreme care should be taken in when considering disc puncture in poorly validated diagnostic or therapeutic disc injections [6].

Trivial findings and the "pseudo-diagnosis"

Too often, as a matter of convenience or poor understanding of common degenerative pathology, patients are given anatomic diagnoses that may be anatomically true but unrelated or weakly contributing to the pain syndrome. Except in cases of fulminant degenerative processes (e.g. complete disc collapse with instability or facets degeneration with loss of stabilizing function) there is little supporting evidence for diagnoses such as "discogenic pain" or "facet syndrome" [3, 7, 8]. These diagnoses are often made on the basis of minor facet or disc abnormalities or unvalidated diagnostic injections, but are almost never corroborated (Table 29.2). These findings are very frequently seen in asymptomatic individuals. Only a small minority of persons with these findings will present with serious LBP. Attributing a patient's illness to the presence of those anatomic diagnoses with little supporting evidence diverts the attention of the patient and family from other possible causes or contributors of persistent LBP illness. This is particularly true in the patient with multiple chronic pain problems, psychological distress, compensation disputes and substance abuse disorders that frequently complicate the treatment of this condition and are associated with a prolonged clinical course and potentially misdirected and risky interventions (e.g. escalating opioid analgesics, spinal fusion, etc.) [2],

Natural history

The natural history of LBP is well described in the literature. Although the lifetime adult prevalence of LBP presenting for clinical evaluation is estimated to be 80% or greater, the majority of patients eventually have significant recovery. In those patients, however, recurrences are common. The point prevalence of LBP with any impairment is estimated at 15–30%. Most of these patients will typically have pain lasting less than 6 weeks. However, 10–15% of patients annually report chronic LBP as the duration of the back pain persists longer than 3 months [9]. Not all patients with persistent LBP have serious impairment. Carragee *et al.* [10] reported on a large cohort of subjects with varying degrees of back pain and found that 10% had persistent LBP but denied functional loss, seeking medical care or activity modification. Conversely, few persons reporting no history of LBP on annual surveys will in fact continue without reported back pain when monthly surveys are performed [11]. Thus, it appears many episodes of LBP are poorly recalled and few people go more than 1 year without one or more episodes. As a burden of disease, LBP illness has increased globally in the last 2 decades. It now ranks as the fourth most common cause of disability in working people with nearly twice the prevalence of 10 years ago.[12].

This phenomenon of poor historical recall of previous low back pain episodes has been well documented in the setting of compensable injuries. In Canada, persons reporting pain after motor vehicle accidents reported far less axial pain prior to the MVA than the general population [13]. Similarly people in MVA's also reported far less psychological distress the same general population. In the US, it was found that subjects perceiving the MVA was due to the fault of the other vehicle, systematically reported much less pre-injury back and neck pain, psychological distress, alcohol problems and mental health problems then were discovered on audit of the patients' actual medical records. In fact, the chances that a subject who expected compensation after a MVA, was more likely than not to mis-report significant pre-existing conditions [14]. These data suggest that the medical history of patients after MVA, especially in litigation, should be viewed with similar skepticism as are self-reported histories in other medical settings such as potential "accidental" gunshot injuries, venereal disease, domestic violence, child-abuse, elder neglect and so on.

Progression to chronic low back pain

Risk factors for the development of chronic LBP may be categorized into morphologic, demographic, psychosocial and genetic factors. Radiographs are poor predictors of prognosis. [8] Magnetic resonance imaging (MRI) studies of asymptomatic adults demonstrate herniated discs in up to 70% of subjects, degenerative discs in 50% and annular fissures in 20% [3,5,16]. Multiple MRI studies have failed to demonstrate causality or even high correlations of these common structural abnormalities with chronic LBP. Only weak associations with LBP progression were demonstrated with the presence of a high intensity zone (HIZ) within the disc and stronger associations are seen with moderate or severe vertebral endplate changes, severe degenerative disc disease and canal stenosis [3].

Studies of asymptomatic subjects with baseline MRI demonstrated that repeat MRI with a new LBP episode did not commonly discover new or progressive structural changes [3, 16,17]. Carragee *et al.* [18] found that 86% of subjects with repeat MRI at mean 6 weeks after a new LBP episode did not demonstrate any new findings other than those associated with aging or a slowly evolving process. Furthermore, minor trauma has not been significantly correlated with progression of LBP nor has minor trauma been found to be the cause of clinically significant structural changes on MRI [3].

Of the demographic risk factors predicting progression to chronic LBP, age over 30 years old, smoking, depression/anxiety diabetes (in men) and obesity are consistently associated with development of debilitating chronic LBP [12,15]. Very heavy labor at young age also predicts higher risk of LBP later in life [19]. Typically, the incidence of disabling back pain diminishes after age 50. Comparative population studies of low and high income countries demonstrated that populations in affluent countries are 2–4 times more likely to have the diagnosis of LBP, despite the high proportion of low-income populations performing heavy physical labor [12, 20]. In addition, the prevalence of clinically reported LBP is higher in urban populations and those working in enclosed workshops than in rural populations. Employment in jobs in certain areas, such as work in enclosed workshops, manual and psychologically stressful work, is a significant risk factor for reporting occupational disability due to persistent back pain [20].

Much research has been dedicated to the interplay of psychological risk factors with progression of chronic LBP. Coexisting depression and anxiety has a significant role in the development of chronic LBP. Jarvik *et al.* [21] demonstrated that depression was a stronger predictor for chronic LBP, as depressed patients were 2.3 times more likely to have persistent LBP. A review of the scientific literature found strong evidence for psychological distress and depressive mood as predictors for the transition from acute to chronic LBP [3, 18, 15].

Multiple studies pointed to other social or neurophysiological factors, such as chronic non-lumbar pain issues, smoking history and worker's compensation cases, as primary predictors of progression to chronic LBP disability [3, 15]. These factors were much stronger predictors of LBP persistence than common degenerative structural findings [3]. Minor traumatic events that incited chronic LBP were highly correlated persistence of LBP only when associated with compensation claims [3]. Boos *et al.* [22] found that psychosocial aspects of work, such as physical job characteristics, adverse work influence on personal life and the quality of social support at the workplace, played a more important role in the duration of LBP than MRI identified disc abnormalities.

Multiple genetic, epigenetic and selective expression factors may contribute to the development of chronic LBP in certain susceptible individuals by affecting the structure of the intervertebral disc, influencing the inflammatory response and abnormally modulating pain perception [19, 20]. Genes responsible for the structural integrity of the intervertebral disc may play a part by affecting the rate of disc degeneration. Although genetic associations with disc degeneration have been described, association with chronic LBP, per se, has been less clear or absent.

Genetic variations in cytokine genes, specifically the interleukin-1 (IL-1) gene locus may have a role in development of LBP by creating a pro-inflammatory milieu that sensitizes nociceptors innervating the discs and surrounding spinal tissue. Polymorphisms of IL-1α, IL-1β and IL-1 receptor antagonist have been shown to affect bone mineral density and promote degenerative disc disease. Inflammatory mediators such as IL-1, IL-6 and tumor necrosis factor α (TNFα) are key factors in propagating the inflammatory response that may become enhanced and difficult to control with certain genetic polymorphisms[23].

Treatment of chronic LBP with only common degenerative changes

Treatment of the major structural pathology (e.g. infection, tumor) is disease-specific. However, common degenerative findings themselves seldom account for the totality of the illness observed. It is highly likely that significant psychological, social or neurophysiological factors contribute to the problem and treatment should be directed at the whole person.

Most people with LBP do not seek medical care. Many persons will self-treat with over-the-counter medications and activity modification. In patients with persistent LBP with only common degenerative findings, reassurances that a serious underlying disease is not present and that the spine is not "fragile" or unstable are critical interventions that are often neglected. The best evidence for treatment indicates a multimodal regimen that includes a psychological support, regular exercise program, weight loss and medications, can be beneficial [24, 25]. Cognitive behavioral approaches have been proven more effective than primary pain-directed approaches. Remarkably, recent work has shown that very short course of cognitive behavioural therapy (CBT) or cognitive functional therapy (CFT) may be as or more effective than the less available long course CBT [26, 27]. Injections, percutaneous interventions and surgery are best indicated for patients with primary radiculopathy, not those with predominant chronic LBP alone. Radiofrequency ablation of lumbar facets has been shown in randomized clinical trials to be weakly or completely ineffective [28, 29].

Pharmacotherapy

There is good evidence that non-steroidal anti-inflammatory drugs (NSAIDs) are effective for chronic LBP but the effect size is very small. Recent evidence suggest NSAIDs are superior to acetaminophen although it is not proven that one NSAID is superior to others [24, 25].

Although non-benzodiazepine muscle relaxants appear useful in patients with acute non-specific back pain, the evidence supporting muscle relaxants for chronic LBP is less convincing [30]. Similarly, very short course opioids may be a reasonable treatment option for severe acute back injuries, but the evidence supporting their routine use or any indication for chronic LBP is poor. In a meta-analysis examining the role of opioid treatment for chronic LBP, the authors concluded that opioids provided only a "non-significant" reduction in pain scores at the price of very significant risks [31]. Significantly, concurrent substance misuse disorders were found in up to 43% of patients receiving opioid treatment for chronic back pain and aberrant medication-taking behavior was reported to range 5–25%. Finally, no functional benefit has been found for long-term opioid treatment (>16 weeks) while complications and risk of death increases.

Tricyclic antidepressants, but not selective serotonin reuptake inhibitors, have been reported to be more effective than placebo for chronic non-specific LBP [28, 29]. This may have to do with better sleep on low doses of tricyclics such as amitriptyline.

Alternative therapies

Chiropractic and other alternative treatment modalities are frequently used and in some LBP patient subgroups this may exceed 50% utilization rates [24,25]. Chou [24] and Qaseem (25), in their guidelines by the American College of Physicians, found fair to good evidence supporting myriad alternative treatments for chronic LBP including heat, acupuncture, yoga, massage and spinal manipulation.

Percutaneous injections, nerve ablation and heating techniques

Unlike for radicular pain processes, percutaneous interventions for LBP alone are poorly supported by available evidence. In patients with suspected facet joint or sacroiliac joint pain, there is very little evidence to support corticosteroid injections and very weak evidence for radiofrequency denervation as described above [28].

For suspected "discogenic pain" a variety of intradiscal measures have been suggested but none have proven efficacy. While intra-discal treatments have anecdotal successes, they also appear to pale with more rigorous scrutiny. An example was the widespread use of intradiscal electrothermal therapy (IDET). The best evidence available regarding intradiscal electrothermal therapy (IDET) was from 3 randomized controlled trials (RCTs) that contradicted the original "highly effective" conclusions from early studies. One RCT showed no benefit. Another RCT conducted in a highly selected patient population (without compensation claims, psychological distress or other comorbidities) showed no benefit in most patients, but a small subgroup (20%) showed a minor effect. A third RCT was discontinued before the study was completed because of the early successes in the placebo group, ensuring a positive effect in the treatment group would be impossible had the study completed [32].

Surgery

Surgical interventions for LBP secondary to major pathologies such as infections, tumors and fractures are often effective in protecting neurologic structures, preventing deformity and relieving pain. In patients with persistent radiculopathy from common degenerative conditions, surgery can reduce pain and improve function. In patients with chronic LBP illness who present with common degenerative changes seen on imaging, surgical interventions (fusion or disc arthroplasty) are less effective. It is not clear that surgical interventions in this group provide a better outcome over a comprehensive rehabilitation program with cognitive behavioral therapy or other modalities. Only 15–40% of patients can expect a highly functional outcome after fusion or disc replacement when patients are highly selected, excluding those with psychological problems, compensation issues or other comorbidities [9, 33, 34]. In patients with abnormal psychological testing, compensation issues, other chronic pain processes and / or opioid dependency, it is clear that fusion or artificial disc replacement is extremely unlikely to result in meaningful functional improvement.

Conclusions

Chronic LBP represents a large spectrum of disorders, ranging from minimal to severe disability. In the absence of serious pathologic findings (e.g. fracture, tumor, instability), serious reported disability is usually associated with psychological, social or neurophysiological comorbidities. The presence of multiple chronic pain problems, psychological distress, compensation disputes and substance abuse disorders frequently complicate the treatment of this condition and are associated with a prolonged clinical course. Specific spinal treatments are most effective when clear pathological causes are found. Treatment efforts directed at the whole person with a cognitive behavioral approach are most effective in patients in whom only common degenerative changes are found and comorbid psychosocial or pain processes are found.

References

1 Mafi JN, Reid RO, Baseman LH *et al.*(2021) Trends in low-value health service use and spending in the US Medicare fee-for-service program, 2014-2018. *JAMA Netw Open* **4(2)**:e2037328.

2 Gray BM, Vandergrift JL, Weng W, Lipner RS, Barnett ML. (2021) Clinical knowledge and trends in physicians' prescribing of opioids for new onset back pain, 2009-2017. *JAMA Netw Open* **4(7)**:e2115328.

3 Carragee E, Alamin T, Cheng I *et al.* (2006) Does minor trauma cause serious low back illness? *Spine* **31(25)**:2942–9.

4 Henschke N, Maher CG, Refshauge KM *et al.* (2009) Prevalence of and screening for serious spinal pathology in patients presenting to primary care settings with acute low back pain. *Arthritis Rheum* **60(10)**:3072–80.

5 Cohen SP, Argoff CE, Carragee EJ. (2008) Management of low back pain. *BMJ* **337**:a2718.

6 Cuellar JM, Stauff MP, Herzog RJ, Carrino JA, Baker GA, Carragee EJ. (2016) Does provocative discography cause clinically important injury to the lumbar intervertebral disc? A 10-year matched cohort study. *Spine J* **16(3)**:273–80.

7 Jarvik JG, Meier EN, James KT *et al.* (2020) The effect of including benchmark prevalence data of common imaging findings in spine image reports on health care utilization among adults undergoing spine imaging: a stepped-wedge randomized clinical trial. *JAMA Netw Open* **3(9)**:e2015713.

8 Chen L, Perera RS, Radojcic MR *et al.* (2021) Association of lumbar spine radiographic changes with severity of back pain-related disability among middle-aged, community-dwelling women. *JAMA Netw Open* **4(5)**:e2110715.

9 Carragee EJ. (2005) Clinical practice: persistent low back pain. *N Engl J Med* **352(18)**:1891–8.

10 Carragee EJ, Alamin TF, Miller J *et al.* (2002) Provocative discography in volunteer subjects with mild persistent low back pain. *Spine J* **2**:25–34.

11 Carragee EJ, Cohen SP. (2009) Lifetime asymptomatic for back pain: the validity of self-report measures in soldiers. *Spine* **34(9)**:978–83.

12 GBD 2019 Diseases and Injuries Collaborators. (2020) Global burden of 369 diseases and injuries in 204 countries and territories, 1990-2019: a systematic analysis for the Global Burden of Disease Study 2019. Lancet **396(10258)**:1204–22. Erratum in: *Lancet* (2020) **396(10262)**:1562.

13 Carragee EJ. (2009) Great expectations. *J Rheumatol* **36(5)**:869–71.

14 Don AS, Carragee EJ. (2009) Is the self-reported history accurate in patients with persistent axial pain after a motor vehicle accident? *Spine J* **9(1)**:4–12.

15 Stevans JM, Delitto A, Khoja SS *et al.* (2021) Risk factors associated with transition from acute to

chronic low back pain in US patients seeking primary care. *JAMA Netw Open* **4(2)**:e2037371.

16 Jarvik JG, Deyo RA. (2002) Diagnostic evaluation of low back pain with emphasis on imaging. *Ann Intern Med* **137(7)**:586–97.

17 Borenstein DG, O'Mara JW Jr, Boden SD *et al.* (2001) The value of magnetic resonance imaging of the lumbar spine to predict low-back pain in asymptomatic subjects: a seven-year follow-up study. *J Bone Joint Surg Am* **83-A**:1306–11.

18 Carragee E, Alamin T, Cheng I *et al.* (2006) Are first-time episodes of serious LBP associated with new MRI findings? *Spine J* **6(6)**:624–35.

19 Heuch I, Heuch I, Hagen K, Sørgjerd EP, Åsvold BO, Zwart JA. (2019) Does diabetes influence the probability of experiencing chronic low back pain? A population-based cohort study: the Nord-Trøndelag Health Study. *BMJ Open* **9(9)**:e031692.

20 Volinn E. (1997) The epidemiology of low back pain in the rest of the world: a review of surveys in low- and middle-income countries. *Spine* **22(15)**:1747–54.

21 Jarvik, JG, Hollingworth W, Heagerty PJ *et al.* (2005) Three-year incidence of low back pain in an initially asymptomatic cohort: clinical and imaging risk factors. *Spine* **30(13)**:1541–8.

22 Boos N, Semmer N, Elfering A *et al.* (2000) Natural history of individuals with asymptomatic disc abnormalities in magnetic resonance imaging: predictors of low back pain-related medical consultation and work incapacity. *Spine* **25(12)**: 1484–92.

23 Videman T, Saarela J, Kaprio J *et al.* (2009) Associations of 25 structural, degradative, and inflammatory candidate genes with lumbar disc desiccation, bulging, and height narrowing. *Arthritis Rheum* 60(**2**):470–81.

24 Chou, R, Deyo Rm Friedly J *et al.* (2017) Systemic pharmacologic therapies for low back pain: a systematic review for an American College of Physicians clinical practice guideline. *Ann Intern Med* **166**:480–92.

25 Qaseem, A, Wilt TJ, McLean RM *et al.* (2017) Noninvasive treatments for acute, subacute, and chronic low back pain: a clinical practice guideline from the American College of Physicians. *Ann Intern Med* **166**:514–30.

26 Darnall BD, Roy A, Chen AL *et al.* (2021) Comparison of a single-session pain management skills intervention with a single-session health education intervention and 8 sessions of cognitive behavioral therapy in adults with chronic low back pain: a randomized clinical trial. *JAMA Netw Open* **4(8)**:e2113401

27 Hadley G, Novitch MB. (2021) CBT and CFT for chronic pain. *Curr Pain Headache Rep* **25(5)**:35.

28 Juch JNS, Maas ET, Ostelo RWJG *et al.* (2017) Effect of radiofrequency denervation on pain intensity among patients with chronic low back pain: the Mint randomized clinical trials. *JAMA* **318(1)**:68–81

29 Buchbinder R, Underwood M, Hartvigsen J, Maher CG. (2020) The Lancet Series call to action to reduce low value care for low back pain: an update. *Pain* **161 Suppl 1(1)**:S57–64.

30 Van Tulder MW, Touray T, Furlan AD *et al.* (2003) Muscle relaxants for nonspecific low back pain: a systematic review within the framework of the Cochrane collaboration. *Spine* **1**:1978–92.

31 Martell BA, O'Connor PG, Kerns RD *et al.* (2007) Systematic review. Opioid treatment for chronic back pain: prevalence, efficacy, and association with addiction. *Ann Intern Med* **146**:116–27.

32 Urrútia G, Kovacs F, Nishishinya MB *et al.* (2007) Percutaneous thermocoagulation intradiscal techniques for discogenic low back pain. *Spine* **32(10)**:1146–54.

33 Mirza SK. (2005) Point of view: commentary on the research reports that led to Food and Drug Administration approval of an artificial disc. *Spine* **30**:1561–4.

34 Carragee EJ, Lincoln T, Parmar VS, Alamin T. (2006) A gold standard evaluation of the "discogenic pain" diagnosis as determined by provocative discography. *Spine* **31(18)**:2115–23.

Chapter 30

Fibromyalgia syndrome and myofascial pain syndromes

Winfried Häuser[1,2] & Mary-Ann Fitzcharles[3,4]

[1] *Department Internal Medicine I and Interdisciplinary Center of Pan Medicine, Klinikum Saarbrücken, Germany*
[2] *Department of Psychosomatic Medicine and Psychotherapy, Technische Universität München, Germany*
[3] *Division of Rheumatology, McGill University Health Centre, Montréal, Québec, Canada*
[4] *Alan Edwards Pain Management Unit, McGill University Health Center, Montréal, Québec, Canada*

Introduction

Musculoskeletal pain is the most prevalent pain type occurring in the general population and in the clinical setting. Musculoskeletal pain can be classified as localized (a single pain site), regional (several pain sites in one body region) or widespread. There has been debate over the years regarding the best criteria to identify widespread or multisite pain, such as the requirement of a minimum of four of five pain regions [1] or more recently at least six of nine body sites [2].

Other than disease localized to the joints or soft tissues around the joints, most musculoskeletal pain syndromes are not associated with any specific organ pathology. The two most common musculoskeletal pain conditions are: (a) myofascial pain syndrome (MPS), a non-specific local and regional chronic musculoskeletal pain condition; and (b) fibromyalgia syndrome (FMS), characterized by chronic widespread pain and associated with other symptoms such as fatigue, sleep disturbance, cognitive difficulties amongst others. MPS and FMS can be overlapping disorders.

The exact underlying pathogenic mechanisms of both MPS and FMS are currently not fully clarified. There is considerable evidence pointing to the role of central sensitization in FMS, but peripheral pain generators may also be operative in perpetuating ongoing pain in a subgroup of patients. Some authors have even suggested that FMS pain may at least be partially initiated by pain arising from trigger points (TrPs). In contrast, MPS is believed to originate at the motor endplate of muscle, with some studies reporting histological, biochemical and electromyographic abnormalities [3].

Recommendations for the management of FMS are derived from the updated interdisciplinary German guideline on the classification, pathophysiology and management of FMS [4] and on the updated recommendations of the European League Against Rheumatism [EULAR] [5]. There are no current guidelines for the management of MPS, with recommendations based on a selective literature search in PubMed using the terms "myofascial pain syndrome" AND "systematic review".

Clinical Pain Management: A Practical Guide, Second Edition. Edited by Mary E. Lynch, Kenneth D. Craig, and Philip W. Peng.

Definitions

Criteria for FMS must be viewed as classification criteria, used to identify homogenous patient groups for study, or diagnostic criteria that can be much more appropriately applied to an individual patient in the clinical setting. Classification criteria for FMS were first developed by the American College of Rheumatology (ACR) in 1990 and defined FMS as chronic (>3 months) widespread pain (including pain on both sides of the body, above and below the waist, and axial pain) and tenderness on manual palpation in at least 11 out of 18 defined tender points [6].

FMS is not a distinct nosological entity and the clinical presentation of patients is heterogenous. It is now recognized that FMS presents as a spectrum of symptoms along a continuum, with variable expression in severity at different time points. FMS should therefore not be ruled as a binary condition as either present or absent, but rather as a condition with mild, moderate or severe expression at a specific time. Within this context FMS can be conceptualized as a cluster of symptoms which are somatic (mainly pain and physical fatigue) and psychological (mainly sleeping and cognitive problems) within a continuum of distress. The heterogeneity of FMS is further exemplified by the fact that patients have differences in their ability to use coping strategies to deal with psychosocial stressors, and manifest differing mental and somatic comorbidities. There are also differences in the impact of FMS on level of function such as ability to work [7].

MPS is characterized by the presence of TrPs, but there is no consensus on the essential diagnostic criteria for diagnosing a TrP. An expert panel has provided the following definitions: a) TrPs are identified when stimulation reproduces any symptom experienced by the patient (e.g. pain, tenderness, paraesthesia), either partially or completely, whereby the symptom is recognized as a familiar experience by the patient, even though it may not be present at the moment of the examination. b) Latent TrPs are identified when stimulation fails to reproduce any symptom experienced by a subject (symptomatic or asymptomatic) and the subject does not recognize the elicited symptom as familiar [8]. Active TrP are classified as those that cause spontaneous pain, whereas latent TrP have all the same clinical features without being responsible for the pain complaint [9].

Active myofascial TrPs may have a role in patients with FMS, tension headache, neck and low back pain, temporomandibular disorders, extremity pain (shoulder, hip, limb), abdominal, thoracic and pelvic/urogenital pain syndromes [9]. Tender point (TP) examination is no longer required for recent diagnostic criteria of FMS [2, 16, 17]. The main difference between TPs and TrPs is that TPs can only be defined in terms of their localization, whereas TrPs can be found upon palpation which may cause a specific referred pain pattern.

Prevalence

A systematic review reported a prevalence of FMS in the general population to be 1.8% (95% confidence interval 1.7 to 1.9). The sex ratio for females vs. males is 2–21: 1. Most patients with FMS are in the age range of 40–60 years, but FMS can also be diagnosed in children, adolescents and the elderly [10].

There are no data on the prevalence and sex ratio of MPS in representative samples of the general population. In clinical samples MPS is most common in women and those of middle age.

It is plausible that there will be clinical overlap of FMS and MPS in some patients, but due to inconsistencies in diagnostic criteria for FMS and MPS, there are no reliable data on the overlap. It has been estimated that 18-40% of patients diagnosed with MPS also met the ACR 1990 classification criteria for FMS, and up to 75% of patients with FMS could be diagnosed with MPS [11].

Course and prognosis

Longitudinal studies of FMS have demonstrated that symptoms persist in nearly all patients. Some patients do adapt sufficiently to ongoing symptoms and the associated limitations and indeed report a better long-term satisfaction with their health status. FMS is not associated with a reduced life expectancy overall [12].

There are no longitudinal outcome studies for MPS. It has been observed in the clinical setting that some patients with MPS might remit spontaneously or resolve with appropriate correction of predisposing factors and therapy. MPS that has been present for longer than 6 months or has followed a chronic relapsing course tends to be continuous. Localized myofascial pain can spread and evolve to regional chronic pain or to chronic widespread pain (CWP) and/or FMS [9].

Diagnosis of fibromyalgia syndrome

History

A pain diagram can be helpful to identify patients pain location in FMS, but it is not uncommon for patients to report "pain all over." Some key points to consider when taking the history from a patient suspected of having FMS include the following:

1 Family history of chronic pain (e.g. low back pain, "rheumatism").

2 Personal history of pain (head, abdomen, joints) in childhood and adolescence.

3 History of physical or psychosocial stressors, especially in childhood (e.g. child abuse).

4 Prolonged local or regional pain.

5 Onset of widespread pain related to physical and/or psychosocial stressors.

6 General hypersensitivity to touch, smell, noise, taste.

7 Hypervigilance.

8 Multiple somatic symptoms (gastrointestinal, urological, gynecological, neurological) with previous diagnosis of functional dyspepsia, irritable bowel syndrome, painful bladder syndrome, tension headache, migraine, temporomandibular disorder.

9 High symptom-related emotional strain.

Physical examination

It can be expected that the physical examination will be within normal limits for the age of the patient for most patients with FMS. Some may demonstrate mild pressure allodynia on palpation of muscles, and in a third of patients there is a report of dysesthesia on light touch. Tender point examination is not required by the new diagnostic criteria (see below). Irrespective of whether a tender point examination is performed, a complete physical examination including musculoskeletal and neurological examination is required to ensure that no underlying condition can be masquerading as CWP in the context of FMS [13].

Blood tests and diagnostic imaging

The following routine blood tests are recommended for the initial evaluation of patients with CWP to screen for somatic diseases which might mimic or contribute to CWP and fatigue:

1 Sedimentation rate, C-reactive protein, red and white cell blood count (polymyalgia rheumatica, inflammatory rheumatic disease, malignancy).

2 Creatine kinase (muscle disease).

3 Calcium (hypercalcemia or hypocalcaemia).

4 Thyroid-stimulating hormone (hypothyroidism).

5 Any further blood testing or diagnostic procedures should be dependent on a suspicion of some other condition/diagnosis based on findings of the clinical history and physical examination.

Unnecessary laboratory and radiographic studies are strongly discouraged (e.g. testing for rheumatoid factor or antinuclear antibodies without clinical justification [14].

Differential diagnosis

Chronic pain of various degrees is a common symptom of patients presenting to internal medicine and neurologists. Physicians must be aware that many medical conditions can present with diffuse body pain and masquerade as FMS. Early inflammatory rheumatic diseases, endocrine diseases, malignancies, myopathies and polyneuropathies might cause or contribute to CWP and fatigue [13].

With the recognition that localized areas of pain, such as osteoarthritis of a knee, may act as a peripheral pain generator, attention should be paid to this localized pain, in the hopes that there could be attenuation of the widespread pain. In contrast, comorbid FMS in well-defined and controlled somatic diseases such as inflammatory rheumatic diseases will require treatments focused toward FMS rather than changes in treatments for the underlying primary disease [15]. Medications should always be remembered as a potential cause of widespread body pain that can be confused with FMS. These include lipid lowering agents in the category of statins, aromatase inhibitors, bisphosphonates and paradoxically – even opioids that can induce a hyperalgesic syndrome [13].

Table 30.1 The 2010 ACR preliminary and 2016 Revisions to the 2010/2011 fibromyalgia diagnostic criteria and the AAPT diagnostic criteria

Criteria (reference)	Diagnostic items	Comments
ACR 2010 preliminary diagnostic criteria [16]	Widespread pain and substantial somatic symptoms Symptoms present for ≥3 months No other disorder that could explain the pain	Pain is scored by the physician according to the number of affected areas, widespread pain index (WPI) (score: 0–19) and symptom severity (SSS) measured in four domains of fatigue, unrefreshing sleep, cognitive and somatic symptoms with ranges from no problem (0) to severe symptoms (3)(score: 0–12). Total score: is the sum of WPI and SSS 0–31; Criteria are met if WPI is 3-6 and SSS ≥9 or of WPI is ≥7 and SSS is ≥5
2016 Revisions to the 2010/2011 fibromyalgia diagnostic criteria [17]	Modified version of research (survey/2011 criteria (entirely self-reported assessment of symptoms)	Widespread Pain Index (WPI) is scored by the patient according to the number of affected areas (total score: 0–19). The SSS is modified to include headaches, pain or cramps in the lower abdomen and depression (score: 0–12). Total score is the sum of WPI and SSS: 0–31 (see Table 30.2) Criteria are met if WPI 4-6 and SSS ≥9 or of WPI is ≥7 and SSS is ≥5 and there is generalized pain sites in at least four of five body regions (four quadrants and axial) except the face and the abdomen
AAPT Diagnostic Criteria for fibromyalgia [2]	Manikin with 9 pain sites History taking of symptoms	Symptoms present for 3 months: a) multisite pain (MSP) defined as 6 or more pain sites from a total of 9 possible sites and b) Moderate to severe sleep problems and /OR fatigue as assessed by the physician

Diagnosis

Although the diagnosis of FMS is clinical, based on a comprehensive history and physical examination, diagnostic criteria may be used to reassure the clinician. Some of the recent proposed diagnostic criteria are outlined below (Table 30.1)

Assessment of severity of FMS

To help direct treatments, classifying patients as having mild, moderate or severe FMS provides a simple and clinically applicable starting point. There are generic, e.g. Patient Health Questionnaire 15 [18] and diseases specific instruments, e.g. Fibromyalgia Impact Scale [19] and Polysymptomatic Distress Scale [17] available to assess the amount of the somatic and psychological symptom burden and thus the severity of FMS.

Diagnosis of myofascial pain syndrome

History

Patients with MPS report a deep aching sensation, often with a feeling of stiffness in the involved area. Pain is aggravated by use of involved muscles, psychological stress, cold temperatures and postural imbalance. Radiation from a myofascial TrP can be described as a sensation of paresthesiae. Myofascial TrP activity may lead to the development of various autonomic changes such as lacrimation, regional

Table 30.2 Fibromyalgia survey questionnaire [17]

Symptom Severity Score			
I. Using the following scale, indicate for each item the level of severity **over the past week** by checking the appropriate box. 0: No problem 1: Slight or mild problems; generally mild or intermittent 2: Moderate; considerable problems; often present and/or at a moderate level 3. Severe: continuous, life-disturbing problems			
Fatigue	☐ 0	☐ 1	☐ 2	☐ 3
Trouble thinking or remembering	☐ 0	☐ 1	☐ 2	☐ 3
Waking up tired (unrefreshed)	☐ 0	☐ 1	☐ 2	☐ 3
II. During the **past 6 months** have you had any of the following symptoms?				
Pain or cramps in lower abdomen:	☐ Yes		☐ No	
Depression:	☐ Yes		☐ No	
Headache:	☐ Yes		☐ No	
Widespread pain index Please indicate below if you have had pain or tenderness over the past 7 days in each of the areas listed below. Please make an X in the box if you have had pain or tenderness. Be sure to mark both right side and left side separately				
☐ Shoulder, left	☐ Upper leg, left	☐ Lower back		
☐ Shoulder, right	☐ Upper leg, right	☐ Upper back		
		☐ Neck		
☐ Hip, left	☐ Lower leg, left			
☐ Hip, right	☐ Lower leg, right			
☐ Upper am, left	☐ Jaw, left	☐ No pain in any of these areas		
☐ Upper arm, right	☐ Jaw, right			
☐ Lower arm, left	☐ Chest			
☐ Lower arm, right	☐ Abdomen			
IV. Overall, were the symptoms listed in I - III above generally present for at **least 3 months**?				
	☐ Yes			☐ No

excessive coldness or vertigo. Motor dysfunction includes restricted range of motion, local weakness, reduced coordination and spasms in other muscles. After prolonged myofascial pain there may be general weakness, reduced work tolerance, fatigue and sleep disturbances [9].

Physical examination

The physical examination for MPS is focused to identify pain on soft tissue palpation. A tender point is a discreet area in the soma which is more tender to the application of pressure than the immediate surrounding tissue. The tenderness is the key feature of a myofascial TrP, but is not exclusive to myofascial TrPs. When an active myofascial TrP is palpated, a patient may wince, give an involuntary jerk referred to as the "jump sign". The patient may report a pattern of pain radiation, with radiation patterns characteristic of particular muscle groups. A taut band may be identified by gentle palpation perpendicular to the direction of the muscle fibers in order to identify a longitudinal region of nodularity. Firm pressure over the taut band is painful and reproduces the patient's pain complaint. Continuous pressure > 5 seconds may reproduce the pattern of referred pain. When the palpating finger is snapped around the taut band, a local contraction of the muscle may be observed in superficial muscles or felt by the examiner in deep muscles (i.e. the twitch response). Neighboring joints should be examined for any abnormality of mobility or local tenderness [9].

Blood tests and diagnostic imaging

Blood tests and diagnostic imaging are not necessary for the diagnosis or exclusion of MPS. In case of poor rapid response to treatment, borderline hypothyroidism or nutritional deficiencies can be considered as a differential diagnosis [20].

Final diagnosis

A cluster of three diagnostic criteria have been proposed as essential for the diagnosis of MPS; these include identification of MTrPs: a taut band, a hypersensitive spot and referred pain [8].

Basic mechanisms

Risk factors

Risk factors for FMS have been identified by population-based longitudinal studies or systematic reviews of cross-sectional studies as follows [21]:

1 *Biological:* family aggregation; inflammatory rheumatic diseases.

2 *Psychological:* Adverse childhood events including sexual and physical abuse; occupational and psychological stressors; depressed mood; sleep problems.

3 *Life style factors:* Smoking; obesity; physical inactivity.

4 *Social:* occupational mechanical burdens.

The following factors are commonly cited but not proven by cross-sectional or longitudinal studies to predispose to development of MPS:

1 *Biological:* Deconditioning, poor posture, repetitive mechanical stress, physical trauma, mechanical imbalance, muscle wasting or ischemia, visceral referred pain, joint disorders, vitamin deficiencies, climatic conditions (damp, draughts, excessive cold or heat).

2 *Psychological*: Non-restorative sleep, psychological stressors[9].

Pathophysiology

Several potential pathophysiological mechanisms in FMS have been described, but their causal relationship is unclear because of the cross-sectional nature of studies. Potential mechanisms include central nervous system pain processing abnormalities (central sensitization), hyporeactivity of the hypothalamic-pituitary-adrenal (HPA) axis causing a fragile stress response system, small fiber pathology and disturbances in the dopaminergic and serotonergic systems. At present, consistent or specific structural or biochemical abnormalities in the muscles or tender points of FMS patients have not been demonstrated. The biopsychosocial model of FMS postulates that there is heterogeneity in the genetic and psychological predispositions as well as in the reactions of the vegetative, endocrine and central nervous system. Different etiological factors and pathophysiological mechanisms lead to a common pathway of the phenotypic expression that is currently classified as FMS [21].

The key pathophysiological abnormalities associated with MPS appear to be principally located at the center of a muscle in its motor endplate zone. Histological, biochemical and electromyographic abnormalities in myofascial TrPs have been reported, but these findings are not specific and require further study [22]. Active myofascial TrPs may serve as one of the sources of noxious input leading to the sensitization of spinal and supraspinal pain pathways that can lead to FMS [23].

Treatment of fibromyalgia syndrome

General principles of management of fibromyalgia syndrome

Patient education: Patients should be educated about the condition and treatment options discussed. The diagnostic label "FM" or "FMS" should be communicated to patients after initial diagnosis and patients should be provided with a clear explanation of the nature of the disorder, planned treatment strategy and expected outcome. Realistic outcome goals should be set in a shared-decision model between patient and physician. This approach is intended to reduce anxiety, which inherently accompanies chronic pain. Patients should be introduced to the concept and importance of understanding the biopsychosocial model for FMS whereby biological factors (e.g., genetic predisposition) and psychosocial factors (e.g., stress) contribute to the predisposition, triggering and perpetuation of symptoms. Reassurance should be given that the symptoms are acknowledged to be real and are not caused by an organic disease (such as abnormality of muscles or joints), but are instead based on a functional disorder of the nervous system (altered processing of pain and other external stimuli) with emphasis on the following:

1 The symptoms are persistent in most adult patients.

2 Total relief of symptoms is seldom achieved.

3 The symptoms should not lead to disablement and do not shorten life expectancy.

4 Most patients learn to adapt to the symptoms over time.

5 The patient can learn to improve symptoms and health-related quality of life via self-management strategies.

Patients should be provided with information (including written material) about the condition [4,5].

Defining individual and realistic goals of treatment: Goals of treatment are to improve quality of life, maintain function (functional ability in everyday situations) and reduce symptoms. Some patients may have unrealistic expectations such as complete symptom relief. Individualized and realistic outcome goals should be developed together with the patient, such as improved daily functioning or symptom reduction (e.g. 30% pain relief). Another important aspect is management of activity and energy, also termed pacing, that aims to avoid excessive activity or inadequate rest [4].

Individualized approach: Identifying the symptom of major importance to an individual patient can help the physician to develop an anchor on which to base a treatment strategy. Treatment modalities should be tailored according to pain intensity, function, associated features (such as depression), fatigue, sleep disturbance and patient preferences and comorbidities [5].

Interventions strongly supported by evidence

First, second and third line treatments for FMS cannot be derived from the multiple systematic reviews and meta-analyses of randomized controlled trials available. A network meta-analysis has concluded that the following interventions hold greatest promise for the management of FMS: pregabalin or serotonin norepinephrine reuptake inhibitors (SNRIs) as pharmacological interventions; multicomponent therapy, aerobic exercise and CBT as non-pharmacological interventions [24].

Non-pharmacological therapies

Evidence for sustained effects following an intervention are only available for cognitive- behavioral therapies (operant therapies; classical cognitive-behavioral therapies, acceptance-based cognitive therapies) [25], aerobic exercise [26], mixed exercise [aerobic, resistance, flexibility] [27] and multicomponent therapies (combination of psychological therapies with at least one physical therapy) [28]. Aerobic exercise should be started at a low level and increased slowly. The final recommended level of aerobic exercise (e.g. aquatic jogging, walking, cycling) is 2–3 times a week for 30 minutes at a moderate intensity (60–75% of the age-adjusted maximum heart rate) [29].

Pharmacological therapies

Of the pharmacological treatments, only duloxetine, milnacipran and pregabalin have approval by the US Food and Drug Administration for use in FMS in the USA, but do not have approval by the European Medicines Agency for use in Europe.

All drug treatments must balance efficacy and adverse effects, especially for those that may cause problems with cognition and fatigue. Drug treatments must be re-evaluated to ensure the need for continuation and should be prescribed at the lowest effective dose, which is often lower than doses reported for clinical trials, and ideally for a limited time.

Graduated approach

Recent guidelines recommend that treatment should focus first on non-pharmacological modalities with active patient participation championing self-management strategies. This is based on availability, cost and safety issues and also patient preferences [5].

Stepwise and individualized treatment according to the European League Against Rheumatism (EULAR) recommendations for the management of FMS are outlined in Figure 30.1 [5].

Treatment of myofascial pain syndrome

Acupuncture may be a good treatment option for MPS. A systematic review and network meta-analysis with 33 studies and 1692 participants concluded that most acupuncture therapies, including acupuncture combined with other therapies, were effective in decreasing pain and in improving physical function in MPS [30]. analgesic medication intake and sleep quality [31].

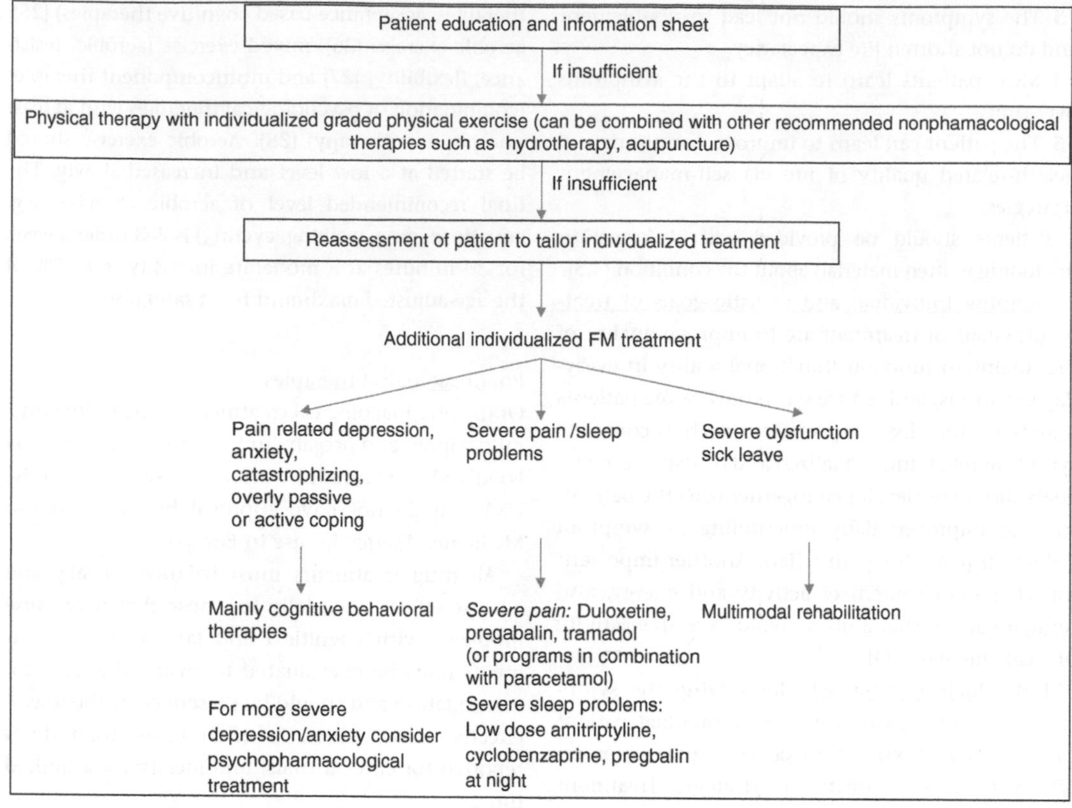

Figure 30.1 Stepwise and individualized treatment according to the European League Against Rheumatism (EULAR recommendations for the management of fibromyalgia [5]

Dry needling is another treatment option with promise. A systematic review included 15 trials and reported that dry needling is effective in the short term for pain relief, increased range of motion and improved quality of life when compared to no intervention/sham/placebo. There is, however, insufficient evidence for the effect of dry needling on disability, analgesic medication intake and sleep quality [31].

Dry needling improves pain following the intervention. In two systematic reviews, one of patients with low back pain and one of patients with neck and shoulder pain with the presence of myofascial TrPs, dry needling of myofascial TrPs, especially if associated with other therapies, relieved pain intensity following the intervention. However, the clinical superiority of dry needling for improvement in functional disability and follow-up effects remain unclear [23, 33].

In contrast to the above treatments, there is inconclusive evidence to support the use of botulinum toxin in MPS according to the results of a systematic review of 4 RCTs with 233 participants [34].

Conclusions

FMS and MPS are the most common musculoskeletal pain conditions and can be associated with significant suffering and associated disability. Empathetic clinical care and patient support should be provided in a non-judgmental way for patients with FMS. As with other chronic pain conditions, effective management must emphasize the importance of a biopsychosocial approach. Treatment of FMS should be individualized and tailored to the severity of FMS and its key symptoms. Education and non-pharmacological therapies are the first line treatment for FMS, with recognition that medications mostly provides only a modest effect for some patients. FMS is likely to be a lifelong complaint, with patients seldom reporting complete symptom relief. In contrast to FMS, MPS may more likely be self-limited and may be amenable to physical interventions such as acupuncture or dry needling, but further study is required.

References

1 Wolfe F, Butler SH, Fitzcharles M *et al.* (2019) Revised chronic widespread pain criteria: development from and integration with fibromyalgia criteria. *Scand J Pain* **20(1)**: 77–86.

2 Arnold LM, Bennett RM, Crofford LJ *et al.* (2019) AAPT Diagnostic Criteria for Fibromyalgia. *J Pain* **20(6)**:611–28.

3 Fernández-de-Las-Peñas C, Arendt-Nielsen L. (2016) Myofascial pain and fibromyalgia: two different but overlapping disorders. *Pain Manag* **6(4)**:401–8.

4 Petzke F, Brückle W, Eidmann U *et al.* (2017) General treatment principles, coordination of care and patient education in fibromyalgia syndrome: Updated guidelines 2017 and overview of systematic review articles]. *Schmerz* **31(3)**:246–54.

5 Macfarlane GJ, Kronisch C, Dean LE *et al.* (2017) EULAR revised recommendations for the management of fibromyalgia. *Ann Rheum Dis* **76(2)**:318–28.

6 Wolfe F, Smythe HA, Yunus MB *et al.* (1990) The American College of Rheumatology criteria for the classification of fibromyalgia: report of the multicenter criteria committee. *Arthritis Rheum* **33**:160–72

7 Häuser W, Perrot S, Clauw DJ, Fitzcharles MA. (2018) Unravelling fibromyalgia-steps toward individualized management. *J Pain* **19(2)**:125–134.

8 Fernández-de-Las-Peñas C, Dommerholt J. (2018) International consensus on diagnostic criteria and clinical considerations of myofascial trigger points: A Delphi study. *Pain Med* **19(1)**:142–50.

9 Cummings M, Baldry P. (2007) Regional myofascial pain: diagnosis and management. *Best Pract Res Clin Rheumatol* **21**: 367–87.

10 Heidari F, Afshari M, Moosazadeh M. (2017) Prevalence of fibromyalgia in general population and patients, a systematic review and meta-analysis. *Rheumatol Int* **37(9)**:1527–39.

11 Bourgaize S, Janjua I, Murnaghan K, Mior S, Srbely J, Newton G. (2019) Fibromyalgia and myofascial pain syndrome: two sides of the same coin? A scoping review to determine the lexicon of the current diagnostic criteria. *Musculoskeletal Care* **17(1)**:3–12.

12 Eich W, Bär KJ, Bernateck M *et al.* (2017) Definition, classification, clinical diagnosis and prognosis of fibromyalgia syndrome: Updated guidelines 2017 and overview of systematic review articles. *Schmerz* **31(3)**:231–8.

13 Häuser W, Perrot S, Sommer C, Shir Y, Fitzcharles MA. (2017) Diagnostic confounders of chronic widespread pain: not always fibromyalgia. *Pain Rep* **2(3)**:e598.

14 Fitzcharles MA, Shir Y, Ablin JN *et al.* (2013) Classification and clinical diagnosis of fibromyalgia syndrome: recommendations of recent evidence-based interdisciplinary guidelines. *Evid Based Complement Alternat Med* **2013**:528952.

15 Fitzcharles MA, Perrot S, Häuser W. (2018) Comorbid fibromyalgia: A qualitative review of prevalence and importance. *Eur J Pain* **22(9)**:1565–76.

16 Wolfe F, Clauw DJ, Fitzcharles MA *et al.* (2010) The American College of Rheumatology preliminary diagnostic criteria for fibromyalgia and measurement of symptom severity. *Arthritis Care Res* **62(5)**:600–6

17 Wolfe F, Clauw DJ, Fitzcharles MA **et al.** (2016) Revisions to the 2010/2011 fibromyalgia diagnostic criteria. *Semin Arthritis Rheum* **46(3)**:319–29.

18 Häuser W, Schmutzer G, Brähler E, Wolfe F. (2014) Patient Health Questionnaire 15 as a generic measure of severity in fibromyalgia syndrome: Surveys with patients of three different settings. *J Psychosom Res* **76**:307–11.

19 Schaefer C, Chandran A, Hufstader M *et al.* (2011) The comparative burden of mild, moderate and severe fibromyalgia: results from a cross-sectional survey in the United States. *Health Qual Life Outcomes* **9**:71

20 Gerwin RD. (2014) Diagnosis of myofascial pain syndrome. *Phys Med Rehabil Clin N Am* **25(2)**:341–55.

21 Üçeyler N, Burgmer M, Friedel E *et al.* Etiology and pathophysiology of fibromyalgia syndrome: updated guidelines 2017, overview of systematic review articles and overview of studies on small fiber neuropathy in FMS subgroups. *Schmerz* **31(3)**:239–45.

22 Basford JR, An KN. (2009) New techniques for the quantification of fibromyalgia and myofascial pain. *Curr Pain Headache Rep* **13**:376–813.
23 Ge HY, Nie H, Madeleine P *et al.* (2009) Contribution of the local and referred pain from active myofascial trigger points in fibromyalgia syndrome. *Pain* **147**:233–40.
24 Nüesch E, Häuser W, Bernardy K, Barth J, Jüni P. (2013) Comparative efficacy of pharmacological and non-pharmacological interventions in fibromyalgia syndrome: network meta-analysis. *Ann Rheum Dis* **72(6)**:955–62.
25 Bernardy K, Klose P, Welsch P, Häuser W. (2018) Efficacy, acceptability and safety of cognitive behavioural therapies in fibromyalgia syndrome - a systematic review and meta-analysis of randomized controlled trials. *Eur J Pain* **22(2)**:242–60.
26 Bidonde J, Busch AJ, Schachter CL *et al.* (2017) Aerobic exercise training for adults with fibromyalgia. *Cochrane Database Syst Rev* **6(6)**:CD012700.
27 Bidonde J, Busch AJ, Schachter CL *et al.* Mixed exercise training for adults with fibromyalgia. *Cochrane Database Syst Rev* **5(5)**:CD013340.
28 Häuser W, Bernardy K, Arnold B, Offenbächer M, Schiltenwolf M. (2009) Efficacy of multicomponent treatment in fibromyalgia syndrome: a meta-analysis of randomized controlled clinical trials. *Arthritis Rheum* **61(2)**:216–24.
29 Häuser W, Klose P, Langhorst J *et al.* (2010) Efficacy of different types of aerobic exercise in fibromyalgia syndrome: a systematic review and meta-analysis of randomised controlled trials. *Arthritis Res Ther* **12(3)**:R79.
30 Li X, Wang R, Xing X *et al.* (2017) Acupuncture for myofascial pain syndrome: a network meta-analysis of 33 randomized controlled trials. *Pain Physician* **20(6)**:E883–902.
31 Espejo-Antúnez L, Tejeda JF, Albornoz-Cabello M *et al.* (2017) Dry needling in the management of myofascial trigger points: a systematic review of randomized controlled trials. *Complement Ther Med* **33**:46–57.
32 Liu L, Huang QM, Liu QG *et al.* (2015) Effectiveness of dry needling for myofascial trigger points associated with neck and shoulder pain: a systematic review and meta-analysis. *Arch Phys Med Rehabil* **96(5)**:944–55.
33 Liu L, Huang QM, Liu QG *et al.* (2018) Evidence for dry needling in the management of myofascial trigger points associated with low back pain: a systematic review and meta-analysis. *Arch Phys Med Rehabil* **99(1)**:144–52.
34 Soares A, Andriolo RB, Atallah AN, da Silva EM. (2014) Botulinum toxin for myofascial pain syndromes in adults. *Cochrane Database Syst Rev* **2014(7)**:CD007533

Chapter 31

Clinical pain management in the rheumatic diseases

Amir Minerbi[1] & Mary-Ann Fitzcharles[2,3]

[1] *Institute for Pain Medicine, Rambam Health Campus, Haifa, Israel*
[2] *Division of Rheumatology, McGill University Health Centre, Montréal, Québec, Canada*
[3] *Alan Edwards Pain Management Unit, McGill University Health Center, Montréal, Québec, Canada*

Introduction

Rheumatic diseases include inflammatory arthritis (IA). of which rheumatoid arthritis (RA) is the most common, as well as degenerative arthritis including peripheral and spinal osteoarthritis (OA) and the spectrum of soft tissue rheumatic complaints of tendonitis and bursitis [1].

Pain associated with rheumatic diseases typically arises from non-infectious inflammation of joints and/or soft tissues, from degenerative pathologies of joints and from sensitization of nociceptive pathways leading to nociplastic pain. Fibromyalgia (FM), previously considered to be a rheumatic disease involving soft tissues, is now considered a nociplastic disorder, as evidence points to dysregulation of pain-processing mechanisms as its main pathophysiologic mechanism [2–4]. The most common presenting symptom of each of these conditions is pain.

Rheumatic conditions are threefold more common today than 40 years ago, with a further future expected increase due to the prevalence of OA as populations age [5]. Some form of arthritis currently affects at least 50% of individuals over the age of 65 years, with doctor-diagnosed arthritis present in more than 21% of adults at any one time. Rheumatic pain, among the most prevalent pain syndromes worldwide, is the leading cause of disability in the USA, and will be experienced by almost all persons at some time during their lifetime [6]. While rheumatic diseases are a prevalent cause of chronic pain, pain is the most common symptom in rheumatic diseases [7–10], and its alleviation is considered by patients as a primary treatment priority (11). The Pain Management Task Force of the American College of Rheumatology has acknowledged pain management as a critical aspect of the medical management of patients with rheumatic diseases [9].

As there is no imminent cure for either IA or OA, the pain associated with these conditions will continue to require attention. As with other painful conditions, rheumatic pain has important negative consequences to overall health with impaired quality of life and poor functional outcome. Therefore, healthcare professionals should be sensitive to the complaint of pain in patients with arthritis and soft tissue rheumatism and should assess and treat pain in parallel with management of the underlying disease.

Clinical Pain Management: A Practical Guide, Second Edition. Edited by Mary E. Lynch, Kenneth D. Craig, and Philip W. Peng.

Basic mechanisms in rheumatic pain

Rheumatic pain has previously been categorized as predominantly nociceptive, arising from activation of nociceptors at peripheral sites of tissue damage or inflammation. A primary inflammatory process initiates the pain message, which is conducted via first order sensory neurons through relays in the dorsal horn to the somatosensory cortex. However, in recent years there is growing appreciation of the pertinence of other pain mechanisms, which have been implicated in the pathophysiology of pain in rheumatic diseases.

1 Inflammation of joints and soft tissues causes pain, with typical inflammatory features. This pain is typically relapsing and remitting in temporal correlation with the level of inflammatory activity, aggravated by rest, alleviated by movement and accompanied by morning stiffness [7].

2 Degenerative changes of joints and tendons may elicit pain which is mechanical in nature. This pain typically appears later in the course of the disease, is aggravated by activity and is affected to a lesser degree by the level of active inflammation [7].

3 Nociplastic pain may develop as a result of alterations in pain processing and modulation systems, leading to increased spontaneous and evoked pain around affected joints but also to widespread pain that may persist even when the inflammatory process has remitted. The most recognized nociplastic pain condition is FM characterized by chronic widespread pain. Nociplastic pain is frequently accompanied by symptoms of fatigue, sleep disturbance and other somatic symptoms. It may occur as a unique condition, as in FM, or be a comorbid associate with autoimmune disorders and various types of arthritis in up to 20% of patients [12–14. Meeting diagnostic criteria for FM, these patients are now identified as having comorbid (or secondary) FM [15].

4 Other types of pain are seen at increased prevalence among individuals with rheumatic diseases, including (but not limited to) comorbid myofascial pain [16] and neuropathic pain [17].

In the context of a purely nociceptive pathogenesis, treatments were previously focused on use of anti-inflammatory drugs and simple analgesics. Now, as the involvement of more pain mechanisms in rheumatic pain is recognized, a wider choice of treatment modalities is available and can be tailored to the needs of the individual patient.

Anatomic considerations

With the exception of healthy cartilage, all joint structures are richly innervated with sensory neurons, which can mediate the pain response [17]. Under normal circumstances, the structures of the joint are not sensitive to strong pressure or even vigorous movement. In contrast, diseased joints that have been primed by inflammatory molecules, develop sensitivity to seemingly benign movements and have a low threshold of activation to noxious stimuli.

Pathogenic mechanisms in IA and OA show considerable similarities with both demonstrating variable degrees of inflammation and structural tissue damage. IA has a more pronounced inflammatory phase than OA, with synovial infiltration of immune cells, leading to invasion of ligaments, cartilage and bone. Structural changes occur in both with time, with radiographic erosions present in IA and subchondral sclerosis and osteophyte formation in OA. Changes in juxta-articular bone, bone marrow edema and bone marrow vascular stasis all play a part in pain generation [18]. Ongoing inflammatory as well as degenerative articular processes sensitize the peripheral and central nervous systems, leading to decreased pain thresholds, increased nociceptor receptive fields and altered pain-modulation activity [19]. Extra-articular soft tissues such as muscles, fascia and ligaments are prone to chronic pain in inflammatory and degenerative rheumatic diseases. Soft-tissue pain is not only common but also an important contributor to the symptomatic burden in rheumatic diseases [16].

The active inflammatory setting

The major stimulus initiating pain in an active inflammatory process is the outpouring of inflammatory molecules at the local tissue site [19, 20]. This occurs to a lesser degree in OA. This neuroactive and inflammatory milieu lowers the firing threshold of high threshold nociceptors to mechanical, thermal or chemical stimuli and a cycle of pain is set in motion. The success of the numerous NSAIDs can be attributed to the importance of inflammatory mechanisms in rheumatic pain.

The chronic rheumatic process

In contrast, chronic pain resulting from tissue destruction and mechanical changes to cartilage, bone and soft tissues is mostly sustained by activation of neurogenic mechanisms. Peripheral and central sensitization contribute to the chronicity of pain [21]. Afferent neuronal pathways are in turn influenced by descending neuron projections, synapsing in the laminae of the dorsal horns, with messages mediated by molecules such as serotonin, norepinephrine, endogenous opioids and cannabinoids. For these reasons, the management of chronic pain is more challenging and often less successful than that of acute pain. Furthermore, chronic pain differs from acute pain not only in the underlying pathophysiologic processes, but also in the psychosocial burden that it imposes on the lives of affected individuals [8, 22].

Clinical practice

A specific diagnosis is the first step to effective management, as early disease-modifying treatment may have important prognostic value in certain inflammatory diseases [23, 24]. IA encompasses a wide spectrum of connective tissue diseases occurring mainly in the middle years of life. Although RA is the most readily recognized IA, other conditions of equal importance are seronegative arthritis, with a negative rheumatoid factor, including psoriatic arthritis, inflammatory spondyloarthritis and reactive arthritis. There is also an array of immunological diseases that have an arthritis component, such as systemic lupus erythematosus, scleroderma, Sjogren's syndrome and others. Crystal-induced inflammation due to gout or pseudogout, a cause of acute joint inflammation, is seen in the older population and presents with acute pain and swelling localized to one or a few joint or tendon sites (Table 31.1).

Next, the mechanisms underlying the patient's pain should be identified. Active inflammation can be inferred based on the history, physical examination, laboratory tests and imaging [24]. Similarly, degenerative, nociplastic, neuropathic and myofascial components should be identified. The level of disability is gauged, as well as potential psycho-social factors that may play a role in the burden of symptoms. In the setting of continued pain there is often an associated sleep disturbance, fatigue and mood disorder, all well described components of FM [3], which must be addressed.

The first goal of treatment for IA must be to control the disease process, reduce the inflammatory activity and prevent chronic joint damage. This is usually achieved to a moderate degree with the use of disease-modifying agents (DMARDs) which may be synthetic such as methotrexate, hydroxychloroquine and others or a biologic such as the tumor necrosis factor targeted molecules and others [24]. Failure to address the global disease will result in continued symptoms, even with the best attention to pain. In contrast, there is no DMARD available for treatment of OA, which is therefore treated symptomatically (25).

Musculoskeletal pain is described as dull and aching, interfering with daily function and sleep, but seldom extreme, except for severe inflammation of infection or crystal arthritis. Inflammatory pain

Table 31.1 Classification of rheumatic painful conditions.

Inflammatory arthritis	Rheumatoid arthritis Seronegative arthritis: psoriatic arthritis, inflammatory spondyloarthritis, reactive arthritis, other connective tissue diseases Crystal-related arthritis: gout, pseudogout Infectious arthritis
Osteoarthritis	Peripheral osteoarthritis: small joints hands, large joints (mostly weight-bearing) Spinal osteoarthritis
Soft tissue rheumatism	Tendonitis, bursitis

generally improves with gentle exercise and is aggravated by immobility. Morning stiffness lasting for over an hour is common. OA pain can be associated with stiffness, but usually lasting minutes rather than hours. Rheumatic pain can vary considerably from day to day and can also be influenced by various environmental factors. One example is the effect of weather on rheumatic pain, which is a matter of ongoing controversy. Weather-related changes are more prevalent in women than in men, are not well understood and apply to temperature, barometric pressure and precipitation changes [26, 27]. Intrinsic factors, such as mood, sleep and physical activity also have an important role in pain variability.

Treatment

Pain management must be tailored to the individual patient, taking into account age, comorbidity, specific rheumatic process, involved pain mechanisms and personal beliefs of the patient. Pain control for one individual may be facilitated by reduction of anxiety, whereas for another it may be simply the advice to use an assistive device such as a cane or supportive pillow. Not every pain requires treatment with a pill and patients should be informed that most pain-relieving drug treatments offer only a modest effect for some patients, with adverse effects often outweighing the beneficial effects [28].

Any pain management strategy must begin with non-pharmacologic management. Patients should be encouraged to develop an internal locus of control and become active participants in their healthcare. There should be emphasis on the importance of good lifestyle practices that include sufficient health-related physical activity, good eating habits and weight control and attention to sufficient sleep. Mood disorders should be addressed as persistent poor mood will be a barrier to effective care. Realistic treatment goals should be identified with the objective to reduce the pain as well as to improve function. Treatment modalities include lifestyle and self-help interventions, physical measures, pharmaceutical measures and psycho-social interventions. An effective treatment plan typically includes more than one modality [28].

Accompanying symptoms of sleep disturbance, mood disorder and fatigue need also to be addressed. The efficacy of any treatment should be carefully balanced with treatment-related side effects and the need for continued treatment must be carefully evaluated. Treatment of pain should also occur in parallel with the best management of the underlying rheumatologic process.

1. Lifestyle and self-help measures

Exercise

Exercise is considered one of the most effective, low-cost and safe interventions for both IA and OA. Physical activity has been shown to improve pain, function and quality of life of affected individuals [29]. In addition, the direct anti-inflammatory effect of physical exercise, putatively mediated by the secretion of anti-inflammatory myokines from skeletal muscles, is thought to attenuate the elevated cardiovascular risk associated with IA [30]. Benefits of physical activity include stimulation of reparative processes in cartilage, maintenance of muscle tone and activation of the natural descending inhibitory pain pathway, via release of endogenous opioids and activation of (supra)spinal nociceptive inhibitory mechanisms orchestrated by the brain [31]. Recent research has, however, shown dysfunction of this endogenous analgesic response to exercise in some patients with chronic pain (i.e.with FM) with a report that exercise induces more pain. Therefore, exercise therapy should be tailored to the specific patient needs, with care to avoiding flares of pain. Exercise should be part of a normal healthy lifestyle routine, appropriate for the patient's age and physical condition and enjoyable to encourage adherence.

Both traditional exercise modalities, such as strengthening, aerobics and flexibility and non-traditional modalities including Tai-Chi, yoga and aquatic training, have been shown to be effective, whether supervised, semi-supervised or unsupervised [32]. Tai chi or a water exercise program are acceptable forms of exercise for many patients. Some people may prefer the slightly more active program of yoga or a low impact exercise program. Exercise combined with weight reduction improves symptoms of arthritic pain in the lower limbs, with one unit of body weight translated into a 4-unit load through the knee joints with every step taken.

Diet

A frequent question by patients with rheumatic pain is whether dietary manipulation could have impact on their pain. This has been the subject of debate for decades [33]. In recent years, there is growing appreciation of the role of the gut microbiome in the development and severity of certain rheumatic diseases including RA [34], spondyloarthropathies [35] and OA [36]. The composition and function of the gut microbiome is readily affected by dietary intake, rendering dietary interventions biologically plausible [37]. Mediterranean diet and fish-oil-rich diets have been shown to improve symptomatic burden in patients with RA, although the level of evidence remains limited [38, 39]. It is yet premature to suggest that alteration of diet will have meaningful effect on musculoskeletal pain. The most reasonable advice at this time is to recommend a diet with reduced fats and sugars and increased fiber to move nutrition closer to a Neolithic type diet with reduced global health risks of obesity and inflammatory disease [40, 41].

Health practitioner administered treatments

Treatments by healthcare practitioners should be focused toward education and providing patients with strategies to manage their pain. Prolonged and unnecessary interventions may have a negative consequence by medicalizing the patient and fostering the sickness role. Patients should learn techniques to modulate pain, rather than develop a dependence on the healthcare provider, which promotes passive behaviors [42, 43]. Advice regarding muscle strengthening and joint protection by a physiotherapist or occupational therapist is ideal but is still unfortunately unrealistic for many. Treatments such as relaxation, meditation, hypnosis, massage, chiropractic and others, have mostly been categorized as complementary therapies [42]. Activation of descending inhibitory pathways is believed to be the mechanism of action for pain relief for many of these treatments, but further study is needed. Heating, cooling and paraffin treatments may provide temporary symptomatic relief.

2. Pharmacotherapy

Topical treatments

Topical applications provide an attractive alternative to oral treatments for patients with musculoskeletal conditions. Good tissue levels of drug are achieved, especially when the painful area is close to the skin, such as in tendonitis in the elbow or wrist region, OA of the finger joints and OA of the knee. Although some systemic absorption does occur, plasma levels of drug are extremely low, contributing to tolerability of treatment and low level of side effects. Topical agents that have been studied include nonsteroidal anti-inflammatory drugs (NSAIDs) [44], capsaicin [45], local anesthetics and others (Chapter 19). Topical NSAIDs appear to be significantly more effective in acute pain conditions than in chronic ones [44].

Systemic pharmacologic treatments

NSAIDs and simple analgesics

NSAIDs are efficacious in mild to moderate rheumatic pain. Considering the toxicity related to gastrointestinal, renal and cardiac effects, it is currently recommended that NSAIDs be used in the lowest doses and for the shortest period of time possible [46]. In light of concerns regarding side effects of the NSAIDs, acetaminophen and dipyrone (where available) may be considered for short-term relief of milder pain [47] (see also Chapter 21).

Opioids

Opioids may be safe and effective for short-term use in the setting of acute inflammatory episode of IA or crystal arthritis [48]. However in chronic pain, the efficacy of opioids typically wanes and important safety concerns rise. Strong opioids (morphine, hydromorphone, oxycodone, fentanyl) are not superior to non-opioid analgesics in the treatment of chronic hip and knee OA pain [49], while being associated with considerable risks. Transdermal buprenorphine, while possibly safer than strong opioids, is not associated with significant pain relief in patients with OA [50]. A 2014 Cochrane review of opioids for knee and hip OA demonstrated a statistically significant improvement in pain relief, but with failure to meet the minimal clinically significant difference [51]. Furthermore, while traditionally considered a safer alternative to strong opioids, tramadol has recently been shown to be associated with increased mortality in a retrospective cohort of individuals with OA [52]. Taken together, these data suggest that opioids should probably be considered only in a small subset of patients where other treatment options have been ineffective or are contraindicated, preferably for the shortest period of time possible. Tramadol should be conditionally preferred over non-tramadol opioids [25].

Corticosteroids

Corticosteroids can be a useful adjunct to pain management in the rheumatic diseases in a few settings. Either an intramuscular injection of a depot preparation of methylprednisolone or a short sharp course of oral corticosteroid for a few days to a few weeks can be used to settle a flare of IA or to treat an acute attack of crystal arthritis. In view of toxicity associated with prolonged use, the treatment strategy should be similar to that for NSAIDs, use of the lowest dose for the shortest period of time possible. Low dose oral corticosteroids, equivalent to less than 7.5 mg/day prednisolone, may be used concomitantly with a DMARD in IA and usually give excellent symptom relief. However, the risk–benefit ratio of long-term corticosteroid use needs to be evaluated for each patient. The notable exception is polymyalgia rheumatica, where low-dose corticosteroid is the treatment of choice.

Adjuvant drugs

Use of antidepressants as pain modulators has been reported in small trials of patients with arthritic disease, with improvements noted in about half of patients treated [53]. Duloxetine, a selective serotonin and noradrenaline reuptake inhibitor (SNRI), has been shown to have modest positive effects on pain and function in patients with knee OA [54]. The anticonvulsants gabapentin and pregabalin, acting on voltage-gated and ligand-gated ion channels and other receptors, are often prescribed for patients with OA, despite limited evidence for their efficacy in pain associated with rheumatic diseases [55]. Nevertheless, in the context of comorbid nociplastic pain (i.e. FM), SNRI, tricyclic antidepressants (TCA) and gabapentinoids may prove moderately effective [56]. Use of adjuvant drugs in treatment of rheumatic pain are mostly off-label, except for indications for pregabalin, duloxetine and milnacipran for FM and the latter two for limb OA or chronic back pain.

Cannabinoids

The medical use of cannabis and cannabinoids is a source of ongoing debate. When considering the possible mechanistic role of cannabinoids on pain and inflammation, there are a number of factors relevant to the rheumatic diseases that pertain to the cannabinoid system. The cannabinoid receptors, of which there are two known to date, are distributed not only throughout the nervous system, but also in the periphery at sites that include the skin, joint tissue and cartilage. The CB1 receptor is mostly associated with neural tissue, whereas the CB2 receptor is found on immunologic cells as well as chondrocytes and osteoclasts. Well-controlled studies examining cannabinoids in treatment of rheumatic pain are lacking; however, modest analgesic effects have been demonstrated in other types of non-cancer pain. The limited study of medical cannabis and cannabis-based medicines in patients with rheumatic diseases has led many groups to advise against use. In the setting of easier access to cannabis in many jurisdictions, patients are either self-medicating with cannabis or requesting information. Much information about medical cannabis is based on anecdote or studies of suboptimum quality. Rather than advise against use, physicians should enter into a respectful dialogue with patients regarding the current state-of-the-art and offer pragmatic advice as has been suggested by the Canadian Rheumatology Association [57]. It should be noted that the absence of sufficient evidence for efficacy of cannabinoids does not infer inefficacy. Indeed, individual patients occasionally seem to derive considerable symptomatic benefit from cannabinoids. (See also Chapter 20).

Choosing the right analgesic

When choosing a pharmaceutical analgesic for a patient with a rheumatic disease one should consider the modest long-term clinical efficacy of most agents, including simple analgesics [58], opioids [49], NSAIDs and cannabinoids [59]. In terms of safety profile, despite the cardiovascular and renal risks associated with the use of NSAIDs, they seem to have a superior safety profile as compared to opioids [60], with comparable efficacy [61]. The clinical choice should be based on individual patient variables such as comorbidities, risk factors and individual preferences. Given the high number-needed-to-treat of most agents, a sequential trial of several agents is common.

Herbal medicine and food supplements

Complementary treatments in many forms have been used for years, often on the basis of hearsay and tradition rather than scientific rigor but should not be immediately discarded for want of evidence. Patients with rheumatic pain use herbal products and dietary interventions extensively. There is increasing evidence that some agents modulate pain or have anti-inflammatory effects such as Borago officinalis, Nigella sativa, Oenothera biennis (evening primrose oil) and curcuma (turmeric) [62]. Several lines of evidence show that dietary omega-3 polyunsaturated fatty acids (e.g. alfa-linolenic acid) possess anti-inflammatory properties [62]. The healthcare professional should acknowledge that disclosure by the patient of use of complementary products speaks to a trusting doctor–patient relationship.

3. Invasive procedures

Injections into joints and soft tissues

Injections into joints, bursae and peri-ligamentous structures remains a useful therapeutic measure. Risks are low, infection is rare and treatment is cheap. Injection of corticosteroids is particularly useful in inflammatory conditions such as crystal arthritis (gout or chondrocalcinosis), single active joint in IA or a painful sacroiliac joint in spondyloarthritis. Corticosteroids are also commonly used in degenerative joint and tendon diseases although their effect is typically short and the level of evidence is low [63, 64]. Nevertheless, they may be useful to treat OA flares. The general rule of thumb, without an evidence base, is to administer no more than three injections per joint per year, with the objective for at least 3 months of pain relief. Care should be taken to avoid repeated peri-tendinous injection of corticosteroids, as this may increase the risk of tendon rupture. Intra-articular hyaluronic acid and platelet rich plasma may provide moderate symptomatic relief in the treatment of knee OA [65, 66]. However, in light of the low level of evidence, the American College of Rheumatology 2019 guidelines for the management of hip and knee OA recommend against injections of hyaluronic acid and prolotherapy in these indications [42].

Nerve blocks, radiofrequency ablation and surgery

Degenerative joint pain can sometimes be temporarily relieved by selective nerve blocks. When a block provides significant short-term symptomatic relief, radiofrequency ablation of the involved nerves may provide a longer clinical effect. Common targets of radiofrequency treatment are the genicular nerves for knee pain, lateral sacral branches for sacroiliac pain, medial branches for facet pain and the suprascapular nerve for shoulder pain [25].

Surgery is typically reserved for severe OA, where functional capacity is impaired and symptoms are poorly controlled by more conservative measures.

4. Physical therapy

Physical and occupational therapy may aid in preserving and improving function, strengthening muscles and improving the ranges of motion. Assistive devices and technologies may also be fitted to the patient. Generally, treatment regimens in which the patient is active should be preferred over passive treatment modalities such as massage and manual therapy without exercise [42].

5. Psycho-social interventions

Individuals with rheumatic diseases are at increased risk for psychiatric comorbidity, specifically affective disorders. In addition to chronic pain and disability, the psychological burden may lead to important social consequences including occupational challenges, interpersonal conflicts and social isolation. It is thus a clinical priority to identify patients at risk of psychosocial distress and to offer treatments that increase active coping strategies and

Table 31.2 Barriers to pain management.

Patient concerns	Side effects of medications
	Dislike of too many pills
	Treatments may not be effective when needed
	Masking disease process
	Fear of addiction
Physician	Additional time required
	Discomfort with treatments
	Lack of education
	Regulatory bodies

address affective distress, self-efficacy and supportive social relationships [67].

Obstacles to optimal pain management

Barriers to optimal pain management exist for patients with rheumatic pain from both the patient's as well as the healthcare professional's perspective (Table 31.2)[68]. Patients often believe that pain is a normal part of the rheumatic disease and that pain management will mask the disease process. There is fear and distrust of medications because of side effects, concerns about loss of efficacy of pain treatments and risks of addiction. Compliance is poor with many studies reporting only 50% adherence to treatments. Physicians have also been remiss in neglecting optimal pain management, as this adds an extra dimension to patient care which is time-consuming, associated with concerns about regulatory scrutiny and has in the past been assigned as having secondary importance to management of the primary rheumatic disease [68].

Conclusions

Current treatment for rheumatic pain must address both disease-modifying (for IA) and pain management approaches. This will include the use of appropriate DMARDs along with approaches for general pain management. Treatment is typically multimodal (Figure 31.1) and should include healthful living such as healthy diet, exercise and weight control as well as quitting smoking. It is also appropriate to add additional analgesic agents, physical and psychological and specific complementary therapies to target the pain following the same principles reviewed in this and other chapters in this volume. Given that the pain leads to significant disability and compromise in quality of life, it is time for clinicians to give priority to the management of pain in rheumatic disease as well as targeting the disease process in order to reduce the inflammatory activity and prevent chronic joint damage.

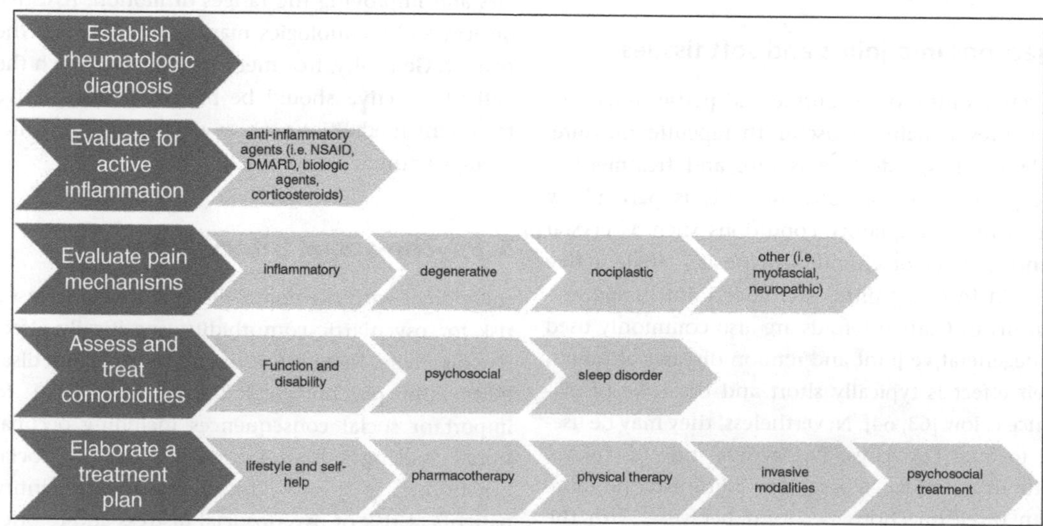

Figure 31.1 a schematic approach to the treatment of pain in individuals with a rheumatologic disease

References

1 Al Maini M, Adelowo F, Al Saleh J *et al.* (2015) The global challenges and opportunities in the practice of rheumatology: white paper by the World Forum on Rheumatic and Musculoskeletal Diseases. *Clin Rheumatol* **34(5)**:819–29.

2 Kosek E, Cohen M, Baron R *et al.* (2016) Do we need a third mechanistic descriptor for chronic pain states? *Pain* **157(7)**:1382–6.

3 Arnold LM, Bennett RM, Crofford LJ *et al.* (2019) AAPT Diagnostic criteria for fibromyalgia. *J Pain Off J Am Pain Soc* **20(6)**:611–28.

4 Maixner W, Fillingim RB, Williams DA, Smith SB, Slade GD. (2016) Overlapping chronic pain conditions: implications for diagnosis and classification. *J Pain Off J Am Pain Soc* **17(9 Suppl)**:T93–107.

5 Hootman JM, Helmick CG, Barbour KE, Theis KA, Boring MA. (2016) Updated projected prevalence of self-reported doctor-diagnosed arthritis and arthritis-attributable activity limitation among US adults, 2015-2040. *Arthritis Rheumatol* **68(7)**:1582–7.

6 Fitzcharles M-A, Shir Y. (2008) New concepts in rheumatic pain. *Rheum Dis Clin North Am* **34(2)**:267–83.

7 Borenstein DG, Hassett AL, Pisetsky D. (2017) Pain management in rheumatology research, training, and practice. *Clin Exp Rheumatol* **35 Suppl 107(5)**:2–7.

8 Edwards RR, Cahalan C, Calahan C, Mensing G, Smith M, Haythornthwaite JA. (2011) Pain, catastrophizing, and depression in the rheumatic diseases. *Nat Rev Rheumatol* **7(4)**:216–24.

9 American College of Rheumatology Pain Management Task Force. (2010) Report of the American College of Rheumatology Pain Management Task Force. *Arthritis Care Res* **62(5)**:590–9.

10 Rifbjerg-Madsen S, Christensen AW, Christensen R *et al.* (2017) Pain and pain mechanisms in patients with inflammatory arthritis: A Danish nationwide cross-sectional DANBIO registry survey. *PLoS ONE* **12(7)**:e0180014.

11 Walsh DA, McWilliams DF. (2014) Mechanisms, impact and management of pain in rheumatoid arthritis. *Nat Rev Rheumatol* **10(10)**:581–92.

12 Clauw DJ, Witter J. (2009) Pain and rheumatology: thinking outside the joint. *Arthritis Rheum* **60(2)**:321–4.

13 Phillips K, Clauw DJ. (2013) Central pain mechanisms in the rheumatic diseases: future directions. *Arthritis Rheum* **65(2)**:291–302.

14 Gwilym SE, Keltner JR, Warnaby CE *et al.* (2009) Psychophysical and functional imaging evidence supporting the presence of central sensitization in a cohort of osteoarthritis patients. *Arthritis Rheum* **61(9)**:1226–34.

15 Fitzcharles M-A, Perrot S, Häuser W. (2018) Comorbid fibromyalgia: A qualitative review of prevalence and importance. *Eur J Pain Lond Engl* **22(9)**:1565–76.

16 Vulfsons S, Minerbi A. (2020) The case for comorbid myofascial pain—a qualitative review. *Int J Environ Res Public Health* **17(14)**:5188.

17 McWilliams DF, Walsh DA. (2018) Pain mechanisms in rheumatoid arthritis. *Clin Exp Rheumatol* **35 Suppl 107(5)**:94–101.

18 O'Neill TW, Felson DT. (2018) Mechanisms of osteoarthritis (OA) pain. *Curr Osteoporos Rep* **16(5)**:611–6.

19 Zhang A, Lee YC. (2018) Mechanisms for joint pain in rheumatoid arthritis (RA): from cytokines to central sensitization. *Curr Osteoporos Rep* **16(5)**:603–10.

20 Krock E, Jurczak A, Svensson CI. (2018) Pain pathogenesis in rheumatoid arthritis-what have we learned from animal models? *Pain 159* **Suppl 1**:S98–109.

21 Lampa J. (2019) Pain without inflammation in rheumatic diseases. *Best Pract Res Clin Rheumatol* **33(3)**:101439.

22 Vilen L, Baldassari AR, Callahan LF. (2017) Socioeconomic burden of pain in rheumatic disease. *Clin Exp Rheumatol* **35 Suppl 107(5)**: 26–31.

23 American College of Rheumatology Ad Hoc Committee on Clinical Guidelines. (1996) Guidelines for the initial evaluation of the adult patient with acute musculoskeletal symptoms. *Arthritis Rheum* **39(1)**:1–8.

24 Ledingham J, Snowden N, Ide Z. (2017) Diagnosis and early management of inflammatory arthritis. *BMJ* **358**:j3248.

25 Kolasinski SL, Neogi T, Hochberg MC *et al.* (2020) 2019 American College of Rheumatology/Arthritis Foundation Guideline for the Management of Osteoarthritis of the Hand, Hip, and Knee. *Arthritis Care Res* **72(2)**:149–62.

26 McAlindon T, Formica M, Schmid CH, Fletcher J. (2007) Changes in barometric pressure and ambient temperature influence osteoarthritis pain. *Am J Med* **120(5)**:429–34.

27 Smedslund G, Hagen KB. (2011) Does rain really cause pain? A systematic review of the associations between weather factors and severity of pain in people with rheumatoid arthritis. *Eur J Pain Lond Engl* **15(1)**:5–10.

28 Kudrina I, Shir Y, Fitzcharles M-A. (2015) Multidisciplinary treatment for rheumatic pain. *Best Pract Res Clin Rheumatol* **29(1)**:156–63.

29 Metsios GS, Kitas GD. (2018) Physical activity, exercise and rheumatoid arthritis: Effectiveness, mechanisms and implementation. *Best Pract Res Clin Rheumatol* **32(5)**:669–82.

30 Benatti FB, Pedersen BK. (2015) Exercise as an anti-inflammatory therapy for rheumatic diseases-myokine regulation. *Nat Rev Rheumatol* **11(2)**:86–97.

31 Nijs J, Kosek E, Van Oosterwijck J, Meeus M. (2012) Dysfunctional endogenous analgesia during exercise in patients with chronic pain: to exercise or not to exercise? *Pain Physician* **15(3 Suppl)**:ES205–213.

32 Wellsandt E, Golightly Y. (2018) Exercise in the management of knee and hip osteoarthritis. *Curr Opin Rheumatol* **30(2)**:151–9.

33 Panush RS. (1984(Controversial arthritis remedies. *Bull Rheum Dis* **34(5)**:1–10.

34 Larsen JM. (2017) The immune response to Prevotella bacteria in chronic inflammatory disease. *Immunology* **151(4)**:363–74.

35 Gilis E, Mortier C, Venken K, Debusschere K, Vereecke L, Elewaut D. (2018) The role of the microbiome in gut and joint inflammation in psoriatic arthritis and spondyloarthritis. *J Rheumatol Suppl* **94**:36–9.

36 Biver E, Berenbaum F, Valdes AM *et al.* (2019) Gut microbiota and osteoarthritis management: An expert consensus of the European society for clinical and economic aspects of osteoporosis, osteoarthritis and musculoskeletal diseases (ESCEO). *Ageing Res Rev* **55**:100946.

37 Guerreiro CS, Calado Â, Sousa J, Fonseca JE. (2018) Diet, microbiota, and gut permeability-the unknown triad in rheumatoid arthritis. *Front Med* **5**:349.

38 Petersson S, Philippou E, Rodomar C, Nikiphorou E. (2018) The Mediterranean diet, fish oil supplements and rheumatoid arthritis outcomes: evidence from clinical trials. *Autoimmun Rev* **17(11)**:1105–14.

39 Paolino S, Pacini G, Patanè M *et al.* (2019) Interactions between microbiota, diet/nutrients and immune/inflammatory response in rheumatic diseases: focus on rheumatoid arthritis. *Reumatologia* **57(3)**:151–7.

40 Cordain L, Eaton SB, Sebastian A et al. (2005) Origins and evolution of the Western diet: health implications for the 21st century. *Am J Clin Nutr* **81(2)**:341–54.

41 Minerbi A, Fitzcharles M-A. (2020) Gut microbiome: pertinence in fibromyalgia. *Clin Exp Rheumatol* **38 Suppl 123(1)**:99–104.

42 Kolasinski SL, Neogi T, Hochberg MC *et al.* (2020) 2019 American College of Rheumatology/ Arthritis Foundation Guideline for the Management of Osteoarthritis of the Hand, Hip, and Knee. *Arthritis Care Res* **72(2)**:149–62.

43 Yocum DE, Castro WL, Cornett M. (2000) Exercise, education, and behavioral modification as alternative therapy for pain and stress in rheumatic disease. *Rheum Dis Clin North Am* **26(1)**: 145–59, x–xi.

44 Derry S, Wiffen PJ, Kalso EA *et al.* (2017) Topical analgesics for acute and chronic pain in adults - an overview of Cochrane Reviews. *Cochrane Database Syst Rev* **5**:CD008609.

45 Guedes V, Castro JP, Brito I. (2018) Topical capsaicin for pain in osteoarthritis: A literature review. *Reumatol Clin* **14(1)**:40–5.

46 Scarpignato C, Lanas A, Blandizzi C et al. (2015) Safe prescribing of non-steroidal anti-inflammatory drugs in patients with osteoarthritis--an expert consensus addressing benefits as well as gastrointestinal and cardiovascular risks. *BMC Med* **13**:55.

47 Machado GC, Maher CG, Ferreira PH *et al.* (2015) Efficacy and safety of paracetamol for spinal pain and osteoarthritis: systematic review and meta-analysis of randomised placebo controlled trials. *BMJ* **350**:h1225.

48 Day AL, Curtis JR. (2019) Opioid use in rheumatoid arthritis: trends, efficacy, safety, and best practices. *Curr Opin Rheumatol* **31(3)**:264–70.

49 Krebs EE, Gravely A, Nugent S et al. (2018) Effect of opioid vs nonopioid medications on pain-related function in patients with chronic back pain or hip or knee osteoarthritis pain: the SPACE randomized clinical trial. *JAMA* **319(9)**:872–82.

50 da Costa BR, Nüesch E, Kasteler R *et al.* (2014) Oral or transdermal opioids for osteoarthritis of the knee or hip. *Cochrane Database Syst Rev* **(9)**:CD003115.

51 Toupin April K, Bisaillon J, Welch V et al. (2019) Tramadol for osteoarthritis. *Cochrane Database Syst Rev* **5**:CD005522.

52 Zeng C, Dubreuil M, LaRochelle MR *et al.* (2019) Association of tramadol with all-cause mortality among patients with osteoarthritis. *JAMA* **321(10)**:969–82.

53 Loveless MS, Fry AL. (2016) Pharmacologic therapies in musculoskeletal conditions. *Med Clin North Am* **100(4)**:869–90.

54 Chen L, Gong M, Liu G, Xing F, Liu J, Xiang Z. (2019) Efficacy and tolerability of duloxetine in patients with knee osteoarthritis: a meta-analysis of randomised controlled trials. *Intern Med J* **49(12)**:1514–23.

55 Appleyard T, Ashworth J, Bedson J, Yu D, Peat G. (2019). Trends in gabapentinoid prescribing in patients with osteoarthritis: a United Kingdom national cohort study in primary care. *Osteoarthritis Cartilage* **27(10)**:1437–44.

56 Argoff CE, Emir B, Whalen E, Ortiz M, Pauer L, Clair A. (2016) Pregabalin improves pain scores in patients with fibromyalgia irrespective of comorbid osteoarthritis. *Pain Med Malden Mass* **17(11)**:2100–8.

57 Fitzcharles M-A, Niaki OZ, Hauser W, Hazlewood G, Canadian Rheumatology Association. (2019) Position statement: a pragmatic approach for medical cannabis and patients with rheumatic diseases. *J Rheumatol* **46(5)**:532–8.

58 Leopoldino AO, Machado GC, Ferreira PH *et al.* (2019) Paracetamol versus placebo for knee and hip osteoarthritis. *Cochrane Database Syst Rev* **2**:CD013273.

59 Fitzcharles M-A, Baerwald C, Ablin J, Häuser W. (2016) Efficacy, tolerability and safety of cannabinoids in chronic pain associated with rheumatic diseases (fibromyalgia syndrome, back pain, osteoarthritis, rheumatoid arthritis): a systematic review of randomized controlled trials. *Schmerz* **30(1)**:47–61.

60 Solomon DH, Rassen JA, Glynn RJ, Lee J, Levin R, Schneeweiss S. (2010) The comparative safety of analgesics in older adults with arthritis. *Arch Intern Med* **170(22)**:1968–76.

61 Smith SR, Deshpande BR, Collins JE, Katz JN, Losina E. (2016) Comparative pain reduction of oral non-steroidal anti-inflammatory drugs and opioids for knee osteoarthritis: systematic analytic review. *Osteoarthritis Cartilage* **24(6)**: 962–72.

62 Chen L, Michalsen A. (2017) Management of chronic pain using complementary and integrative medicine. *BMJ* **357**:j1284.

63 Jüni P, Hari R, Rutjes AWS *et al.* (2015) Intra-articular corticosteroid for knee osteoarthritis. *Cochrane Database Syst Rev* **(10)**:CD005328.

64 Kane SF, Olewinski LH, Tamminga KS. (2019) Management of chronic tendon injuries. *Am Fam Physician* **100(3)**:147–57.

65 Altman R, Hackel J, Niazi F, Shaw P, Nicholls M. (2018) Efficacy and safety of repeated courses of hyaluronic acid injections for knee osteoarthritis: a systematic review. *Semin Arthritis Rheum* **48(2)**:168–75.

66 Dai W-L, Zhou A-G, Zhang H, Zhang J. (2017) Efficacy of platelet-rich plasma in the treatment of knee osteoarthritis: a meta-analysis of randomized controlled trials. *Arthrosc J Arthrosc Relat Surg Off Publ Arthrosc Assoc N Am Int Arthrosc Assoc* **33(3)**:659–670.e1.

67 Sturgeon JA, Finan PH, Zautra AJ. (2016) Affective disturbance in rheumatoid arthritis: psychological and disease-related pathways. *Nat Rev Rheumatol* **12(9)**:532–42.

68 Fitzcharles M-A, Almahrezi A, Shir Y. (2005) Pain: understanding and challenges for the rheumatologist. *Arthritis Rheum* **52(12)**:3685–92.

Further reading

Kolasinski SL, Neogi T, Hochberg MC et al. (2020) 2019 American College of Rheumatology/Arthritis Foundation Guideline for the Management of Osteoarthritis of the Hand, Hip, and Knee. *Arthritis Care Res* **72(2)**:149–62.

Chapter 32

Headache

Stephen D. Silberstein

Jefferson Headache Center, Thomas Jefferson University, Philadelphia, Pennsylvania, USA

Introduction

Headache is one of the most common medical complaints of humankind, accounting for more than 18 million outpatient visits per year in the United States. The International Headache Society (IHS) classification system (ICHD-3) [1] divides headache into primary and secondary disorders. In a primary headache disorder, headache is the disorder. In a secondary headache disorder, headache is attributable to another disorder.

Evaluation and diagnostic testing

Headache diagnosis is based on a history, physical and neurologic examination. Characteristics helpful in diagnosis include age at onset; headache frequency, duration, location and severity; factors associated with initiation, exacerbation or remission; accompanying symptoms; and preceding conditions.

Recurrent episodic severe headaches with onset in adolescence or early adulthood suggests a primary headache disorder. A sudden-onset severe (thunderclap) headache suggests a subarachnoid hemorrhage (SAH) or reversible cerebral vasoconstriction syndrome (RCVS) if recurrent. In patients over 50 years of age, tenderness on palpation of the temporal arteries accompanied by scalp tenderness, jaw claudication or visual changes suggests giant cell arteritis (GCA). Neck stiffness may indicate meningeal irritation due to infection or SAH hemorrhage. Papilledema indicates increased intracranial pressure. Focal neurologic symptoms or mental status changes typically accompany structural lesions. History may suggest the cause of headache: for example, recent head trauma, hemophilia, alcoholism or anticoagulant therapy may suggest a subdural hematoma.

Testing serves to exclude organic causes of headache, rule out coexistent diseases that could complicate treatment and establish a baseline for and exclude contraindications to drug treatment.

Patients require urgent neuroimaging [computed tomography (CT) or magnetic resonance imaging (MRI)] when any of the following is present:

1 Sudden-onset thunderclap headache;
2 Altered mental status
3 New seizure
4 Focal neurologic deficits;
5 Papilledema; or
6 Severe hypertension.

Except in an emergency situation or when an MRI cannot be done, MRI is preferred to CT. In addition, an anormal CT scan does not rule out SAH, meningitis or encephalitis; lumbar puncture is indicated when they are suspected. Patients with unusual persistent headaches may also require lumbar puncture.

Clinical Pain Management: A Practical Guide, Second Edition. Edited by Mary E. Lynch, Kenneth D. Craig, and Philip W. Peng.

Symptoms requiring prompt imaging include a change in prior headache pattern, new-onset headache after age 55, systemic symptoms (e.g. weight loss), secondary risk factors (e.g. cancer, HIV, head trauma) or chronic unexplained headache. MRI, magnetic resonance angiography (MRA) and/or magnetic resonance venography (MRV) are preferred; these tests can show many causes of headache (e.g. carotid dissection, cerebral vein thrombosis, pituitary apoplexy, vascular malformations, cerebral vasculitis, Chiari type I malformation) that can be missed on CT.

Other tests are used if specific disorders are suspected (e.g. erythrocyte sedimentation rate for GCA).

Migraine

Migraine is a chronic neurologic disease characterized by episodic attacks of headache and associated symptoms [2]. In the United States about 17.6% of women and 6% of men had one migraine attack in the previous year [3].

Description of the migraine attack

The migraine attack can consist of premonitory, aura, headache and postdrome phases. Premonitory symptoms may include psychological, neurologic, constitutional or autonomic features (depression, cognitive dysfunction and food cravings) and can occur hours to days before headache onset.

The migraine aura consists of focal neurologic symptoms that precede, accompany or (rarely) follow an attack. Aura usually develops over 5–20 minutes, lasts less than 60 minutes, can be visual, sensory or motor and may involve language or brainstem disturbances [1]. Headache usually follows within 60 minutes of the end of the aura.

The typical headache is unilateral, of gradual onset, throbbing, moderate to marked in severity and aggravated by movement [1]. It lasts 4–72 hours in adults and 2–48 hours in children [1].

Anorexia is common. Nausea occurs in almost 90% of patients, while vomiting occurs in about one-third. Sensory hypersensitivity results in patients seeking a dark quiet room [2,4]. Patients may experience blurry vision, nasal stuffiness, anorexia, hunger, tenesmus, diarrhea, abdominal cramps, polyuria, facial pallor, sensations of heat or cold and sweating. Depression, fatigue, anxiety, nervousness, irritability and impairment of concentration are common.

The ICHD-3 divides migraine into migraine without aura (Table 32.1) and migraine with aura (Table 32.2) [1]. Migraine persisting for more than 3 days defines "status migrainosus." Migraine occurring 15 or more days per month is called chronic migraine (CM) (Table 32.2).

Basilar-type migraine aura features brainstem symptoms: ataxia, vertigo, tinnitus, diplopia, nausea and vomiting, nystagmus, dysarthria, bilateral

Table 32.1 Migraine without aura.

A	At least five attacks
B	Headache attacks last 4–72 hours and occur <15 days/month or unsuccessfully treated
C	Headache has at least two of the following characteristics: 1. Unilateral location 2. Pulsating quality 3. Moderate or severe intensity 4. Aggravation by or causing avoidance from routine physical activity
D	During headache at least one of the following: 1. Nausea and/or vomiting 2. Photophobia and phonophobia
E	Not attributed to another ICHD-3 diagnosis

Table 32.2 Migraine with typical aura.

A	At least two attacks
B	One or more of the following fully reversible aura symptoms: 1. visual 2. sensory 3. speech and/or language 4. motor 5. brainstem 6. retinal
C	At least three of the following six characteristics: 1. at least one aura symptom spreads gradually over 5 minutes 2. two or more aura symptoms occur in succession 3. each individual aura symptom lasts 5–60 minutes 4. at least one aura symptom is unilateral 5. at least one aura symptom is positive 6. the aura is accompanied, or followed within 60 minutes, by headache
D	Not better accounted for by another ICHD-3 diagnosis.

paresthesia, or a change in level of consciousness and cognition [1]. Hemiplegic migraine can be sporadic or familial [2,4]. Familial hemiplegic migraine (FHM) is an autosomal dominant disorder associated with attacks of migraine, with and without aura, and hemiparesis.

Pathophysiology

The migraine aura is believed to be caused by cortical spreading depression (CSD). Headache probably results from activation of meningeal and blood vessel nociceptors combined with a change in central pain modulation. Headache and its associated neurovascular changes are subserved by the trigeminal system. Stimulation results in the release of substance P and calcitonin gene-related peptide (CGRP) from sensory C-fiber terminals and neurogenic inflammation. Neurogenic inflammation sensitizes nerve fibers (peripheral sensitization), which now respond to previously innocuous stimuli, such as blood vessel pulsations, causing, in part, the pain of migraine. Brainstem activation also occurs in migraine without aura, in part because of increased activity of the endogenous anti-nociceptive system. The migraine aura can trigger headache: CSD activates trigeminovascular afferents. In the absence of aura, CSD may occur in silent areas of the cortex or the cerebellum.

Treatment

Migraine treatment begins with making a diagnosis, explaining it to the patient and developing a treatment plan that considers comorbid conditions [2,4]. Treatment may be acute or preventive and patients may require both approaches. Acute treatment attempts to relieve the pain and impairment once an attack has begun. Preventive therapy is given to reduce the frequency, duration or severity of attacks. Additional benefits include improved responsiveness to acute attack treatment, improved function and reduced disability. In addition, lifestyle changes are also important, including healthy diet, regular physical exercise and relaxation strategies.

Acute treatment can be specific (dihydroergotamine [DHE], triptans, gepants and ditans) or non-specific (analgesics and opioids). Non-specific medications control the pain of migraine or other pain disorders, while specific medications are effective in migraine (and certain other) headache attacks but are not useful for non-headache pain disorders. Analgesics are used for mild to moderate headaches. Triptans or DHE are first line drugs for severe attacks and for less severe attacks that do not adequately respond to analgesics.

Gepants (small molecule CGRP antagonists and ditans (selective serotonin 1F agonists) can be used when triptans or DHE are contraindicated or have intolerable side effects. Early intervention prevents escalation and may increase efficacy. Limiting acute treatment to 2–3 days a week can prevent medication overuse headache. When headaches are very frequent, early intervention may not be appropriate.

Treatment occasionally fails and patients need to have rescue medications (opioids, neuroleptics and corticosteroids) available. These provide relief, but often limit function because of sedation or other adverse events.

Preventive treatment

Preventive treatment may prevent the progression of episodic to chronic migraine. However, prevention is not being utilized to nearly the extent it should be; only 5% of all migraineurs currently use preventive therapy to control their attacks [5].

Indications for preventive treatment include the following:

1 Migraine that significantly interferes with the patient's daily routine despite acute treatment.

2 Failure of, contraindication to, or troublesome adverse events from acute medications.

3 Acute medication overuse.

4 Very frequent headaches (>1 per week).

5 Patient preference.

6 Special circumstances, such as hemiplegic migraine.

Preventive medication groups include beta-adrenergic blockers, antidepressants, calcium channel antagonists, anticonvulsants and non-steroidal anti-inflammatory drugs (NSAIDs). In addition, the mAbs directed against CGRP and its receptor are now available. onabotulinum toxin is approved for the treatment of chronic migraine. Choice is based on efficacy, adverse events and coexistent conditions. The drug is started at a low dose and increased slowly until therapeutic effects develop or the ceiling dose is reached. A full therapeutic trial may take 2–6 months. If headaches are well controlled, medication can be tapered and discontinued. The preventive medications with the best documented efficacy are beta-blockers, valproic acid, topiramate, all the mAbs and onabotulinum toxin (for CM)

Although monotherapy is preferred, it is sometimes necessary to combine preventive medications. Antidepressants are often used in combination with the other effective medications. Coexistent diseases have important implications for treatment. In some instances, two or more conditions may be treated with a single drug.

Behavioral and psychological interventions used for prevention include relaxation training, thermal biofeedback combined with relaxation training, electromyography biofeedback and cognitive behavioral therapy.

Chronic daily headache

Chronic daily headache (CDH) refers to headache disorders experienced 15 or more days a month [1]. The major primary disorders are chronic migraine (CM) (Table 32.3), hemicrania continua (HC), chronic tension-type headache (CTTH) (Table 32.4) and new daily persistent headache (NDPH).

Most patients with CM are women. Patients often report a process of transformation characterized by headaches that become more frequent over months to years, with the associated symptoms of photophobia, phonophobia and nausea becoming less severe and less frequent. The headaches resemble a mixture of tension-type headache and migraine.

Table 32.3 Chronic migraine.

A Headache on 15 or more days per month for at least 3 months
B Occurring in a patient who has had at least five attacks fulfilling criteria B–D for migraine without aura and/or criteria B and C for Migraine with aura)
C On 8 days/month for >3 months, fulfilling any of the following 2:
1. criteria C and D for migraine without aura
2. criteria B and C for migraine with aura
3. believed by the patient to be migraine at onset and relieved by a triptan or ergot derivative

D Not better accounted for by another ICHD-3 diagnosis

Table 32.4 Tension-type headache.

Frequent episodic tension-type headache
A At least 10 episodes of headache occurring on 1–14 days/month on average for >3 months
B Headache lasting from 30 minutes to 7 days
C At least two of the following characteristics:
1. Bilateral location
2. Pressing/tightening (non-pulsating) quality
3. Mild or moderate intensity
4. No aggravation by walking stairs or similar routine physical activity

D Both of the following:
1. No nausea or vomiting (anorexia may occur)
2. Photophobia and phonophobia are absent, or one but not the other may be present

E Not better accounted for by another ICHD-3 diagnosis

Chronic tension-type headache
A Headache occurring on ≥15 days/month on average for >3 months
B Lasts hours to days, or unremitting
C At least two of the following characteristics:
1. Bilateral location
2. Pressing/tightening (non-pulsating) quality
3. Mild or moderate intensity
4. No aggravation by walking stairs or similar routine physical activity

D Both of the following:
1. No more than one of the following: photophobia, phonophobia or mild nausea
2. No moderate or severe nausea and no vomiting

E Not better accounted for by another ICHD-3 diagnosis

Medication overuse headache

Patients with frequent headaches often overuse analgesics, opioids, ergotamine and triptans (Table 32.5). Although stopping the acute medication may result in withdrawal symptoms and increased headache, subsequent headache improvement usually occurs. Acute drug overuse may interfere with the effectiveness of preventive headache medications. Prolonged use of large amounts of medication may cause renal or hepatic toxicity in addition to tolerance, habituation or dependence.

Treatment

Patients with CDH can be difficult to treat, especially when complicated by medication overuse. First, exclude secondary headache disorders; second,

Table 32.5 Headache attributed to medication overuse.

A	Headache occurring on 15 days/month in a patient with a pre-existing headache disorder
B	Regular overuse for >3 months of one or more acute and/or symptomatic treatment drugs 1. Ergotamine, triptans, opioids or combination analgesic medications on ≥10 days/month on a regular basis for >3 months 2. Simple analgesics or any combination of ergotamine, triptans, analgesics opioids on ≥15 days/month on a regular basis for >3 months without overuse of any single class alone
C	Not better accounted for by another ICHD-3 diagnosis.

diagnose the specific primary headache disorder; and third, identify comorbid conditions and exacerbating factors. Limit acute medications and start preventive medication, with the understanding that the drugs may not become fully effective until medication overuse has been eliminated. Detoxification options include outpatient infusion in an ambulatory infusion unit if available. If outpatient treatment proves difficult or is dangerous, hospitalization may be required.

Tension-type headache

Tension-type headache (TTH) (Table 32.6) is very common, with a lifetime prevalence of 69% in men and 88% in women. Episodic TTHs (ETTH) are now classified as either infrequent (<1 day/month or 12 days/year) or frequent (>1 but <15 days/ month or >12 but <180 days/year) [6]. The pain is a dull achy non-pulsatile feeling of tightness, pressure or constriction and it is usually mild to moderate in intensity. Most patients have bilateral pain; some have neck or jaw discomfort. There is no prodrome and, with the exception of occasional anorexia, there are no associated autonomic or gastrointestinal symptoms. Many TTH patients also have migraine [1].

Management

Patients with TTH usually self-medicate with over-the-counter analgesics, with or without caffeine. If they are not effective, prescription NSAIDs or combination analgesic preparations can be used. Patients

Table 32.6 Cluster headache.

A	At least five attacks fulfilling
B	Severe or very severe unilateral orbital, supraorbital and/or temporal pain lasting 15–180 minutes if untreated
C	Either or both of the following: 1. at least one of the following symptoms or signs, ipsilateral to the headache: a. conjunctival injection and/or lacrimation b. nasal congestion and/or rhinorrhea c. eyelid edema d. forehead and facial sweating e. miosis and/or ptosis 2. a sense of restlessness or agitation
D	Occurring with a frequency between one every other day and eight per day
E	Not better accounted for by another ICHD-3 diagnosis

with both migraine and TTHs benefit from specific migraine medications [6].

Medications used for TTH prevention include antidepressants, beta-blockers and anticonvulsants. Antidepressants, the medication of first choice, should be started at a low dose and increased slowly every 3–7 days. The addition of biofeedback therapy or beta-blocking agents may improve its therapeutic benefit [6].

Cluster headache and other trigeminal autonomic cephalgias

The short-lasting primary headache syndromes with autonomic activation include cluster headache (Table 32.6), paroxysmal hemicrania (episodic or chronic) and short-lasting unilateral neuralgiform headache with conjunctival injection and tearing (SUNCT syndrome).

With an incidence of 0.01–1.5% in various populations, cluster headache prevalence is lower than that of migraine or TTH and more common in men than women. The most common form of cluster headache is episodic cluster. Cluster headache generally begins in the late twenties.

Patients with cluster headache have multiple episodes of short-lived but severe, unilateral, orbital, supraorbital or temporal pain. Either or both of the following associated symptoms must occur: 1) conjunctival injection, lacrimation, nasal congestion, rhinorrhea, facial sweating, miosis, ptosis or eyelid edema 2) a sense of restlessness or agitation. Episodic cluster consists of headache periods of 1 week to 1 year, with remission periods lasting at least three months, whereas chronic cluster headache has either no remission periods or remissions that last less than three months.

The pain of a cluster attack rapidly increases to excruciating levels within 15 minutes. The attacks often occur at the same time each day and frequently awaken patients from sleep. The attacks usually last from 30–90 minutes. During an attack, patients often feel agitated or restless. The attack frequency varies from one every other day to eight a day, occurring in periods that last a week to a year. Remissions between cluster periods generally last 6 months to 2 years.

Management

Effective acute treatments include oxygen, sumatriptan and DHE. Inhaled oxygen, 7–10 L/ min for 10 minutes following headache onset, is 70% effective and is often the first choice treatment. Parenteral injections of sumatriptan or DHE provide significant relief for about 80% of patients [7,8,9]. Percutaneous vagal nerve stimulation has been approved for the treatment of episodic cluster headache.

Cluster headaches require preventive treatment; drugs include calcium channel blockers, lithium, corticosteroids, topiramate, melatonin and capsaicin. Recently galcanezumab, a mAb, has been approved for the treatment of episodic cluster headache If medical therapy fails completely, surgical intervention may be beneficial. The surgery consists of neuronal ablation procedures directed toward the sensory input of the trigeminal nerve and autonomic pathways [10].

Trigeminal neuralgia

Trigeminal neuralgia is a painful disorder occurring in the maxillary and mandibular divisions of the trigeminal nerve. It is typically evoked by trivial stimuli. It is a disorder of the elderly, often causes severe disability and has a relapsing remitting course. It is characterized by brief severe electric shock-like pain and is limited to one or more divisions of the trigeminal nerve. The pain generally lasts seconds, although it can last up to 2 minutes. Multiple attacks may occur daily. Most individuals have short periods of pain-free time between spikes of pain. Symptomatic trigeminal neuralgia is caused by a structural lesion, such as an acoustic neuroma, or multiple sclerosis. Demyelination of primary sensory trigeminal afferents in the root entry zone is the predominant pathophysiological mechanism in nonsymptomatic cases. Patients are usually started with a drug regimen that includes phenytoin, carbamazepine, oxcarbazepine and baclofen. Candidates for surgical therapy are patients who have failed medical therapy (which occurs approximately 30% of the time) or who became intolerant to medical therapy. In medically refractory patients, with a neurovascular conflict, microvascular decompression (MVD) is the first-choice treatment. (11)

Conclusions

Headache is one of the most common medical complaints of humankind. Headache diagnosis is based on a history, physical and neurologic examination. Testing serves to exclude organic causes of headache. Migraine is a chronic neurologic disease characterized by episodic attacks of headache and associated symptoms. Migraine treatment begins with making a diagnosis, explaining it to the patient and developing a treatment plan. Acute treatment attempts to relieve or stop the progression of an attack or the pain and impairment once an attack has begun. Preventive therapy is given in an attempt to reduce the frequency, duration or severity of attacks. Preventive treatment may prevent episodic migraine's progression to chronic migraine. CDH refers to headache disorders experienced 15 or more days a month. Patients with frequent headaches often overuse analgesics, opioids, ergotamine and triptans. TTH is the most common type of headache disorder. Patients with TTH usually self-medicate with over-the-counter analgesics. Patients with cluster headache have multiple episodes of short-lived but severe, unilateral, orbital, supraorbital or temporal pain. The pain of a cluster attack rapidly increases to excruciating levels within 15 minutes. Effective acute treatments include oxygen, sumatriptan and DHE. Most patients with cluster headache require preventive treatment. Trigeminal neuralgia is a painful disorder in the distribution of the trigeminal nerve that is typically evoked by trivial stimuli. Both medical and surgical modalities may be used as treatment. Approximately 50% of patients with trigeminal neuralgia will require surgery.

References

1 Headache Classification Committee of the International Headache Society. (2018) International Classification of Headache Disorders, 3rd edn. *Cephalalgia* **38(1)**:1–2110.

2 Lipton RB, Scher AI, Silberstein SD *et al.* (2008) Migraine diagnosis and comorbidity. In: Silberstein SD, Lipton RB, Dodick DW, eds. *Wolff's Headache and Other Head Pain*, 8th edn. Oxford University Press, New York. pp. 153–76.

3 Lipton RB, Diamond S, Reed M *et al.* (2001) Migraine diagnosis and treatment: results from the American Migraine Study II. *Headache* **41**:638–45.

4 Silberstein SD, Freitag FG, Bigal ME. (2008) Migraine treatment. In: Silberstein SD, Lipton RB, Dodick DW, eds. *Wolff's Headache and Other Head Pain*, 8th edn. Oxford University Press, New York. pp. 177–292.

5 Burch R C, Buse DC, Lipton RB (2019) Migraine epidemiology, burden, and comorbidity. *Neurologic Clinics* **37(4)**:631–49

6 Silberstein SD. (2005) Transformed and chronic migraine. In: Goadsby PJ, Silberstein SD, Dodick DW, eds. *Chronic Daily Headache for Clinicians*. BC Decker, Hamilton. pp. 21–56.

7 Silberstein SD. (1994) Pharmacological management of cluster headache. *CNS Drugs* **2(3)**:199–207.

8 Goadsby PJ, Tfelt-Hansen P. (2009) Cluster headaches: introduction and epidemiology. In: Olesen J, Goadsby PJ, Ramadan N *et al.*, eds. *The Headaches*, 3rd edn. Lippincott, Williams & Wilkins, Philadelphia. pp. 743–5.

9 Brandt, R.B., Doesborg, P.G.G., Haan, J. *et al.* (2020) Pharmacotherapy for Cluster Headache. *CNS Drugs* **34**:171–184

10 Jarrar RG, Black DF, Dodick DW *et al.* (2003) Outcome of trigeminal nerve section in the treatment of chronic cluster headache. *Neurology* **60(8)**:1360–2.

11 Maarbjerg, S., Di Stefano, G., Bendtsen, L., & Cruccu, G. (2017). Trigeminal neuralgia – diagnosis and treatment. *Cephalalgia* **37(7)**:648–65.

Chapter 33

Orofacial pain

Barry J Sessle[1], Lene Baad-Hansen[2,3], Fernando Exposto[2,3], & Peter Svensson[2,3,4]

[1] *Faculties of Dentistry and Medicine, University of Toronto, Toronto, Ontario, Canada*
[2] *Section for Orofacial Pain and Jaw Function, Aarhus University, Aarhus, Denmark*
[3] *Scandinavian Center for Orofacial Neurosciences (SCON), Aarhus University, Aarhus, Denmark*
[4] *Faculty of Odontology, Malmø University, Malmø, Sweden*

Introduction

The orofacial region is the site of some of the most common acute and chronic pain conditions. This region also has special psychological, social and emotional meaning and importance in eating, drinking, sexual behaviour, speech and expression of emotions. The orofacial tissues are densely innervated by nociceptive afferents and have an extensive somatosensory representation in the central nervous system (CNS). These features may also account for why many people find it unpleasant and painful to go for a routine dental examination.

This chapter first highlights the peripheral and central neurobiological mechanisms underlying orofacial pain and then outlines the clinical features of some of the most common or perplexing chronic orofacial pain conditions.

Orofacial nociceptive processes

Primary afferent mechanisms

The rich innervation of the orofacial region is almost exclusively by branches of the trigeminal nerve. Many trigeminal primary afferent fibers terminate in these tissues as free nerve endings and function as nociceptors. The nociceptive afferents are either small-diameter, myelinated (A-delta) afferents or even smaller (and slower conducting) unmyelinated (C) afferents. Their primary afferent cell bodies occur in the trigeminal ganglion.

Like analogous afferent endings and ganglion cell bodies of spinal nerves (see Chapter 3), trigeminal nociceptive afferents are subject to considerable modulation because a peripheral substrate exists for complex interactions between the neural, immune, cardiovascular and endocrine systems [1-7]. Tissue damage, and inflammation if present, cause the release of chemical mediators, some of which can enhance the excitability of the nociceptive endings (e.g. prostaglandins, interleukins, ATP, glutamate). The increased excitability can be expressed as outright activation or as so-called nociceptor or peripheral sensitization. This sensitization can be reflected in a lowered activation threshold, increased responsiveness to subsequent noxious stimuli and spontaneous activity of the nociceptive endings that contribute, respectively, to the allodynia, hyperalgesia and spontaneous pain that are features of acute and many persistent orofacial pain conditions [1-7]. The chemical mediators may also spread through the tissues and act on the endings of adjacent nociceptive afferents and thus contribute to the spread of orofacial pain. Injury or inflammation of peripheral tissues, including nerves, may also lead to phenotypic

Clinical Pain Management: A Practical Guide, Second Edition. Edited by Mary E. Lynch, Kenneth D. Craig, and Philip W. Peng.

changes, sprouting or abnormal discharges of the nociceptive afferents and be of pathophysiological significance in certain chronic pain conditions. It is also notable that some of the chemical mediators may reduce the excitability of the nociceptive afferent endings. Peripherally acting analgesic drugs may act by counteracting the effects of mediators that enhance afferent excitability; for example, aspirin affects the synthesis of prostaglandins. It is also noteworthy that some of these effects of orofacial injury or inflammation may also be expressed in the neuronal cell bodies of the primary afferents in the trigeminal ganglion and involve several mediators and non-neural cells in the ganglion (e.g. satellite glial cells) [3, 5]. Interestingly, the excitability changes induced in the ganglion neurons by these factors may occur not only in the neurons innervating the injured or inflamed tissues but also other ganglion neurons innervating non-injured or non-inflamed tissues. Many of these neuronal excitability changes are excitatory and, as a result, abnormal ectopically evoked afferent inputs may project into the brainstem and contribute to the spread, poor localization and ectopic sensations that occur in some orofacial pain conditions.

Facial skin, oral mucosa, temporomandibular joint (TMJ), craniofacial muscle and periodontal tissues are supplied by nociceptive afferents with properties generally analogous to those of spinal nociceptive afferents although corneal and cerebrovascular nociceptive afferents do have some special properties as do those supplying the tooth pulp [2, 5, 7]. The tooth pulp is a highly vascular and richly innervated tissue which is exceptionally sensitive to stimulation and a frequent source of dental pain. The dentine encasing the pulp is also very sensitive despite its sparse innervation and it appears that activation of intradentinal afferents is brought about by a hydrodynamic mechanism; non-neural cells in the pulp (e.g. odontoblasts) are also involved. Injury to the tooth and pulpal inflammation (e.g. as a result of dental caries) can induce peripheral sensitization of intradental afferents, which may result in extremely intense toothache, because inflammation of the pulp occurs in a non-compliant environment (it is encased by dentine) with a high extracellular tissue pressure. This is thought to be an important factor accounting for the great sensitivity of pulp afferents when the pulp is inflamed [2].

Brainstem mechanisms

From the trigeminal ganglion, trigeminal afferents project into the brainstem and terminate on neurons especially in the trigeminal brainstem sensory nuclear complex. Here they release neurochemicals (e.g. glutamate, neuropeptides) that can activate the neurons. The trigeminal brainstem sensory nuclear complex consists of the trigeminal main sensory and the trigeminal spinal tract nucleus. The latter is subdivided into three subnuclei: oralis, interpolaris and caudalis (Figure 33.1). The subnucleus caudalis is a

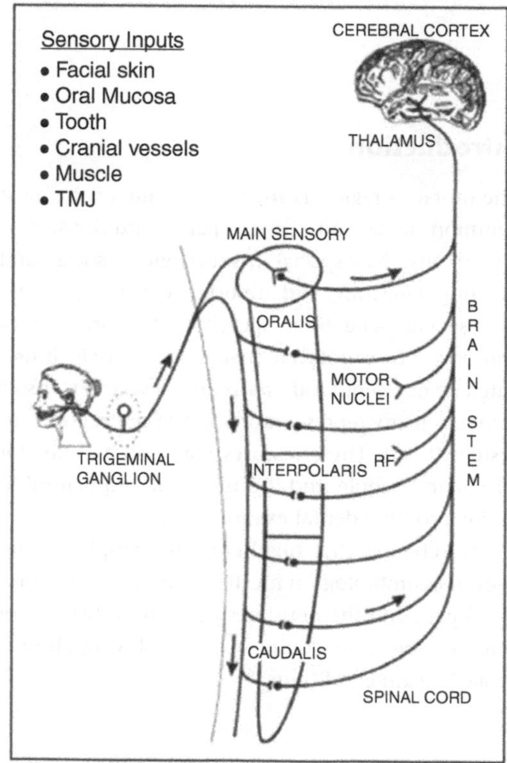

Figure 33.1 Major somatosensory pathway from the orofacial region. Trigeminal primary afferents project via the trigeminal ganglion to second-order neurons in the trigeminal brainstem sensory nuclear complex comprising the main sensory nucleus and the subnuclei oralis, interpolaris and caudalis of the spinal tract nucleus. These neurons may project to neurons in higher levels of the brain (e.g. thalamus) or in brainstem regions such as cranial nerve motor nuclei, autonomic nuclei or the reticular formation (RF). Not shown are the projections of some cervical nerves and cranial nerve VII, X and XII afferents to the trigeminal complex and the projection of many VII, IX and X afferents to the solitary tract nucleus. TMJ, temporomandibular joint. *Source*: Reproduced with permission from Sessle [4].

laminated structure with many morphological and functional similarities to the dorsal horn of the spinal cord; indeed, it is often termed the medullary dorsal horn. Based on its anatomic, neurochemical and physiological features and the effects of brainstem lesions, caudalis is now considered the principal although not exclusive brainstem relay site of trigeminal nociceptive information. Indeed, the other subnuclei (oralis, interpolaris), the so-called transition zone between subnuclei caudalis and interpolaris, and even the upper cervical spinal dorsal horn (which itself receives some trigeminal afferent inputs), may contribute to the brainstem mechanisms of orofacial pain [3-7].

Some caudalis nociceptive neurons respond only to stimulation of a cutaneous or mucosal mechanoreceptive field and can do so in a graded manner as stimulus intensity is increased. As a consequence, they are thought to have an important role in our ability to localize, detect and discriminate superficial noxious stimuli and their intensity. However, most neurons can also be activated by peripheral afferent inputs from other tissues (e.g. tooth pulp, TMJ, jaw muscle or cerebrovasculature) innervated by trigeminal nerve branches and some by afferent inputs from tissues supplied by non-trigeminal nerves (e.g. upper cervical nerves). Such features are thought to contribute to the very common clinical findings of poor localization and referral of pain from deep tissues or from one tooth to another.

Neurons in caudalis and other components of the trigeminal brainstem complex project to the thalamus either directly or indirectly by polysynaptic pathways (e.g. via the reticular formation) (Figure 33.1). Some of the latter projections, as well as those to the cranial nerve motor nuclei and brainstem autonomic nuclei, provide part of the central substrate underlying autonomic, endocrine and muscle reflex responses to orofacial stimuli. Some neurons have only intrinsic projections such that their axons do not leave the trigeminal brainstem complex but instead terminate within it (e.g. interneurons in lamina II of caudalis, the so-called substantia gelatinosa).

Thalamocortical mechanisms

Orofacial somatosensory information is relayed from the brainstem to the lateral thalamus (e.g. ventrobasal complex; the ventroposterior nucleus in humans) and medial thalamus (e.g. medial nuclei) which contain nociceptive neurons with properties generally similar to those described for nociceptive neurons in the subthalamic relays such as subnucleus caudalis [4-7]. Those in ventrobasal thalamus have properties and connections with the overlying somatosensory cerebral cortex which point to a role in localization and discrimination of orofacial noxious stimuli, whereas those in the more medial thalamic nuclei project to other higher brain areas (e.g. hypothalamus, anterior cingulate cortex) which are involved more in the affective or motivational dimensions of pain, by analogy with the spinothalamic system and its presumed functional aspects.

Modulatory influences

Pain is modulated by a variety of influences that regulate perceptual, emotional, autonomic and neuroendocrine responses to noxious stimuli by utilizing several excitatory and inhibitory neuro-chemicals. Some of these modulatory influences may be expressed at thalamic and cortical levels, but the intricate organization of each subdivision of the trigeminal brainstem complex, coupled with the variety of inputs to each of them from peripheral tissues or descending from some parts of the brain (e.g. in the thalamus, reticular formation, limbic system and cerebral cortex), provides a rich substrate for numerous and complex interactions between the various inputs that can result in the modulation of orofacial nociceptive transmission [3-7]. This means that the neural circuitry underlying nociceptive transmission, including that in the trigeminal system, is "plastic" and not "hard-wired" which may be a significant feature in the chronification of orofacial pain.

The descending influences are activated by a variety of behavioral and environmental events and can modify pain. Orofacial nociceptive transmission is also subject to modulation by so-called segmental or afferent influences, which can be evoked by peripheral stimulation and involve the interneuronal circuitry existing within subnucleus caudalis and adjacent brainstem areas. Segmental or descending inhibitory substrates are thought to contribute to the efficacy of several analgesic approaches (e.g. deep brain stimulation; drugs such as morphine, carbamazepine, tricyclic antidepressants [TCAs]).

As in the spinal system, nociceptive transmission in the trigeminal system can also be enhanced by alterations to the peripheral afferent inputs to the CNS as a result of trauma or inflammation to peripheral tissues or nerves. Trauma or inflammation produces a barrage of nociceptive primary afferent inputs into the CNS that may lead to neuroplastic alterations in subnucleus caudalis (and spinal dorsal horn) and/or higher-order neurons; processes which collectively have been termed central sensitization. Trigeminal central sensitization is reflected in an increased excitability of caudalis nociceptive neurons, manifested as an increase in spontaneous activity, mechanoreceptive field expansion, lowering of activation threshold and enhancement of peripherally evoked nociceptive responses of the neurons [3-7]. These neuroplastic changes can be prolonged and contribute to the development and maintenance of persistent and chronic orofacial pain and its common characteristics of spontaneous pain, pain spread and referral, allodynia and hyperalgesia. Several membrane receptor mechanisms, ion channels and intracellular signaling processes are involved in trigeminal central sensitization and include purinergic and neurokinin as well as N-methyl-D-aspartate (NMDA) and non-NMDA (e.g. metabotropic) glutamatergic receptor processes. Non-neural cells (especially astroglia and microglia) in subnucleus caudalis have been shown to be key players in the development and maintenance of trigeminal central sensitization Trigeminal central sensitization occurs not only in subnucleus caudalis but also in subnucleus oralis and higher brain regions such as ventrobasal thalamus; nonetheless, caudalis has been shown to be responsible for the expression of central sensitization in these structures by way of its projections to both. Several currently used analgesic approaches (e.g., opioids, pregabalin) have been shown to act by counteracting the processes underlying central sensitization [4, 5, 7] and the standard approach in dentistry of using local anesthesia to minimize pain before, during and after an operative procedure is effective because it blocks the nociceptive afferent inputs from the operative site that otherwise would induce trigeminal central sensitization. This brings us to consider other clinical aspects bearing on orofacial pain and in particular its more chronic manifestations.

Clinical aspects

Orofacial pain covers a wide range of conditions with different clinical manifestations. Recently, a comprehensive classification of all types of orofacial pain was published based on an international multidisciplinary collaboration, the International Classification of Orofacial Pain (ICOP) [8]. The following sections focus on some of the most common and most perplexing of these conditions. Because of their complexity, plus the special emotional and psychosocial meaning of the orofacial region, the diagnostic work-up and management strategy will often require a substantial interdisciplinary approach between the medical profession, dentists, psychologists and specialists in orofacial pain.

Temporomandibular disorders

Temporomandibular disorders (TMD) cover an umbrella of common and related pain conditions in the jaw muscles, TMJ and associated structures. A milestone paper in the field suggested that these conditions could be divided into three main categories [9]: 1). Myofascial pain; 2). Disc displacements; and 3). TMJ arthralgia, osteoarthrosis and osteoarthritis. Perhaps more important than this physical axis (axis I) was the introduction of an axis II to cover the disability and pain-related distress of the patient [9]. A follow-up on this classification - the so-called Diagnostic Criteria for TMD (DC/TMD) [10] proposed a reorganization into 1). Muscle disorders (myalgia and myofascial pain) 2). TMJ disorders (arthralgia, disc displacements, degenerative joint diseases and dislocation and 3). Headache attributed to TMD. The recent release of the ICOP mentioned above integrates the DC/TMD with the International Association for the Study of Pain and International Classification of Diseases (ICD11) [11] and the International Classification of Headache Disorders (ICHD-3) [12]. An important aspect of these classifications are the introduction of primary and secondary pains. Chronic primary pain is pain that persists greater than 3 months and cannot be explained by another chronic pain condition - pain as a disease in its own right. Secondary chronic pain is pain linked to other diseases as the underlying cause and may initially be regarded as a symptom. Thus, for all TMD pain conditions, there are now operationalized and specific criteria to help in phenotyping the specific subtype of TMD pain on two axes.

TMD pain is very common in the population (3–15%) and is 1.5–2 times more prevalent in women than in men, with a peak around 20–45 years [13]. Degenerative TMJ conditions generally increase over the lifespan. The incidence of TMD pain is 2–4%, with the incidence of persistent types being 0.1%. Generalized pain conditions such as fibromyalgia, whiplash-associated disorders, tension-type headache/migraine, low-back pain, irritable bowel syndrome and general joint laxity, as well as sleep disturbances, depression and anxiety, have all been found to be often comorbid with TMD pain conditions [13].

Overall, there are three cardinal symptoms of TMD:

1 Pain in the jaw muscles and/or TMJ.

2 Sounds from the TMJ (clicks, crepitation).

3 Limitation in range of jaw motion [14].

Pain is typically reported to be moderate to intense and fluctuating during the day with exacerbations during jaw movements. The basic features mentioned above with spontaneous pain, pain spread and referral, deep tissue allodynia and hyperalgesia can readily be observed in painful TMD conditions. For example, myofascial TMD pain is described as a deep ache, tender and diffuse, often with referral to the TMJ, ear, temple and teeth. TMJ arthralgia is more localized around the TMJ, with a sharp component and pain referrals to the ear region. It is important to note the frequency of pain (e.g. infrequent episodes, frequent episodes or highly-frequent episodes) is in line with the ICOP. Typically, the jaw muscles and the TMJ will be painful on palpation which should be standardized according to duration and pressure applied. Clicking in the TMJ is rarely a problem in itself but may be unpleasant for the patient. The TMJ disc position may cause limitation in the range of motion (TMJ locking). TMD diagnosis is based on a systematic history and clinical examination as per the DC/TMD and ICOP classifications. Imaging of the TMJ (e.g. magnetic resonance imaging [MRI] for disc displacements with persisting reduction in jaw opening or computed tomography [CT] for TMJ progressing degenerative changes) is only required in some cases [10].

The pathophysiology of TMD pain is unclear but both peripheral sensitization and central sensitization are believed to be involved, with contributions from anatomic, psychological–psychosocial and neurobiological factors (see above). There is also some evidence of a less effective activation of endogenous pain-inhibitory systems in TMD patients and recent studies suggest that there may be genetic risk factors involved in complex TMD pain conditions. Stochastic interaction models between multiple risk factors may be needed to help explain the pain trajectories of individual patients [15].

Most primary TMD pain conditions cannot be causally treated but only managed with the important goal of pain alleviation and restoration of function [16]. Various physical strategies (e.g. stretching, relaxation oral splints) can be used but generally, their efficacy is only modest and non-specific. The number-needed-to-treat (NNT) values for oral splints range from 3–4 for management of myofascial TMD and around 5–6 for TMJ arthralgia and there is good evidence that self-care instructions and monitoring can provide at least as good pain relief as usual dental approaches. Evidence-driven recommendations for pharmacological approaches are also needed (for a review see 17). Non-steroidal anti-inflammatory drugs (NSAIDs) such as ibuprofen in combination with diazepam can be used for short-term management of TMD pain. Gabapentin appears to have some effect on myofascial TMD pain and tenderness, as does cyclobenzaprine or flupirtine. Low doses of TCAs may be an option for persistent TMD pain. Naproxen appears to be effective in the management of TMJ arthralgia and intra-articular injections with corticosteroid and hyaluronate may also be useful [17]. Intra-articular morphine increases the pressure pain thresholds and jaw-opening capacity and reduces TMJ pain but probably has limited clinical application. Botulinum toxin and acupuncture cannot at present be recommended as first lines of management because of inconclusive evidence. Management of TMD pain should adhere to the general principle "primum non nocicere" (first do no harm) and irreversible treatment should be avoided [17].

Tooth pain

Tooth pain is a very common and is usually an acute condition [8]. Prevalence estimates range from 7–66%, depending on criteria and the population studied [18]. The most frequent local causes are presented in Table 33.1 Acute tooth pain may be very intense, disturbs sleep and may be confused with trigeminal neuralgia and various headache conditions such as migraine (see Chapter 33).

Tooth pain can also become chronic after dental procedures or oral surgery and as with all postoperative pain must be managed using appropriate analgesia to maximize pain control which will facilitate comfort and healing. As with other postsurgical pain states, it is probable that better pain control at the time of the procedure will diminish the chances of persistent postsurgical pain.

Post-traumatic trigeminal neuropathic pain

Traumatic injury to trigeminal nerve branches may occasionally result in post-traumatic trigeminal neuropathic pain (PTNP) [8]. The trigeminal system is often stated to have unique features compared to the spinal system with respect to its lower propensity to develop neuropathic pain following a nerve injury [19]; however, direct comparative studies are lacking.

Tooth extraction or root canal treatment entails injury and deafferentation of the nerve supply to the tooth pulp [20] and may lead to development of PTNP. The presence of chronic infections and inflammatory reactions in the tooth pulp or periapical region may in some cases increase the risk. Third molar surgery results in 4–6% of patients having somatosensory disturbances involving the inferior alveolar or lingual nerves after 1 week, but these persist only in 0.7–1% after 2 years (for review see Svensson & Baad-Hansen [18] and Baad-Hansen & Benoliel [19]). Orthognathic surgery is used for correction of craniofacial abnormalities and many patients develop injuries to the maxillary or mandibular divisions of the trigeminal nerve. Depending on the specific type of osteotomy, patient age, intraoperative variables and somatosensory assessment techniques, nerve injury prevalence data vary from 10–85%, but less than 5% of such cases eventually develop PTNP [18, 19]. Dental implant insertion and other surgical procedures may also contribute to risk for trigeminal nerve injuries [21]. Zygomatico-orbital fractures are common facial injuries and occur in about 1 of every 10,000 people, with frequent (~ 50%) acute involvement of the somatosensory function of the infraorbital nerve but only 3–4% develop chronic PTNP [18, 19]. Dental injections carry a very small risk (e.g. 1 out of 26,762 mandibular blocks) for the development of PTNP; the proposed mechanisms are direct needle trauma, formation of hematoma or neurotoxicity of the local anesthetic [18].

Patients with PTNP often report a constant burning, dull aching or sharp and/or shooting pain in a neuroanatomically relevant area [8]. The pain debut is in close temporal relation to a traumatic event as revealed in the patient history [8]. Pain may also be triggered by mechanical stimuli applied to the skin or oral mucosa or by normal oral functions. Clinical inspection reveals no signs of inflammation but there is detectable somatosensory dysfunction within the same neuroanatomically relevant region [22, 23]. Quantitative sensory testing (QST) may reveal both hypoesthesia and hyperesthesia. Advanced electrophysiological tests are also of potential diagnostic value according to the grading system for neuropathic pain [20, 22, 24]. In the differential diagnosis, it is crucial to rule out odontogenic pains, sinusitis, sialoadenitis, persistent idiopathic facial pain and persistent idiopathic dento-alveolar pain (please see below). It has been suggested that QST could be important to differentiate between some of these conditions.

Trigeminal neuralgia must also be considered but the clinical presentation is usually very different (Chapter 33). Trigeminal post-herpetic neuralgia (PHN) may also be considered if the pain occurs in temporal relation to an acute Herpes Zoster infection affecting the trigeminal region [8].

The pathophysiology of PTNP is likely to involve basic mechanisms similar to those linked with spinal nerve lesions [19]. However, recovery appears to be faster in the trigeminal system, autonomic responses differ (e.g. no sprouting of sympathetic terminals on trigeminal ganglion cells) and the neuropeptide content and the specific patterns of upregulation and downregulation of sodium channels are different between the two systems and these differences have potential implications for clinical characteristics [25]. Trigeminal central sensitization likely underlies or at least contributes to PTNP and other conditions involving injury to branches of the trigeminal nerve since animal models of trigeminal nerve injury have documented the development and persistence of a central sensitization state [4, 6, 25].

Table 33.1 Common causes and features of acute tooth pain.

Condition	Features	Cause/comments	Treatment
Pulpal pain attributed to hypersensitivity (Dentine hypersensitivity)	Sharp or shooting pain with mechanical or thermal stimulation of dentinal surface	Caused by hydrodynamic activation of intradental afferents	Local application of fluoride gel or a desensitizing agent [24] Use of a soft toothbrush
Pulpal pain attributed to a crack in the enamel (Cracked tooth syndrome)	Sharp, poorly localized pain evoked by mastication, simple test is to have patient bite on a cotton roll	Incomplete fracture of a vital tooth that may extend into the pulp. Radiography does not reveal the pathology	Restorative dental procedure If severe: endodontic treatment or extraction
Pulpal pain attributed to reversible pulpitis	No spontaneous pain. Pain evoked by hot or cold liquids or food items	Caused by pulpal inflammation which resolves with treatment or time	Treat the pain evoking stimulus (e.g. carious lesion). If NSAIDs are ineffective a stronger analgesic may be required
Pulpal pain attributed to irreversible pulpitis	Intense spontaneous pain and pain evoked by hot or cold liquids or food items	Caused by pulpal inflammation with changes in pulpal nociceptors and central connections resulting in sensitization	Endodontic treatment and appropriate analgesia*
Periodontal pain attributed to apical periodontitis due to endodontic disease	Often asymptomatic but when present, symptoms include pain, tooth elevation, sensitivity to percussion and swelling	An inflammatory condition of the apical periodontium caused by necrosis of the tooth pulp with accumulation of bacteria and inflammatory mediators in the root canal with spread into periapical tissues	Endodontic treatment. If an abscess is present it must be drained and systemic antibiotics may be indicated
Referred pain	Experienced as pain involving the teeth and surrounding tissues	Pain can be referred to the teeth from structures outside of the mouth: • maxillary sinuses • jaw muscles • heart/angina	Rule out dental pathology and TMD. Image sinuses, perform ECG, refer to specialist as appropriate
Postoperative periodontal pain	Iatrogenic pain due to surgically induced tissue damage and subsequent inflammation	Pain is typically mild to moderate and may be accompanied by clinically observable swelling and, occasionally, pus formation	If normal physiological (primary) healing occurs, pain duration is typically a maximum of 2 weeks

ECG, electrocardiogram; NSAID, non-steroidal anti-inflammatory drug; TMD, temporomandibular disorders.

*Appropriate analgesia refers to treatment required to assist the patient with adequate pain control and is reviewed in chapters on pharmacotherapy.

In the absence of specific guidelines for management of PTNP, the same principles as for other neuropathic pain conditions should be followed (see Chapter 37). However, an important point is to avoid further trauma to the area (e.g. by avoiding further explorative oral surgery).

Idiopathic Orofacial Pain

In addition to the more common types of orofacial pain described above, the patient may present with a number of less common but nonetheless very challenging types of pain due to diagnostic issues and poor response to treatment.

The ICOP divides idiopathic orofacial pain into four different types: 1) Burning Mouth Syndrome (BMS); 2) Persistent Idiopathic Facial Pain (PIFP); 3) Persistent Idiopathic Dentoalveolar Pain and 4) Constant Unilateral Facial Pain with Additional Attacks (CUFPA).

Burning mouth syndrome

Burning mouth syndrome (BMS) is an intraoral burning or dysesthetic sensation for which no dental or medical cause is evident and recurs daily for at least 2 hours for more than 3 months [8]. Other terms such as glossodynia and stomatodynia have been used [26]. Its prevalence is estimated to be between 0.1-3.9% but may be confounded by a considerable variability in its definition (Ariyawardana et al.). BMS increases with age and women aged 60-69 have the highest prevalence [27, 28]. BMS is characterized by daily moderate to severe burning pain, sometimes with dysesthetic qualities, in the mouth (tongue, palate, lips, gingiva) that persists for most of the day. The oral mucosa looks normal and no obvious pathology can be detected. Symptoms are usually bilateral and may be associated with taste changes, xerostomia and hyposalivation. There is significant comorbidity with depression and anxiety but for most patients these are likely the result of persistent pain rather than a risk factor for BMS [29]. Furthermore, a high percentage of patients with BMS have been shown to have significant sleep disturbances that seem to correlate with the above-mentioned depression and anxiety [30].

The etiology and pathophysiology of BMS are unknown; however, recent studies have demonstrated intraoral small-fiber changes, (subclinical) somatosensory changes and abnormal brainstem reflex responses, which suggest dysfunction in the peripheral and/or central nervous system [31].

In the differential diagnosis, it is important to appreciate that burning mouth symptoms could be caused by systemic or local conditions, including vitamin B, folic acid or iron deficiency, untreated diabetes, hormonal disturbances, anemia, oral candidiasis, hyposalivation, Sjögren's syndrome, oral lichen planus, systemic lupus erythematosus, medication side effects and certain allergies [28]. As such, BMS is a diagnosis of exclusion and other causes should be ruled out before diagnosing BMS.

Management consists of patient education and avoidance of spicy foods; some patients experience pain relief while sucking (sugar-free) pastilles. Pharmacological treatment of BMS generally has a modest effect. A recent systematic review showed that the best available evidence for effective BMS management pertains to alpha-lipoic acid, capsaicin and clonazepam; systemic and local forms are equally effective but systemic medications show more side-effects [32]

Persistent Idiopathic Facial Pain and Persistent Idiopathic Dentoalveolar Pain

Persistent idiopathic facial pain (PIFP) is described as "persistent facial pain, with variable features, recurring daily for more than 2 hours per day for more than 3 months, in the absence of clinical neurological deficit or preceding causative event" [8]. Whereas Persistent idiopathic dentoalveolar pain (PIDAP) is described in the same terms, the pain however is located in a dentoalveolar site. Both of these conditions may or may not be accompanied by somatosensory changes.

In previous classifications, PIFP was combined with atypical odontalgia (AO) which was considered a subtype. In the ICOP, these have been separated and AO has been renamed PIDAP.

The incidence of PIFP is estimated to be 4.4 per 100,000 person years [33] and to have a prevalence of 0.03% [34] within the general population. On the other hand, the prevalence of PIDAP is more obscure but may in combination with PTNP (please see above) occur in 3–12% of patients having undergone endodontic treatment [35, 36]. Clinically, PTNP and PIFP/PIDAP may seem very similar and to distinguish the conditions, diagnostic criteria should be followed closely. Hence, PIFP and PIDAP may occur without a history of trauma to the nerve, whereas a diagnosis of PTNP requires such trauma [8]. Also, PTNP requires the pain and somatosensory disturbances to be neuroanatomically plausible [8]. If this is not the case, i.e. if the pain crosses boundaries between relevant nerve branches, the diagnosis is PIFP or PIDAP [8]. PIFP particularly affects middle-aged or older women, whereas PIDAP affects both sexes and all adult ages, although with a predominance of women in their mid-forties. The symptoms can be pain that is deep, poorly localized, mostly unilateral (in two-thirds of patients) in the mid-face or intra-orally but the pain can also be superficial [37, 38]. The pain is often reported to start in relation to dental surgery or other orofacial trauma, in a specific area but usually spreads diffusely not following the distribution of the trigeminal nerve. Words like dull, drawing, burning, stabbing or throbbing are used by patients to characterize PIFP and PIDAP [39, 40]. There is a marked comorbidity especially with psychiatric disorders and other pain conditions (e.g. headache and back pain [41].

PIFP and PIDAP are conditions with suggested risk factors that include psychological factors, hormonal factors, minor nerve trauma and infection of the sinuses or teeth. Tooth related pathology is excluded by oral and dental examinations with relevant radiography. Diagnostic local anesthetic blocks can be useful when dental pathology is suspected. Pain originating from the maxillary sinuses, can be ruled out by nasal endoscopy, radiography or computerized tomography (CT) of the sinuses. TMD pain also needs to be considered. Trigeminal neuralgia can usually be distinguished from PIFP and PIDAP by the symptomatology: patients with trigeminal neuralgia are pain-free most of the time and have attacks with short-lasting shock-like pain, whereas PIFP and PIDAP pain is constant and non-paroxysmal. Patients with some forms of primary headaches may also present with symptoms like PIFP and PIDAP [42].

The management of PIFP and PIDAP is challenging. The first step is to educate the patient to accept the fact that there is no infection or "bad tooth" causing the pain. The next step is pharmacological treatment where the first choice is TCAs such as amitriptyline. Anticonvulsants such as gabapentin may also be useful. Other types of treatments (e.g. acupuncture, transcutaneous electrical nerve stimulation [TENS], biofeedback) lack sufficient evidence, whereas hypnosis appears effective [43]. Opioids and NMDA receptor antagonists are not promising agents in PIFP and PIDAP treatment [44]. The fact that no treatment has been shown to have even a moderate effect on PIFP or PIDAP, is most likely due to different pain conditions being included in studies under the umbrella of idiopathic pains [39].

Constant Unilateral Facial Pain with Additional Attacks

Constant Unilateral Facial Pain with Additional Attacks (CUFPA) is a new diagnostic category that has been included in the ICOP and was first proposed by Ziegeler and May [45]. Patients describe "constant unremitting and full unilateral facial pain of mild to moderate intensity, accompanied by distinct attacks of moderate to severe pain in the same location lasting 10-30 minutes [8]. Furthermore, no autonomic or migrainoid features are present, which distinguishes CUFPA from the trigeminal autonomic cephalalgias (TAC). Because CUFPA is a newly described entity, there is no information available of its pathophysiology. Regarding management, there have been reports that indomethacin, pregabalin, ibuprofen and metamizole may be at least partially effective [45]. However, these were anecdotal reports and randomized clinical trials are needed to confirm which medications may help patients with CUFPA.

Orofacial Pains Resembling Presentations of Primary Headaches

Primary headaches are defined as head pain that is a disorder in itself and not attributed to another disorder. The most common of these are migraine, tension-type headache and the TAC. Each one of these present with specific characteristics that allow a diagnosis according to the ICHD-3. However, when a headache naïve patient experiences pain attacks that resemble these primary headaches in character, duration, intensity as well as accompanying symptoms but are located in the orofacial region, they should be diagnosed as one of the orofacial pains resembling presentations of primary headaches [8]. Briefly, the ICOP has divided these conditions into orofacial migraine, tension-type orofacial pain, trigeminal autonomic orofacial pain and neurovascular orofacial pain. These disorders are very rare and most of the evidence for their management comes from a few case reports or case series [45, 46]. It is generally recommended that the management of these conditions should be the same as for their counterparts presenting in the head [47]. As an example, if a patient presents with intraoral pain attacks, with no head pain, that last around 10 hours, are pulsating in quality, unilateral in location, exacerbated by physical activity, severe in intensity and are accompanied by nausea, photophobia and phonophobia the diagnosis of orofacial migraine should be given [8]. In this case, management should be the same as for a migraine diagnosis [48]. For example, sumatriptan could be used to abort an attack and in case the frequency or the burden of attacks is high prophylactic management with for example propranolol is warranted.

Summary

This chapter has briefly summarized the physiology and pathophysiology of nociception and pain processing in the trigeminal system. Outlines are also provided of the many pain conditions that are manifested in the orofacial region. Substantial progress of knowledge regarding the basic neurobiological mechanisms have been made in the last 2-3 decades and has served as a stepping stone for the improvements in diagnostic systems of orofacial pain conditions and their management. Emphasis now needs to be on further development of individualized and mechanism-centered diagnosis and treatment for more efficient management and rational rehabilitation of the patient with an orofacial pain complaint.

References

1 Ringkamp M, Raja SN, Campbell JN, *et al.* (2013) Peripheral mechanisms of cutaneous nociception. In: McMahon SB, Koltzenburg M, Tracey I, *et al.*, eds. *Wall and Melzack's Textbook of Pain*, 6 edn. Saunders, Philadelphia. pp.1–30.

2 Matthews B, Sessle BJ. (2020) Peripheral mechanisms of orofacial pain. In: Sessle BJ, Lavigne GJ Lund JP, eds. *Orofacial Pain.* 2nd edn. Quintessence Publishing Co., Inc., Batavia. pp.27–43.

3 Iwata K, Imamura Y, Honda K, *et al.* (2011) Physiological mechanisms of neuropathic pain: The orofacial region. *Int Rev Neurobiol* **97**: 227–50.

4 Sessle BJ. (2000) Acute and chronic craniofacial pain: Brainstem mechanisms of nociceptive transmission and neuroplasticity, and their clinical correlates. *Crit Rev Oral Biol Med* **11**:57–91.

5 Sessle BJ, ed. (2014) *Orofacial Pain: Recent Advances in Assessment, Management and Understanding of Mechanisms.*: IASP Press, Baltimore.

6 Woda A. (2003) Pain in the trigeminal system: from orofacial nociception to neural network modeling. *J Dent Res* **82**:764–8.

7 Chichorro JG, Porreca F, Sessle B. (2017) Mechanisms of craniofacial pain. *Cephalalgia* **37**:613–26.

8 International classification of orofacial pain, 1st edition (ICOP). (2020) *Cephalalgia* **40**:129–221.

9 Dworkin SF, LeResche L. (1992) Research diagnostic criteria for temporomandibular disorders: Review, criteria, examinations and specifications, critique. *J Craniomandib Disord* **6**:301–55.

10 Schiffman E, Ohrbach R, Truelove E *et al.* (2014) Diagnostic criteria for temporomandibular disorders (DC/THD) for clinical and research applications: Recommendations of the international RDC/TMD Consortium Network* and Orofacial Pain Special Interest Group. *J Oral Facial Pain Headache* **28**:6–27.

11 Treede RD, Rief W, Barke A *et al.* (2019) Chronic pain as a symptom or a disease: The iasp classification of chronic pain for the international classification of diseases (ICD-11). *Pain* **160**:19–27.

12 Headache Classification Comitee of the International Headache Society (HIS). (2018) The international classification of headache disorders, 3rd edition (ICHD-3). *Cephalalgia* **38**:1–211.

13 Macfarlane T. (2014) Epidemiology of orofacial pain. In: Sessle BJ (ed) *Orofacial Pain: Recent*

Advances in Assessment, Mmanagement, and Understanding of Mechanisms, 1st edn. IASP Press, Baltimore. pp. 33–51.

14 Okeson JP, ed. (2014) *Bell's Oral and Facial Pain*. Quintessence Publishing, Batavia.

15 Svensson P, Kumar A. (2016) Assessment of risk factors for oro-facial pain and recent developments in classification: Implications for management. *J Oral Rehabil* **43**:977–89.

16 Schindler H, Svensson P. (2007) Myofascial temporomandibular disorder pain. In: Turp JC, Sommer C, Hugger A, eds. *The Puzzle of Orofacial Pain: Pain and Headache*. Karger Publishers, Basel. pp.91–123.

17 Häggman-Henrikson B, Alstergren P, Davidson T *et al.* (2017) Pharmacological treatment of oro-facial pain - health technology assessment including a systematic review with network meta-analysis. *J Oral Rehabil* **44**:800–26.

18 Svensson P, Baad-Hansen L. (2008) Facial pain. In: Wilson PR, Watson PJ, Haythornthwaite JA *et al.*, eds. *Clinical pain management: Chronic pain*. Hodder Arnold, London. pp.467–483.

19 Baad-Hansen L, Benoliel R. (2017) Neuropathic orofacial pain: facts and fiction. *Cephalalgia* **37**:670–9.

20 Svensson P, Sessle BJ. (2004) Orofacial pain. In: Miles TS, Nauntofte B, Svensson P, eds. *Clinical Oral Physiology* pp.93–139.

21 Vázquez-Delgado E, Viaplana-Gutiérrez M, Figueiredo R *et al.* (2018) Prevalence of neuropathic pain and sensory alterations after dental implant placement in a university-based oral surgery department: a retrospective cohort study. *Gerodontology* **35**:117–22.

22 Pillai RS, Pigg M, List T *et al.* (2020) Assessment of somatosensory and psychosocial function of patients with trigeminal nerve damage. *Clin J Pain* **36**:321–35.

23 Melek LN, Smith JG, Karamat A et al. (2019) Comparison of the neuropathic pain symptoms and psychosocial impacts of trigeminal neuralgia and painful posttraumatic trigeminal neuropathy. *J Oral Facial Pain Headache* **33**:77–88.

24 Finnerup NB, Haroutounian S, Kamerman P *et al.* Neuropathic pain: An updated grading system for research and clinical practice. *Pain* **157**:1599–1606.

25 Sessle BJ. (2009) Role of peripheral mechanisms in craniofacial pain conditions. In: Cairns BE, ed. *Peripheral Receptor Targets for Analgesia: Novel Approaches to Pain Management*. John Wiley & Sons, Inc., Hoboken. pp. 3–20.

26 Forssell H and Svensson P. (2006) Atypical facial pain and burning mouth syndrome. *Handb Clinl Neurol* **81**:597–608.

27 Bergdahl M, Bergdahl J. (1999) Burning mouth syndrome: Prevalence and associated factors. *J Oral Pathol Med* **28**:350–4.

28 Klasser GD, Grushka M, Su N. (2016) Burning mouth syndrome. *Oral and Maxillofacial Surgery Clinics of North America* **28**:381–96.

29 Jääskeläinen SK, Woda A. (2017) Burning mouth syndrome. *Cephalalgia* **37**:627–47.

30 Adamo D, Sardella A, Varoni E, *et al.* (2018) The association between burning mouth syndrome and sleep disturbance: a case-control multicentre study. *Oral Dis* **24**:638–49.

31 Imamura Y, Shinozaki T, Okada-Ogawa A, *et al.* (2019) An updated review on pathophysiology and management of burning mouth syndrome with endocrinological, psychological and neuropathic perspectives. *J Oral Rehabil* **46**:574–87.

32 Kisely S, Forbes M, Sawyer E (2016) A systematic review of randomized trials for the treatment of burning mouth syndrome. *J Psychosom Res* **86**:39–46.

33 Koopman JS, Dieleman JP, Huygen FJ *et al.* (2009) Incidence of facial pain in the general population. *Pain* **147**: 122–7.

34 Mueller D, Obermann M, Yoon M-S *et al.* (2011) Prevalence of trigeminal neuralgia and persistent idiopathic facial pain: a population-based study. *Cephalalgia* **31(15)**:1542–8.

35 Woda A, Pionchon P. (2000) A unified concept of idiopathic orofacial pain: Pathophysiologic features. *J Orofac Pain* **14**:196–212.

36 Clark GT. (2006) Persistent orodental pain, atypical odontalgia, and phantom tooth pain: ahen are they neuropathic disorders? *J Calif Dent Assoc* **34**:599–609.

37 Marbach JJ, Raphael KG. (2000) Phantom tooth pain: a new look at an old dilemma. *Pain Med* **1**: 68–77.

38 Polycarpou N, Ng YL, Canavan D *et al.* (2005) Prevalence of persistent pain after endodontic treatment and factors affecting its occurrence in cases with complete radiographic healing. *Int Endod J* **38**:169–78.

39 Benoliel R, Gaul C. (2017) Persistent idiopathic facial pain. *Cephalalgia* **37**:680–91.
40 Baad-Hansen L, Leijon G, Svensson P *et al.* (2007) Comparison of clinical findings and psychosocial factors in patients with atypical odontalgia and temporomandibular disorders. *Journal of Orofacial Pain* **22**:7–14.
41 Baad-Hansen L. (2008) Atypical odontalgia – pathophysiology and clinical management. *Journal of Oral Rehabilitation* **35**:1–11.
42 Obermann M, Mueller D, Yoon MS *et al.* (2007) Migraine with isolated facial pain: a diagnostic challenge. *Cephalalgia* **27**:1278–82.
43 Abrahamsen R, Baad-Hansen L, Svensson P. (2008) Hypnosis in the management of persistent idiopathic orofacial pain--clinical and psychosocial findings. *Pain* **136**:44–52.
44 Baad-Hansen L, Juhl GI, Jensen TS *et al.* (2007) Differential effect of intravenous s-ketamine and fentanyl on atypical odontalgia and capsaicin-evoked pain. *Pain* **129**:46–54
45 Ziegeler C, May A. (2019) Facial presentations of migraine, tacs, and other paroxysmal facial pain syndromes. *Neurology* **93**: e1138–47.
46 Benoliel R, Birman N, Eliav E *et al.* (2008) The international classification of headache disorders: accurate diagnosis of orofacial pain? *Cephalalgia* **28**:752–62.
47 Sharav Y, Katsarava Zm Charles A. (2017) Facial presentations of primary headache disorders. *Cephalalgia* **37**:714–19.
48 Evers S, Afra J, Frese A *et al.* (2009) EFNS guideline on the drug treatment of migraine--revised report of an EFNS task force. *Eur J Neurol* **16**:968–81.

Chapter 34

Visceral pain

Klaus Bielefeldt[1,2] & Gerald F. Gebhart[3]

[1] *George E. Wahlen Veterans Administration (VA) Medical Center, Salt Lake City, Utah, USA*
[2] *Department of Medicine, University of Utah, Salt Lake City, Utah, USA*
[3] *Carver College of Medicine, University of Iowa, Iowa City, Iowa, USA*

Introduction

Visceral pain is a common clinical problem and manifests in a wide spectrum of illnesses from acute myocardial infarction to dysmenorrhea or irritable bowel syndrome. Not surprisingly, severity, duration, location and character of pain as well as associated symptoms vary widely. Despite these obvious differences, visceral pain syndromes share some characteristics. Sherrington defined visceral sensations as interoceptive. Such interoceptive signals provide important homeostatic information and are closely linked to autonomic function. Interoception is also associated with a strong motivational dimension. For example, hunger triggers complex behavioral responses that ultimately result in food intake. The level of complexity increases even further as motivation and emotion are closely related, which may explain why humans rate the unpleasantness of visceral events (e.g. rectal distension) higher than that of similarly intense non-visceral stimuli (e.g. local pressure) [1].

Visceral pain is associated with changes in autonomic function that may be cause and/or consequence of the underlying painful disorder and often complicate treatment. This interrelationship affects pain management, as medications may also influence organ function (e.g. constipation with opioids). The affective dimensions of pain are quite prominent, especially if essential and typically pleasant activities of daily life such as eating become triggers of pain or other unpleasant sensations.

Basic mechanisms of visceral pain

Investigating pain mechanisms largely focuses on nociception, the neural process of encoding noxious stimuli, usually – but not necessarily - linking a noxious stimulus to perception and behavioral responses. This concept is useful, even if not entirely accurate, because it enables us to investigate and treat components that contribute to visceral pain. Those components include the sensory afferent nerves that innervate visceral organs, the second order spinal or brainstem neuronal targets upon which the afferents terminate and the supraspinal sites in brain that process, interpret and modulate visceral input.

Molecular mechanisms of visceral sensation

Based on the link between activation of peripheral afferents and perception, we should be able to blunt or even block pain by interfering with the molecules that translate a noxious stimulus into action potentials discharged by nociceptive neurons. Many candidate molecules have been identified and new ones

Clinical Pain Management: A Practical Guide, Second Edition. Edited by Mary E. Lynch, Kenneth D. Craig, and Philip W. Peng.

continue to emerge. Using pharmacologic tools or experiments with genetically modified animals, three members of the transient receptor potential family of ion channels (TRPV1, TRPV4, TRPA1) appear to have an important role in responses to chemical signals, such as acid, and to high intensity mechanical stimulation during visceral distension [2]. Purinergic receptors, which are activated by ATP, may also contribute to visceral sensation and pain. These receptors require ATP release from neighboring cells, thus functionally linking the nervous system to other structures, such as the epithelium. The importance of epithelial signals has long been recognized in gastrointestinal physiology, with specialized enteroendocrine cells releasing mediators, which in turn activate primary afferent neurons. The best-characterized signaling cascade involves the release of serotonin, which initiates local reflexes and activates extrinsic afferents that may lead to conscious perception of visceral stimuli [3]. Other evidence points to endocannabinoids as another signaling system that modulates visceral sensation and function. Animal experiments and human data have clearly established a role for cannabinoid receptors in regulation of gastrointestinal motility and transit, which may have therapeutic potential but also contribute to adverse effects. While effective as antiemetics, cannabinoid agonists have not yet demonstrated analgesic properties in visceral pain in humans [4]. More recently, changes in luminal content (e.g. trypsin, metabolites of the gut microbiome) have been shown to activate afferent pathways and contribute to visceral pain, potentially opening up new treatment options for colonic visceral pain conditions [5].

Structural elements of visceral sensation

Most viscera are derived from midline structures and consequently are innervated bilaterally and thus activate both hemispheres of the brain. Despite the bilateral innervation, the density of the visceral afferent innervation is sparse relative to the afferent innervation of non-visceral tissues (principally skin) that convey input to the spinal cord. Unlike sensory neurons innervating non-visceral tissues, many sensory neurons have multiple receptive fields within an organ. Most visceral afferents are polymodal, meaning they respond to more than one stimulus modality. These and other anatomic and physiologic findings described below correlate well with the clinical observation that visceral sensations are poorly localized and do not reliably reflect the underlying stimulus modality.

Except for pelvic structures, all viscera receive a dual sensory innervation from spinal and vagal afferents. Pelvic organs are also innervated by two distinct sensory pathways, both of which project to the spinal cord via the lower splanchnic and pelvic nerve, respectively. The cell bodies of vagal sensory fibers are located in the nodose and the slightly more rostral jugular ganglion, with central terminations projecting directly to brainstem nucleus of the solitary tract and from there via the parabrachial nucleus and ventromedial thalamus to the insular cortex. Vagal afferent input has a role in the regulation of autonomic and homeostatic functions and is important in nausea, cough and dyspnea or complex sensations, such as hunger and satiety, but likely contributes little to acute pain. Spinal afferents have their cell bodies in dorsal root ganglia and project to second order neurons within the spinal cord, which send information rostrally through the spinothalamic tract and dorsal column. Second order neurons in the spinal cord typically receive convergent input from cutaneous sites, which provides the structural basis for pain referral to cutaneous as well as to other, typically nearby viscera, thus contributing to organ cross-sensitization (see [6] for a recent review).

Central processing of visceral sensation

Perception requires the activation of higher cortical structures. Detailed psychophysical experiments coupled with functional brain imaging reveal a matrix of structures activated by painful stimuli, discussed in more detail in Chapter 3. Functional brain imaging has not, however, demonstrated striking qualitative differences between the processing of visceral and non-visceral sensations. Notably, visceral pain more strongly activates the perigenual portion of the anterior cingulate cortex, while non-visceral pain is primarily represented in the mid-cingulate cortex [7].

Sensitization and visceral pain

The relationship between stimulus intensity and the related sensory response, whether neuronal or perceptual, is represented as a stimulus-response function. In 1973, James Ritchie first demonstrated in clinical studies in patients with irritable bowel syndrome (IBS) a left-ward shift of this stimulus–response function to *greater* sensitivity [8] (e.g. Figure 34.1). The increase in sensitivity to a stimulus, and the left-ward shift of the stimulus-response function, operationally defines sensitization. Many studies have since documented that sensitization of sensory pathways and sensory processing contributes to the pathogenesis of chronic visceral pain syndromes. Sensitization can be caused by peripheral and/or central mechanisms. Experimentally induced gastric, urinary bladder, colonic or other organ inflammation increases the excitability of primary afferent neurons. A variety of endogenous mediators have been identified as likely contributors, including prostaglandins, bradykinin, interleukins, cytokines as well as several neurotrophic factors, which are important in maintaining or modulating the function of nerve cells and thus may have a role in chronic pain syndromes. Extensive experimental data show changes in the properties of second order spinal neurons and more rostrally located areas of the central nervous system, which are at least in part mediated through glutamate acting on N-methyl -D-aspartate (NMDA) receptors.

Pain without peripheral input

The mechanisms of peripheral and central sensitization described above are all based on shifts in the causal relationship between a stimulus, its perception and the reaction of the organism. However, the model fails to explain chronic pain that is present without apparent peripheral input. While such a scenario runs counter to our training and practice, it is clinically quite relevant. For example, patients with IBS reported visceral pain in response to a visual stimulus that had previously been linked to painful colorectal distension. Functional brain imaging performed during such "conditioned" pain showed activation patterns that were quite like those seen during actual painful visceral stimulation [9]. Neuroaxial blocks to the point of complete surgical anesthesia eliminated pain in less than 50% of patients with chronic pancreatitis. These examples demonstrate the importance of 'top-down' mechanisms, which modulate afferent input through descending inhibition or facilitation or even generate the above-mentioned pain perception without any peripheral input. Anxiety with heightened attention (hypervigilance) to and altered processing of visceral input (catastrophizing) play key roles as central drivers of such pain experiences and may contribute to functional changes and structural remodeling that has been shown in brain imaging studies.

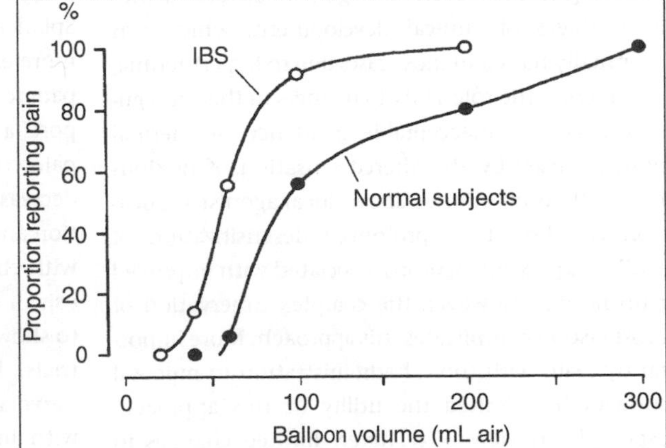

Figure 34.1 Ritchie first showed the clinical importance of sensitization with a lowering of pain thresholds during rectal distension in patients with irritable bowel syndrome. Source: Adapted from Ritchie J (1973).

Evidence-based treatment strategies

The multiple organ systems that may be directly or indirectly involved in visceral pain syndromes often lead to different symptoms, from palpitations or shortness of breath to nausea or constipation. Despite the resulting complexity, several strategies have been tested across different patient groups. We will discuss approaches based on mechanisms and common clinical scenarios.

Interventions targeting peripheral pathways

A variety of strategies have been developed to block afferent signal transduction and thus transfer of information to second-order central nociceptive neurons, with mixed and inconclusive results. One strategy is to non-selectively suppress afferent input using local anesthetics. Instillation of lidocaine into the urinary bladder or rectum can reduce ongoing discomfort as well as pain reports in response to experimental distension, suggesting that visceral afferent drive contributes to pain in many if not all affected persons. Despite this potential benefit, the need for repeated administration (e.g. lidocaine enemas) limits its utility in the management of chronic visceral pain syndromes [10]. Alternatively, more selective strategies to target peripheral pathways have been tested. Considering the preferential distribution of the vanilloid receptor TRPV1 on peripheral nociceptive neurons, antagonists and receptor desensitization through agonist application have been used in preclinical studies and/or small clinical studies [11, 12]. Several antagonists advanced into early stages of clinical development, which was eventually halted in most cases due to hyperthermia, considering the role TRPV1 channels in thermoregulation, or an unacceptable incidence of thermal burns, caused by the altered sensation of noxious heat [13]. As mentioned above, local agonist application can lead to a prolonged desensitization of TRPV1-expressing neurons associated with improved pain ratings. However, the complex innervation of most viscera complicates this approach. More importantly, pain with topical administration to mucosal surfaces has limited the utility of this approach, especially in view of relatively limited changes in global improvement ratings [14].

Peripherally acting k-opioid receptor agonists of the arylamide family have been shown to block sodium channels and decrease visceral hypersensitivity in animal studies. However, clinical studies do not show a convincing analgesic effect in patients with visceral pain. Eluxadoline is a peripherally restricted agent with mixed effects on opioid receptors, including the k-opioid receptor. Eluxadoline has been approved for the treatment of diarrhea-predominant irritable bowel syndrome based on an improved composite endpoint that includes bowel pattern and pain. However, it is unclear if the agent has direct analgesic properties or whether the benefit is primarily driven by changes in bowel patterns. More importantly, effects on the sphincter of Oddi triggered episodes of acute pancreatitis with several reported fatal outcomes.

Pregabalin and gabapentin interact with the $\alpha_2\delta$ subunit of voltage-sensitive calcium channels and thus target peripheral and central nociception. Despite their increasing use, available evidence remains inconclusive, with some positive data in pain management of chronic pancreatitis but inconsistent findings in irritable bowel syndrome and chronic pelvic pain [15, 16].

The complexity of visceral innervation with bilateral afferent input and spinal as well as vagal sensory pathways complicates the practical use of regional blocks. Depending on the primary location and presumed etiology of the pain syndrome, three anatomically distinct areas are currently treated through regional blocks, even though evidence supporting their efficacy is still limited. Small case series suggest a potential benefit of stellate ganglion block in select patients with refractory angina symptoms. Splanchnic or celiac blocks have been examined more extensively, mostly in patients with advanced pancreatic adenocarcinoma. Current evidence supports a significant, albeit transient, improvement in pain control after such blocks, which translates into decreased opioid requirements. Uterine nerve ablation and/or presacral neurectomy are used in women with chronic pelvic pain associated with endometriosis or dysmenorrhea. Uterine nerve ablation failed to show consistent benefit in appropriately designed trials. The alternative surgical procedure, presacral nerve ablation, has been examined in several trials with inconsistent results. A meta-analysis did not find sufficient evidence supporting efficacy [17].

While non-operative approaches have been developed, we still lack data comparing their impact on pain and quality of life to control interventions.

Interventions targeting luminal contents

The secretagogues linaclotide and plecanatide activate the generation of cyclic GMP, triggering secretion, which alleviates constipation and decreases associated pain [18]. The cyclic nucleotide is also released on the basolateral side, suggesting a potential inhibitory effect on afferent nerve endings located in the proximity. While in vitro experiments support such a mechanism, meta-analyses suggest a more indirect effect due to the laxative effects of these agents [19].

The gut, more specifically the colon, contains the highest concentration of microbes colonizing the human body. Complex interactions between dietary factors, host factors, the microbiome and its metabolome affect gastrointestinal function and sensation [20]. Differences between healthy controls are emerging, but often leave us with the question whether specific patterns of microbial colonization drive illness processes or, alternatively, whether altered host-factors, such as dietary choices or medical treatments, favor these shifts in microbiome. Mechanistic studies suggest a causal role, as the changes in microbiome are associated with other changes in luminal contents, such as higher protease activity, which can affect gut functions, such as epithelial permeability and sensory function, and thus lead to pain [21]. Dietary interventions with a reduction of poorly absorbed foods lowered colonic fermentation and reduced symptoms [22]. Attempts to alter the microbial flora within the gut have used pro- and antibiotics with variable results. Despite their widespread use, probiotics at best provide some relief in diarrhea predominant irritable bowel syndrome [23]. The poorly absorbed antibiotic rifaximin decreased overall symptom severity when given for a period of 2 weeks [24]. However, symptoms recurred in two thirds of the responders within less than 4 months. While repeated treatment cycles can restore the response in many patients, a repeated use of antibiotics for a chronic benign illness seems questionable in an era of increasingly antibiotic-resistant organisms. Nonetheless, the microbiome, especially the high number of microorganisms in the gut, is an important target for interventions that will directly or indirectly influence visceral sensation and pain.

Interventions targeting visceral contractions

Intermittent visceral pain is often associated with changes in smooth muscle activity, which may secondarily increase afferent input. Reducing contractility, for example with anticholinergics, such as dicyclomine, hyoscyamine or scopolamine, has demonstrated some benefit in patients with IBS. Considering the importance of prostaglandins in uterine contractions, non-steroidal anti-inflammatory drugs (NSAIDs) are helpful in alleviating uterine cramps, although about 20% of women with dysmenorrhea appear to be NSAID-resistant. One trial showed benefit of inhaled beta-adrenergic agonists in proctalgia fugax, a disorder characterized by intense anal pain, mediated by internal anal sphincter contractions. Considering the importance of serotonin in gastrointestinal physiology, several drugs interfering with serotonin receptor signaling have been examined, but none demonstrated convincing effects on visceral pain.

Interventions targeting central processing

Centrally acting analgesics: Opioids certainly blunt visceral pain. Yet, concerns about dependence, abuse and long-term effects argue against their widespread use in common benign disorders. In addition, opioid side effects from nausea to constipation target visceral function. Despite concerns about the opioid epidemic in the United States, opioids are commonly used to prevent visceral pain during medical procedures and treat acute visceral pain. Clinicians and investigators increasingly explore alternative approaches to avoid or at least limit opioid use in diseases associated with chronic pain, such as chronic pancreatitis or pancreatic cancer.

Antidepressants: Based on studies showing a potential benefit in neuropathic pain, tricyclic antidepressants (TCAs) and later selective serotonin reuptake inhibitors (SSRIs) were employed in patients with visceral pain syndromes. While several studies reported changes in sensory thresholds or global improvement, results varied. The largest trial did not show a significant benefit of desimpramine for patients with IBS when examined based on an intention-to-treat analysis, partly due to a high incidence of adverse effects and patient withdrawals. Meta-analyses suggest benefits over placebo, providing a rationale for their use in clinical practice [25]. For patients with functional dyspepsia, a similarly mixed picture emerges with systematic reviews supporting the use of antidepressants [26]. The serotonin/norepinephrine reuptake inhibitor (venlafaxine) has been systematically examined in patients with functional dyspepsia and was found not to be superior to placebo [27]. Duloxetine has not been appropriately evaluated in gastrointestinal disorders associated with pain. However, small studies suggest a benefit when the agent is combined with an alpha-receptor blocker to treat chronic prostatitis [28].

Psychologically based interventions: Based on the importance of anxiety and depression in chronic visceral pain syndromes, psychological interventions may have an important role in their management and have become an integral part of comprehensive multidisciplinary approaches. Several studies have examined the effects of cognitive behavioral therapy, mindfulness and hypnotherapy in different patient groups. While the effects on pain ratings vary, most investigations demonstrate an improvement in global well-being scores that may be maintained for years after completion of treatment [25]. However, treatments by appropriately trained providers may not be available or may not be covered by insurances. Recent developments with shortened therapy courses, group sessions and web-based interactions are effective and may overcome these barriers.

Alternative and complementary therapies

With the limited treatment options and often persistent symptoms, the use of alternative medical approaches from dietary changes to therapeutic writing is widespread in patient groups suffering from chronic pain. Very few studies have systematically evaluated the effectiveness of these interventions in visceral pain. Of the different herbal remedies, ginger, peppermint oil, capsaicin and some herbal combination therapies have some empiric support, suggesting utility in IBS or functional dyspepsia, respectively [29]. While many case series indicate a potential benefit of acupuncture, a large and well-designed trial did not demonstrate any benefit compared to sham treatment [30]. Other complimentary approaches including mind-body treatments, such as yoga, have been used in different settings but are still awaiting more rigorous assessment. Current evidence suggests that these treatments give patients a sense of control, which may improve quality of life independent of potential effects on pain.

Management of common visceral pain syndromes

By the time patients seek specialized help to manage pain or discomfort most of the affected individuals have already been evaluated extensively and tried a variety of different treatment approaches. Consensus or evidence-based treatments have typically been exhausted. Nevertheless, we outline algorithms for the more common visceral pain syndromes to provide some guidance for a rational approach in these patients.

Non-cardiac chest pain

Non-cardiac chest pain (NCCP) is typically an intermittent non-exertional pain that is not associated with dyspnea or other symptoms suggesting a cardiac etiology. The most common cause of NCCP is gastroesophageal acid reflux. Thus, the most cost-effective approach is an empiric trial of high dose acid suppression, which may even function as a diagnostic tool. If this step fails, compliance, appropriate dosing and timing of medication use should be checked before contemplating further steps, which will depend on the presence of associated symptoms (Figure 34.2) [31].

Functional dyspepsia

Dyspeptic symptoms are quite common with an estimated prevalence of up to 15% in the general population. Pain or discomfort are primarily localized in the

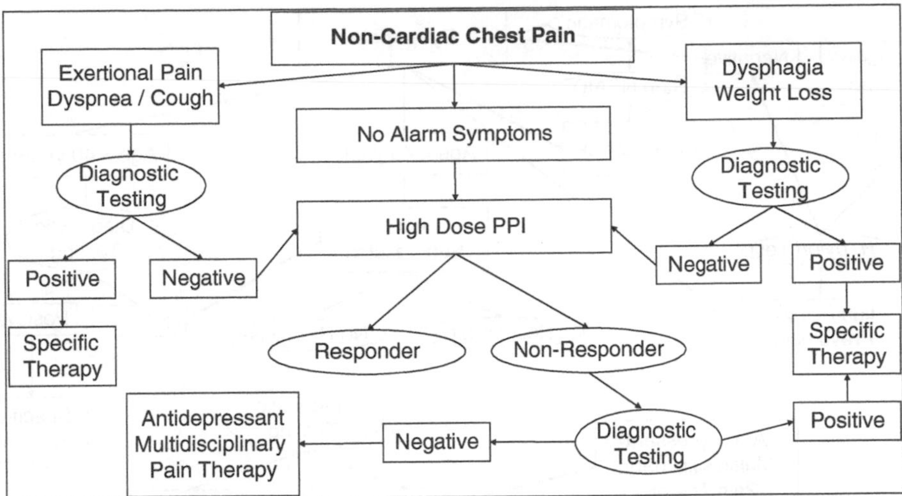

Figure 34.2 Diagnostic and therapeutic approach in patients with non-cardiac chest pain. PPI, proton pump inhibitor.

epigastric area and typically show an association with food intake. Considering the importance of gastric acidity in foregut disorders, therapies primarily rely on empiric acid suppression. While alarm symptoms, such as weight loss or bleeding typically trigger diagnostic testing, such alarming features have a limited positive predictive value for underlying problems, most importantly ulcer disease or gastric cancer[26]. Age is a key factor that should influence the approach to patients with dyspeptic symptoms, as the prevalence of potentially relevant diseases, most importantly cancer, increases with age. With fullness and nausea as predominant symptom, prokinetic agents, such as metoclopramide could be tried. While infections with *Helicobacter pylori* may contribute to chronic dyspeptic symptoms and associated illnesses, such as peptic ulcer disease, testing should be considered, especially if the background prevalence in the area is higher than 10% (Figure 34.3) [26].

Chronic pancreatitis

Chronic pancreatitis typically causes significant pain, which may decrease with the development of atrophy during disease progression. Assessment in specialized centers should first determine if there are anatomic causes that should be addressed with endoscopic or surgical treatment, such as large pseudocysts or obstructing stones within the ductal system. If such options do not exist, management often relies on opioids, which is problematic considering the opioid epidemic and the importance of substance abuse (i.e. alcoholism) as a common cause for chronic pancreatitis in Western countries. Antioxidants have shown promise with significant benefit in a cohort with patients suffering from idiopathic or tropic forms of chronic pancreatitis. Results were not replicated in subsequent studies conducted in Western countries. Strategies to improve pain by inhibiting pancreatic stimulation through oral administration of pancreatic enzymes are often used but have not consistently shown benefit. While localized nerve blocks can be performed relatively easily, they only provide transient if any benefit. Uncontrolled studies reported benefit from operative interventions, such as implantation of a spinal cord stimulator or even total pancreatectomy with islet cell transplantation. However, pain relief may be incomplete or transient only, highlighting the need for additional studies before adopting these approaches in clinical practice [32].

Irritable bowel syndrome

Irritable bowel syndrome (IBS) is the most common gastrointestinal disease associated with discomfort and pain. The clinical manifestations vary substantially, including patients with severe diarrhea as well as individuals with significant constipation. Independent of

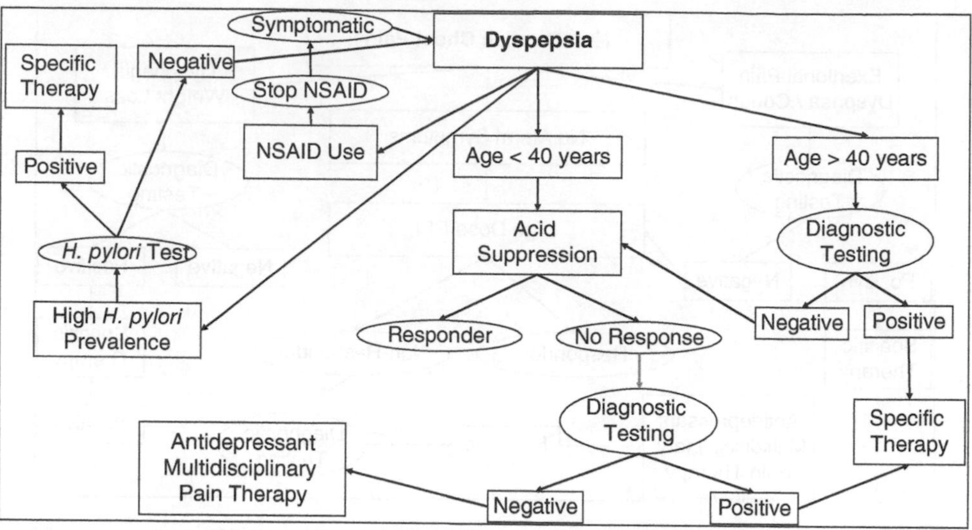

Figure 34.3 Diagnostic and therapeutic approach in patients with dyspeptic symptoms in countries with reference to prevalence of *Helicobacter pylori* infection. NSAID, non-steroidal anti-inflammatory drug.

the clinical scenario, dietary adjustments with a healthy diet and focus on water soluble fiber and lifestyle modification with an emphasis on stress management may benefit patients with IBS. While this consensus is largely based on expert opinion, costs and risks of thorough dietary assessment and counseling are minimal. Beyond such general advice, most specific treatment strategies should be based on the dominant complaint and primary treatment goals defined in a shared decision-making process with the patient.

Well-designed trials and meta-analyses support the use of antidepressants, which may also affect bowel patterns due to their anticholinergic (tricyclic antidepressants) or serotoninergic (selective serotonin reuptake inhibitors) effects. Psychological treatments from mindfulness to cognitive behavioral or hypnotherapy improve overall symptom severity. Innovative approaches with internet- or group-based interventions may overcome constraints due to cost or limited availability. Cramps or spasms respond to peppermint oil preparations or anticholinergics. Changing the microbiome with probiotics is a widespread clinical practice with still limited support, but likely benefit for diarrhea-predominant symptoms. For this subgroup, a diet low in poorly absorbed and hence fermentable foods (FODMAP diet) is often helpful. The poorly absorbed antibiotic rifaximin, eluxadoline, a peripherally restricted agent targeting κ opioid receptors, and the serotonin receptor antagonist alosetron all show efficacy in IBS with diarrhea, but should be reserved for otherwise refractory patients due to costs or potential adverse effects. In IBS associated with constipation, such second-tier treatment options include the secretagogues lubiprostone, linaclotide and plecanatide and prokinetics, such as prucalopride (Figure 34.4) [33].

Inflammatory bowel disease

Pain is a common problem in patients with Crohn's disease and ulcerative colitis. About two thirds of the affected individuals will experience pain in the course of their illness, with pain intensity and character largely reflecting the severity of their underlying inflammatory condition [34]. With the introduction of anti-TNF and other biological agents, mucosal healing has become an important treatment endpoint for many clinicians. The more frequent endoscopic reassessment blurred the dichotomy between structural and functional illnesses, as ongoing symptoms are often not explained by persistent inflammation. While scarring with obstruction or fistulizing disease may account for some of this discrepancy in Crohn's disease, such changes are not seen in ulcerative colitis. Persistent symptoms with pain and bowel changes in about 20% of the affected individuals led some experts to

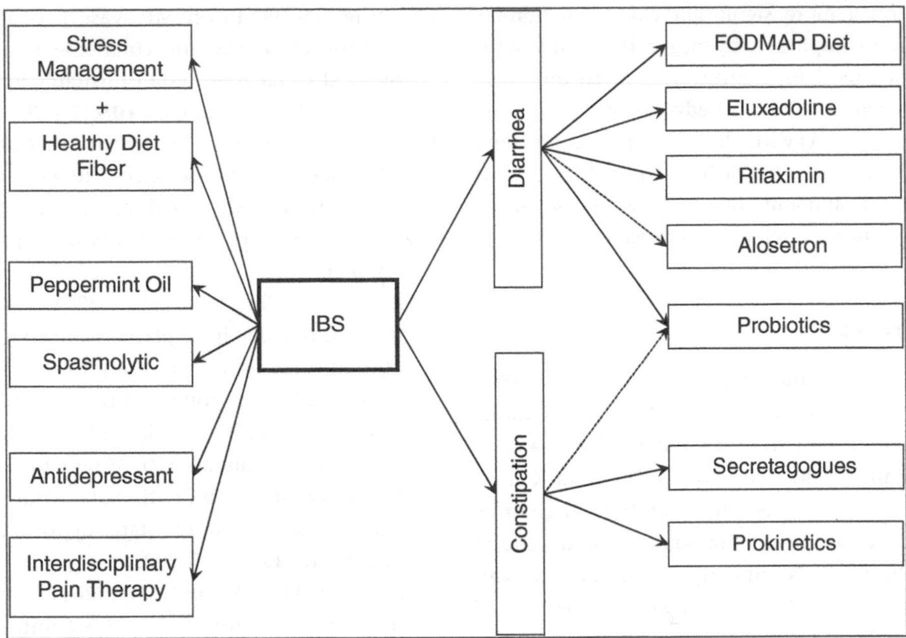

Figure 34.4 Diagnostic and therapeutic approach in patients with irritable bowel syndrome (IBS).

conclude that we are dealing with a post-inflammatory sensitization of afferent pathways and or sensory processing [35]. Management of these patients is more complex, as ongoing active inflammation or the consequences of a chronic inflammatory process on gut structure and function confound the picture. Most clinicians apply approaches used in individuals with IBS, even though the supporting evidence is often limited or even lacking [36]. Beyond relying on overlapping symptoms and perhaps even mechanisms, pain management should clearly avoid NSAIDs, which can trigger exacerbation of the underlying inflammation [37]. Opioids may similarly have a detrimental effect with increasing hospitalization rates and higher mortality [38]. This negative impact does not seem to be driven by effects on the disease process but may be due to unintentional overdoses and the correlation between illness severity, related complications and pain.

Chronic pelvic pain

Chronic pelvic pain encompasses multiple different disorders from myofascial pain to dysmenorrhea, endometriosis and painful bladder syndrome. Further detail will be covered in Chapter 33 on pelvic and urogenital pain. Overall, relatively few well-designed trials have been conducted to examine the efficacy of different diagnostic or therapeutic strategies in patients with chronic pelvic pain and the best approach is to follow the general principles of chronic pain management found in other chapters in this book utilizing a multidisciplinary biopsychosocial approach. If diagnostic evaluations suggest an inflammatory component (e.g. chronic prostatitis), NSAIDs may be beneficial. Although operative interventions are often used, the true efficacy of surgical approaches is often limited. In painful bladder syndrome and chronic prostatitis, approaches targeting bladder dysfunction, such as botulinum toxin injection or alpha receptor blockade combined with duloxetine, can improve global symptom scores without directly affecting pain mechanisms [39. 40].

Conclusions

Chronic visceral pain, from non-cardiac chest pain to IBS, is common. The underlying cause and/or associated changes in visceral function vary tremendously. Compared with somatic pain syndromes, visceral pain carries a more significant emotional burden. Treatment is complicated by the fact that many of the medications used for management of chronic pain exhibit a high incidence of adverse effects on autonomic function. As with all chronic pain conditions, a multidisciplinary approach is required in treating the pain, clinical manifestation of organ or organ system dysfunction as well as psychosocial factors.

References

1 Strigo IA, Bushnell MC, Boivin M *et al.* (2002) Psychophysical analysis of visceral and cutaneous pain in human subjects. *Pain* **97**:235–46.

2 Balemans D, Boeckxstaens GE, Talavera K *et al.* (2017) Transient receptor potential ion channel function in sensory transduction and cellular signaling cascades underlying visceral hypersensitivity. *Am J Physiol Gastrointest Liver Physiol* **312**:G635–48.

3 Gershon MD, Tack J. (2007) The serotonin signaling system: from basic understanding to drug development for functional GI disorders. *Gastroenterology* **132**:397–414.

4 Fioramonti J, Bueno L. (2008) Role of cannabinoid receptors in the control of gastrointestinal motility and perception. *Expert Review of Gastroenterology & Hepatology* **2**:385–97.

5 Jimenez-Vargas NN, Pattison LA, Zhao P *et al.* (2018) Protease-activated receptor-2 in endosomes signals persistent pain of irritable bowel syndrome. *Proc Natl Acad Sci USA* **115**:E7438–47.

6 Gebhart GF, Bielefeldt K. (2016) Physiology of visceral pain. *Compr Physiol* **6**:1609–33.

7 Kano M, Dupont P, Aziz Q, *et al.* (2018) Understanding neurogastroenterology from neuroimaging perspective: a comprehensive review of functional and structural brain imaging in functional gastrointestinal disorders. *J Neurogastroenterol Motil* **24**:512–27.

8 Ritchie J. (1973) Pain from distension of the pelvic colon by inflating a balloon in the irritable colon syndrome. *Gut* **14**:125–32.

9 Yágüez L, Coen S, Gregory LJ *et al.* Brain response to visceral aversive conditioning: a functional magnetic resonance imaging study. *Gastroenterology* **128**:1819–29.

10 Verne GN, Robinson ME, Vase L *et al.* (2003) Reversal of visceral and cutaneous hyperalgesia by local rectal anesthesia in irritable bowel syndrome (IBS) patients. *Pain* **105**:223–30.

11 Arsenault P, Chiche D, Brown W *et al.* (2018) NEO6860, modality-selective TRPV1 antagonist: a randomized, controlled, proof-of-concept trial in patients with osteoarthritis knee pain. *Pain Rep* **3**:e696.

12 Lee J, Kim BH, Yu KS *et al.* (2017) A first-in-human, double-blind, placebo-controlled, randomized, dose escalation study of DWP05195, a novel TRPV1 antagonist, in healthy volunteers. *Drug Des Devel Ther* **11**:1301–13.

13 Moran MM, Szallasi A. (2018) Targeting nociceptive transient receptor potential channels to treat chronic pain: current state of the field. *Br J Pharmacol* **175**:2185–203.

14 Zhang W, Deng X, Liu C *et al.* (2017) Intravesical treatment for interstitial cystitis/painful bladder syndrome: a network meta-analysis. *Int Urogynecol J* **28**:515–25.

15 Olesen SS, Graversen C, Bouwense SA *et al.* (2013) Quantitative sensory testing predicts pregabalin efficacy in painful chronic pancreatitis. *PLoS One* **8**:e57963.

16 Pontari MA, Krieger JN, Litwin MS *et al.* (2010) Pregabalin for the treatment of men with chronic prostatitis/chronic pelvic pain syndrome: a randomized controlled trial. *Arch Intern Med* **170**:1586–93.

17 Proctor ML, Latthe PM, Farquhar CM *et al.* (2005) Surgical interruption of pelvic nerve pathways for primary and secondary dysmenorrhoea. *Cochrane Database Syst Rev* **(4)**: Cd001896.

18 Layer P, Stanghellini V. (2014) Review article: linaclotide for the management of irritable bowel syndrome with constipation. *Alimentary Pharmacology & Therapeutics* **39**:371–84.

19 Black CJ, Burr NE, Quigley EMM *et al.* (2018) Efficacy of secretagogues in patients with irritable bowel syndrome with constipation: systematic review and network meta-analysis. *Gastroenterology* **155**:1753–63.

20 Weersma RK, Zhernakova A, Fu J. (2020) Interaction between drugs and the gut microbiome. *Gut* **69**:1510–19.

21 Edogawa S, Edwinson AL, Peters SA *et al.* (2020) Serine proteases as luminal mediators of intestinal barrier dysfunction and symptom severity in IBS. *Gut* **69**:62–73.

22 Halmos EP, Power VA, Shepherd SJ *et al.* (2014) A diet low in FODMAPs reduces symptoms of irritable bowel syndrome. *Gastroenterology* **146**:67–75.e5.

23 Ford AC, Harris LA, Lacy BE *et al.* (2018) Systematic review with meta-analysis: the efficacy of prebiotics, probiotics, synbiotics and antibiotics in irritable bowel syndrome. *Aliment Pharmacol Ther* **48**:1044–60.

24 Pimentel M, Lembo A, Chey WD *et al.* (2011) Rifaximin therapy for patients with irritable bowel syndrome without constipation. *N Engl J Med* **364**:22–32.

25 Ford AC, Lacy BE, Harris LA *et al.* (2019) Effect of antidepressants and psychological therapies in irritable bowel syndrome: an updated systematic review and meta-analysis. *Am J Gastroenterol* **114**:21–39.

26 Moayyedi PM, Lacy BE, Andrews CN *et al.* (2017) ACG and CAG clinical guideline: management of dyspepsia. *Am J Gastroenterol* **112**:988–1013.

27 van Kerkhoven LAS, Laheij RJF, Aparicio N *et al.* (2008) Effect of the antidepressant venlafaxine in functional dyspepsia: a randomized, double-blind, placebo-controlled trial. *Clinical Gastroenterology and Hepatology* **6**:746–52.

28 Giannantoni A, Porena M, Gubbiotti M *et al.* (2014) The efficacy and safety of duloxetine in a multidrug regimen for chronic prostatitis/chronic pelvic pain syndrome. *Urology* **83**:400–5.

29 Deutsch JK, Levitt J, Hass DJ. (2020) Complementary and alternative medicine for functional gastrointestinal disorders. *Am J Gastroenterol* **115**:350–64.

30 Lembo AJ, Conboy L, Kelley JM *et al.* (2009) A treatment trial of acupuncture in IBS patients. *Am J Gastroenterology* **104**:1489–97.

31 Fass R, Shibli F, Tawil J. (2019) Diagnosis and management of functional chest pain in the Rome IV era. J *Neurogastroenterol Motil* **25**:487–98.

32 Gardner TB, Adler DG, Forsmark CE *et al.* (2020) ACG clinical guideline: chronic pancreatitis. *Am J Gastroenterol* **115**:322–39.

33 Ford AC, Moayyedi P, Lacy BE *et al.* (2014) American College of Gastroenterology monograph on the management of irritable bowel syndrome and chronic idiopathic constipation. *American Journal of Gastroenterology* 109:S2–26.

34 Kochar B, Martin CF, Kappelman MD *et al.* (2018) Evaluation of Gastrointestinal Patient Reported Outcomes Measurement Information System (GI-PROMIS) symptom scales in subjects with inflammatory bowel diseases. *Am J Gastroenterol* **113**:72–9.

35 Grover M, Herfarth H, Drossman DA. (2009) The functional-organic dichotomy: postinfectious irritable bowel wyndrome and inflammatory bowel disease-irritable bowel syndrome. *Clinical Gastroenterology and Hepatology* **7**:48–53.

36 Thorkelson G, Bielefeldt K, Szigethy E. (2016) Empirically supported use of psychiatric medications in adolescents and adults with IBD. *Inflamm Bowel Dis* **22**:1509–22.

37 Habib I, Mazulis A, Roginsky G *et al.* (2014) Nonsteroidal anti-inflammatory drugs and inflammatory bowel disease: pathophysiology and clinical associations. *Inflamm Bowel Dis* **20**:2493–502.

38 Lichtenstein GR, Feagan BG, Cohen RD *et al.* (2006) Serious infections and mortality in association with therapies for Crohn's disease: TREAT registry. *Clinical Gastroenterology and Hepatology* **4**:621–30.

39 Cheong YC, Smotra G, Williams AC. (2014) Non-surgical interventions for the management of chronic pelvic pain. *Cochrane Database Syst Rev***(3)**:Cd008797.

40 Mahran A, Baaklini G, Hassani D *et al.* (2019) Sacral neuromodulation treating chronic pelvic pain: a meta-analysis and systematic review of the literature. *Int Urogynecol J* **30**:1023–35.

Chapter 35

Pelvic and urogenital pain

Anjali Martinez
Obstetrics and Gynecology, George Washington University, Washington, DC, USA

Introduction

Chronic pelvic pain is a common disorder in women, with a prevalence of about 4% [1]; similar to the prevalence of migraine headaches and asthma. It is a frequent reason for outpatient visits to doctors. Women with chronic pelvic pain not infrequently also have limited function or disability, marital problems or divorce, and often have been subjected to multiple surgical treatments without much benefit.

Chronic pelvic pain is defined as non-cyclic pelvic or lower abdominal pain of greater than 3–6 months' duration. Traditionally, chronic vulvar pain is not included based on its anatomic location, but it is discussed in this chapter as part of genital pain. Note that a specific diagnosis is not necessary for the diagnosis of chronic pelvic pain, and indeed sometimes chronic pain itself is the only or best diagnosis. Chronic pelvic or urogenital pain may have multiple etiologies, and often multiple etiologies exist at once. Some of these disorders have no cure so naturally lead to the chronic nature of chronic pelvic pain, but why other etiologies lead to chronic pain are less understood. Although most etiologies of pelvic pain may start as visceral or somatic nociceptive pain, neuropathic pain or centralization of pain may occur, so that the pain is maintained regardless of the status of the original source of pain.

Etiology

The differential diagnoses of the disorders associated with chronic pelvic pain are very broad. Visceral sources of pain include the gastrointestinal tract, the urologic system and the reproductive system. Somatic sources of chronic pain in this area include the musculoskeletal system and the neurologic system. In a large British primary care study, chronic pelvic pain was more often related to the gastrointestinal tract and urinary system than to the reproductive system [1]. Although many etiologies of chronic pelvic pain are not gender-specific, this discussion focuses on chronic pelvic pain in women. Disorders that have strong evidence of a causal relationship with chronic pelvic pain include interstitial cystitis/bladder pain syndrome, irritable bowel syndrome (IBS), constipation, endometriosis and abdominal wall myofascial pain. For many disorders, there is only limited evidence that the disease leads to chronic pain. For a list of diagnoses commonly associated with chronic pelvic pain see Table 35.1.

Evaluation

Diagnosis is mostly based on a thorough history and physical examination. Because the etiologies of pain are diverse, both the history and examination must

Clinical Pain Management: A Practical Guide, Second Edition. Edited by Mary E. Lynch, Kenneth D. Craig, and Philip W. Peng.

Table 35.1 Conditions that may cause or exacerbate pelvic and urogenital pain, by level of evidence.

Level of evidence	Gastrointestinal	Gynecologic	Urologic	Musculoskeletal
Level A	Irritable bowel syndrome	Endometriosis	Interstitial cystitis	Abdominal wall Myofascial pain (trigger points)
			Bladder Pain syndrome	
	Constipation	Gynecologic malignancies	Bladder malignancy	Pelvic floor tension myalgia
	Inflammatory bowel disease	Ovarian retention syndrome (residual ovary syndrome)	Radiation Cystitis	Neuralgia of iliohypogastric, ilioinguinal, and/or genitofemoral nerve
	Carcinoma of the colon	Ovarian remnant syndrome		Peripartum pelvic pain syndrome
		Pelvic congestion syndrome		
		Pelvic inflammatory disease		
		Vestibulodynia		
		Vulvodynia		
Level B		Adhesions	Urethral diverticulum	Neoplasia of spinal cord or sacral nerve
		Benign cystic mesothelioma		Coccydynia
		Leiomyomata		Lumbar disk herniation
		Postoperative peritoneal cysts		
Level C	Colitis	Adenomyosis	Chronic urinary tract infection	Compression of lumbar vertebrae
	Chronic intermittent bowel obstruction	Atypical dysmenorrhea	Recurrent acute cystitis	Degenerative joint disease
	Diverticulosis	Adnexal cysts	Recurrent acute urethritis	Hernias (ventral, inguinal, femoral, spigelian)
		Cervical stenosis	Urolithiasis	Thoracolumbar facet syndrome
		Chronic endometritis		
		Residual accessory ovary		
		Genital prolapse		
		Endosalpingiosis		

Level A: good and consistent scientific evidence of causal relationship to chronic pelvic pain.
Level B: limited or inconsistent scientific evidence of causal relationship to chronic pelvic pain.
Level C: causal relationship to chronic pelvic pain based on expert opinions.

cover multiple organ systems. A good history will include details of the pain itself including quality, severity, timing and location, preferably mapped by the patient on a diagram of the body; a psychosocial history; questions regarding bowel and bladder symptoms and a depression screen. Details in the patient's history often suggest which organ systems are involved (gastrointestinal, urologic, musculoskeletal, gynecologic, neuropathic) and can guide further evaluation and care. Depression or anxiety often co-exist with chronic pelvic pain [2], and psychosocial factors may contribute to a patient's interpretation of pain and response to treatment.

The physical examination is performed to identify any anatomic sources of the patient's pain. It is important to isolate and examine the musculoskeletal, gastrointestinal, urinary, reproductive and neurological systems during the evaluation to pinpoint specific diagnoses if present. In particular, the pelvic examination for chronic pelvic pain is different from the traditional bimanual pelvic examination in that it is performed with one finger of one hand so that focal areas of tenderness that reproduce the patient's baseline pain can be sought in bony, nervous, muscular and visceral structures (referred to as a "pain-mapping exam"). For details on conducting the physical examination, see Chronic Pelvic Pain in Adult Females: Evaluation [3].

Presentations of some of the most common disorders associated with chronic pelvic pain are outlined here.

Irritable Bowel Syndrome

IBS is the most common diagnosis in women with chronic pelvic pain. Diagnosis is based on history but laboratory data may help differentiate it from an infectious or inflammatory process. Symptoms must include chronic abdominal pain and abnormal bowel habits. Because these symptoms are often subjective and vary greatly among individuals, it may be useful to use standardized criteria for the diagnosis of IBS such as the Rome criteria. The most recent criteria (Rome IV) are recurrent abdominal pain or discomfort for at least one day per week (on average) in the last 3 months associated with two or more of the following: pain is related to defecation, pain is associated with a change in frequency of stool, or pain is associated with a change in form or appearance of stool [4].

Interstitial Cystitis or Bladder Pain Syndrome

The current American Urologic Association defines Interstitial Cystitis or Bladder Pain Syndrome as "An unpleasant sensation (pain, pressure, discomfort) perceived to be related to the urinary bladder, associated with lower urinary tract symptoms of more than six weeks duration, in the absence of infection or other identifiable causes" [5, 6]. Patients tend to have more discomfort with a full bladder and voiding provides relief.Diagnosis used to be based on cystoscopy with hydro-distention or a potassium sensitivity test, but these tests are not sensitive or specific and are not usually used anymore.

Endometriosis

Endometriosis is the presence of histologically confirmed endometrial glands and/or stroma outside of the endometrium and myometrium. Endometriosis-associated pelvic pain usually begins as cyclic menstrual pain or dysmenorrhea but can progress to constant pain with premenstrual and menstrual exacerbations. Patients may also present with an adnexal mass (endometrioma) or infertility. Physical examination is often normal, but sometimes shows evidence of scarring with malposition of the uterus or cervix, palpable tender endometriotic nodules or an adnexal mass.

Vulvodynia

Vulvodynia is a chronic recurrent vulvar pain with at least three months duration with no other known cause. It can involve localized or generalized vulvar symptoms that occur spontaneously or be provoked. The timing of symptoms can vary. Frequently, the woman is unable to use tampons and unable to have coitus because of pain. Pain with speculum insertion is almost always present. Diagnosis is based on history and with abnormal tenderness on the vulvar vestibule to cotton-tip applicator palpation (positive "Q-tip test"). The vulvar vestibule is medial to the labia minora but external to the hymeneal ring.

Myofascial pain

Myofascial pain of the abdominal muscles or the pelvic floor is a significant cause of chronic pelvic pain. Muscular pain may be due to injury, tension, and/or trigger points. Evaluation is based on physical exam findings.

Many of the diagnoses associated with chronic pelvic pain need no diagnostic laboratory or imaging studies, so routine testing, such as barium enemas, colonoscopy, laparoscopy or intravenous pyelography, is not usually necessary. Diagnostic testing should be based on the history and physical examination. For example, diagnostic laparoscopy may be valuable if chronic pain is thought to be caused by endometriosis or pelvic adhesive disease, but not if interstitial cystitis or IBS seem to be the most likely associated disorder. A negative laparoscopy should never be used to tell a patient that she has no diagnosis or that her pain is not real.

Treatment

Like many sources of chronic pain, treatment options for chronic pelvic or urogenital pain are usually not curative. Instead, the goal of treatment is control of symptoms and for improved function and activity. Treatment can be disease-specific, meaning it targets the diagnoses that are contributing to the patient's pain, or be pain-specific for chronic pain itself. A patient's treatment regimen may often include both of these treatment options.

Disease-specific treatment

For brevity, specific treatment options for only the most common disorders causing chronic pelvic or urogenital pain are discussed here and the focus is on first line treatments that providers from any specialty can offer.

Endometriosis

Endometriosis can be treated medically and/or surgically. Many providers follow the American Society of Reproductive Medicine's principle that "Endometriosis should be viewed as a chronic disease that requires a lifelong management plan with the goal of maximizing the use of medical treatment and avoiding repeated surgical procedures [7]."

Medical treatment usually involves suppressing growth and activity of endometriosis lesions. This can be done with hormonal suppression of ovarian cycling using combination estrogen-progestin contraceptives or gonadotropin releasing hormone agonists (GnRH-a). Progestin only contraceptives can also be used, as progestins inhibit endometrial growth. The most extensively studied medical treatment for endometriosis is of gonadotropin releasing hormone agonists (GnRH-a) but the duration of treatment is limited to about six months due to the association with loss in bone mineral density [8] and is associated with menopausal side effects. Combination oral contraceptives are often used to treat endometriosis in either cycling or continuous form; recent studies suggest that continuous administration may be more effective [9]. Progestin only treatment such as norethindrone acetate and medroxyprogesterone acetate may also be used for the treatment of endometriosis-associated pelvic pain [10] and is especially useful if estrogen use is contraindicated. These contraceptive options can also be used as a treatment for any cyclic pain symptoms, not just endometriosis, but are only appropriate if the patient is not actively trying to conceive.

Surgical treatment should be limited to those who have had extensive evaluation of their chronic pain and who are not responding well to medical therapy in order to limit exposing people to the risks of surgery. The mainstay of surgical treatment is laparoscopic ablation or excision of endometriosis because it improves pain scores for mild-moderate endometriosis [11] but a recent update on that meta-analysis states that the evidence is not clear compared to diagnostic laparoscopy alone [12]. Although excision is not clearly better than ablation, excision does provide the opportunity for definitive pathologic diagnosis.

Performing presacral neurectomy at the time of endometriosis surgery has been shown to slightly improve pain relief with conservative surgery in patients with severe dysmenorrhea and centralized pain [13]. Uterosacral nerve ablation has not been shown to improve pain symptoms compared to traditional surgical treatment [14, 15].

Irritable bowel syndrome

Dietary and lifestyle modification are usually recommended as first line therapy for IBS [4]. A trial of eliminating lactose should be attempted because of the similar symptoms of lactose intolerance and IBS and their frequent overlap. General recommendations such as regular meals, limiting caffeine and alcohol, maintaining adequate hydration and avoidance of processed foods are reasonable suggestions. Patients with gas and bloating symptoms should limit the intake of gas-producing foods such as beans or pulses. In these patients, fiber may exacerbate symptoms, while in patients with predominant constipation increased soluble fiber may help. Medical management targets the patient's most bothersome symptoms. Antispasmodics such as peppermint oil or dicyclomine can help with gas and bloating and antidiarrheals such as loperamide are helpful in patients with predominantly symptoms of diarrhea for short periods of time but long-term use has not been adequately studied. Additional approaches targeting specific symptoms in IBS are presented in Chapter 34.

Interstitial cystitis/Bladder Pain Syndrome

Behavioral and diet modifications are often the first recommended treatments for painful bladder syndrome. Foods or beverages such as alcohol, caffeine and acidic foods that exacerbate symptoms should be avoided. Pelvic floor relaxation techniques or physical therapy may help, while pelvic floor strengthening exercises should be avoided. Medications such as analgesics, amitriptyline, cimetidine, hydroxyzine, or sodium pentosan polysulfate may help [5].

Vulvodynia/Vestibulodynia

Conservative treatment of vulvodynia includes lifestyle changes such as vulvar hygiene habits, symptom relief, and stress reduction. Some of The National Vulvodynia Association's recommendations include: all-white cotton underwear, loose fitting clothing, unscented/undyed detergents, avoiding scented bath soaps, and using lukewarm sitz baths to relieve symptoms [16]. Pelvic floor physical therapy is often effective at decreasing symptoms [17]. Medical management options include topical lidocaine, or oral medication like hormones, antidepressants, or neuropathic agents. Vulvar vestibulectomy is a surgery that removes the portion of the vestibule that contributes to pain and is most effective in those with localized, provoked vestibulodynia who have not responded sufficiently to more conservative options [17]. A long term follow up study showed that over 90% of people with provoked vestibulodynia were satisfied with their surgery over 10 years later [18].

Myofascial Pelvic Pain

The first line treatment for myofascial pelvic pain is physical therapy. If the pain involves the pelvic floor, it is important to specifically have pelvic floor physical therapy. If trigger points are involved, trigger point injections with local anesthetic may provide added benefit.

Pain-specific treatment

Education, reassurance and a good patient– physician relationship go a long way in treating chronic pain conditions. Often, a patient with chronic pelvic pain has been to many doctors and simply listening to their story and believing their symptoms benefits them. Medical treatment for chronic pain includes analgesics such as aspirin, acetaminophen, and nonsteroidal anti-inflammatory medications (NSAIDs). NSAIDs are usually the best first line agent for many of the etiologies of chronic pelvic pain. Opiates are generally not recommended to manage chronic pain.

Management may also include treatment of mood disorders since depression and anxiety often co-exist with chronic pain. Cognitive behavioral therapy may be helpful as part of a multidisciplinary approach to treatment and will help with a goal-oriented care plan [19, 20]. Antidepressants can also improve quality of life in patients with neuropathic pain [21]. Tricyclic antidepressants can help improve pain tolerance and sleep habits separately from their anti-depressive qualities. Anticonvulsants such as gabapentin have also been shown to decrease pain in women with chronic pelvic pain [22].

Conclusions

Because chronic pelvic pain is relatively common among women and the differential diagnoses are so broad, it is important for healthcare providers across many specialties to be familiar with the commonly associated disorders that contribute to chronic pelvic pain. The pain itself may be the most important aspect to address and in this case the general principles of pain management presented in other chapters of this book are appropriate. Having a physician listen and then validate the patient's chronic pelvic pain is an important component of treatment. Finally, first line treatment may often be offered regardless of the provider's specialty, decreasing the time the woman searches for care before she starts getting help for her chronic pain.

Acknowledgments

We acknowledge Fred M. Howard as co-author of the previous version of this chapter.

References

1 Zondervan KT, Yudkin PL, Vessey MP *et al.* (1999) Patterns of diagnosis and referral in women consulting for chronic pelvic pain in UK primary care. *Br J Obstet Gynaecol* **106**:1156–61.

2 Bryant C, Cockburn R, Plante AF, Chia A. (2016) The psychological profile of women presenting to a multidisciplinary clinic for chronic pelvic pain: high levels of psychological dysfunction and implications for practice. *J Pain Res.* **9**:1049–1056.

3 Tu, F and AS-Sanie, S. (2020) Chronic pelvic pain in Adult females: Evaluation. In: UpToDate. Sharp, H (Ed), UpToDate Waltham 2020. https://www.uptodate.com/contents/chronic-pelvic-pain-in-adult-females-evaluation. Accessed January 2021.

4 Mearin F, Lacy BE, Chang L, Chey WD, Lembo AJ, Simren M, Spiller R. (2016) Bowel disorders. *Gastroenterology*. **150(6)**:1393–1407.

5 Hanno P, Burks D, Clemens J *et al.* (2011) AUA guideline for the diagnosis and treatment of interstitial cystitis/bladder pain syndrome. *J Urol* **185(6)**: 2162–70

6 Hanno PM, Erickson D, Moldwin R et al. (2015). Diagnosis and treatment of interstitial cystitis/bladder pain syndrome: AUA guideline amendment. J Urol **193**:1545–53.

7 Practice Committee of the American Society for Reproductive Medicine. (2014) Treatment of pelvic pain associated with endometriosis: a committee opinion. *Fertil Steril* **101(4)**:927–35. Erratum in: *Fertil Steril*. 2015 **104(2)**:498.

8 Brown J, Pan A, Hart RJ. (2010) Gonadotrophin-releasing hormone analogues for pain associated with endometriosis. *Cochrane Database Syst Rev* **2010(12)**:CD008475.

9 Zorbas KA, Economopoulos KP, Vlahos NF. (2015) Continuous versus cyclic oral contraceptives for the treatment of endometriosis: a systematic review. *Arch Gynecol Obstet* **292(1)**:37–43.

10 Brown J, Kives S, Akhtar M. (2012) Progestagens and anti-progestagens for pain associated with endometriosis. *Cochrane Database Syst Rev* **2012(3)**:CD002122.

11 Duffy JM, Arambage K, Correa FJ *et al.* (2014) Laparoscopic surgery for endometriosis. *Cochrane Database Syst Rev* **(4)**:CD011031. Update in: *Cochrane Database Syst Rev*. 2020 **10**:CD011031.

12 Bafort C, Beebeejaun Y, Tomassetti C, Bosteels J, Duffy JM. (2020) Laparoscopic surgery for endometriosis. *Cochrane Database Syst Rev* **10**:CD011031.

13 Zullo F, Palomba S, Zupi E *et al.* (2003) Effectiveness of presacral neurectomy in women with severe dysmenorrhea caused by endometriosis who were treated with laparoscopic conservative surgery: a 1-year prospective randomized double-blind controlled trial. *Am J Obstet Gynecol* **189(1)**:5–10.

14 Sutton CJG, Ewen SP, Whitelaw N *et al.* (1994) Prospective, randomized, double-blind trial of laser laparoscopy in the treatment of pelvic pain associated with minimal, mild and moderate endometriosis. *Fertil Steril* **62**:696–700.

15 Vercellini P, Aimi G, Busacca M *et al.* (2003) Laparoscopic uterosacral ligament resection for dysmenorrhea associated with endometriosis: results of a randomized, controlled trial. *Fertil Steril* **80(2)**:310–9.

16 Self-Help Tips. [Internet]. 2021. Available at: https://www.nva.org/for-patients/self-help-tips . Accessed January 2021.

17 Goldstein AT, Pukall CF, Brown C, Bergeron S, Stein A, Kellogg-Spadt S. (2016) Vulvodynia: assessment and treatment. *J Sex Med* **13(4)**:572–90.

18 David A, Bornstein J. (2020) Evaluation of long-term surgical success and satisfaction of patients after vestibulectomy. *J Low Genit Tract Di* **24(4)**:399–404.

19 Chronic Pelvic Pain: ACOG Practice Bulletin, Number 218. *Obstet Gynecol* **135(3)**:e98–109.

20 Twiddy H, Lane N, Chawla R et al. (2015) The development and delivery of a female chronic pelvic pain management programme: a specialised interdisciplinary approach. *Br J Pain* **9(4)**:233–40.

21 Caruso R, Ostuzzi G, Turrini G et al. (2019)Beyond pain: can antidepressants improve depressive symptoms and quality of life in patients with neuropathic pain? A systematic review and meta-analysis. *Pain* **160(10)**:2186–98.

22 AbdelHafeez MA, Reda A, Elnaggar A, El-Zeneiny H, Mokhles JM. (2019) Gabapentin for the management of chronic pelvic pain in women. *Arch Gynecol Obstet* **300(5)**:1271–77.

Chapter 36

Neuropathic pain

Maija Haanpää[1] & Rolf-Detlef Treede[2]

[1] *Department of Neurosurgery, Helsinki University Hospital, Helsinki, Finland*
[2] *Medical Faculty Mannheim, University of Heidelberg, Mannheim, Germany*

Introduction

Neuropathic pain (NP), defined as "pain arising as a direct consequence of a lesion or disease affecting the somatosensory system" [1] is a challenge to healthcare providers as it is common, often under-diagnosed, under-treated and, when severe, associated with suffering, disability and impaired quality of life. Standard treatment with conventional analgesics does not typically provide effective relief of pain.

The most common reasons for NP are radiculopathy, diabetic polyneuropathy and nerve trauma including postoperative neuralgia. Population prevalence of pain with neuropathic characteristics is 6.9–10% [2]. Incidences of painful diabetic neuropathy, postherpetic neuralgia and trigeminal neuralgia are 5.3–72.3/100,000 person-years (PY), 3.9–42.0/100,000 PY and 0.2–0.4/100,000 PY, respectively [2]. NP follows spinal cord injury in 53 % of patients [3] and stroke in 11 % of patients [4]. As the population is aging and the prevalence of diabetes is increasing, prevalence of NP is expected to rise.

In the ICD-11 classification, NP is first organized into peripheral and central neuropathic pain based on the location of the lesion or disease in the peripheral or central somatosensory nervous system [5]. Within each of these categories, pain is classified into different NP conditions based on the underlying disease. Peripheral NP includes: (1) trigeminal neuralgia, (2) NP after peripheral nerve injury, (3) painful polyneuropathy, (4) postherpetic neuralgia, (5) painful radiculopathy and 6) other specified and unspecified peripheral NP. Central NP includes: (1) central NP associated with spinal cord injury, (2) central NP associated with brain injury, (3) central post-stroke pain, (4) central NP caused by multiple sclerosis and (5) other specified and unspecified central NP. This classification covers the epidemiologically most relevant conditions and provides clear diagnostic criteria that are backed by literature [5].

Unlike nociceptive pain, which is caused by physiological activation of peripheral nociceptive nerve terminals in response to tissue damage or threat of such damage, chronic NP has no beneficial effect. It can arise from damage to the nerve pathways at any point from the terminals of the peripheral nociceptors to the cortical neurons in the brain. It is not known why the same condition is painful in some patients and painless in others. Currently, a mechanism-based classification of NP is not possible, as the detailed pain mechanisms in an individual case cannot be identified. Furthermore, one mechanism can be responsible for many different symptoms and the same symptom in two patients can be caused by different mechanisms [6]. Our understanding of the underlying pathophysiology has increased considerably in the last decades, although not to the extent that treatment has improved [7]. As NP can coexist with nociceptive pain, clinicians should try to identify different pain components and treat each of them according to the best available evidence.

Clinical Pain Management: A Practical Guide, Second Edition. Edited by Mary E. Lynch, Kenneth D. Craig, and Philip W. Peng.

Basic mechanisms

Damage to the somatosensory system leads to negative sensory symptoms (feeling of numbness) and signs (sensory loss to the somatosensory submodalities touch, proprioception, thermoreception, nociception or visceroreception). Damaged neurons, however, can also develop spontaneous activity (e.g. by altered expression of ion channels at a neuroma or in the dorsal root ganglion). When ectopically generated action potentials are transmitted to the nociceptive network in the brain, this results in a pain sensation that is projected to the receptive field of the damaged neural structure (Figure 36.1). Peripheral nerve damage can also lead to secondary changes within the central nervous system, including altered synaptic connectivity and receptive field reorganization. These secondary changes involve local excitatory and inhibitory neurons, ascending and descending pathways, as well as microglia and astrocytes [8]. When the neural damage is partial, the remaining neural connections may be facilitated as a result of these secondary changes, leading to positive sensory symptoms (paraesthesia and spontaneous pain) and signs (hyperalgesia and allodynia, mostly to mechanical or cold stimuli) (For further discussion of mechanisms see Chapter 3).

The coexistence of negative and positive sensory phenomena within the same region is prototypical for patients with NP. The spatial distribution of these symptoms and signs and the distribution of the projected pain sensation provide information on the neuroanatomic site of neural damage. Current and future therapies for NP are directed at central and peripheral nociceptive signal processing (centrally and peripherally acting analgesics, modulators of endogenous pain control systems), ectopic impulse generation (local anesthetics) and at the pathophysiological processes of degeneration, regeneration and reorganization [9]. In general, systemic NP medication has to pass the blood–brain barrier in order to reach its target. Such a barrier is also present in the peripheral nervous system, but the blood–nerve barrier is leaky in the dorsal root ganglion and in peripheral nerve inflammation.

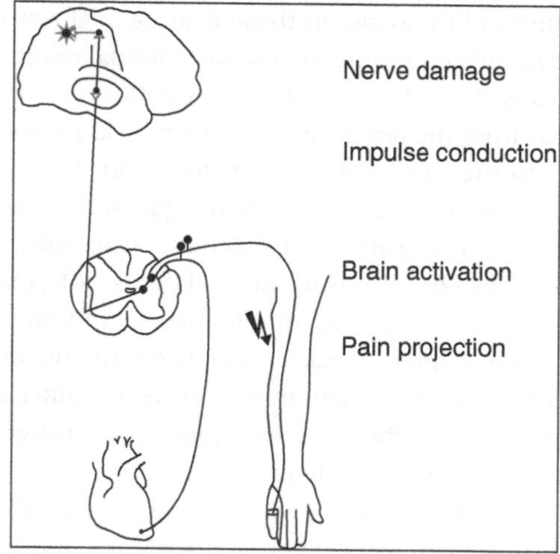

Figure 36.1 Projected pain. Damage to a peripheral nerve may lead to action potential generation at the site of damage. When these action potentials reach the nociceptive network in the brain, the resulting pain sensation is projected into the peripheral receptive field of the damaged nerve, where this activity would normally originate. Thus, pain in a body part may result from damage to that body part itself or to any site along the neural pathways connecting that body part with the brain. Based on Treede (2001) Kapitel A3, In: Zenz, Jurna (Hrsg.) Lehrbuch der Schemerztherapie, Fig. 11.

Clinical picture

NP can be spontaneous (stimulus-independent) or elicited by a stimulus (stimulus-evoked pain). Spontaneous pain is often described as a constant burning sensation, but it may also include intermittent shooting lancinating sensations, electric shock-like pain and dysesthesia (i.e. an unpleasant abnormal sensation). The pain may also be accompanied by paresthesia, an abnormal sensation that is not unpleasant. Stimulus-evoked pains are elicited by mechanical, thermal or chemical stimuli. Hyperalgesia consists of an increased pain response to a stimulus that is normally painful and activates peripheral nociceptive terminals, whereas allodynia has been introduced as a term to describe pain sensation from a stimulus that does not normally provoke pain and that does not activate nociceptors (such as gentle stroking by a brush) and thus implies a change in central neural processing [10]. Additionally, there may be other symptoms and clinical findings (e.g. motor paresis, muscle cramps, autonomic nervous system signs) depending on the site of the lesion. It is not possible to conclude the etiology of NP from the clinical characteristics of pain.

Once present, NP pain tends to be long-lasting. However, some patients may recover from their pain completely and others may obtain relief by pharmacotherapy or learn to cope with their symptoms by attending interdisciplinary treatment or self-management programs.

Clinical examination

Assessment of a patient with suspected NP aims at: (i) recognition of NP; (ii) localizing of the lesion as far as possible (peripheral or central and further whether the lesion is in the brain hemisphere, brainstem, spinal cord, nerve root, plexus, peripheral nerve or its branches); and (iii) diagnosing the causative disease or event. In addition, assessment of psychosocial aspects is necessary for an individually tailored management strategy. Possible comorbidities such as impaired sleep, anxiety, depression, disability and secondary impairment in work, family and social life should also be taken into account [11].

The clinical examination of the patient presenting with NP is the same as that described for any patient presenting with chronic pain (Chapter 8). The neurosensory examination is particularly important. Sensory testing at the bedside can be accomplished with simple tools [12]. Touch is tested with a finger or cotton wool, pinprick with a wooden cocktail stick, warm and cold with a cold and a warm object and vibration with a tuning fork. The response to each stimulus can be graded as normal, decreased or increased. The findings in the painful area are compared with the findings in the contralateral area in unilateral pain and in other sites on the proximal–distal axis in bilateral pain.

Identifying a neurological disease or a nervous system lesion is based on a systematic search of neurological abnormalities in the clinical examination. In the neurological examination the signs are repeatable and the location of lesion is concluded on the basis of the neurological signs. In addition to the sensory examination, the motor assessment (muscle strength, tonus, coordination and fluency of movements), examination of tendon reflexes and examination of cranial nerves are performed. Assessment of the peripheral autonomic nervous function (warmth and color of skin, sudomotor function) is important especially when a complex regional pain syndrome is suspected.

Other diagnostic procedures

Sometimes the diagnosis is straightforward (e.g. NP after an obvious nerve lesion during surgery or postherpetic neuralgia after shingles). In these cases no additional tests are needed. If a patient has stocking and glove-type pain location (Figure 36.2), then one might consider nerve conduction studies (NCS) and electromyography (EMG). As presented in more detail in Chapter 11, EMG and NCS evaluate large myelinated axons and because neuropathic pain is often caused by disease of small myelinated Aδ and C fibers these tests may be normal in patients whose condition principally affects the small fibers. The cause of polyneuropathy may be identified further using laboratory tests (e.g. full blood count, sedimentation rate, glucose, creatinine, alanine transaminase [ALT], glucose tolerance test, vitamin B_{12}, serum protein immunoelectrophoresis and thyroid function). If the NCS and EMG are normal it is possible that the patient may have pure small fiber polyneuropathy. In this case additional investigations include quantitative sensory testing (QST) (Chapter 10), laser evoked potential (LEP) and skin biopsy to assess small-caliber (C, Aδ) sensory fibers. These tests are not yet available in many centers and one must often rely on bedside testing and very good clinical examination to substantiate the diagnosis. The most common cause for small-fiber painful polyneuropathy is impaired glucose tolerance.

In general, the decision about a consultation with a specialist should be individualized and depends on the clinical picture, the experience and training of the clinician and the availability of specialists with relevant expertise. Patients suspected to have NP should be seen by a physician who is experienced in assessing somatosensory system function. When referring to the neurological clinic for further assessment, care should be taken to ask for tests of small peripheral fiber and spinothalamic tract system functions, because these tests are not yet part of their standard repertoire. Tests in a specialized center may include conventional electrophysiological procedures, QST, neuroimaging, blood and cerebrospinal fluid samples and less conventional laboratory tools to assess the nociceptive pathways in the peripheral and central nervous systems. For more detailed information, neurological handbooks and NP guidelines [13] are recommended.

Grading of the certainty of the diagnosis of neuropathic pain

A hierarchical system has been developed, to grade evidence for the presence of NP [14]. This grading system, which is recommended for clinical practice and research, divides NP into three classes: possible, probable, and definite NP. NP is *possible* if history is compatible with a lesion in the nervous system and pain distribution is neuroanatomically plausible (see examples in Figure 36.2). NP is *probable* if pain is associated with sensory signs in the same neuroanatomically plausible distribution on clinical examination and NP is *definite* if diagnostic tests confirm a lesion or disease of somatosensory nervous system explaining the pain.

Management of neuropathic pain

As reviewed in previous chapters, the first step is to educate the patient about the cause of their pain and approaches to management, which include correction of the pathology where possible, self-management strategies, interdisciplinary approaches including therapeutic exercise, addressing of psychosocial issues and pharmacotherapy. As pain is usually regarded as a threat, explaining the character of NP (unnecessary nuisance instead of a warning sign) helps the patient to cope with the situation. The causative disease may warrant specific treatment (e.g. decompression of a peripheral nerve entrapment or a nerve root compression, medication to reach normoglycemia for diabetics to prevent progression of neuropathy and other complications or immunomodulatory treatment of multiple sclerosis) or secondary prevention (e.g. commencement of antithrombotic medication and control of risk factors of atherosclerosis after a stroke).

Pharmacotherapy of neuropathic pain

Pharmacotherapy of NP must be individualized. NP is treated mainly with antidepressants and antiepileptics, whereas simple analgesics have not shown efficacy on NP. Complete pain relief is usually not achieved. In meta-analyses, patients with at least 50% pain relief are classified as responders. Reduction of pain with at least 30% is considered clinically relevant. The etiology of NP, concomitant chronic medical conditions and their medications, individual risks (e.g. previous abuse or suicidal history) and costs of treatment need to be considered. In addition to pain relief, medication may provide better sleep, improved mood or relief of anxiety. In many cases the side effect profile guides drug selection.

Based on a systematic review and meta-analysis of published and unpublished randomized controlled double-blind trials, the Neuropathic Pain Special Interest Group (NeuPSIG) of the International

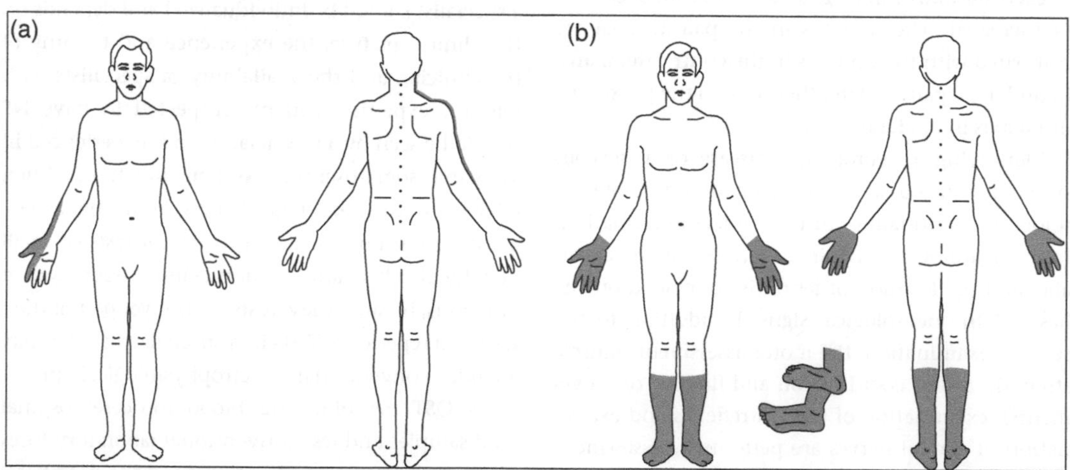

Figure 36.2 Examples of pain drawings of neuropathic pain patients. (a) Radicular pain of the right C6 dermatome. (b) Painful polyneuropathy.

Association for the Study of Pain (IASP) has published recommendations for the pharmacological treatment of neuropathic pain [15]. Drugs with a moderate-to-high quality of evidence and strong recommendation were tricyclic antidepressants, gabapentinoids (gabapentin and pregabalin) and serotonin noradrenaline reuptake inhibitors duloxetine and venlafaxine and these are recommended as first-line drugs. Drugs with a weak recommendation included capsaicin 8% patches, lidocaine 5 % patches and subcutaneous injections of botulinum toxin type A for peripheral neuropathic pain only. The recommendations are summarized in Table 36.1.

In clinical practice one of the first-line drugs is selected and titrated to the effective dose, maximum tolerated dose or recommended maximum dose. If the selected drug fails to provide acceptable pain relief, it is tapered off and another drug is commenced. If the relief is partial, two drugs with different mechanisms of action can be combined (Chapter 22).

Dosing and mechanism of action of the first- and second-line drugs for NP are presented in Table 36.2.

Of note, clear evidence for the efficacy of neuropathic drugs is lacking in painful radiculopathy suggesting that a complex combination of neuropathic, skeletal and myofascial mechanisms is involved in the development radicular pain in many patients.

The role of strong opioids in treatment of NP has been debated due to the increase in opioid abuse and diversion and observations of opioid-induced endocrine changes. NeuPSIG gave a weak recommendation for their use as third-line option with low-to moderate doses [15]. Risk factors for prescription opioid abuse such as a history of substance abuse should be investigated before prescription and signals of misuse should be assessed at each renewal.

NeuPSIG gave a weak recommendation against the use of cannabinoids in NP, mainly because of negative results, potential misuse, diversion and long-term mental health risks of cannabis particularly in susceptible individuals [15]. Since the NeuPSIG publication both positive and negative studies of cannabinoids in NP have been published [17]. The authors of the most recent meta-analysis suggest that reliable evidence is still needed regarding the efficacy and safety of cannabinoids in patients with neuropathic pain [17].

For patients with NP refractory to pharmacological therapy neuromodulation may be considered (Chapter 23).

Treatment of trigeminal neuralgia

Trigeminal neuralgia comprises idiopathic trigeminal neuralgia, classical neuralgia produced by vascular compression of the trigeminal nerve and secondary neuralgias caused by a tumor or cyst at the cerebellopontine angle or multiple sclerosis [18]. Trigeminal neuralgia pain is short-lasting, sharp, shooting, electric shock-like pain and some patients also have a concomitant but less intense continuous pain in the same area as the stabbing pain lasting from hours to days [19, 20]. MRI using specific sequences should be a part of the diagnostic workup to detect a possible neurovascular contact and exclude secondary causes (19, 20).

Treatment guidelines for trigeminal neuralgia recommend carbamazepine or oxcarbazepine as a drug-of-choice (19, 20). Both drugs are effective for the treatment of trigeminal neuralgia pain, but treatment is often hampered by side-effects. Typical daily dose is 200–1800 mg for carbamazepine and 300–2700 mg for oxcarbazepine. Patients should be encouraged to alter the dosage depending on pain severity and side-effects, as periods of partial or complete remission do occur. If carbamazepine and oxcarbazepine are ineffective or poorly tolerated, lamotrigine (typical daily dose 100–400 mg), baclofen (typical daily dose 15–70 mg), gabapentin (typical daily dose 600–3600 mg), pregabalin (typical daily dose 150–600 mg) or phenytoin (typical daily dose 50–300 mg) may be used either alone or as add-on therapy. One treatment option is botulinum toxin A with dose 25–100 units which are injected subcutaneously or submucosally (5 units/injection site) in the painful area every third month [20].

It is recommended that patients should be offered surgery if pain is not sufficiently controlled medically or if medical treatment is poorly tolerated. Microvascular decompression is recommended as first-line surgery in patients with classical TN. Neuroablative treatments should be the preferred choice if MRI does not demonstrate any neurovascular contact [19, 20].

Table 36.1 Summary of GRADE recommendations by NeuPSIG (15).

	Drug	Quality of evidence	Effect size	Tolerability and safety	Values and preferences	Strength of recommend-dation	Neuropathic pain conditions
First line drugs	Duloxetine and venlafaxine	High	Moderate	Moderate	Low -moderate	Strong	All
	Tricyclic anti-depressants	Moderate	Moderate	Low -moderate	Low -moderate	Strong	All
	Gabapentin and pregabalin	High	Moderate	Moderate – high	Low -moderate	Strong	All
Second line drugs	Tramadol	Moderate	Moderate	Low -moderate	Low -moderate	Weak	All
	Capsaicin 8 % patches	High	Low	Moderate – high	High	Weak	Peripheral
	Lidocaine 5 % patches	Weak	Unknown	High	High	Weak	Peripheral
Third line drugs	Strong opioids	Moderate	Moderate	Low - moderate	Low -moderate	Weak	All
	Botulinum toxin A	Moderate	Moderate	High	Moderate – high	Weak	Peripheral

GRADE = Grading of Recommendations Assessment, Development and Evaluation

Table 36.2 Dosing and mechanisms of action of the first-and second-line drugs for neuropathic pain.

Medication	Starting dose	Maximum dose	Mechanism of action	Major side effects
Tricyclic antidepressants (TCAs)				
Nortriptyline, desipramine, (amitriptyline, imipramine)*	10–25 mg at bedtime	150 mg daily[#]	Serotonin and noradrenalin reuptake inhibition, sodium channel block, NMDA-receptor antagonist	Cardiac conduction block, sedation, confusion, anticholinergic effects, orthostatic hypotension, weight gain
Serotonin-noradrenalin reuptake inhibitors				
Duloxetine	30 mg once daily	120 mg daily	Serotonin and noradrenalin reuptake inhibition	Nausea, loss of appetite, constipation, sedation, dry mouth, hyperhidrosis, anxiety
Venlafaxine	37.5 mg once daily	225 mg daily		
Gabapentinoids				
Gabapentin	100–300 mg at bedtime	3600 mg daily	A calcium channel $\alpha_2\delta$ ligand, which reduces release of presynaptic transmitters	Sedation, dizziness, weight gain, edema, blurred vision
Pregabalin	75 mg twice daily	600 mg daily		
Topical lidocaine				
5% lidocaine patch	Maximum 3 patches daily for maximum 12 h		Block of peripheral sodium channels and thus of ectopic discharges	Application site reactions (such as burning, dermatitis, erythema, pruritus, rash, skin irritation and vesicles)
Topical capsaicin				
8 % capsaicin patch	Maximum 4 patches to the painful area for 30–60 min every 3 months		Binding to TRPV1 receptors[¤] leading to transient desensitization and denervation of the skin	Application site reactions (such as pruritus, papules, vesicles, edema and dryness)
Opioid agonists				
Tramadol	50 mg once or twice daily	400 mg daily[##]	μ-opioid receptor agonist and serotonin and noradrenalin reuptake inhibition	Nausea, dizziness, sedation, headache, constipation, dry mouth, hyperhidrosis,

TCAs = tricyclic antidepressants. NMDA = N-methyl-D-aspartate.

* Secondary amine TCAs (notriptyline, desipramine) are preferred because of better tolerability. Use of a tertiary amine TCA (amitriptyline, imipramine) is recommended only if a secondary amine TCA is not available.

[#] For elderly maximum 75 mg daily

[##] For elderly maximum 300 mg daily

[¤] Transient receptor potential vanilloid 1 receptor

Data modified from references [15, 16].

Conclusions

In conclusion, neuropathic pain is caused by a lesion or disease affecting the somatosensory system. It is often under-diagnosed and under-treated and when severe is associated with significant suffering and disability. An approach to the diagnosis and management of NP has been reviewed. The first step is to educate the patient about the cause of their pain as well as possible and review approaches to management which include correction of the pathology where possible, self-management strategies, interdisciplinary approaches including addressing of psychosocial issues, pharmacotherapy and, where appropriate, consideration of neuromodulatory approaches.

References

1 Treede R, Jensen T, Campbell J *et al.* (2008) Redefinition of neuropathic pain and a grading system for clinical use: consensus statement on clinical and research diagnostic criteria. *Neurology* **70**:1630–5.

2 van Hecke O, Austin SK, Khan RA *et al.* (2014) Neuropathic pain in the general population: a systematic review of epidemiological studies. *Pain* **155**:654–662.

3 Burke D, Fullen BM, Stokes D *et al.* (2017) Neuropathic pain prevalence following spinal cord injury: a systematic review and meta-analysis. *Eur J Pain* **21**:29–44.

4 Liampas A, Velidakis N, Georgiou T *et al.* (2020) Prevalence and management challenges in central post-stroke neuropathic pain: a systematic review and meta-analysis. *Adv Ther* **37**:3278–3291.

5 Scholz J, Finnerup NB, Attal N *et al.* (2019) Thee IASP classification of chronic pain for ICD-11: chronic neuropathic pain. *Pain* **160**: 53–59.

6 Woolf CJ, Mannion RJ. (1999) Neuropathic pain: aetiology, symptoms, mechanisms and management. *Lancet* **353**:1959–64.

7 Finnerup NB, Kuner R, Jensen TS. (2021) Neuropathic Pain: From Mechanisms to Treatment. *Physiol Rev* **101**:259–301.

8 Scadding JW, Koltzenburg M. (2005) Neuropathicpain. In: Mc Mahon SB, Koltzenburg M, eds. *Wall and Melzack's Textbook of Pain*. Churchill Livingstone, Edinburgh. pp. 973–99.

9 Campbell JN, Basbaum AI, Dray A *et al.*, eds. (2006) *Emerging Strategies for the Treatment of Neuropathic Pain*. IASP Press, Seattle.

10 Loeser JD, Treede RD. (2008) The Kyoto Protocol of IASP basic pain terminology. *Pain* **137**:473–7.

11 Haanpää M, Backonja M, Bennett M *et al.* (2009) Assessment of neuropathic pain in primary care. *Am J Med* **122**:S13–21.

12 Cruccu G, Anand P, Attal N *et al.* (2004) EFNS guidelines on neuropathic pain assessment. *Eur J Neurol* **11**:153–62.

13 Haanpää M, Attal N, Backonja M *et al.* (2011) NeuPSIG guidelines on neuropathic pain assessment. Pain **152**:14–27.

14 Finnerup NB, Haroutounian S, Kamerman P *et al.* (2016) Neuropathic pain: an updated grading system for research and clinical practice. *Pain* **157**:1599–606.

15 Finnerup NB, Attal N, Haroutounian S *et al.* (2015) Pharmacotherapy for neuropathic pain in adults: a systematic review and meta-analysis. *Lancet Neurol* **14**:162–73.

16 Haanpää M, Gourlay GK, Kent JL *et al.* (2010). Treatment considerations for patients with neuropathic pain with medical comorbidities and other medical conditions. *Mayo Clin Proc* **85(3 Suppl)**:S15–25.

17 Di Stefano G, Di Lionardo A, Di Pietro G *et al.* (2021) Pharmacotherapeutic options for managing neuropathic pain: a systematic review and meta-analysis. *Pain Res Manag* 2021:6656863.

18 Cruccu G, Finnerup NB, Jensen TS *et al.* (2016). Trigeminal neuralgia: New classification and diagnostic grading for practice and research. *Neurology* **87**:220–8.

19 Bendtsen L, Zakrzewska JM, Abbott J *et al.* (2019) European Academy of Neurology guideline on trigeminal neuralgia. *Eur J Neurol* **26**:831–49.

20 Bendtsen L, Zakrzewska JM, Heinskou TB *et al.* (2020) Advances in diagnosis, classification, pathophysiology, and management of trigeminal neuralgia. *Lancet Neurol* **19**:784–96.

Chapter 37

Complex regional pain syndrome

Michael Stanton-Hicks

Pain Management Department, Centre for Neurological Restoration; Children's Hospital CCF Shaker Pediatric Pain Rehabilitation Program, Cleveland Clinic, Cleveland, Ohio, USA

History

Complex Regional Pain Syndrome (CRPS), synonymous with Reflex Sympathetic Dystrophy (RSD), has a long history. Ambrose Pare', surgeon to King Charles IX, provided one of the earliest descriptions of this syndrome in the 16th century after bloodletting in the arm of the Monarch who was suffering from smallpox [1]. Denmark in 1813 provided a similar description following amputation in a soldier during the Peninsula War [2]. In 1900, Sudeck, a German surgeon in Eppendorf, described radiologic changes that were associated with the putative syndrome that bears his name in German-speaking countries [3]. The next major and perhaps the most complete description came from Silas Weir Mitchell, who described what he named causalgia (causa - heat, algia - pain) that developed following a musket shot wound in an extremity of soldiers during the American Civil War [4]. Symptoms were the same; extremely severe burning pain and shiny, red, hot skin. During World War II, James Evans introduced the term RSD [5]. In 1994, a consensus group under the auspices of the International Association for the Study of Pain (IASP) developed the initial criteria that make up the acronym CRPS (Complex Regional Pain Syndrome) [6, 7].

Introduction

CRPS is a painful condition that is invariably a consequence of a sprain, fracture or surgery of an extremity that tends to be distal, but can, less frequently, occur at other sites of the body (e.g. the knee) or, rarely, without any recorded history. In fact, the trigger may be as inconsequential as an insect bite. Two distinct subtypes are described: CRPS I (formally RSD) in which there is no obvious nerve injury and CRPS II (formerly causalgia), where nerve injury has occurred. The clinical presentation includes inflammatory changes, autonomic dysfunction, nervous system sensitization, spontaneous pain, allodynia/hyperalgesia and motor disturbances that are out of proportion with what would be expected from each inciting event. In most cases, the foregoing clinical features are usually found in one extremity but, in a smaller number of patients, they may be expressed in another or multiple extremities [8, 9]. Early or acute CRPS is generally associated with "warm" skin, but a few patients may present with so called-called "cold" CRPS, normally a feature of the chronic syndrome. Secondary structural changes in superficial and deep tissues may develop over time [10].

While our understanding of CRPS epidemiology has improved considerably, there are still distinct anomalies

Clinical Pain Management: A Practical Guide, Second Edition. Edited by Mary E. Lynch, Kenneth D. Craig, and Philip W. Peng.

between study populations, data gathering and countries that highlight the current gaps in our knowledge. The first study of 85 patients from a small community in Rochester, MN, USA, gathered by Sandroni et al in 2003 using IASP criteria, found a prevalence of 21:100,000 with females predominating 3:1 and expression in the upper extremity occurring in more than 60% of all patients [11]. A more recent study of 1043 patients in a regional community in Germany by Ott and Maihöfner has corroborated these results [12]. Most recently, however, Kim et al. used data from the National Health Insurance Service of Korea (74,349 patients) and found a much narrower ratio of female to male prevalence, a reversal of the upper vs. lower limb incidence and a higher age incidence. It should be pointed out, however, that many of the patients in this study were diagnosed using the Persistent Disability and Assessment Guidelines of the American Medical Association (AMA) and not the IASP criteria. In addition, the study population included individuals who were both older and on workers compensation, thereby increasing the proportion of those with lower extremity injuries. These data are not directly comparable because of the different criteria used and the nature of the populations studied [13] In adolescents and children, where the data are more certain, females outnumber males by a ratio of 4:1 [14].

This chapter describes the diagnostic assessment and subsequent management of CRPS based on the best evidence approach. A number of mechanisms underlying sensory, motor, inflammatory, immune/auto immune, autonomic and genetic influences are addressed in the context of treatment and management strategies.

Diagnosis and Influencing Factors

Whereas the initial International Association for the Study of Pain (IASP) diagnostic criteria that were introduced in 1999 lacked clinical validation, their introduction was meant to provide a common descriptive set of clinical signs and symptoms without the suggestion of a purported mechanism that could be applied to the diagnosis of CRPS [6]. Their subsequent validation and acceptance as the Budapest Criteria by the IASP in 2010 now provides a universal clinical tool with a high degree of specificity while still maintaining adequate sensitivity that will avoid the underdiagnosis of CRPS [15, 16]. The phenomenon of Sympathetically Maintained Pain (SMP), previously a requirement for the diagnosis of CRPS, is now acknowledged as being a symptom that may be present in many other neuropathic disorders that is not exclusive to CRPS [17]. The Budapest criteria are shown in Table 37.1.

To improve the integrity of the Budapest criteria and provide both a catalogue of the presenting symptoms from which temporal changes during the course of the syndrome can be quantified, it was necessary to develop a scale that includes elements of the Budapest criteria that express severity of the condition at any time point. Of the previous severity scales, the Impairment Level SumScore (a validated instrument) is one the best and most comprehensive, but does not contain some of the

Table 37.1 Diagnostic critera "Budapest" for CRPS. Patients must exhibit at least 1 SYMPTOM in 3 of 4 categories and 1 SIGN in 2 or more categories (sens. 0.99; spec. 0.68)"

Category	Symptom	Sign
SENSORY	Hyperesthesia, allodynia	hyperalgesia (PP) allodynia – mech. / thermal / deep
VASOMOTOR	Δ skin / color Δ temperature	> 1° C / Δ skin color
SUDOMOTOR EDEMA	Δ sweating / edema	Δ sweating / edema
MOTOR TROPHIC	motor dysfunction ⬇ ROM Δ trophic	motor dysfunction ⬇ ROM (weak, dystonia, tremor) / trophic

elements in the Budapest Criteria and therefore would not be appropriate in this case. To address this issue, Harden et al, 2010 developed the CRPS Severity Score (CSS). The study based on the same 16 signs and symptoms that was subsequently validated was published by Harden et al. in 2017 [18] (Figure 37.1).

A number of recent reports have identified predisposing factors, the nature of injuries and possible biomarkers that would seem to make the development of CRPS more likely. Fractures of the forearm, the so-called antebrachial region or similar injuries of the lower extremity (ankle fracture) are more susceptible to the development of CRPS [19, 20]. Severe fractures and high energy trauma, musculoskeletal disease, rheumatoid arthritis and prolonged general anesthesia (but not regional anesthesia) are all associated with a higher incidence of CRPS [21]. Immobilization is a risk factor for the development of CRPS. Studies of immobilization in humans shown the development of sensitivity to heat and pressure without pain [22].

Finally, the question of whether there is a genetic association in CRPS has been raised. Some smaller studies have described polymorphisms in potential mediators of inflammation such as cytokines and the α1a-adrenoceptor [23]. Many diseases with associated inflammation, such as multiple sclerosis and celiac disease, also have a genetic association with the human leukocyte antigen (HLA) system [24]. Mailis and Wade were the first to implicate the HLA and CRPS (RSD) and drew attention to multiple sclerosis and narcolepsy, which also share the DR2(15) antigen. The HLA-DR13 antigen is associated with dystonia in CRPS and, in a study of genome-wide profiling, certain genes including HLA-related genes are differentially expressed [25]. Another aspect of genetic studies is the identification of specific micro RNAs. As such, these non-coding RNA molecules are "master regulators" that control many proteins and are responsible for translational processes involved in cell-to-cell communication and could ultimately be biomarkers for CRPS soon after injury [26]. A definite genetic underpinning with CRPS therefore remains to be confirmed.

Adjuncts to Diagnosis

Temperature measurement, preferably by thermography, is one of the most useful objective signs and is also a component of the CSS [27]. For some years, bone scintigraphy (3-phase) has been promoted as a useful adjunct to confirm a diagnosis of CRPS. However, although its specificity is high, its sensitivity in relation to the Budapest criteria is poor [28]. Furthermore, a recent metanalysis of bone scintigraphy does not support its use in the diagnosis of CRPS [29].

As a diagnostic tool, electromyography is useful to identify a nerve lesion (CRPS 2). More recently, electromyography has been suggested as a tool to distinguish myoclonus in CRPS patients from other causes [30]. However, because this sign is present in

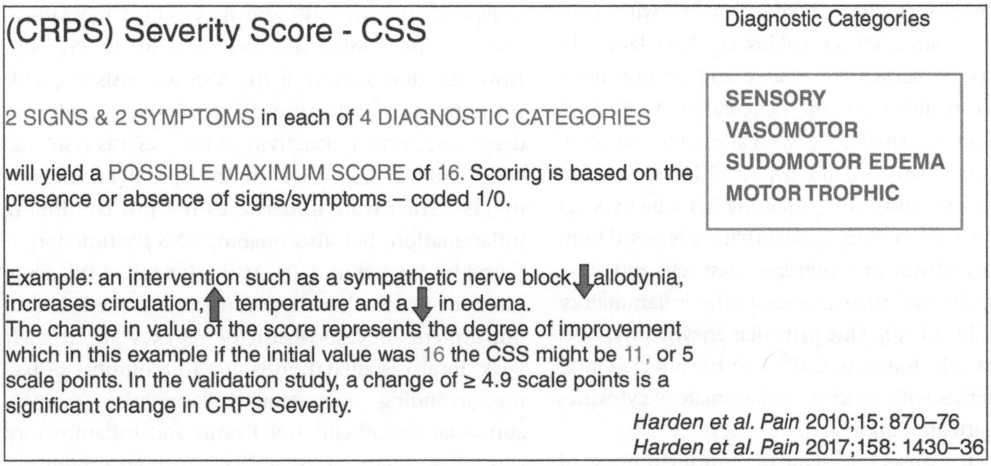

(CRPS) Severity Score - CSS

Diagnostic Categories

SENSORY
VASOMOTOR
SUDOMOTOR EDEMA
MOTOR TROPHIC

2 SIGNS & 2 SYMPTOMS in each of 4 DIAGNOSTIC CATEGORIES

will yield a POSSIBLE MAXIMUM SCORE of 16. Scoring is based on the presence or absence of signs/symptoms – coded 1/0.

Example: an intervention such as a sympathetic nerve block ↓ allodynia, increases circulation, ↑ temperature and a ↓ in edema.
The change in value of the score represents the degree of improvement which in this example if the initial value was 16 the CSS might be 11, or 5 scale points. In the validation study, a change of ≥ 4.9 scale points is a significant change in CRPS Severity.

Harden et al. Pain 2010;15: 870–76
Harden et al. Pain 2017;158: 1430–36

Figure 37.1 (CRPS) Severity Score - CSS.

only 11 - 36 % of cases, it lacks sensitivity to support a clinical diagnosis of CRPS.

Pathophysiology

No unitary pathology is available to explain the onset of CRPS. In fact, it seems to be a combination of an abnormal inflammatory response and peripheral nervous system dysfunction [31].

Underlying the typical features of inflammation, is a complex immune response that includes the proliferation of keratinocytes releasing inflammatory cytokines (an innate-immune response) [32]. Cytokines (including TNFα, IL-6 and IL-8) found in the first 3 months after onset amongst other inflammatory reactions also evoke the release of osteoblasts and osteoclasts that are responsible for the bony changes (osteoporosis) and the proliferation of connective tissue cells that ultimate lead to contractures [33, 34].

The peripheral nervous system both manifests and is impacted by the inflammatory response. Neurogenic inflammation (the term used to describe the release from nociceptors of substance P (SP) and calcitonin gene-related peptide (CGRP), which are neuropeptides that supplement the classical signs of inflammation) added to nociceptor sensitization by inflammatory cytokines leads to pain and hyperalgesia [35]. Additionally, SP underlies increased hair growth, a frequent accompaniment of CRPS and CGRP that can cause hyperhidrosis [36].

CRPS has also been ascribed as having a small-fiber neuropathic etiology [37]. Intraepidural neurites are reduced by 29% in affected skin compared with unaffected control sites [38]. Axonal loss can have far reaching effects in sub-served tissues and absent nervi vasorum can affect the microcirculation indiscriminately causing mismatch between arteriolar and venular flows and increasing the bypass of blood flow via arteriovenous shunts (AVS), resulting in tissue hypoxia and edema. Other neuropeptides that are released from small fibers activate macrophages, mast cells and other immune cells that then exaggerate the inflammatory response [39. 23, 40]. One particular enzyme, tryptase, from mast cells found in CRPS 1 in the affected local tissue together with other pro-inflammatory cytokines promotes inflammation [41].

During the onset and acute (3- 4-month) phase of the syndrome, an adaptive-immunity develops after which there is a tendency for some of the early clinical signs to normalize. However, in many cases temporal changes in the pathophysiology of CRPS can be identified as the syndrome passes through an intermediate (15 month) timeframe before becoming chronic. Some of these reflect autoimmune aspects such as serum autoantibodies against adrenergic and cholinergic receptors [42, 43]. These findings will be discussed below. Although the clinical inflammatory signs are less obvious in cold CRPS, recent studies underscore a continuing but changed type of local inflammation [44].

Autonomic Nervous System and the Immune Response

A disturbance of the sympathetic component of the autonomic nervous system has always been associated with CRPS [45]. The alteration in sweating, vasoconstriction, related fluctuations of temperature and the phenomenon of Sympathetically Maintained pain (SMP) have been considered synonymous with CRPS. Although this viewpoint has taken a back seat to the enormous progress that has been made in our understanding of the combined inflammatory and complex immune processes that constitute CRPS, the recent discovery of agonistic serum auto-antibodies against adrenergic and cholinergic receptors (SNS) suggestive of an autoimmune involvement gives one pause for thought [46]. The relief of pain after sympathetic block suggests a direct or indirect interruption of the SNS [47]. The failure to relieve pain after a sympathetic block however is termed sympathetically independent pain (SIP) and may reflect reorganization of the central nervous system (CNS) [48]. However, dysfunction of the SNS is consistent with the both acute and chronic CRPS. In fact, Gradl et al determined that hypoactivity of the SNS was systemic-wide and not exclusive to the ipsilateral extremity [49]. Their work underscores not just continuing inflammation, but also ongoing SNS dysfunction as found by Vogl et al. [50]. At the height of the acute phase of CRPS when hypofunction of the SNS and impairment of vasoconstrictor reflexes are at their peak, local vasodilatation is due to a number of factors including neurogenic inflammation (above), abnormal endothelin-1/NO ratio and inflammatory cytokines IL-1β, !L-6, TNFα. Antigen-presenting cells (APC) such as dendritic cells (epidermal synonymous with Langerhans cell) are another source of inflammatory cytokines, above [51]. These cells express α1- adrenoceptors, which are also found on lymphoid tissue [52. 53]. The sub-type α1A-adrenoceptor is driven by the expression of inflammatory cytokines TNFα or IL-1β [54].

The two phenotypes, warm and cold CRPS represent not just differences in temperature, but also reflect dissimilar risk factors or mechanisms. Warm CRPS is associated with mechanical hyperalgesia while sensory loss, cold-induced pain and dystonia are clinical features found in cold CRPS [55]. A history of prior chronic pain or severe life events are also more common in patients who present with cold CRPS [47]. Twenty percent of patients with early CRPS present with a cold extremity [56].

The change in temperature and blood flow from acute to chronic CRPS reflects a continuum of vasoactivity and inflammation throughout the early course of the syndrome that trends in most cases toward a cold extremity. In a few patients, however, the limb will remain warm, sometimes for years.

We know from studies that the up-regulation and increasing density of alpha-1 adrenoceptors (α-1 AR's) is also responsible for vasoconstriction and a cold extremity [57, 58]. Beta-2 adrenoceptors (β-2 AR) activated by norepinephrine have also been shown to liberate interleukin-6 (IL-6), which sensitizes nociceptors and thereby amplifies CRPS symptoms, an indirect adrenergic action [59]. Whereas the noradrenergic system in the CNS is normally antinoceptive, with alpha-2 adrenoceptors (α-2 AR) having an inhibitory function at the dorsal horn, this system is compromised after peripheral nerve injury, thereby enhancing excitatory transmission [59].

Autoimmunity

During the past decade, much interest has been generated by autoimmune aspects of CRPS. In their studies of immunoglobulins such as IgG in both animals and patients, Goebel and coworkers have characterized CRPS as a "novel kind of autoimmune disease" [60, 61]. Agonistic autonomic receptor autoantibodies are prevalent in CRPS. Translational studies in rodents have shown that human serum immunoglobulins from patients with long-standing CRPS activate α1A adrenoceptors or muscarinic receptors with high binding affinity [62]. Flow cytometric and spectrofluorometric studies would suggest an antibody-induced α1A adrenoceptor activation. Many CRPS patients also suffer from visceral conditions such as voiding difficulties (Interstitial cystitis (IS)) and irritable bowel syndrome (IBS) - suggestive of a much more widespread autonomic dysregulation [63]. Another example of an autoimmune-related mechanism in CRPS are the results of recent studies by Tajerian et al. who used liquid crystal mass spectrometry to detect increased levels of a large protein Krt16, which is a biomarker for conditions like rheumatoid arthritis. The finding of increased binding of Krt16 on mRNA and protein in mouse skin in their murine fracture immobilization model is suggestive of an autoimmune reactivity in animals and humans with CRPS. These results corroborate the association of CRPS with the HLA system already mentioned above [64].

Central Nervous System

The observation of neuronal plasticity in the CNS during the course of CRPS been greatly facilitated by almost two decades of extraordinary advances in neuro imaging. Cumulative evidence of both structural and functional changes in somatosensory and somatomotor cortical representations, subcortical and autonomic brain regions are reflected during CRPS [65]. The prevalence of motor symptoms including paresis, tremor, dystonia, myoclonus and exaggerated tendon reflexes in CRPS patients is associated with morphological and functional alterations in the primary somatosensory cortex [66, 67]. Weakness, poor coordination and reduced distal arm mobility followed by tremor are the most common impairments [68] and dystonia occurs in more than 50% of patients [69]. Dystonia is related to neuropathological defects in basal ganglia and is manifested by posturing involving the wrist and fingers in the upper extremity with plantar flexion or inversion as the most common signsl in the lower extremity [70]. Dystonia may occur not just in the acute phase, but also during the chronic phase. The disease may spread to involve more than one extremity and dystonia may also occur in more than one limb.

fMRI imaging of CRPS patients has revealed bilateral reduction of putaminal and nucleus acumbens volumes [71]. Similar changes in the ventral striatum would also be consistent with corresponding changes of functional connectivity between these subcortical structures and the ipsilateral somatosensory and association cortices. Such alterations of somatosensory networks have been described in children who avoid movement due to fear of pain. Other CRPS CNS changes that have benefited from brain imaging are the cingulate and amygdala (emotional function), perirhinal and hippocampus (memory). As a research tool, understanding the clinical course of CRPS has benefitted from observing changes in connectivity after different therapeutic interventions [72].

Another direct consequence of somatosensory reorganization is the body midline-shift to the healthy side – distorted image of the affected extremity [73]. Similarities in the perception of their affected extremity are found between patients who have CRPS or stroke. After crossing the unaffected limb to the ipsilateral side, any tactile information will be perceived as arising from the unaffected limb [74]. Application of this phenomenon to the use of mirror therapy will be discussed under clinical management.

Central sensitization (e.g. onset of allodynia) is demonstrated by activation of the "brain matrix" and has been demonstrated by fMRI [75].

Behavioral Aspects

Although several studies and one large metanalysis have not found any predisposing psychological morbidity that might influence the onset and maintenance of CRPS, some factors such as posttraumatic stress disorder (PTSD) after previous injury have been shown to influence the onset of CRPS [76, 77].

Additionally, while there is no evidence to suggest that patients with CRPS are more anxious or more depressed than other patients after trauma, the comparatively severe and relentless nature of symptoms and depersonalization (an attributive behavioral state) has recently undergone evaluation in patients who have continuing chronic pain following trauma. An instrument, the Cambridge Depersonalization Scale, has been used to compare patients with limb trauma and CRPS. Recent results have shown a greater number of depersonalization phenomena in CRPS patients.

An exaggerated negative psychological response to painful stimuli (catastrophizing) could influence the onset of CRPS, although distinguishing this from its natural history is difficult [78]. Catastrophizing in children is associated with altered somatosensory brain volumes leading to chronic pain and impaired motor function [79].

During the past decade several recent studies have addressed how social factors can adversely influence the onset or course of CRPS. These include social status, workers compensation and litigation related to the source of injury [80, 81].

Management of CRPS

From the foregoing description, it is clear that there is no singular approach to treatment. Once an established diagnosis and an CSS have been determined, recognizing that there is no evidence-based treatment, the management of CRPS should follow empirical guidelines that have been developed on the basis of both the pathophysiology described above and the author's more than 4 decades of CRPS management (see Figure 37.1).

The basic principles include:

1 medical and pharmacologic therapy for the acute or chronic phases.

2 occupational and physical therapy together with mirror therapy and graded motor imagery (GMI).

3 behavioral and social therapy (if needed).

4 a sympathetic nerve block (SNB) to determine the presence of SMP.

5 consultation with other medical/surgical disciplines in the event that concurrent care is required.

6 other interventions as deemed appropriate to address particular changes in the disease course and or severity.

Acute phase

The successful use of corticosteroids in early CRPS is supported by randomized controlled trials (RCT) [82, 83]. A significant number of adults and children benefit with an increased range of motion (ROM), reduced swelling and less pain. While an optimal dosage of steroids has not been determined, typically a high starting dose of between 30–100 mg followed with a taper over 10–20 days is described. Similar results are not seen with non-steroidal anti-inflammatory agents (NSAID).

Pain during the onset of acute CRPS may require use of mild to strong opioids. Clear guidelines determining their dosage will depend on the patient's response, namely that at least 50% pain reduction is achieved at the time. Larger dosage is not appropriate and an end point of 2–3 weeks will generally prevent tolerance or dependence from occurring. This approach will prevent the development of opioid hyperalgesia and chronic opioid dependence. The phenomenon of opioid insensitive pain may result from a decreased CNS opioid receptor availability in CRPS [84, 85].

Antioxidant treatment for CRPS was pioneered in the Netherlands. A significant number of patients may benefit from the topical form of dimethyl sulfoxide (DMSO), a treatment that is supported by RCT's. The cream should be applied 3 times daily and is effective against free radicals that have been documented in the inflamed tissues [86].

Prophylactic vitamin C, also having antioxidant properties, may influence the onset of CRPS if given at the time of injury [87]. However, some recent publications have contested this position [88].

Based on an RCT and many clinical studes, the anticonvulsant, gabapentin is effective in reducing sensitivity, treating neuropathic pain and preventing long-term sensory deficits in the chronic phase of CRPS [89]. The newer anti-convulsant pregabalin is equally effective and better tolerated than gabapentin. The effective dose of these drugs is wide-ranging and depends on both the side-effect profile and a stable dose for effect. In the event that a side effect or effects preclude the use of the foregoing class of drugs, "off-label" anticonvulsants such as levetiracetam, lamotrigine or carbamazepine can be substituted to achieve the same desired effect. While gabapentin has a good safety profile, mood disorders and suicidal ideation are rare adverse side-effects. Such side effects are possible with this class of drugs.

Tricyclic antidepressants have an important place in the treatment of CRPS, both for their approved indication and their sedative effects. Nortriptyline and desipramine are good examples. The serotonin-norepinephrine reuptake inhibitors (SNRI) although not as sedating, are a useful alternative if tricyclics are not well tolerated.

Bisphosphonates, also supported by RCTs, clearly benefit CRPS patients, mostly in the acute phase but also with documented success in chronic CRPS patients. They reduce inflammation and inhibit osteoclast activity [90]. Neridronate, recently introduced, has a low side-effect profile and maybe substituted for alendronate or chlodronate, which are well established medications for use in managing pain of CRPS [91].

Patients who have demonstrated a positive response to a sympathetic block with the relief of pain (i.e. SMP) can be tried on an α_1- adrenoceptor blocker such as terazosin or phenoxybenzamine [92]. A small dose of terazosin of 1 mg q.h.s titrating up to 3 mg daily over two weeks is satisfactory in most patients. About 5% of patients may require up to 20 mg daily. These medications are not only efficacious in early CRPS and may obviate the need for any other analgesics, but their mechanism of action (MOA) may enhance the effect of spinal-cord stimulation (SCS), dorsal route ganglion stimulation (DRG) or peripheral nerve stimulation (PNS).

Because the NMDA receptor is upregulated in CRPS, NMDA receptor blocking agents have been used with some success in moderating pain and some of the other side-effects of the syndrome.

Ketamine administered as an infusion daily over seven days or, if under observation, as a continuous 24-hour infusion for 7 days, may result in a complete remission of CRPS symptoms in patients who are otherwise refractory to all other conservative measures. Three RCTs substantiate the use of this medication. Remissions of 4–12 months have been recorded [93]. Side-effects include nausea, vomiting, disorientation, bradycardia, other cardiogenic arrhythmias and, with repeated use, a low incidence of liver failure. Severe dystonia maybe treated with botulinum toxin type A (BTX-A). This requires the injection of multiple muscles in the affected extremity, a procedure that can only be carried out at specialized centers [94]. (BTX-A) can also be used to undertake sympathetic blockade, a procedure that can provide long-term sympathetic blockade [95]. This and the use of baclofen for dystonia is discussed under the section on Interventions in the Management of CRPS.

Chronic CRPS

Except for corticosteroids, many of the foregoing pharmacological approaches described, if successful, will continue to be useful during the chronic phase of CRPS. Likewise, the continued use of successful anti-depression therapy should be continued during the chronic phase. The α_1- adrenoceptor blockers, in particular terazosin or prazosin, are well tolerated and can be maintained for months or years after a successful response to an SNB.

Because of the mineral loss and remodeling that takes place in the CRPS extremity, calcitonin (which promotes osteogenesis) has beneficial effects on the microvasculature and is antinociceptive. Calcitonin may be more effective for treating chronic than acute CRPS pain. The drug is not widely used and, although it has a relatively poor side-effect profile including nausea and vomiting, it is still worth trying for those cases in which pain is proving difficult to manage [96].

The calcium channel blocker nifedipine can be used to manage vasoconstriction in the chronic phase.

Finally, mention should be made of hyperbaric oxygen (HBOT). While this therapy can be used during the acute phase, particularly where skin breakdown is an issue, its anti-nociceptive value in chronic CRPS is often overlooked. Its MOA is via the neural NO-dependent release of dynorphin that then activates μ and κ opioid receptors. The therapy is validated by an RCT and the pain relief is also accompanied by increased ROM and reduction of edema. Pain relief durations of 3-4 months Have been reported [97].

Immunomodulation and the Future

Thalidomide and lenalidomide are two agents with anti-inflammatory and immunomodulatory MOA that are used in oncology and which have recently undergone studies for their potential help in the treatment of CRPS [98]. One study showed that one-third of patients had functional improvement and a reduction of pain after 4-6 weeks by suppressing inflammatory cytokines and promoting anti-inflammatory cytokines such as IL-10. A multicenter RCT (Phase IIb) with lenalidomide vs placebo did not reach significance for many reasons, but the targeted CRPS population may have been lacking specific responders [99]. Interestingly, some patients with the highest pain scores who are refractory to other treatments are more likely to respond to this class of agents. Immunomodulatory effects have recently been reported from interventional therapies such as spinal cord stimulation (SCS) and dorsal root ganglion stimulation (DRG). These will be discussed under Interventional measures.

Functional Restoration

As a severe inflammatory process and because CRPS involves the entire nervous system, it will be associated with measurable Central and Peripheral pathophysiology. Dysfunctional changes in the affected extremity require the immediate application of physiotherapeutic maneuvers in order to preclude any further loss of function. As pain-induced limitation of movement in the affected extremity is anathema to the successful restoration of function, all efforts should therefore be directed towards providing an optimal treatment environment with symptom-directed medications (against the suspected pathophysiology), treatment of any comorbidities, pain-directed procedures (e.g. sympathetic block for SMP) and interdisciplinary management. This latter approach is the sine qua non of CRPS management. Early specialist consultation (e.g. orthopedic) to address some particular pathology (e.g. carpal tunnel) is fundamental to a best outcome.

Psychological management is frequently necessary to overcome a lack of compliance with physical treatment measures, that is in terms of pain and also in the face of neglect. Voluntary use of the extremity, in spite of pain, is encouraged. In fact, knowing the speed with which connective tissue cells proliferate in some patients only early intervention can prevent the evolution of subsequent contractures. Obviously, such measures must be undertaken with a degree of empathy. In such situations, mirror therapy in which the patient adapts to interpreting an image of the contralateral, healthy, extremity as belonging to the CRPS limb can promote and extend the range of movement (ROM) [100]. Graded motor imagery (GMI) is another useful instrument that utilizes images of limb laterality in three stages, moving the limb based on an image and thirdly seeing a reflection of the affected limb moving in a mirror. GMI has been validated by 2 RCTs, but both techniques are complementary and are associated with improvements in pain and function [101]. The Stress-Loading technique developed by Watson and Carlson to support rehabilitation of the upper extremity in patients who developed CRPS after undergoing reconstructive surgery of the hand was highly successful as an occupational therapy instrument at a time when there were no evidence-based procedures [102]. Despite the "low" quality RCTs of occupational and physical therapy for CRPS that were reviewed by the Cochrane Committee, their place in

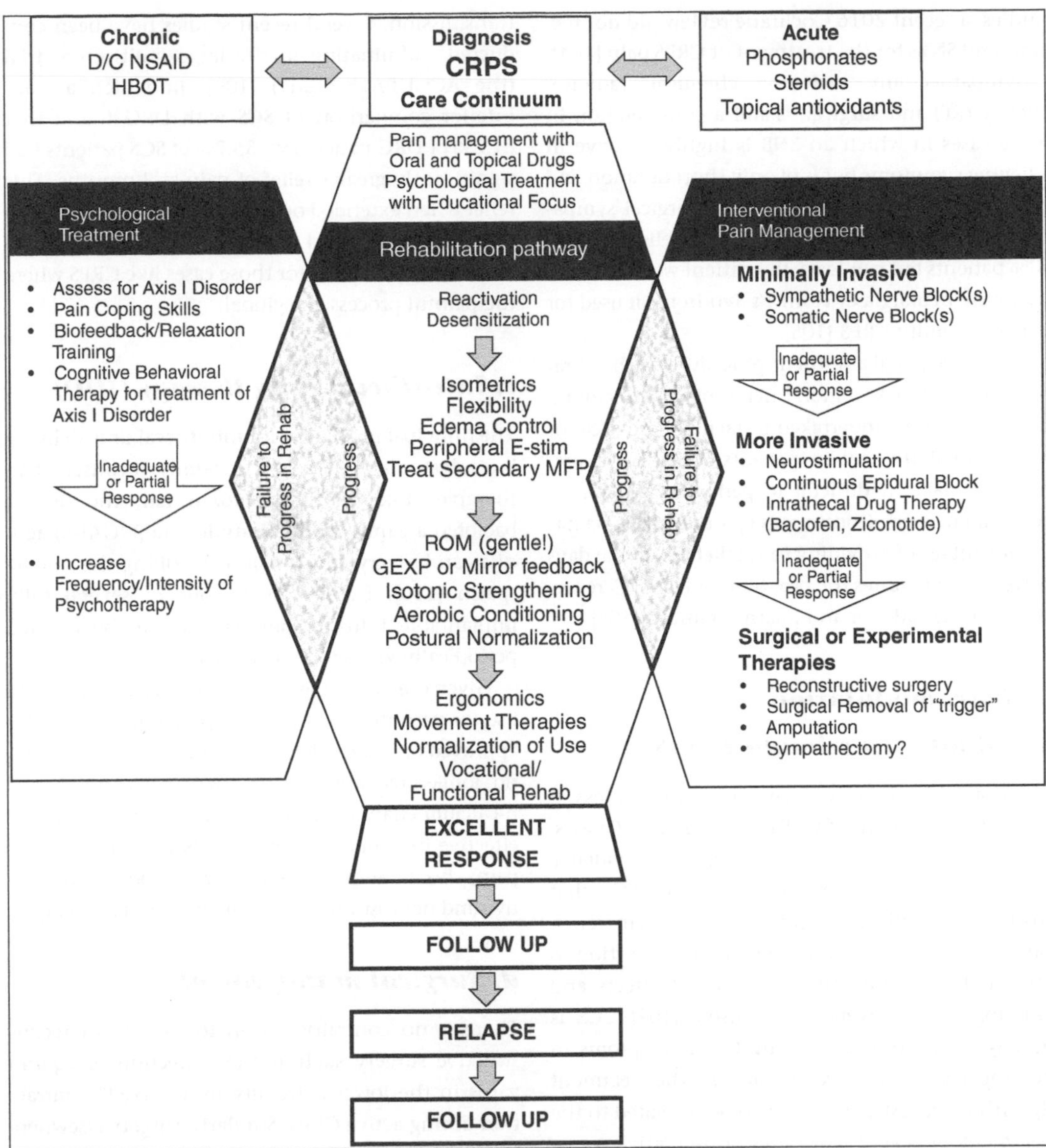

Figure 37.2 The Physiotherapeutic Algorithm

rehabilitation is absolute [103]. The Physiotherapeutic Algorithm is shown in Figure 37.2.

Interventional measures

Depending on the severity and response to the foregoing conservative measures, it may be necessary to utilize more invasive interventions. These can be broken down into regional anesthetic blocks, neuromodulation or surgery.

1. Regional anesthesia

SNBs may be useful in acute CRPS to determine the presence of SMP. Should the patient respond with several days of pain relief, the block can be repeated. This is a good reason to trial an α_1-adrenoceptor blocking agent like terazosin. A non-responder, either technical failure or SIP is a good reason to reevaluate and determine the value of any future SNB. Because of a lack of high-quality studies, a recent 2016 Cochrane review did not recommend SNBs for the treatment of CRPS pain [104].

Sympathectomy including chemical, radiofrequency (RF) and surgical, is still a consideration in those cases in which an SNB is highly effective in relieving symptoms but is of only short duration and is still performed in some centers. Surgical sympathectomy can provide up to 50% pain relief in about 40% patients but can leave the patient with anhidrosis, severe neuralgia or Horner's Syndrome if used for upper extremity CRPS [105].

Certain regional anesthetic procedures such as brachial plexus block, femoral nerve block or epidural analgesia can be undertaken to facilitate physical or occupational therapy in patients whose pain prevents or makes it difficult to perform physiotherapeutic maneuvers. Continuous epidural analgesia has the advantage of providing pain relief for several days or weeks but requires the provision of Home Care servicing of the catheter and pharmaceuticals [106].

2. Neuromodulation

a. Spinal cord stimulation (SCS)

Anecdotal reports have documented the success of SCS in the treatment of CRPS over the past 50 years. There is now, however, supporting (RCT) evidence including a recent review of 19 studies of (SCS) that attributed significant improvement of pain relief, pain scores, quality of life (QOL) and satisfaction to this modality although psychological effects and functional status were inconclusive [107]. SCS is equally effective in addressing CRPS symptoms in the upper and lower extremities. As the treatment algorithm suggests, SCS tends to be relegated to the treatment of severe pain after conservative measures have failed. Recent evidence suggests however that in certain cases, this modality should be employed earlier in the treatment ladder to facilitate rehabilitation and to address severe pain [108].

b. Dorsal root ganglion stimulation (DRG)

This relatively new technology is proving to be very effective in the management of CRPS. Because of its anatomical location in the spinal foramen and its physiological function, the DRG has long been considered an ideal target to interrupt to interrupt pain transmission. Several recent studies have been conducted, culminating in the large multicenter trial (the ACCURATE study) [109], in which a non-inferior comparison of SCS with DRG found that 81.2% of DRG patients vs. 55.7% of SCS patients had significantly greater relief of pain at 3 months. This relief when extended out to 12 months was 74.2% vs 53% in the DRG and SCS groups, respectively. DRG may well replace SCS for those cases like CRPS where the painful process is regional.

c. Intrathecal drug therapy (IDD)

The principal indication for intrathecal drug delivery is for dystonia of the lower extremity. If conservative therapies like botulinum toxin fail, the use of baclofen a gamma aminobutyric acid-β (GABA) agonist can be very effective in controlling the muscle spasm [110]. Delivery is by one of several fully implantable infusion pumps that can be re-filled periodically via percutaneous access.

Given our current experience of long-term μ-opioid use for pain management, morphine, the only FDA-approved opioid for delivery by intrathecal infusion is no longer recommended. However, ziconotide, an n-calcium channel blocking agent that can be highly effective in about 30% of patients with neuropathic pain, should always be considered if both conservative and neurostimulation management fails [111].

d. Surgical management

There is no contraindication to the use of reconstructive surgery such as the correction of equino varus in the lower extremity from "fixed" contraction during active CRPS. Similarly, surgery elsewhere in the body can be safely undertaken in a patient with CRPS. Several recent studies have supported the use of amputation in cases of florid CRPS, severe infection (osteomyelitis) or gangrene [112, 113].

CRPS in children

Recognition of the fact that CRPS can occur in children of all ages is quite a different view from that which was our understanding when the first edition of this book was published. While the acute presentation of CRPS in children resembles that in the adult with the affected extremity tending to be vasodilated and warm, there is a very low prevalence of edema, hyperpathia, hypesthesia, tremor, dystonia and the "cold" form of the syndrome. Pseudoparalysis and myoclonus however are not infrequent. The other characteristic that distinguishes children from adults is the frequent rapid rate of remission with treatment.

Behavioral influences are prominent etiological factors in children due to the confluence of environmental factors (social, school, parental relations, developmental) all of which together, or separately, can have a profound influence on the response to treatment. Whether prepubertal or adolescent, hormone influences likely play a significant role' on the manifestation of the syndrome.

Most children respond to a coordinated exercise [both physical therapy (PT) and occupational therapy (OT)] and behavioral therapy program with in particular an emphasis and reassurance that most cases will be associated with a complete remission. In a few cases, severe hyperpathia and in some, allodynia, can interfere with therapy. Some children will respond to topical treatment containing an antioxidant such as DMSO. Recent studies including an RCT have confirmed pain improvement using topical ketamine. Topical prazosin can also influence pain in children with SMP [114]. Likewise, an SnB block or a regional analgetic procedure can be performed in older children and adolescents who are refractory to therapy.

References

1 Pare' A. (1634) Of the cure of wounds of the nervous system. In: *The Collected Works of Ambroise Pare'*. Milford House, New York.

2 Denmark A. (1813) An example of symptoms resembling tic dolereux produced in a wound in the radial nerve. *Med Chirp Trans* **4**: 48–52

3 Sudeck P. (1900) Über die akute entzündliche Knochenatrophie. *Archiv für klinische Chirurgie* **342**:1012–6

4 Mitchell SW, Morehouse GR, Keen WW. (1864) *Gunshot Wounds and Other Injuries of Nerves*. JB Lippincott, Philadelphia.

5 Evans JA. (1946) Reflex sympathetic dystrophy. *The Surg Clin of North America* **26**:78–90.

6 Stanton-Hicks M, Jänig W, Hassenbusch S *et al.* (1995) Reflex sympathetic dystrophy: changing concepts and taxonomy. *Pain* **63**:127–33.

7 Jänig W, Stanton-Hicks M. (1996) *Reflex Sympathetic Dystrophy: a reappraisal*. IASP Press, Seattle.

8 Veldman PHJM, Reynen HM, Arntz IE *et al.* (1993) Signs and symptoms of reflex sympathetic dystrophy: prospective study of 829 patients. *The Lancet* 342:1012–6.

9 Van Rijn MA, Marinus J, Putter H *et al.* (2011) Spreading of complex regional pain syndrome: not a random process. *J Neural Transm* **118**:1301–9.

10 Marinus J, Moseley GL, Birkllein F *et al.* (2011) Clinical features and pathophysiology of complex regional pain syndrome. *Lancet Neurol* **10**:637–48

11 Sandroni P, Benrud-Larson LM, McClelland RL, Low PA. (2003) Complex regional pain syndrome type I: incidence and prevalence in Olmsted county, a population-based study. *Pain* **103**:199–207.

12 Ott S, Maihofner C. (2018) Signs and symptoms in 1,043 patients with complex regional pain syndrome. *J. Pain* **19**:599–611.

13 Kim H, Lee CH, Kim SH, Kim YD. (2018) Epidemiology of complex regional pain syndrome in Korea: an electronic health data study. *PLoS One* **13**:e0198147.

14 Abu_Arafeh H, Abu-Arafeh I. (2016) Complex regional pain syndrome in children: incidence and clinical characteristics. *Arch Dis Child* **101**:719–23.

15 Harden RN, Bruehl S, Galer BS *et al.* (1999) Complex regional pain syndrome: are the IASP diagnostic criteria valid and sufficiently comprehensive? *Pain* **83**:211–9.

16 Harden RN, BruehL S, Perez RS *et al.* (2010) Validation of proposed diagnostic criteria (the "Budapest Criteria") for Complex Regional Pain Syndrome. *Pain* **150**:268–74.

17 Merskey H, Bogduk N. (1994) *Complex Regional Pain Syndromes (CRPS), Type I (1-4) and Type II (1-5). Classification of Chronic Pain Terms*. IASP Press, Seattle.

18 Harden RN, Maihofner C, Abousaad E *et al* (2017) A prospective, multisite, international validation of the Complex Regional Pain Syndrome Severity Score. *Pain* **158**:1430–6.

19 Bussa M, Mascaro A, Cuffaro L, Rinaldi S. (2017) Adult complex regional pain syndrome type I: a narrative review. *PM R* **9**:707–19.

20 Birklein F, Ajit SK, Goebel A, Perez R, Sommer C. (2018) Complex regional pain syndrome – phenotypic characteristics and potential biomarkers. *Nat Rev Neurol* **14**:27284.

21 Petersen PB, Mikkelsen KL, Lauritzen JB, Krogsgaard MR. (2018) Risk factors for posttreatment complex regional pain syndrome (CRPS): an analysis of 647 cases of CRPS from the Danish Patient Compensation Association. *Pain Pract* **18**:341–9.

22 Terkelsen AJ, Bach FW, Jensen TS. (2008) Experimental forearm immobilization in humans induces cold and mechanical hyperalgesia. *Anesthesiology* **109**:297–307.

23 Herlyn P, Müller-Hilke B, Wendt M, Hecker M, Mittlmeier T, Gradl G. (2010) Frequencies of polymorphisms in cytokines, neurotransmitters and adrenergic receptors in patients with complex regional pain syndrome type I after distal radial fracture. *Clin J Pain* **26**:175–81.

24 Mailis A, Wade J. (1994) Profile of Caucasian women with possible genetic predisposition to reflex sympathetic dystrophy. *Clin J Pain* **10**:210–7.

25 De Mos M, de Brujn AG, Huygen FJ *et al.* (2007) The incidence of complex regional pain syndrome: a population-based study. *Pain* 129:12–20.

26 McDonald MK, Tian Y, Qureshi RA, *et al.* (2014) Functional significance of macrophage-derived exosomes in inflammation and pain. *Pain* **155**:152739.

27 Bruehl S, Maihofner C, Stanton-Hicks M et al. (2016) Complex regional pain syndrome: evidence for warm and cold subtypes in a large prospective clinical; sample. *Pain* **157**: 1674–81.

28 Wertli MM, Brunner F, Steuer J, Held U. (2017) Usefulness of bone scintigraphy for the diagnosis of complex regional pain syndrome I: a systemic analysis and Bayesian meta-analysis. *PLoS One* **12**:e0173688.

29 Ringer R, Wertli M, Bachman LM, Buck FM, Brunner F. (2012) Concordance of qualitative bone scintigraphy results with presence of clinical complex regional pain syndrome I: meta-analysis of test accuracy studies. *Eur J Pain* **16**:1347–56.

30 Munts AG, Van Rootselaar AF, Van der Meer JN Koelman JH, van Hilten JJ, Tijssen MA. (2008) Clinical and neurophysiological characterization of myoclonus in complex regional pain syndrome. *Mov Disord* **23**:581–7.

31 Schwartzman RJ, Alexander GM, Grothusen J. (2006) Pathophysiology of complex regional pain syndrome. *Expert Rev Neurother* **6**:669–81.

32 Birklein F, Drummond PD, Li W, Sclereth T, Finch P, PM, Dawson LF, Clark JD, Kingery WS. (2014) Activation of cutaneous immune responses in complex regional pain syndrome. *J Pain* **15**:485–95.

33 Wehmeyer C, Pap T, Buckley CD, Naylor AJ. (2017) The role of stromal cells in inflammatory bone loss. *Clin Exp Immunol* **189**:1–11.

34 Bianchi E, Taurone S, Bardella L et al. (2015) Involvement of pro-inflammatory cytokines and growth factors in the pathogenesis of Dupytren's contracture: a novel target for a possible future therapeutic strategy? *Clin Sci (Lond)* **129**:711–20.

35 Maihofner C, Handwerker HO, Neundorfer NB, Birklein F. (2005) Mechanical hyperalgesia in complex regional pain syndrome: a role for TNF-alpha? *Neurology* **12**:311–13.

36 Paus R. (1998(Principles of hair cycle control. *J Dermatol* **25**:793–802.

37 Oaklander AL, Fields HL. (2009) Is reflex sympathetic dystrophy/complex regional pain syndrome type I a small fiber neuropathy? *Ann Neurol* **65**:629–38.

38 Rasmussen VF, Karlsson P, Drummond PD et al. (2018) Bilaterally reduces intraepidermal nerve fiber density in unilateral CRPS-1. *Pain Med* **19**:2021–30.

39 Birklein F, Ibrahim A, Sclereth T *et al.* (2018) The rodent tibia fracture model: a critical review and comparison with complex regional pain syndrome literature. *J Pain* **19**:1102.e1–19.

40 Dirckx M, Groeneweg G, van Daele PL *et al.* (2013) Mast cells: a new target in the treatment of complex regional pain syndrome? *Pain Pract* **13**:599–603.

41 Morellini N, Finch PM, Goebel A, Drummond PD. (2018) Dermal nerve fibre and mast cell density, and proximity of mast cells to nerve fibres in the skin of patients with complex regional pain syndrome. *Pain* **159**:2021–29.

42 Knudsen LF, Terkelsen AJ, Drummond PD, Birklein F. (2019) Complex regional pain syndrome: a focus on the autonomic nervous system. *Clin Autonom Res* **29**:457–67.

43 Kohr D, Tschematsch M, Schmitz *et al.* (2009) Autoantibodies in complex regional pain syndrome bind to a differentiation-dependent neuronal surface autoantigen. *Pain* **143**:246–51.

44 Groeneweg JG, Huygen FJ, Heijmans-Antonissen C, Niehof S, Zilstra FG. (2006) Increased endothelin1 and diminished nitric oxide levels in blister fluids of patients with intermediate cold type complex regional pain syndrome type-I. *BMC Musculoskeletal Disord* **7**:91.

45 Birklein F, Riedl B, Claus D, Neundörfer B. (1998) Pattern of autonomic dysfunction in time course of complex regional pain syndrome. *Clin Aut Res* **8**:79–85.

46 Goebel A, Blaes F. (2013) Complex regional pain syndrome, prototype of a novel kind of autoimmune disease. *Autoimmun Rev* **12**:682–6.

47 O'Connell NE, Wand BM, Gibson W, Carr DB, Birklein F, Stanton TR. (2016) Local anesthetic sympathetic blockade for complex regional pain syndrome. *Cochrane Database Syst Rev* **7**:CD004598.

48 Campbell JN, Meyer RA, Raja SN. (1992) Is nociceptor activation by alpha-adrenoceptors the culprit in sympathetically maintained pain. *APS Journal* **1**:3–11.

49 Gradl G, Byer AS, Azad S. (2005) Evaluation of sympathicolysis after continuous brachial plexus analgesia using laser Doppler flowmetry in patients suffering from CRPS (in German) *Anaesthesiol Intensivmed Notfallmed Schmerzther* **40**:345–9.

50 Vogel T, Gradl G, Ockert B *et al.* (2010) Sympathetic dysfunction in long-term complex regional pain syndrome. *Clin J Pain* **26**:128–31.

51 Goyarts E, Matsui M, Mammone T *et al.* (2008) Norepinephrine modulates human dendritic cell activation by altering cytokine release. *Exp Dermatol* **17**:188–96.

52 Seiffert K, Hosoi J, Torii H et al. (2002) Catecholamines inhibit the antigen-presenting capability of epidermal Langerhans cells. *J Immunol* **168**:6128–35.

53 Kavelaars A. (2011) Regulated expression of alpha-1 adrenoceptors in the immune system. *Brain Behav Immun* **16**:799–807.

54 Heijnen CJ, Rouppe van der Voort C, Wulffraat N, van der Net J, Kuis W, Kavelaars A. (1996) Functional alpha 1-adrenergic receptors on leucocytes of patients with polyarticular juvenile arthritis. *J Neuroimmunol* **71**: 223–6.

55 Goh EL, Chidambaram S, Ma D. (2017) Complex regional pain syndrome: a recent update. *Burns Trauma* **5**:2.

56 Bruehl S, Maihöfner C, Stanton-Hicks M *et al.* (2016) Complex regional pain syndrome: evidence for warm and cold subtypes in a large prospective clinical sample. *Pain* **157**:1674–81.

57 Teasel RW, Arnold JM. (2004) Alpha-1 adrenoceptor hyperresponsiveness in three neuropathic pain states: complex regional pain syndrome I, diabetic peripheral neutropathic pain and central pain states following spinal cord injury. *Pain Res Manag* **9**:89–97.

58 Dawson LF, Phillips JK, Finch PM *et al.* (2011) Expression of α1-adrenoceptors on peripheral nociceptive neurons. *Neurosci* **175**:300–14.

59 Rahman W, Suzuki R, Hunt SP. (2008) Selective ablation of dorsal horn in NK1 expressing cells reveals a modulation of spinal alpha-2 adrenergic inhibition of dorsal horn neurons. *Neuropharmacology* **51**:208–14.

60 Goebel A, Shenker N Padfield N *et al.* (2014) Low-dose intravenous immunoglobulin treatment for complex regional pain syndrome (lips): study protocol for a randomized controlled trial. *Trials* **15**:404.

61 Goebel A, Bisla J, Carganillo R *et al.* (2017) Low-dose intravenous immunoglobulin treatment for long-standing complex regional pain syndrome. *Ann Intern Med* **167**:476–83.

62 Dubuis E, Thompson V, Leite MI, Blaes F, Maihöfner C, Greensmith D *et al.* (2014) Longstanding complex regional pain syndrome is associated with activating autoantibodies against alpha-1 adrenoceptors. *Pain 155*:2408–17.

63 Tajerian M, Hung V, Khan H *et al.* (2017) Identification of Krt 16 as a target of an autoantibody response in complex regional pain syndrome. *Experimental Neurology* **287**:14–20.

64 Vartiainen NV, Kirveskari E, Forss N. (2008) Central processing of tactile and nociceptive stimuli in complex regional pain syndrome. *Clin Neurophysiol* **119**:2380–88.

65 Pedersen LH, Scheel-Krüger J, Blackburn-Munro G. (2007) Amygdala GABA-A receptor involvement in mediating sensory-discriminative and affective-motivational pain responses in a rat model of peripheral nerve injury. *Pain* **127**: 17–26.

66 Maihöfner C, DeCol R. (2007) Decreased perceptual learning ability in complex regional pain syndrome. *Eur J Pain* **11**:903–9.

67 DiPietro F, McAuley JH, Parkitny L *et al.* (2013) Primary somatosensory cortex function in complex regional pain syndrome: a systemic review and meta-analysis. *J Pain* **14**:287–93.

68 Van Rijn MA, Marinus J, Putter H *et al.* (2007) Onset and progression of dystonia in complex regional pain syndrome. *Pain* **130**:287–93.

69 Azqueta-Gavaldon M, Sculte-Göcking H, Storz C et al. (2017) Basal ganglia dysfunction in complex regional pain syndrome – a valid hypothesis? *Eur J Pain* **21**:415–24.

70 Azqueta-Galvadon M, Youssef AM, Storz C et al. (2020) Implications of the putamen in pain and motor deficits in complex regional pain syndrome. *Pain* 161:595–608.

71 Simons LE, Erpelding N, Hernandez JM et al. (2016) Fear and reward circuit alterations in pediatric CRPS. *Front Hum Neurosci* **19**:703.

72 Kim JH, Choi SH, Jang JH et al. (2017) Impaired insula functional connectivity associated with persistent pain perception in patients with complex regional pain syndrome. *PLoS One* **10**:e0180479.

73 Moseley GL, Gallace A, Iannetti GD. (2012) Spatially defined modulation of skin temperature and hand ownership of both hands in patients with unilateral complex regional pain syndrome. *Brain* **135**:3676–86.

74 Moseley GL. Gallace A, Spence C. (2009) Space-based, but not arm-based, shift inn tactile processing in complex regional pain syndrome and its relationship to cooling of the affected limb. Brain **132**:3142–51.

75 Maihöfner C, Handwerker HO, Birklein F. (2006) Functional imaging of allodynia in complex regional pain syndrome. *Neurology* **66**:711–17.

76 Speck V, Schlereth T, Birklein F, Maihöfner C. (2017) Increased prevalence of posttraumatic stress disorder in CRPS. *Eur J Pain* **21**:466–73.

77 Urits I, Shen AH, Jones MR, Viswaneth O, Kaye AD. (2018) Complex regional pain syndrome, current concepts and treatment options. *Curr Pain Headache Rep* **22**:10.

78 Sullivan MJL, Bishop SR, Pivik J. (1995) The pain catastrophizing scale: development and validation. *Psychol Assess* **7**:524–32.

79 Erpelding N, Simons L, Lebel A *et al.* (2016) Rapid treatment-induced brain changes in pediatric CRPS. *Brain Struct Funct* **221**:1095–111.

80 Clement ND, Duckworth AD, Wickramasinghe NR, Court-Brown CM, McQueen MM. (2017) Does socioeconomic status influence the epidemiology and outcome of distal radial fractures in adults? *Eur J Orthop Surg Traumatol* 27:1075–82.

81 Lee JY Kim DK, Jung DW Yang JY, Kim DY. (2017) Analysis of disputes regarding chronic pain management in the 2009-2016 period using the Korean Society of Anesthesiologists Database. *Korean J Anesthesiol* **70**:188–95.

82 Christensen K, Jensen EM, Noer I. (1982) The reflex dystrophy syndrome response to treatment with systemic corticosteroids. *Acta Chir Scand* **148**:653–5.

83 Winston P. (2016) Early treatment of acute complex regional pain syndrome after fracture or injury with prednisone: why is there a failure to treat? A case series. *Pain Res Manag* **2016**:7019196.

84 Gustin SM, Schwarz A, Birbaumer N, Sines N *et al.* (2010) NMDA-receptor antagonist and morphine decrease CRPS-pain and cerebral pain representation. *Pain* **151**:6976.

85 Roeckel LAS, Le Coz GM, Gaveriaux-Ruff C, Sinonin F. (2016) Opioid-induced hyperalgesia: cellular and molecular mechanisms. *Neuroscience* **338**:160–82.

86 Perez RS, Zuurmond WW, Bezemer PD Kulik DJ *et al.* (2003) The treatment of complex regional pain syndrome type I with free radical scavengers: a randomized controlled study. *Pain* **102**:297–307.

87 Ekrol I, Duckworth AD, Ralston SH, Court-Brown CM, McQueen MM. (2014) The influence of vitamin C on the outcome of distal radial fractures: a double-blind, randomized controlled trial. *J Bone Jt Surg Am* **96**:1451–9.

88 Evaniew N, McCarthy C, Kleinlugtenbelt YV, Ghert M, Bhandari M. (2015) Vitamin C to prevent complex regional pain syndrome in patients with distal radius fractures: a meta-analysis of randomized controlled trials. *J Orthop Trauma* **29**:e235–41.

89 Van de Vusse AC, Stomp-van den Berg SG, Kessels AH, Weber WE. (2004) Randomized controlled trial of gabapentin in complex regional pain syndrome type I. *BMC Neurol* **4**:13.

90 Caroll I, Curtin CM. (2013) Management of chronic pain following nerve injuries/CRPS type II. Peripheral nerve conditions: using evidence to guide treatment, **29**:401–8.

91 Chevreau M, Romand X, Gaudin P, Juvin R, Baillet A. (2017) Biphosphonates for treatment of complex regional pain syndrome type I: a systematic review

and meta-analysis of randomized controlled trials versus placebo. *Jt Bone Spine* **84**:393–9.

92 Inchiosa MA Jr. (2013) Phenoxbenzamine in complex regional pain syndrome: potential role and novel mechanisms. *Anesthesiol Res Pract* **2013**:978615.

93 Schwartzman RJ, Alexander GM, Grothusen JR, Paylor T *et al.* The use of ketamine for the treatment of complex regional pain syndrome: a double-blind placebocontrolled study. *Pain* **147**:107–15.

94 Schilder JC, van Dijk JG, Dressler D, Koelman JH, Marinus J, van Hilten JJ. (2014) Responsiveness to botulinum toxin type A in muscles of complex regional pain patients with tonic dystonia. *J Neural Transm (Vienna)* **121**: 761–7.

95 Lee Y, Lee CJ, Choi E, Lee PB, Lee HJ, Nahm FS. (2018) Lumbar sympathetic block with botulinum toxin Type A and Type B for complex regional pain syndrome. *Toxins (Basel)* **19**:E164.

96 Bickerstaff DR, Kanis JA, (1991) The use of nasal calcitonin in the treatment of traumatic algodystrophy. *Br J Rheumatol* **30**:291–4.

97 Kiralp MZ, Yildiz S, Vural D, Keskin I, Ay H, Dursun H (2004) Effectiveness of hyperbaric oxygen therapy in the treatment of complex regional pain syndrome. *J Int Med Res* **32**:258–62.

98 Schwartzman RJ, Chevlan K, Bengston K. (2003) Thalidomide has activity in treatment of complex regional pain syndrome. *Arch Int Med* **163**:1487–8.

99 Manning DC, Alexander G, Arezzo JC et al. (2014) Lenalinamide for complex regional pain syndrome type I: lack of efficacy in a phase II randomized study. *J Pain* **15**:1366–76.

100 McCabe C. (2011) Mirror visual feedback therapy. A practical approach. *J Hand Ther* **99**:170–8.

101 Moseley GL, (2004) Graded motor imagery is effective for long-standing complex regional pain syndrome: a randomized controlled trial. *Pain* **108**:192–8.

102 Watson HK, Carlson L. (1987) Treatment of reflex sympathetic dystrophy of the hand with an active: stress loading: program. *J Hand Surg Am* **12**:779–85.

103 O'Connell NE, Wand BM, McAuley J, Marston L, Moseley GL. (2013) Interventions for treating pain and disability in adults with complex regional pain syndrome. *Cochrane database Syst Rev* **7**:CD009416.

104 O'Connell NE, Wand BM, Carr DB, Birklein F, Stanton TR. (2016) Local anesthetic sympathetic blockade for complex regional pain syndrome. *Cochrane Database Syst Rev* **28**:CD004598.

105 Forouzanfer T, van Kleef M, Weber WE. (2000) Radiofrequency lesions of the stellate ganglion in chronic pain syndrome type I: retrospective analysis of clinical efficacy in 86 patients. *Clin J Pain* **16**:164–8.

106 Zyluk A, Puchalski P. (2018) Successful treatment of paedriatric lower limb CRPS by continuous epidural anaesthesia: a report of 2 cases. *Handchir Mikrochir Plast Chir* **50**:359–62.

107 Kemler MA, deVet HC, Barendse GA, van den Wildenberg FA, van Kleef M. (2008) Effect of spinal cord stimulation for chronic complex regional pain syndrome type I: five-year final follow-up of patients in a randomized controlled trial. *J Neurosurg* **108**:2978.

108 Poree L, Krames E, Pope J, Deer TR, Levy R, Schultz I. (2013) Spinal cord stimulation as treatment for complex regional pain syndrome should be considered earlier than last resort therapy. Neuromodulation **16**:125–41.

109 Deer TR, Levy RM, Kramer J *et al.* (2017) Dorsal root ganglion stimulation yielded higher treatment success rate for complex regional pain syndrome and causalgia at 3 and 12 months: a randomized comparative trial. *Pain* **158**:669–81.

110 VanHilten BJ, van de Beek WJ, Hoff JL, Voormolen JH, Delhass EM. (2000) Intrathecal baclofen for the treatment of dystonia in patients with reflex sympathetic dystrophy. *N Engl J Med* **343**:625–30.

111 Herring EZ, Frizon LA, Hogue O et al. (2018) Long-term outcomes using intrathecal drug delivery systems in complex regional pain syndrome. *Pain Med* **20**:515–20.

112 Bodde MI, Dijkstra PU, den Dunnen WF, Geetzen JH. *2011) Therapy-resistant complex regional pain syndrome type I: to amputate or not. *J Bone Joint Surg Am* **93**(19):1799–805.

113 Finch PM, Knudsen L, Drummond PD. (2009) Reduction of allodynia in patients with complex regional pain syndrome: a double-blind placebo-controlled trial of topical ketamine. *Pain* **146**:18–25.

114 Drummond ES, Maker G, Birklein F, Finch PM, Drummond PD. (2016) Topical prazosin attenuates sensitivity to tactile stimuli in patients with complex regional pain syndrome. *Eur J Pain* **20**:926–35.

Chapter 38

Cancer pain management

Amy Swan & Eduardo Bruera

Department of Palliative Care and Rehabilitation Medicine Unit 1414, University of Texas M.D. Anderson Cancer Center, Houston, Texas, USA

Introduction

Pain is one of the most common and distressing symptoms among cancer patients, with increasing frequency and severity as disease progresses. Approximately 30–50% of newly diagnosed cancer patients report having pain. This proportion increases to 35–96% in terminally ill cancer patients [1]. Despite significant progress in research and education on pain management, there remain multiple barriers to effective pain control. These include inconsistent pain assessment, insufficient training and knowledge, misconceptions about opioids and financial challenges [2]. In addition to overcoming these obstacles, it is important to recognize that the diagnosis of cancer is associated with significant physical, psychological and spiritual distress, all of which can contribute to worsening pain. Thus, effective management of cancer pain necessitates an interprofessional approach customized to the individual's needs.

Basic mechanisms

Patients with cancer may experience pain from progressive disease, diagnostic procedures, cancer treatments and/or other comorbidities. Table 38.1 provides an overview of cancer pain mechanisms. The basic mechanism of nociception is reviewed in Chapter 3 and is not discussed in this chapter. Cancer is a life-threatening disease and is frequently associated with psychosocial distress. Although the pathway of neurotransmission from noxious stimuli to somatosensory cortex is similar between cancer pain and non-cancer pain, how cancer patients perceive, and ultimately express, their pain may be quite different from patients with non-cancer Diagnoses (Figure 38.1).

An understanding of the unique circumstances associated with the diagnosis of cancer has important implications for both assessment and treatment of cancer pain. Cancer patients typically have a heavy symptom burden as a result of progressive cancer, cancer treatments and/or comorbidities. Using the Memorial Symptom Assessment Scale, one study demonstrated that advanced cancer patients have an average of 11 ± 6 symptoms [3]. Because many of these symptoms are closely related, effective management of pain in the context of malignancy requires concurrent management of other complaints (e.g. coughing and chest pain, vomiting and abdominal pain). Also, polypharmacy is a common issue among cancer patients, with a high potential for drug interactions. For instance, the level of methadone may be affected by concurrent use of various CYP3A4 inducers and/or inhibitors.

Clinicians caring for cancer patients should be cognizant of the concept of "total pain," defined as the sum of four components: physical, psychological, social and spiritual. This framework highlights the

Clinical Pain Management: A Practical Guide, Second Edition. Edited by Mary E. Lynch, Kenneth D. Craig, and Philip W. Peng.

Table 38.1 Cancer pain mechanisms.

Type	Clinical features	Examples
Nociceptive-somatic	Well localized	Bone metastasis Pathologic fracture Surgical incision pain
Nociceptive-visceral	Poorly localized Deep, squeezing, pressure, referred pain	Liver metastasis Pancreatitis Bowel obstruction
Neuropathic	Poorly localized Dysesthetic, constant burning, radiating pain Neuralgic/lancinating	Compression of nerve roots by tumor Spinal cord compression Chemotherapy-induced peripheral neuropathy Radiation-induced brachial plexopathy

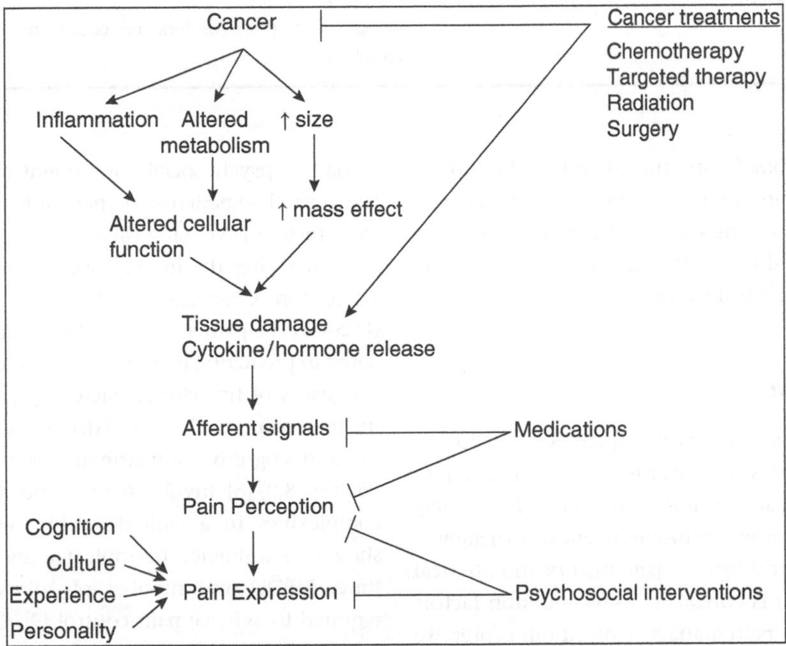

Figure 38.1 Pathophysiology of cancer pain. Cancer progression can result in increasing mass effect and altered cellular function, leading to tissue damage and cytokine/hormone release. Afferent signals are transmitted to the central nervous system and eventually the somatosensory cortex where the pain is perceived. In addition to nociceptive input, how the patient expresses his/her symptom(s) is affected by other factors, such as culture, personal experience, personality and cognition. Cancer therapies, various supportive care medications and psychosocial interventions all have a role in alleviation of pain.

complex interconnectedness between the body, mind and spirit. For instance, a patient may experience 4 out of 10 shoulder pain caused by the nociceptive input from bone metastasis, while another patient with similar level of noxious physical stimuli may rate his/her pain as 10 out of 10 because of significant psychosocial (e.g. recent bad news) or spiritual (e.g. punishment from God) distress. Pain for the first patient can easily be managed with analgesics, while pain for the second patient warrants comprehensive assessment with multidisciplinary input.

Poorly controlled pain can result in reduced sleep, decreased function, altered mood and can significantly compromise a patients' quality of life. When a patient requires ever-increasing doses of analgesics without adequate pain control, it is important to

Table 38.2 Risk factors for refractory cancer pain

Risk factors	Specific solutions
Disease-related factors	
Progressive cancer (compression, obstruction, infiltration)	Cancer treatments (radiation, chemotherapy)
Cancer related complications	
Ischemia	Supportive measures
Infections	Antibiotics
Fractures	Surgery
Treatment related complications	Opioid rotation, dose reduction, adjuvants for opioid-sparing effect
Opioid-induced neurotoxicity (e.g. hyperalgesia)	
Patient-related factors	
Delirium	Neuroleptics, non-pharmacologic treatments
Personality	Counseling
Psychosocial stressors	Counseling
Chemical coping	Limit opioids, emphasis on function, counseling
Secondary gain	Counseling

step back and look for specific risk factors (Table 38.2) before prescribing more medications. This not only helps to minimize the amount of analgesics and thus the associated side effects, but also provides a more effective pain control strategy.

Assessment

Effective management of cancer pain begins with regular and frequent screening, which allows clinicians to diagnose pain early, to initiate treatment in a timely fashion and to monitor the effectiveness of therapy.

In addition to a focused pain history and physical examination, it is critical to assess common factors that may affect pain management. At our center, we routinely screen patients for various physical and psychological symptoms, delirium and history of alcoholism, using validated instruments such as the Edmonton Symptom Assessment Scale (ESAS; Figure 38.3) [4], the Memorial Delirium Assessment Scale (MDAS) [5] and the CAGE questionnaire [6], respectively. This information can help clinicians formulate the pain diagnosis and assess the need to utilize specific pain management strategies. For instance, a delirious patient who keeps complaining of pain should be treated with neuroleptics rather than simply escalating the opioid dose. In another example, a patient with 10 out of 10 pain and severe symptoms in multiple other ESAS domains is likely to have a psychosocial component contributing to the overall experience of pain and would benefit from further psychological assessments.

Recognizing the importance of these factors, the Edmonton Classification System for Cancer Pain (ECS-CP) is a pain assessment tool that has been validated in predicting pain management complexity [7]. It consists of five clinical factors: pain mechanisms, incident pain, psychological distress, addictive behavior and cognitive impairment, as outlined below (Figure 38.2) [8]. Involvement of one of more of these complexities in a patient's pain picture has been shown to influence multiple factors including the time, MEDD and number of adjuvant analgesics required to achieve pain control [9]. One important note is that it doesn't take into account addictive behavior if it occurred remotely. Because people tend to employ the same coping mechanisms when dealing with stress, a history of alcoholism any time in the past should be relevant [10-12]. Regular assessment and documentation using ECS-CP will facilitate communication between members of the interprofessional team and help optimize pain control.

Management

In 2018, the World Health Organization updated its guidelines to say that it is appropriate to initiate a pain regimen with opioids in the context of

Edmonton Classification System for Cancer Pain

Patient Name: ______________________________

Patient ID No: ______________________________

For each of the following features, circle the response that is most appropriate, based on your clinical assessment of the patient.

1. Mechanism of Pain

- No No pain syndrome
- Nc Any nociceptive combination of visceral and/or bone or soft tissue pain
- Ne Neuropathic pain syndrome with or without any combination of nociceptive pain
- Nx Insufficient information to classify

2. Incident Pain

- Io No incident pain
- Ii Incident pain present
- Ix Insufficient information to classify

3. Psychological Distress

- Po No psychological distress
- Pp Psychological distress present
- Px Insufficient information to classify

4. Addictive Behavior

- Ao No addictive behavior
- Aa Addictive behavior present
- Ax Insufficient information to classify

5. Cognitive Function

- Co No impairment. Patient able to provide accurate present and past pain history unimpaired
- Ci Partial impairment. Sufficient impairment to affect patient's ability to provide accurate present and/or past pain history
- Cu Total impairment. Patient unresponsive, delirious or demented to the stage of being unable to provide any present and past pain history
- Cx Insufficient information to classify.

ECS-CP profile: N__ I__ P__ A__ C__ ***(combination of the five responses, one for each category)***

Assessed by: ______________ **Date:** ______________

Figure 38.2 The Edmonton Classification System for Cancer Pain (ECS-CP). Presence of any of its elements - neuropathic pain, incident pain, psychological distress, addictive behavior or impaired cognitive function -complicates management of pain. Incident pain is a sudden, significant increase in pain level, often related to a known trigger (urination, dressing changes, swallowing, etc).

moderate to severe cancer-related pain, alone or in combination with non-steroidal anti-inflammatory drugs (NSAIDs) and/or acetaminophen. This is a change from their previous recommendation to initiate all patients on non-opioid therapies, regardless of their pain level. However, this should be done on a case-by-case basis and other factors, such as risk of non-medical opioid use, should be taken into account (to be discussed later). Adjuvant treatments such as antidepressants, anticonvulsants, bisphosphonates, steroids, radiation and chemotherapy may be added to the pain regimen at any time if indicated.

Opioid mechanism of action

Details of opioid action have been reviewed in Chapter 19. Opioids exert their analgesic effect through binding to various μ-, δ- and κ-receptors, both centrally and peripherally. Activation of μ1-receptors is responsible for the analgesic and

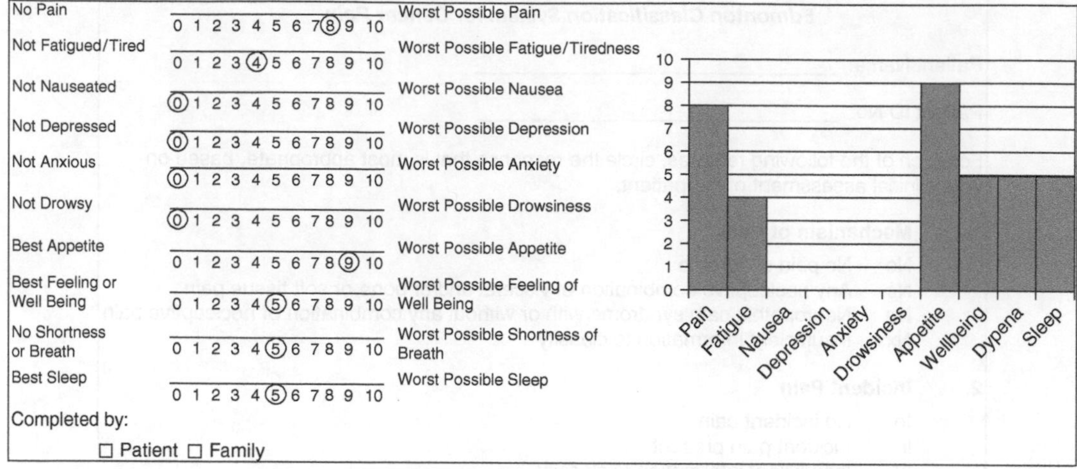

Figure 38.3 The Edmonton Symptom Assessment Scale (ESAS). ESAS documents the average intensity of 10 symptoms over the past 24 hours. It has been validated in cancer populations and is useful for both screening purposes as well as longitudinal assessments. The right panel is a plot of a patient's ESAS score, which allows a quick visual examination of the patient's symptom profile and facilitates comparison between assessments.

euphoric effects of the opioid, while interaction with μ2-receptors is associated with various opioid-induced side effects such as respiratory depression, nausea and sedation. Methadone also has N-methyl-D-aspartate (NMDA) antagonist activity, which is associated with a theoretical benefit for neuropathic pain and opioid resistance.

There is great interindividual variation in the degree of responsiveness to opioids, which is dependent on various pharmacodynamic and pharmacokinetic factors. These in turn are affected by the patient's age, sex, genetic makeup (i.e. opioid receptor expression and sensitivity, P450 enzymes), organ function, comorbidities, diet and concurrent medications. For instance, 8–10% of the Caucasian population have an inactive CYP2D6 variant and cannot convert codeine from its prodrug form to the active metabolite. The pharmacogenomics of opioid agents represents an area of active research.

Because pain expression is a subjective measure, psychosocial factors such as personality, past experience, culture and placebo effect may also affect the response.

Clinical use of opioids

Patients with moderate to severe cancer pain can be started on conservative doses of short-acting opioids around the clock if appropriate with their pain picture, with as needed opioid (usually 10% –15% of total daily dose) every 2–4 hours for breakthrough pain. While each opioid has a variable potency and activity spectrum, there is no evidence that any opioid is superior to another as first line therapy for cancer pain.

Because of the need to titrate the opioid dose initially, the use of long-acting formulations and transdermal fentanyl should be avoided until the pain is stabilized. In general, patients who require three or more breakthroughs per day should have their scheduled dosage increased, whereas patients who do not require any breakthrough medications may benefit from a dosage reduction. Once a stable dosage of pain medication has been achieved, a long-acting formulation may be added for convenience. Immediate release opioid every 4 hours, slow release formulations every 12–24 hours and transdermal fentanyl every 72 hours have similar efficacy. For patients who require parenteral opioids, continuous intravenous infusion, continuous subcutaneous infusion and intermittent subcutaneous injections all represent effective models of pain control [13, 14].

Adverse effects of opioids

Common opioid-related adverse effects include sedation, nausea and vomiting, which tend to resolve within a few days as patients develop tolerance to opioids. However, constipation is likely to continue for the duration of treatment. Patients should be counseled regarding these common side effects and prescribed antiemetics (e.g. metoclopramide 10 mg orally every 4 hours) and laxatives (e.g. 2 senna tablets orally at bed time) for prophylaxis. For patients with severe opioid-induced constipation, the use of μ-antagonists such as methylnaltrexone can be useful.

QTc prolongation may develop in patients on high doses of methadone or with pre-existing risk factors, such as structural cardiac diseases, electrolyte abnormalities or other medications associated with QTc prolongation. These individuals are at risk for development of torsade de pointes, ventricular arrhythmia and sudden cardiac death and would benefit from regular electrocardiogram monitoring. Other adverse effects associated with long-term opioid use include hypogonadism, osteoporosis, sexual dysfunction, immunosuppression, altered renal function and peripheral edema [15].

Opioid-induced neurotoxicities (OIN) include delirium (agitation, tactile and visual hallucination), nightmares, myoclonus, hyperalgesia and seizures. Risk factors for OIN include high doses of opioids for prolonged periods of time, pre-existing cognitive impairment, renal failure and infections. Hyperalgesia should be suspected if patients have severe pain despite rapid escalation of opioid doses and should be distinguished from inadequately controlled pain. The former is characterized by the presence of pain sensitivity, delirium and other OIN symptoms. Management of hyperalgesia includes opioid rotation, reduction of total opioid dose and use of other non-opioid analgesics such as acetaminophen, dexamethasone, lidocaine and ketamine [16].

Opioid rotation

Opioid rotation, the practice of switching from one opioid to another, is indicated for two reasons:

1 When pain persists despite escalating doses of an opioid; or

2 When opioid-induced neurotoxicity develops.

Because each opioid has a different spectrum of opioid receptor affinity and sensitivity, switching to a new opioid may allow for more effective pain control, taking advantage of incomplete cross-tolerance. By reducing the concentration of the previous opioid and its metabolites, opioid rotation can also help to mitigate neurotoxicity.

A Cochrane review on opioid rotation included 14 prospective uncontrolled studies, 15 retrospective studies/audits and 23 case reports [19]. No randomized controlled trials were available. The majority of the studies used morphine as the first line opioid and methadone as the second line opioid. All reports except one concluded that opioid switching is a useful clinical maneuver for improving pain control and/or reducing opioid-related side-effects.

Opioid rotation is performed by determining the total PO morphine equivalent daily dose (MEDD), then calculating the dose of the new opioid using equianalgesic ratios (Table 38.3). A 30% dose reduction of the new opioid is generally applied, taking into account the incomplete cross-tolerance. However, for patients who require opioid rotation for uncontrolled pain, no change in the total MEDD dose may be necessary. For patients who require opioid rotation for OIN, reduce the MEDD dose by 50%.

Prescribing opioids during an opioid epidemic

In light of the opioid epidemic, the role of the physician becomes two-fold: to advocate for and provide adequate access to opioids while at the same time, to increase vigilance and enhance safe prescribing of opioids. Even though many of the prescribing restrictions and guidelines that have been put in place since 2016 [20] have excluded cancer/palliative care patients, it has resulted in untoward decrease of opioid availability to this population, as well as a decreased willingness to prescribe opioids by their oncologists [21].

Opioids remain the gold standard for treatment of cancer-related pain and the clinician should not hesitate to prescribe them when they are needed, but it must be done so safely and responsibly. Providers should have a discussion with every patient considering opioid therapy regarding risks, benefits and alternate therapies. It should be explained that opioids are not the sole modality of treatment, but will be combined with adjuvant medication/nonpharmacologic approaches of pain management. Proper

Table 38.3 Equianalgesic table.

Opioid	From Parenteral Opioid to Parenteral Morphine	From Same Parenteral Opioid to Oral Opioid	From Oral Opioid to Oral Morphine	From Oral Morphine to Oral Opioid
Morphine	1	2-3	1	1
Hydrocodone	N/A	N/A	1*	1*
Hydromorphone	5	2.5	5	0.2
Oxycodone	1.5	2–3	1.5	0.7
Oxymorphone	0.10	10	3	0.3
Fentanyl**		See notes		
Methadone†		1–2	See notes	

* For hydrocodone doses <40 mg/day, conversion factor to morphine of 1.5 is recommended.

** For fentanyl patch, consider use of the table included in the package insert (though in some cases this may be too conservative). This is a unidirectional chart for starting a fentanyl patch only; to go from fentanyl patch to MEDD, multiply by 2.5; Fentanyl 15 µg IV is equivalent 1 mg IV morphine.

† To convert to methadone, a conversion ratio of 10:1 should be used for MEDD < 199 mg and a conversion ratio of 20:1 should be used for MEDD > 199 mg. If patient is older than 65, used a conversion ratio of 20:1. Note this is a one-way conversion from MEDD to methadone only. Methadone has complicated pharmacologic properties and should be managed by an experienced provider [17].

To calculate the equianalgesic dose

1. Obtain the MEDD by taking the total amount of opioid that effectively controls pain in 24 hours and convert to PO morphine.
2. Multiply by conversion factor in table. Give 30% less of the new opioid to avoid partial cross-tolerance.
3. Divide by the number of doses/day.

Source: Modified from Heung *et al* [18].

use, storage and disposal of opioids should be reviewed as well as appropriate handling/sorting of the medication, especially if there are children in the home. Risks of self-titration and education on how to handle situations that require changes in medications and dosing should be explained and it should be stressed to never share opioids with anyone. Much of the harm done from opioids is a result of re-starting a previous dose of opioid before tolerance is re-built. How to recognize and treat a case of suspected overdose should be discussed, with consideration of a prescription for intranasal naloxone, especially if the patient is on other potentially sedating medications, has a high MEDD, or other medical conditions that could contribute to central nervous system (CNS) depressions, such as sleep apnea.

Non-Medical Opioid Use and Substance Use Disorder

Non-medical opioid use (NMOU) and substance use disorder (SUD) are common concerns among patients and clinicians and represent a key barrier to appropriate opioid use. It has been previously believed that those with cancer pain carry a relatively lower risk than the general population, but in light of the current opioid epidemic, new research has indicated that this is not the case [22, 23].

Dependence is a normal pharmacophysiologic effect that manifests as development of withdrawal symptoms (e.g. agitation, pain, fever, sweats, tremor and tachycardia) if opioids are stopped abruptly after a prolonged period of use, while addiction or SUD is an abnormal psychopathological compulsion to use a substance affecting daily function. A diagnosis of SUD begins with behaviors worrisome for non-medical opioid use, which has emerged as a preferred term over 'abuse' or 'aberrant behavior.'

All patients should be screened on initial consult and again periodically to assess risk of developing opioid addiction. A positive history of abuse of any substance (i.e. alcohol or illicit drug use) indicates that there is also a risk of developing addiction to opioids. The CAGE questionnaire is a validated tool for alcoholism and consists of four questions: Have you felt you needed to cut down on your drinking? Have you felt annoyed by criticism of your drinking? Have you felt guilty about drinking? Have you felt you needed a drink first thing in the morning (eye-opener)? An affirmative response to two or more questions indicates a high likelihood of alcoholism and therefore a higher likelihood of opioid misuse.

Specific opioid risk tools, such as the SOAPP (Screener and Opioid Assessment for Patients with Pain), is another recommended screening tool for opioid misuse. This is a validated tool with 14 questions that render a score from 0–56, with a cutoff value of 7 or higher representing an increased risk of opioid misuse. Other risk factors of opioid misuse are younger age, male gender, anxiety diagnosis or financial distress and history of tobacco use [24, 25].

Increased risk for an opioid use disorder should heighten the awareness of the provider to monitor closely for behaviors that could be indicative of NMOU. If a patient starts to show signs that are consistent with NMOU, the provider must employ increased supervision, education and boundaries. If unrecognized, these patients may be prescribed ever-escalating doses of opioid without adequate pain control, with increased risk of opioid-induced delirium, myoclonus, hyperalgesia and grand mal seizures. While there is not a consensus on specific recommendations, emerging research indicates there are several things that the provider can do to minimize the risks.

Use of intermittent urine drug screens can help to identify use of illicit substances or opioids that have not been prescribed. They are also useful to identify patients that could be diverting their opioid medication. Careful review of the prescription drug monitoring program is also helpful in determining if a patient is being truthful about past or current prescriptions and to find cases where opioids are being prescribed by multiple providers or "doctor shopping". Patients that exhibit behaviors consistent with NMOU can be asked to return for more frequent provider or nursing visits, to bring their pills with them when they come in order to perform a pill count and can be given shorter than standard quantities of pills for a given amount of time. It is also useful to emphasize the use of opioids for improving function rather than pain control and is extremely important to provide interdisciplinary patient and family support.

Predisposition to development of opioid addiction is related to a combination of genetic and environmental factors. It is important to remember that while part of the problem is a result of the patient's poor choices and subsequent behaviors, there is also a certain degree of misfortune that has fallen on these patients with respect to genetics and exposure. Therefore it is important to provide a straightforward and compassionate approach when assisting these patients. One study found a decrease in number of aberrant behaviors from 3 to 0.4 as well as a decrease in MEDD from 165 to 112 after the use of a specialized interdisciplinary approach for patients identified as misusing opioids. The approach consisted of an intervention involving an honest discussion detailing opioid risks, the team's concerns regarding the patient behavior and realistic goals of opioid therapy [26].

Lastly, take pseudoaddiction into account. Pseudoaddiction is a situation that arises from undertreated pain, in this case a patient's efforts to obtain a higher dose of opioid are related to attempts to find relief from the pain. If the patient exhibits some behaviors consistent with NMOU but overall their pain picture makes sense, it could be that their opioid dose is not yet high enough. The difference here will usually be that increases in opioids are somewhat helpful and that after several increases, reasonable pain control is able to be ultimately achieved.

Adjuvant therapies

While opioids are effective for management of cancer pain, adjuvant therapies or co-analgesics are indicated for specific pain syndromes for two reasons:

1 To enhance pain control through different mechanisms of action; and

2 To reduce the amount of opioid required (i.e. "opioid sparing").

Table 38.4 highlights a number of adjuvant therapies for common pain syndromes.

For selected patients with good performance status and treatment sensitive disease, cancer therapies such as radiation, chemotherapy and targeted agents represent feasible options for effective pain control. However, tumor response is usually not observed until weeks later and any clinical benefit tends to be for a short duration only. Furthermore, cancer therapies can be associated with significant morbidities.

Table 38.4 Adjuvant treatments for specific cancer pain syndromes.

	Good evidence	Limited evidence
Bone pain	NSAIDs, COX-2 inhibitors Bisphosphonates (Cochrane) Palliative radiation (Cochrane) Radionuclides (Cochrane)	Steroids
Neuropathic pain	Gabapentin Tricyclic antidepressants Serotonin-noradrenaline reuptake inhibitors (venlafaxine, duloxetine) Lidocaine	Steroids SSRI
Pancreatic cancer pain	Celiac axis block	
Bowel obstruction	Anticholinergic agents Octreotide	Steroids
Oral mucositis		Lidocaine viscous

COX, cyclo-oxygenase; NSAID, non-steroidal anti-inflammatory drug; SSRI, selective serotonin reuptake inhibitor.

Thus, judicious use of antineoplastic therapies after careful consideration of the risks and benefits is warranted.

For neuropathic pain, tricyclic antidepressants, opioids, gabapentin/pregabalin, venlafaxine/duloxetine, topical lidocaine and topical capsaicin have all been shown to have some benefit. Most if not all of the evidence for these is based on non-cancer pain syndromes [27]. Of these, TCAs have some of the best evidence for use but given their increased side effect profile including anticholinergic and sedating effects, they should be used with more caution in the cancer and palliative population. Opioids are sometimes used more for neuropathic pain in these patients because many cancer patients are already on them. Given the wide selection of co-analgesics, the agent of choice depends on the patient's comorbidities and the agent's side effect profile.

Ketamine is an NMDA antagonist which represents an emerging option for cancer pain, although evidence supporting its efficacy is still limited [28]. Ketamine is typically given as a subcutaneous infusion though may also be administered orally. Patients on ketamine should be monitored for excessive secretions, hallucinations and changes in heart rate/rhythm. Cannabinoids have also been used for selected patients with some effect (Chapter 20).

A number of complementary treatments such as music therapy and touch therapies also have an adjunctive role in cancer pain management. Involvement of other specialties such as intervention radiologists and anesthesiologists may also be indicated in specific circumstances, such as vertebroplasty/kyphoplasty for vertebral fractures, celiac plexus block for visceral abdominal pain and superior hypogastric plexus block for pelvic pain. Neurosurgery consultation for cordotomy may be considered for severe unilateral pain that has proven difficult to treat.

Continuity of care and multidisciplinary management

In addition to timely diagnosis and treatment of pain, it is important to provide continual education and counseling, to assess patients' adherence to the pain regimen, to follow-up on response to analgesics and to monitor side effects.

Throughout this chapter we emphasized that analgesics alone may not be adequate for pain management, particularly for patients who have complex psychosocial needs and existential suffering. A detailed review of psychological assessment and counseling in cancer is beyond the scope of this chapter. However, consultation of palliative care specialists, psychiatrists, clinical psychologists and other members of the interprofessional team in a timely fashion may help to minimize medication use and to optimize pain control.

References

1 Solano JP, Gomes B, Higginson IJ. (2006) A comparison of symptom prevalence in far advanced cancer, AIDS, heart disease, chronic obstructive pulmonary disease and renal disease. *J Pain Symptom Management* **31(1)**:58–69.

2 Oldenmenger WH, Sillevis Smitt PA, van Dooren S *et al.* (2009) A systematic review on barriers hindering adequate cancer pain management and interventions to reduce them: a critical appraisal. *Eur J Cancer* **45(8)**:1370–80.

3 Portenoy RK, Thaler HT, Kornblith AB *et al.* (1994) Symptom prevalence, characteristics and distress in a cancer population. *Qual Life Res* **3(3)**:183–9.

4 Bruera E, Kuehn N, Miller MJ *et al.* (1991) The Edmonton Symptom Assessment System (ESAS): a simple method for the assessment of palliative care patients. *J Palliat Care* **7(2)**:6–9.

5 Breitbart W, Rosenfeld B, Roth A *et al.* (1997) The Memorial Delirium Assessment Scale. *J Pain and Symptom Management* **13(3)**:128–37.

6 Ewing JA. (1984) Detecting alcoholism. The CAGE questionnaire. *JAMA* **252(14)**:1905–7.

7 Fainsinger RL, Nekolaichuk CL. (2008) A "TNM" classification system for cancer pain: the Edmonton Classification System for Cancer Pain (ECS-CP). *Support Care Cancer* **16(6)**:547–55.

8 Fainsinger R, Nekolaichuk C, Lawlor P *et al.* (2019) Edmonton Classification System for Cancer Pain (ECS-CP) Administration Manual Available at: https://www.albertahealthservices.ca/assets/info/peolc/if-peolc-ed-ecs-cp-admin-manual.pdf. Accessed March 4, 2021.

9 Fainsinger RL, Nekolaichuk C, Lawlor P *et al.* (2010) An international multicentre validation study of a pain classification system for cancer patients. Eur J of Cancer **46(16)**:2896–904.

10 Bruera E, Moyano J, Seifert L *et al.* (1995) The frequency of alcoholism among patients with pain due to terminal cancer. *J Pain Symptom Management* **10(8)**:599–603.

11 Poulin C, Webster I, Single E. (1997) Alcohol disorders in Canada as indicated by the CAGE questionnaire. CMAJ **157(11)**:1529–35.

12 Moore RD, Bone LR, Geller G *et al.* (1989) Prevalence, detection, and treatment of alcoholism in hospitalized patients. *JAMA* **261(3)**:403–7.

13 Watanabe S, Pereira J, Tarumi Y *et al.* (2008) A randomized double-blind crossover comparison of continuous and intermittent subcutaneous administration of opioid for cancer pain. *J Palliative Med* 11(**4**):570–4.

14 Parsons HA, Shukkoor A, Quan H *et al.* (2008) Intermittent subcutaneous opioids for the management of cancer pain. *J Palliat Med* 11(**10**):1319–24.

15 Harris JD. (2008) Management of expected and unexpected opioid-related side effects. *Clin J Pain* **24 Suppl 10**:S8–s13.

16 de Leon-Casasola OA. (2008) Current developments in opioid therapy for management of cancer pain. *Clin Journal Pain* **24 Suppl 10**:S3–7.

17 McPherson ML, Walker KA, Davis MP *et al.* (2019) Safe and appropriate use of methadone in hospice and palliative care: expert consensus white paper. *J Pain Symptom Management* **57(3)**:635–645.e634.

18 Heung Y, Reddy A, Reddy S. (2018) Pain Management. In: Dalal S, Bruera E, (Eds). *The MD Anderson Supportive and Palliative Care Handbook*, 6th edn. The University of Texas MD Anderson Cancer Center, Houston.pp. 30.

19 Quigley C. (2004) Opioid switching to improve pain relief and drug tolerability. Cochrane Database Syst Rev**(3)**:Cd004847.

20 Dowell D, Haegerich TM, Chou R. (2016) CDC guideline for prescribing opioids for chronic pain--United States, 2016. *JAMA* **315(15)**:1624–45.

21 Haider A, Zhukovsky DS, Meng YC *et al.* (2017) Opioid prescription trends among patients with cancer referred to outpatient palliative care over a 6-year period. *J Oncol Practice* **13(12)**:e972–81.

22 Arthur JA, Edwards T, Lu Z *et al.* (2016) Frequency, predictors, and outcomes of urine drug testing among patients with advanced cancer on chronic opioid therapy at an outpatient supportive care clinic. *Cancer* **122(23)**:3732–9.

23 Kwon JH, Tanco K, Park JC *et al.* (2015) Frequency, predictors, and medical record documentation of chemical coping among advanced cancer patients. *Oncologist* **20(6)**:692–7.

24 Yennurajalingam S, Edwards T, Arthur JA *et al.* (2018) Predicting the risk for aberrant opioid use behavior in patients receiving outpatient supportive care consultation at a comprehensive cancer center. *Cancer* 124(**19**):3942–9.

25 Arthur J, Bruera E. (2019) Balancing opioid analgesia with the risk of nonmedical opioid use in patients with cancer. *Nat Rev Clin Oncol* **16(4)**:213–26.
26 Arthur J, Edwards T, Reddy S *et al*. (2018) Outcomes of a specialized interdisciplinary approach for patients with cancer with aberrant opioid-related behavior. *Oncologist* **23(2)**:263–70.
27 Finnerup NB, Attal N, Haroutounian S *et al*. (2015) Pharmacotherapy for neuropathic pain in adults: a systematic review and meta-analysis. *Lancet Neurol* **14(2)**:162–73.
28 Bell RF, Eccleston C, Kalso EA. (2017) Ketamine as an adjuvant to opioids for cancer pain. *Cochrane Database Syst Rev* **6(6)**:Cd003351.

Chapter 39

Pain and addiction

Douglas L. Gourlay[1], Howard A. Heit[2], & Andrew J. Smith[3]

[1] *Educational Consultant, Hamilton, Ontario, Canada*
[2] *Private Practice, Reston, Virginia, USA*
[3] *Interprofessional Pain and Addiction Recovery Clinic, Centre for Addiction and Mental Health, Toronto Academic Pain Medicine Institute, Toronto, Ontario, Canada*

Pain and addiction

This chapter will focus on two important topics: the basic science of substance use disorders (SUDs) from a neurobiologic perspective and how to apply this to the clinical assessment and management of the high-risk patient.

This is hardly a complete exploration of the subject but should give the reader a practical approach to the clinical care of this challenging population of patients. It is the authors' sincere hope that all pain practitioners will become talented amateurs in the field of addiction medicine [1].

Neurobiology of addiction

Addiction is a treatable chronic neurobiological disease influenced by genetic, psychosocial and environmental factors. It involves brain centers that normally mediate arousal and reward in situations that enhance the growth and survival of the person, such as food, sex, social interactions and unexpected novel stimuli. Prescribed opioids and drugs of abuse activate these circuits to a much greater extent and without reaching satiety compared to normal stimuli. They tend to serve the individual no useful purpose.

Exciting advances in neuroscience and functional imaging research are beginning to clarify the pathophysiology of addiction as developing through a framework of three recurring stages: binge and intoxication; withdrawal and negative affect; and preoccupation and anticipation (or craving) [2]. Each stage involves activation of specific neural pathways with behavioral correlates which worsen with repeated exposure to a reinforcing substance as neuroplastic changes occur to brain systems that mediate reward, stress and executive function. These behavioral manifestations form the basis of the diagnosis of a SUD with hallmarks of continued use of a substance despite harm, impaired control over use, compulsive use and cravings [3].

In the initial stage [2], the substance (or prescribed medication) will cause release of dopamine and other neurotransmitters (endorphins, serotonin, GABA, acetylcholine) into the ventral striatum. This results in the subjective experience of reward or a "high" (or relief of pain in patients with a chronic pain condition), that positively reinforces their use.

At the same time, normally countervailing circuits maintain proper inhibition and decision making, motivation, stress reactivity and awareness of inner body states. These "braking" circuits become less effective with ongoing use of the drug – there is no satiety as with normal stimuli like food or sex.

Over time, less dopamine is released with repeated exposure to the drug itself, but more in anticipation

Clinical Pain Management: A Practical Guide, Second Edition. Edited by Mary E. Lynch, Kenneth D. Craig, and Philip W. Peng.

of the reward, a process known as conditioned reinforcement [4]. A previously neutral stimulus (e.g. a pharmacy) becomes more rewarding through its association with the drug and becomes a reinforcer in its own right.

This "cuing" is a normal evolutionary adaptation meant to provide us more triggers to engage in rewarding/adaptive behaviors and involves the same molecular mechanisms underpinning learning and memory via synapse formation. For example, we feel a sense of wellbeing not just at the thought of our favourite meal, but when we think of where and with whom we ate that meal.

The ***withdrawal and negative affect stages*** [5] occurs when drug use is stopped or precipitously reduced. The symptoms vary depending on the substance used and the extent of use and are thought to result from two processes: reduced activation of the reward circuitry and activation of the stress of "anti-reward" systems in the greater amygdala.

Tolerance [6]

Tolerance is defined by either of the following:

1 a need for markedly increased amounts of a substance to achieve intoxication or a desired effect.

2 markedly diminished effect with continuous use of the same amount of a substance.

The important point here is that tolerance is an expected, neuroadaptive response to chronic agonist exposure. Whether this is good or bad depends on perspective. Tolerance to the cognitive impairment associated with opioids occurs relatively quickly and is considered a good thing; tolerance to the analgesic effects of an opioid is generally considered a bad thing. In a similar fashion, a person can lose tolerance, especially to the respiratory depressant effects of this class of drug, relatively quickly, increasing the risk of overdose and death, substantially [7].

Physical dependence/withdrawal

For the most part, physical dependency is an expected consequence of exposure to many agonist agents, including the opioid class of drugs. It is characterized as a "class-specific constellation of symptoms associated with abrupt discontinuation of a drug, rapid reduction in drug levels, or administration of an antagonist" [8].

Table 39.1 Opioid withdrawal symptoms.

Aches/pain	Hot flashes/chills
Muscle spasms/twitching/ and tension	Heart pounding
	Lacrimation
Tremor	Sweating
Abdominal cramps	Rhinorrhea
Nausea/vomiting/diarrhea	Pupillary dilatation
Anxiety/restlessness and dysphoria	Yawning
	Gooseflesh
Irritability	
Insomnia	

It is important to remember; withdrawal symptoms are typically the opposite of the therapeutic effect. As an example, sedatives that depress the reticular activating system lead to hyperactivity in that system upon withdrawal. In some cases, seizures may be the result. In the case of the opioid class of drugs, their primary sympatholytic effect leads to sympathetic over activity with multiple resulting symptoms (Table 39.1). As such, one of the common classes of non-opioid agents used to treat opioid withdrawal are the alpha-2-agonists such as clonidine. Their ability to mitigate symptoms of opioid withdrawal is only partial; opioid tapering, with or without substitution remains the gold standard for the acute management of opioid withdrawal.

Interestingly, through the phenomenon of cross tolerance, the symptoms of withdrawal can be reversed or mitigated by the reintroduction of the original drug or a drug of a similar class [8].

As a rule, the more potent, shorter acting agents have a more intense withdrawal syndrome than other, less potent or longer acting agents. It is important to note that withdrawal is less about drug levels than it is about rate of change of drug levels in the physically dependent user.

For example, if a methadone maintenance patient has a peak to trough ratio of 2, 50% of the peak drug level remains prior to administration of the next dose, assuming a "once daily" dosing regimen commonly seen in maintenance treatment.[1] Most patients are quite stable on once-daily dosing, even though the serum level of drug has been reduced by 50%.

Contrast this with an individual who is given an injection of the antagonist, naloxone. In this case, the abrupt reduction in μ agonist effect is generally very poorly tolerated. Unfortunately, individual response to serum levels of drugs is highly variable: generally, the longer the person is on the drug, and the higher the dose, the more severe are the withdrawal symptoms.

In fact, some people on relatively low doses of opioids may experience severe withdrawal; others on much higher doses seem relatively unaffected by relatively large dose reductions. As such, withdrawal symptoms should not be considered a reliable indicator of treatment compliance, even in patients on relatively large doses of medication.

It is also useful to look at opioid withdrawal in terms of early, "subjective" effects and late, "objective" effects. The early, subjective effects include a dysphoric state. The objective signs of withdrawal are typically more intense. For a more complete examination of opioid withdrawal assessment, the reader should review the original paper by Handelsman et al. [9].

With ongoing drug use, less dopamine is released and functional neuroimaging reveals reduced expression of dopamine D2 receptors in the reward circuits, especially in addicted individuals [10]. Both of these phenomena contribute to a reduced responsiveness of the reward system. As a result, normal adaptive behaviors become neglected in favor of the much more rewarding substance [11].

Activation of the "antireward" system in the amygdala also occurs at this stage [12]. Corticotropin-releasing factor (CRF), dynorphin, endocannabinoids and other neurotransmitters become over-expressed, promoting stress reactivity and intense dysphoria. Instead of experiencing the intense reward (i.e *euphoria* or pain relief) when they took the drug in the first stage, patients at this point will obtain diminishing reward over time and instead experience relief from an overwhelmingly negative experience. The quickest way for them to feel "normal" is to take more drug, an intensely powerful negative reinforcer. It is in this stage that patients act as if getting the drug is key to survival and will do "whatever it takes" to escape withdrawal and dysphoria. Thus, the subject is no longer using to get high but rather to feel once again normal. This concept is somewhat paradoxical and difficult to process for many clinicians unfamiliar with SUDs

In those with persistent pain, a parallel neuroplastic process amplifies the negative affect. The brain networks involved with pain shift central processing of pain away from sensory and towards emotional and cognitive brain areas, the same areas being disrupted by anti-reward activation [13]. Seeking pain relief from prescribed opioids AND the elimination of abstinence or withdrawal symptoms (between doses of the prescribed opioids) become strong conditioned reinforcers, as does everything along the way to obtaining that relief [14].

The ***preoccupation and anticipation stage*** occurs when a person may seek substances after a period of abstinence and becomes preoccupied with using again (i.e. craving). It is characterised by disruption of executive functions in the prefrontal cortex (PFC), such as self-regulation, decision making and importantly exercises control over incentive salience, a cognitive process that confers desire and motivation to cues associated with stimuli. Many neuroscientists understand the function of the PFC as a balance between a "Go" system and a "Stop" system [11]. The upregulation of the Go system by the increased activity of glutamate increases cravings and habits associated with substance use, while the downregulated Stop circuits lead to more impulsivity and compulsive drug seeking and less dampening of the stress circuits.

The power of drugs of abuse, including pain medications, to produce feelings of wellbeing and relief from negative feelings (and/or pain) can foster the emergence of compulsive use. The development of addiction requires not only repeated or ongoing exposure to a medication or substance that is potentially addicting, but also must occur in an individual with certain biological, psychological, genetic and sociological susceptibilities. With increased salience (binge/intoxication stage), combined with reduced reward and increased stress sensitivity (withdrawal/negative affect stage) and impaired executive function, a perfect storm of neuroplasticity can result in drug seeking and use especially in those at risk and can become overpowering.

One should understand the difference between addiction and physical dependence. The latter is a

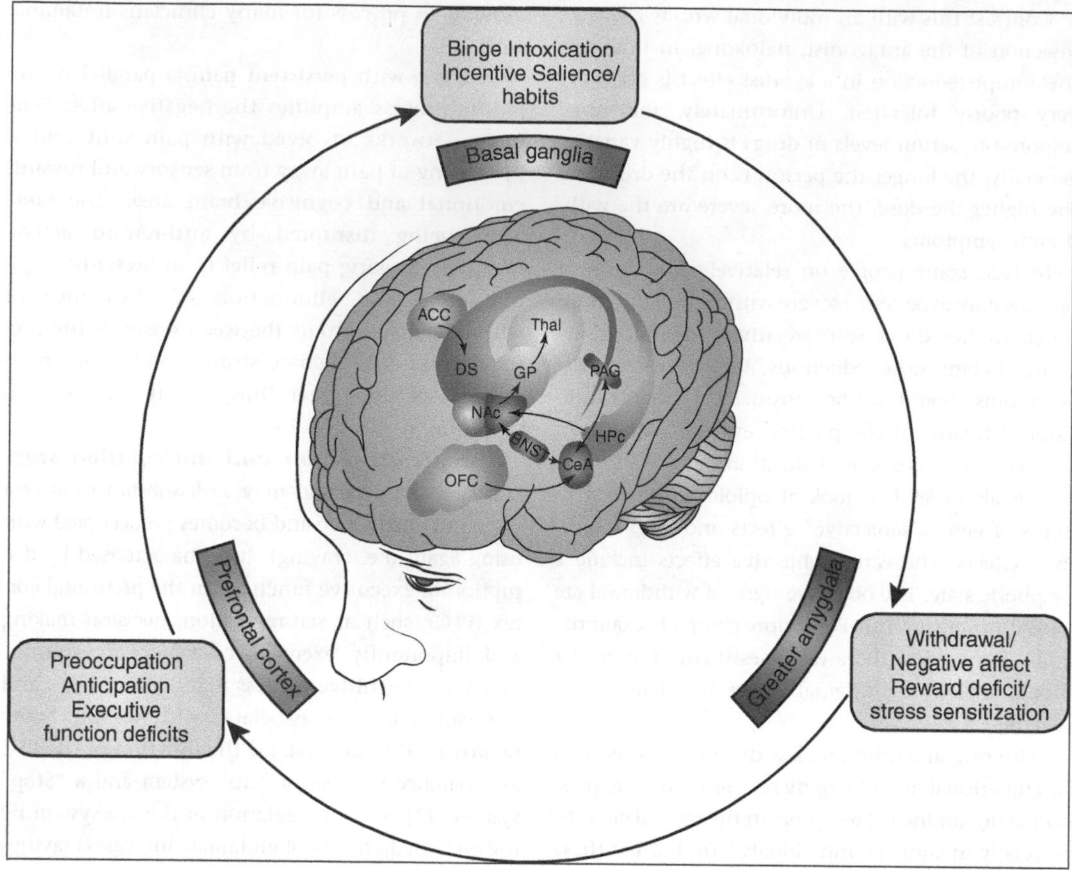

Figure 39.1 Stages of the addiction cycle. During intoxication, drug-induced activation of the brain's reward regions (in blue) is enhanced by conditioned cues in areas of increased sensitization (in green). During withdrawal, the activation of brain regions involved in emotions (in pink) results in negative mood and enhanced sensitivity to stress. During preoccupation, the decreased function of the prefrontal cortex leads to an inability to balance the strong desire for the drug with the will to abstain, which triggers relapse and reinitiates the cycle of addiction. The compromised neurocircuitry reflects the disruption of the dopamine and glutamate systems and the stress-control systems of the brain, which are affected by corticotropin-releasing factor and dynorphin. The behaviors during the three stages of addiction change as a person transitions from drug experimentation to addiction as a function of the progressive neuroadaptations that occur in the brain. ACC, anterior cingulate cortex; BNST, basal nucleus of the stria terminalis; CeA, central nucleus of the amygdala – change to Amyg on diagram (Amyg, central nucleaus of the amygdala); DS, dorsal striatum; GP, globus pallidus; HPC, hippocampus; NAC, nucleus accumbens; OFC, orbitofrontal cortex; PAG, periaqueductal gray; Thal, thalamus (Color Plate 9) [Modified from Koob and Volkow 105].

normal, expected neurophysiological adaptation that occurs with chronic exposure to certain classes of substances, and is manifest by a withdrawal syndrome specific to a class of medication or substance which is abruptly discontinued or reduced. Physical dependence is neither necessary nor sufficient in the diagnosis of an addiction [15], and, in fact, is mediated by different neural pathways than those involved with addiction [8, 16].

The application of our understanding of the neurobiology of addiction to the problematic use of prescribed medications for the legitimate treatment of chronic pain remains a point of constant debate. However, taking a consistent approach to assessing these susceptibilities in all patients before embarking on treatment and all through their trajectory of care will result in less risk and significantly improved outcomes (Figure 39.1).

Approach to clinical care in the physically dependent/substance use disordered pain patient

In recent years, clinical approaches to the chronic use of the opioid class of drugs in the management of pain has fallen out of favor. The early use of opioids, in often excessively high doses has been replaced by a much more cautious and sadly, not always rational use of these potent drugs[17]. Pharmacologic principles such as "full μ agonists have no ceiling" were interpreted as meaning "no limit to clinical dosing", leading to excessive use of medication by some patients with chronic pain. Of course, this pharmacologic principle must always be offset by a careful risk/benefit analysis. Once again, the pendulum has swung from the liberal use of opioids to a much more constrained view of these medications.

As a result, sometimes onerous restrictions have been placed on these opioids, resulting in many legitimate patients with pain, often the more marginalized ones, being subjected to forced dose reductions and, in some cases, "tapers to discontinuation." Unfortunately, this has led some patients to depart from traditional medical sources of these drugs, instead turning to non-medical sources of drugs. Many of these are counterfeit, often laced with high potency opioids such as fentanyl or even carfentanyl, with tragic results.

In this sense, there most certainly is a prescription opioid problem in North America. Unlike previous years where the use was almost ad lib, excessive restrictions are now leading established medical users to find their previously prescribed opioid drugs being supplied by illegitimate sources. In doing so, the illegal drug trade in counterfeit pharmaceuticals blossomed, leaving a trail of despair and death in their wakes [18, 19].

From the previous section on addiction medicine, there is an undeniable but complex difference between simple physical dependency and the complex disease of addiction. This difference becomes more challenging when the agent of misuse is prescribed legally by a medical professional [20].

Ballantyne et al opined that the terms opioid dependence and addiction might essentially be "a distinction without a difference"[21]. Unfortunately, words matter, especially in the context of both social and regulatory scrutiny [6]. While this point would certainly cause significant consternation in traditional addiction medicine circles, it may be a practical approach to take when dealing with the complexities of problematic use of medications. This is especially true in patients who have been legally prescribed these therapeutic agents. If carefully set limits and boundaries are the bulwarks of treatment in both the patient with complex pain and the patient dealing with problematic substance use, it might simply be better to avoid the stigmatizing labels and take a pragmatic approach to this issue.

There is little disagreement within the medical community about the inappropriateness of using cocaine or methamphetamines. There really is no accepted medical purpose in using either for the treatment of chronic pain. In these cases, the diagnosis of a SUD is relatively straightforward.

When there is a therapeutic indication for a drug that is being used problematically, such as the opioid or benzodiazepine class of drugs, these agents may initially be therapeutically effective. Over time, at least for some predisposed individuals, therapeutic use may become problematic and, in some cases, even rising to the level of a SUD. The use may be therapeutically defensible, but no longer appropriate in the full context of careful risk/benefit analysis. In many of these problematic users, there are personal or familial cautionary warning flags that either went ignored or were unelicited. Although there is no firm data in this regard to guide us, it is thought that de novo drug misuse in patients without such risk factors is likely low [22, 23], the fact is we simply do not know. For this reason, application of carefully set limits and boundaries in ALL patients, at least until actual risk is more clearly established, has become a prudent practitioners' safe harbor in these challenging times.

While the above is true, there are practical consequences for a physically dependent patient with chronic pain with inadequate opioid levels. They all will experience some degree of withdrawal. In fact, withdrawal may best be thought of as a progressive state beginning with mild Subjective Symptoms and progressing to a more severe Objective Withdrawal state [24, 25]. In some cases, there may even be a post-acute withdrawal syndrome lasting several months or more [26].

This state of early, subjective withdrawal can lead to a marked increase in the underlaying complaint of pain. It often goes unrecognized by patient and practitioner alike as opioid withdrawal, especially if they have had some personal experience in the past with severe, objective withdrawal. Because the complaints of pain at least partially respond to the correction of the "Opioid Debt" [27, 28] by the addition of the deficient drug, the ongoing use of opioids is further reinforced. Opioid withdrawal is a hypersensitive state leading to an amplification of all types of pain, even with pain mechanisms that would not typically be considered "opioid responsive" [29].

From the patient's perspective, the "opioid medication might just take the edge off their daily pain", but when they miss a dose, the pain is significantly worse. Clearly, the drug seems to be exerting some positive role in the management of their pain. In fact, the ongoing use of opioids may be more for the treatment of a physical dependency, rather than the original intent of providing optimum μ analgesia. This should not be considered as "opioid maintenance treatment" but rather, optimizing μ opioid tone. In some cases, the distinction may seem to be without a difference, but in some jurisdictions, special licensure is required for maintenance agonist treatment. The legal requirements for the use of opioids in the treatment of acute or chronic pain is much less complicated, typically requiring an authorized individual to be operating within the course of their usual and customary medical practice.

Unfortunately, the chronic use of opioids does lead to some unavoidable consequences such as a lowered pain threshold. So, if your patient is not clearly "winning" with chronic opioid therapy, they are likely paying an unacceptable price to continue this course of treatment. It is likely you have a patient in your practice who has a diminished pain tolerance who is physically dependent on their medication and is suffering from all the negative consequences of the chronic use of this class of drug. The fact that pain gets worse when the dose is diminished or discontinued does not support the presence of opioid-responsive pain. Again, it may simply serve to reinforce the fact that virtually all pain gets worse in the context of opioid withdrawal [30].

In a similar way, most chronic pain seems to respond, at least initially to the introduction of opioids. The sustainability of this response will help determine if the pain is in fact truly opioid responsive or simply a case of the novelty of a new therapeutic agent. Dose escalation with the development of tolerance tends to suggest the latter mechanism might at work. It may be useful to apply a "Timeline Followback" [31] approach to help clarify the pro and con of continued reliance on the current medication regimen. Of course, getting onto agonist therapy is typically much easier than reducing or discontinuing these agents.

While it is true that all withdrawal symptoms can be mitigated, it is impossible to eliminate all withdrawal symptoms even in the most cleverly designed taper protocols. "Beware of the agonist debt"[20] (i.e. worsening pain that results from inadequate agonist levels in a physically dependent patient) is an important warning that many clinicians seem unaware of even today.

More recently, micro doses of buprenorphine (with or without naloxone) has been found to be an effective method to transition from the full mu agonist class of drugs. Traditionally, conventional wisdom has been that buprenorphine should not be introduced to a fully mu dependent patient without a preceding period of abstinence. While it is true that the addition of milligram doses of a partial mu agonist to a fully mu dependent subject can precipitate acute withdrawal, this is not necessarily the case when the crossover is started with microdoses [32-35] of the partial agonist. Again, withdrawal is more about rate of change of drug levels rather than absolute levels of drug.

A detailed exploration of this process is beyond the scope of this chapter, however interested readers may find a recent review article by T Kosten et al on the subject useful [36].

Pain and chemical dependency: not an either/or proposition

Despite the many papers published about the prevalence of addiction within the population of patients with chronic pain, there really is no widespread agreement between either the addiction medicine community or pain management clinicians of the actual magnitude of the problem. Clearly, aberrant behavior may be present in situations of undertreated pain or where there is a SUD; it is important to take steps to distinguish the two.

To address some of these issues, the concept of "Universal Precautions in the management of chronic pain" was introduced in 2005 [28, 37, 38]. The novelty of the paper was to suggest that the 10 steps of risk assessment, mitigation and management be applied to ALL patients. This risk is also dynamic. In other words, an apparently lower risk patient may, under stress exhibit at-risk behaviors that normalize with more structure and support in the treatment plan.

In practical terms, it is helpful to remember that a SUD (for the prescribed medication) is often best diagnosed prospectively in people with chronic pain, over time, through systematic monitoring for aberrant drug-related behaviors in the context of reasonably set limits and boundaries. In fact, some patterns of patient behavior may be iatrogenically driven. This is commonly seen with excessively tight limits and boundaries that even healthy patients would likely transgress. Regardless of etiology, aberrant behavior is unacceptable. As such, it should be identified, where it exists, discussed with the patient and steps taken to address this behavior.

Legitimate versus appropriate factors in considering a trial of opioid therapy [39]

Many patients with chronic pain still consider the opioid class of drugs as the "Holy Grail" of pain management. For some, it represents the belief that their clinician "takes their pain, seriously". For others, the use of potent opioids gives them a sense of control[40]; sometimes, even in the absence of objective improvement of pain or function. While this is certainly the case in acute, severe pain it is becoming apparent that this is not the case for most patients with chronic pain.

In most cases of chronic unremitting pain, the decision to initiate a trial of opioid therapy, assuming all state and federal regulations are met, can be considered a legitimate therapeutic choice. Unfortunately, a legitimate indication may not be sufficient to support this choice. The appropriateness of any therapeutic treatment plan depends on much more than what is required for legitimate use. It must also meet the test of "appropriateness." Some of the added issues to consider include a personal and family history of risk. Social circumstances of the patient such as homelessness or concurrent illicit drug use must also be considered to mention only two factors. In fact, there are both patient and prescriber issues to consider.

For the prescriber, it may be legitimate to prescribe 500 tablets of a controlled substance to be dispensed at one time, but it would rarely be appropriate, regardless of the apparent benefit to the patient. The regulatory scrutiny that would result, would be both unwelcomed and unnecessary. As well, patients tend to have less trouble adhering to treatment plans with smaller quantities of medications than with a seemingly inexhaustible supply [28].

Similarly, a palliative care patient may have a legitimate indication for chronic opioid therapy, but it may not be appropriate for a community-based prescriber to continue this therapy with evidence of ongoing cocaine use. These risks are often better managed through referral.

As stated previously, the basic tenet of Universal Precautions is that you "Can't judge a book by its cover". In this regard, the following 10 principles are worth considering in the treatment of any chronic condition, especially chronic pain.

Universal precautions in pain medicine [37]

The following universal precautions are recommended as a guide for all healthcare professionals who prescribe opioid medications to treat chronic pain. As with universal precautions in infectious diseases [41], applying the following recommendations can result in improved patient care, stigma reduction and lower overall risk.

The 10 steps of universal precautions in pain medicine:

1 Make a diagnosis with an appropriate differential. Treatable causes for pain should be identified when they exist and therapy should be directed to the cause of pain. Any comorbid conditions, including SUDs and other psychiatric illnesses, must also be addressed.

2 Perform a psychological assessment, including risk of addictive disorders. A complete inquiry into past personal and family history of substance misuse is essential to adequately assess any patient. A sensitive and respectful assessment of risk should not be seen in any way as diminishing a patient's complaint of pain. Patient-centered urine drug testing should be discussed with all patients regardless of the medications that they are currently taking [42, 43]. Patients found to be using illicit or unprescribed licit drugs should be offered further assessment for possible SUDs. Those refusing such assessment should be considered unsuitable for pain management with a controlled substance.

3 Obtain tnformed consent. The healthcare professional must discuss the proposed treatment plan with patients and answer any questions that they may have about its anticipated benefits and foreseeable risks.

4 Develop a treatment agreement. The expectations and obligations of both the patient and the treating practitioner need to be clearly set forth in writing or by verbal agreement. Combined with informed consent, the treatment agreement forms the basis of the therapeutic trial. A carefully worded treatment agreement will help to clarify appropriately set boundary limits making possible early identification and intervention around aberrant behaviors [44, 45].

5 Assess pre- and post-intervention pain level and function. It must be emphasized that any treatment plan must begin with a trial of therapy. This is particularly true when controlled substances are contemplated or used. Without a documented assessment of preintervention pain scores and level of function, it will be difficult to assess success in any medication trial. The ongoing assessment and documentation of successfully met clinical goals will support the continuation of any mode of therapy. Failure to meet these goals will necessitate re-evaluation and possible change in the treatment plan.

6 Use an appropriate trial of opioid therapy with or without adjunctive medication. Pharmacologic regimens must be individualized on the basis of subjective as well as objective clinical findings. The appropriate combination of agents, including opioids and adjunctive medications, may be seen as "rational pharmacotherapy" and provide a stable therapeutic platform from which to base treatment changes.

7 Reassess pain score and level of function. Regular reassessment of the patient combined with corroborative support from family or other knowledgeable third parties will help document the rationale to continue or modify the current therapeutic trial.

8 Regularly assess the "4 A's" of pain medicine. Routine assessment of analgesia, activity, adverse effects and aberrant behaviors will help to direct therapy and support pharmacologic options taken [46].

9 Periodically review pain diagnosis and comorbid conditions, including addictive disorders. Underlying illnesses evolve. Diagnostic tests change with time. As a result, treatment focus may need to change over the course of time. If an addictive disorder predominates, aggressive treatment of an underlying pain problem will likely fail if not coordinated with treatment for the concurrent addictive disorder.

10 Complete thorough documentation. Careful and complete recording of the initial evaluation and each follow-up is both medicolegally indicated and in the best interest of all parties. Thorough documentation combined with an appropriate clinician-patient relationship will reduce medicolegal exposure and risk of regulatory sanction.

In the assessment of any patient with chronic pain, especially those considered to be at elevated risk, the following approach may be useful in treating this often-challenging patient population.

In the context of risk management, three important clinical determinations are key:

1 Does the patient have a pain problem? It is generally wise to accept this at face value.

2 Is there a SUD? The answer may be "possibly."

3 If both a pain problem and a SUD are present (i.e. pain and a high risk of SUD), which is dominant?

Remember, you cannot solve a chronic pain condition in the face of an active, untreated addiction. Of course, this does not mean you cannot treat pain in a patient with a SUD, it simply reminds the reader of the increased challenges they are likely to face.

Monitoring and medical necessity

[42, 47]. It is important to accept that ALL chronic use of the opioid class of drugs carries with it a degree of risk. ALL patients on chronic therapy should be

provided with varying degrees of structure and support that reflect this risk. Examples include more frequent in-person follow-ups, drug testing, "do not fill until" prescriptions, the use of "pill counts" are all useful tools to credibly address this perceived risk. As time progresses, a more accurate assessment of actual risk will become apparent.

Unfortunately, risk is not static and can change over time. A high-risk patient can, with treatment move into a moderate risk categorization but they cannot move into a low-risk classification. Elevated risk once identified cannot be eliminated, only managed. It is always easier to loosen tight limits and boundaries that were appropriate during the initial assessment and management period than it is to tighten lax boundaries in response to problematic behavior.

It is important to remember that drug testing is not a treatment for a SUD. However, it is a good way to remind the patient and others who might review your clinical treatment plan, that you have an appreciation of, and a commitment to managing risk.

There is a misconception that in a perfect world, where drug testing incurred no costs, all patients should be tested all the time. The fact is that you can test too frequently. There is no evidence, even in high-risk patients, that more frequent testing leads to better outcomes. Medically necessary drug testing should include the following 3 points:

1 The clinician has a clinical reason for doing the test.

2 The results obtained are discussed with the patient and clinical decisions are made to reflect this risk.

3 This is all appropriately documented in the patient's medical record.

Failure to apply rational clinical judgement to drug testing may lead to a variety of patient care issues that negatively impact treatment outcomes.

The following clinical pearls may be useful to remember when treating chronic pain.

Aberrant behavior

Why the patient is behaving aberrantly is often less important than focusing on the behavior itself – i.e., it might not be addiction driving it, but the behavior is unacceptable. As such it must be documented and treatment plans adjusted accordingly. Never forget the immutables. Missed appointments; emergency refills at the end of the day; ad abnormal or missed drug tests should never be ignored. While there are many appropriate courses of action to take in the context of an abnormal urine drug test (UDT) result or abnormal pattern of behavior, there is one absolutely incorrect thing to do, whicht is to ignore it!

Patient risk

"If your patient has a pulse, they have risk." It may be low, moderate or high, but risk is there. It cannot be eliminated, only managed.

Drug testing

UDT is not therapeutic in and of itself. Its use should be predicated on "medical necessity". A UDT result cannot diagnose a SUD, physical dependence or diversion. However, it may be a useful adjunct to the assessment of all these problems.

The Golden Moment

Never miss the Golden Moment when the patient begins to see things the way they are, not the way that they wished that things were [43]. For some patients, struggling with problematic use of their medications, a brief intervention from a compassionate caregiver may be all that is needed to plant the seeds of change. Assessment of a "possible" SUD must be clearly framed in terms of a possible complication, not a dismissal of any underlying complaint of pain.

Identify, stabilize, refer:

As needed, patients should be referred either to a pain management specialist or, in more severe cases, to a specialist in addiction medicine.

Patient selection

Know which patients can be safely managed as low risk, patients at added risk needing co-management with a specialist and those patients at such high risk they might need transfer to someone with more experience and more resources to safely care for them.

Diagnosing addiction

The diagnosis of addiction is most often made, prospectively over time [39]. A patient who continues to step out of reasonably set boundaries despite the appropriate management of their pain is likely suffering from another, as yet unidentified disorder, which could include SUD.

Time management

It takes 30 seconds to say "Yes" and 30 minutes to say "No" when writing a prescription, use your time wisely! Giving a patient a prescription you are uncomfortable with may seem, at the time, to temporize a difficult situation. Making the wrong decision in the interest of expediency may at best compromise patient care. At worst, it might result in a patient's death.

Conclusions

The management of any patient with chronic pain is often time-consuming and complex. Not all clinicians have the experience or resources to safely treat this challenging population. In pain management it is important to identify co-morbid SUDs when present as well as patterns of problematic medication use to insure appropriate support and treatment in the overall treatment plan. This chapter has presented an approach to guide the front-line clinician on how to approach this complex area.

References

1 Heit AH, Gourlay DL (2018) The treatment of chronic pain in patient's with a history of substance abuse. In: *Bonica's Management of Pain*, 5th edn. Ballantyne JF, Fishmann SM, ds. Lippincott Williams and Wilkins, Philadelphia. pp. 1001-11.

2 Volkow ND, Koob GF, McLellan AT. (2016) Neurobiologic Advances from the Brain Disease Model of Addiction. *N Engl J Med* **374**(4):363-71.

3 American Society of Addiction Medicine. (2011) Public Policy Statement : Definition of Addiction. Available at: https://www.asam.org/Quality-Science/definition-of-addiction. Accessed Nov 7, 2021.

4 Volkow N.D, Morales M. (2015) The brain on drugs: from reward to addiction. *Cell* **162**(4):712-25.

5 Koob GF and Volkow ND. (2016) Neurobiology of addiction: a neurocircuitry analysis. *Lancet Psychiatry* **3**(8):760-773.

6 Heit HA and DL Gourlay. (2009) DSM-V and the definitions: time to get it right. *Pain Med* **10**(5):784-6.

7 Joudrey PJ, Khan MR, Wang EA *et al.*, (2019) A conceptual model for understanding post-release opioid-related overdose risk. *Addict Sci Clin Pract* **14**(1):17.

8 Savage SR, Joranson DE, Covington EC, Schnoll SH, Heit HA, Gilson AM *et al.* (2003) Definitions related to the medical use of opioids: evolution towards universal agreement. *J Pain Symptom Manage* **26**(1):655-67.

9 Handelsman L, Cochrane JK, Aaronson MJ, Ness R, Rubenstein KJ, Kanof PD *et al.* (1987) Two new rating scales for opiate withdrawal. *Am J Drug Alcohol Abuse* **13**(3):293-308.

10 Volkow ND, Tomasi D, Wang G-J *et al.* (2014) Stimulant-induced dopamine increases are markedly blunted in active cocaine abusers. *Mol Psychiatry* **19**(9):1037-43.

11 Koob GF, Le Moal M. (2001) Drug addiction, dysregulation of reward, and allostasis. *Neuropsychopharmacology* **24**(2):97-129.

12 Koob GF. (2020) Neurobiology of opioid addiction: opponent process, hyperkatifeia, and negative reinforcement. *Biol Psychiatry* **87**(1):44-53.

13 Kucyi A, Davis KD. (2017) The neural code for pain: from single-cell electrophysiology to the dynamic pain connectome. *Neuroscientist* **23**(4):397-414.

14 Ewan EE, Martin TJ. (2013) Analgesics as reinforcers with chronic pain: evidence from operant studies. *Neurosci Lett* **557 Pt A**:60-4.

15 Wise RA Koob GF. (2014) The development and maintenance of drug addiction. *Neuropsychopharmacology* **39**(2):254-62.

16 Heit, H.A. (2003) Addiction, physical dependence, and tolerance: precise definitions to help clinicians evaluate and treat chronic pain patients. *J Pain Palliat Care Pharmacother* **17**(1):15-29.

17 Bohnert ASB, Guy, Jr GP, Losby JL. (2018) Opioid prescribing in the United States before and after the Centers for Disease Control and Prevention's 2016 opioid guideline. *Ann Intern Med* **169**(6):367-75.

18 Green TC Gilbert M. (2016) Counterfeit medications and fentanyl. *JAMA Intern Med* **176**(10):1555-7.

19 Blackstone EA, Fuhr, Jr JP, Pociask S. (2014) The health and economic effects of counterfeit drugs. *Am Health Drug Benefits* **7**(4):216-24.

20 Gourlay DL Heit HA. (2008) Pain and addiction: managing risk through comprehensive care. *J Addict Dis* **27**(3):23-30.

21 Ballantyne JC, Sullivan MD, Kolodny A. (2012) Opioid dependence vs addiction: a distinction without a difference? *Arch Intern Med* **172**(17):1342-3.

22 Hojsted J, Sjogren P. (2007) Addiction to opioids in chronic pain patients: a literature review. *Eur J Pain* **11**(5):490-518.

23 Milledge JS. (2001) Opioids in chronic non-malignant pain. Opioids can cause addiction even in patients with pain. *BMJ* **323**(7312):571-2.

24 Bergeria CL, Huhn HL, Tompkins DA, Bigelow GE, Strain EC, Dunn Ke. (2019) The relationship between pupil diameter and other measures of opioid withdrawal during naloxone precipitated withdrawal. *Drug Alcohol Depend* **202**:111-4.

25 Malcolm BJ, Polanco M, Barsuglia JP. (2018) Changes in withdrawal and craving scores in participants undergoing opioid detoxification utilizing ibogaine. *J Psychoactive Drugs*. **50**(3):256-65.

26 Jasinski DR. (1981) Opiate withdrawal syndrome: acute and protracted aspects. *Ann N Y Acad Sci* **362**:183-6.

27 Wilson JL, Poulin PA, Sikorski R, Nathan HJ, Taljaard M, Smyth C. (2015) Opioid use among same-day surgery patients: prevalence, management and outcomes. *Pain Res Manag* **20**(6):300-4.

28 Gourlay DL, Heit HA. (2009) Universal precautions revisited: managing the inherited pain patient. *Pain Med* **10** Suppl 2: S115-23.

29 Indelicato RA, Portenoy RK. (2002) Opioid rotation in the management of refractory cancer pain. *J Clin Oncol* **20**(1):348-52.

30 Younger J, Barelka P, Carroll I *et al.* (2008) Reduced cold pain tolerance in chronic pain patients following opioid detoxification. *Pain Med* **9**(8):1158-63.

31 Sobell LC, Brown J, Leo GI, Sobell MB. (1996) The reliability of the Alcohol Timeline Followback when administered by telephone and by computer. *Drug Alcohol Depend* **42**(1):49-54.

32 Wong, J.S.H., et al., Comparing rapid micro-induction and standard induction of buprenorphine/naloxone for treatment of opioid use disorder: protocol for an open-label, parallel-group, superiority, randomized controlled trial. *Addict Sci Clin Pract*, 2021. **16**(1): p. 11.

33 Ahmed, S., et al., Microinduction of Buprenorphine/Naloxone: A Review of the Literature. *Am J Addict*, 2020.

34 Moe J, O'Sullivan F, Hohl CM *et al.* (2021) Short communication: systematic review on effectiveness of micro-induction approaches to buprenorphine initiation. *Addict Behav* **114**:106740.

35 De Aquino JP, Fairgrieve C, Klaire S, Garcia-Vassallo G. (2020) Rapid transition from methadone to cuprenorphine utilizing a micro-dosing protocol in the outpatient Veteran Affairs setting. *J Addict Med* **14**(5):e271-3.

36 Kosten TR, Baxter LE. (2019) Review article: effective management of opioid withdrawal symptoms: a gateway to opioid dependence treatment. *Am J Addict* **28**(2):55-62.

37 Gourlay DL, Heit HA, Almahrezi A. (2005) Universal precautions in pain medicine: a rational approach to the treatment of chronic pain. *Pain Med* **6**(2):107-12.

38 Gourlay DL, Heit HA. (2011) Universal precautions: it's not about the molecule! *J Pain* **12**(6):722; author reply 723-4.

39 Heit AH, Gourlay DL (2018) The treatment of chronic pain in patient's with a history of substance abuse. In: *Bonica's Management of Pain*, 5th edn. Ballantyne JF, Fishmann SM, ds. Lippincott Williams and Wilkins, Philadelphia. pp. 1896.

40 Ljungvall H, Rhodin A, Wagner S, Zetterberg H, Åsenlöf P *et al.* (2020) "My life is under control with these medications": an interpretative phenomenological analysis of managing chronic pain with opioids. *BMC Musculoskelet Disord* **21**(1):61.

41 Broussard IM, Kahwaji CI. (2020) Universal precautions. StatPearls Publishing, Treasure Island.

42 Gourlay D, Heit H, Caplan YH. (2012) *Urine Drug Testing in Clinical Practice - The Art and Science of Patient Care,* 5th edn. Johns Hopkins University School of Medicine, Baltimore.

43 Heit HA, Gourlay DL. (2015) Using urine drug testing to support healthy boundaries in clinical care. *J Opioid Manag* **11**(1):7-12.

44 Nikulina V, Guarino H, Acosta MC *et al.* (2016) Patient vs provider reports of aberrant medication-taking behavior among opioid-treated patients with chronic pain who report misusing opioid medication. *Pain* **157**(8):1791-8.

45 Starrels JL, Becker WC, Alford DP, Kapoor A, Williamson AR, Burner BJ. (2010) Systematic review: treatment agreements and urine drug testing to reduce opioid misuse in patients with chronic pain. *Ann Intern Med* **152**(11):712-20

46 Passik SD, Weinreb HJ. (2000) Managing chronic nonmalignant pain: overcoming obstacles to the use of opioids. *Adv Ther* **17**(2):70-83.

47 Practice Guidelines for Ordering Urine Testing for Drugs-of-Abuse: Targeted and Screening Tests (CLP013). Ontario Association of Medical Laboratories. https://oaml.com/wp-content/uploads/2016/05/OAMLGUIDELINEFOR-ORDERINGDOAFINALMarch142013.pdf. Accessed April 9, 2021.

Notes

1 The duration of action of methadone as a maintenance drug is substantially different from that typically needed as an analgesic. This requires 2- or 3-times daily dosing for methadone when used as an analgesic. When once daily dosing of methadone results in 24 hr pain relief, consideration of a withdrawal-mediated mechanism of pain should be considered.

Part 9

Special Populations

Chapter 40

Pain in older adults: a brief clinical guide

Thomas Hadjistavropoulos[1] **& Una E. Makris**[2]

[1] *Department of Psychology and Centre on Aging and Health, University of Regina, Saskatchewan, Canada*
[2] *University of Texas Southwestern Medical Center, Dallas, Texas, USA*

Epidemiology

Pain affects people of all ages with epidemiological studies reporting exceedingly high prevalence rates of pain in general community samples and even higher rates in institutional settings. The absolute prevalence figures for persistent pain in the general population vary widely and depend upon the sample being examined (community, hospital, outpatient settings etc), the severity of pain to classify a case (i.e. any, bothersome, disabling, significant), the time interval sampled (i.e. right now, past week or months, etc.), the time in pain during this interval (i.e. every day, most days, or any pain during the period), and the sampling technique (i.e. telephone survey, interview, questionnaire etc) (e.g. [1, 2]). Specifically for older adults, the prevalence of bothersome pain over the last month in a sample of over 7,000 adults 65 years of age or older was estimated as being greater than 52%; 74% of those with pain endorsed multiple pain sites [3]. Patel et al. [3] also showed that pain reports were strongly associated with decreased physical function.

Examining chronic pain (defined as duration for at least three months), Larsson et al. [4] estimated a 38.5% prevalence in people who were at least 65 years of age. Pain in long-term care environments appears to be even more common. Although estimates vary from study to study, they have been found to be as high as 83% [5, 6]. Females are more likely to suffer from pain than males, although the magnitude of gender difference may decrease in very old age.

The Undertreatment of Pain Among Older Adults

When considering the high prevalence of pain in later life and the potentially taxing implications for health service delivery, it is important to understand that not all persistent pain will be bothersome or of high impact. Indeed, many older adults will not seek treatment for pain and will manage pain symptoms without help. That said, a survey of members of the American Academy of Pain Medicine and the American Pain Society [7] identified the undertreatment of pain among older adults and the inadequate pain assessment among persons with dementia as being among the most pressing ethical concerns for pain clinicians. More recent evidence suggests that the issue of pain undertreatment in the general older adult

Clinical Pain Management: A Practical Guide, Second Edition. Edited by Mary E. Lynch, Kenneth D. Craig, and Philip W. Peng.

population continues to be an issue [8, 9] although better quality studies assessing the extent of pain undertreatment in community dwelling dementia patients are still needed [10]. Pain undertreatment appears to be substantial for patients with cognitive impairments who reside in long-term care (LTC) facilities [11]. Specifically, it has been demonstrated in several studies that patients with cognitive impairments tend to receive considerably less pain medication than their cognitively intact counterparts, despite a similar prevalence of pain problems [12, 13]. A Canadian study suggests that patients with pain, who have cognitive impairments, are often likely to be prescribed psychotropic rather than analgesic medications [14]. It is noted, however, that recent investigations from Denmark and Norway suggest that the frequency of pain undertreatment may be decreasing in those countries [15, 16].

In addition to challenges that are common among most age groups, the assessment of older adults is complicated further by the entrenched but misleading notion that having pain is "natural" in old age [17, 18]. While pain problems are frequent in this population, if we think of pain as being "natural" for this age group, we would be less likely to treat it than we would be for younger persons. Pain results from pathology rather than from old age per se and, as such, should not be considered to be natural. Other factors that have been cited as contributing to the undertreatment of pain among older adults include sensory (e.g. a patient may not be able to hear staff questions about his or her functioning due to hearing loss) and cognitive impairments that affect some older individuals, concerns about the risk of addiction to opioids and a possible stoicism may make many older adults less likely to report pain [18, 19]. Moreover, nurses identify insufficient access to available assessment methodologies, inadequate pain education, and insufficient time as being barriers to adequate pain management in older adults [18, 20], despite advances of pain assessment methodologies for seniors with dementia [21–23]. Other research has raised concerns about inadequate communication between long-term care facility nurses and family physicians of patients with some physicians not having adequate trust in LTC nurses for making decisions about narcotics and other pain medications [24].

Age-related Change in Pain Sensitivity and Nociceptive Processing

Experimental studies have shown small, although somewhat inconsistent, increases in pain threshold with advancing age (i.e. a reduced sensitivity to faint pain) [25–27]. Age-related threshold changes may be specific to certain stimulus modalities. For example, El Tumi et al. [28] found age-related reductions in pressure pain thresholds but no age differences in contact heat thresholds. Recent meta-analytic research has casted doubt on earlier claims that there are age-related reductions in ability to tolerate pain [27]. Moreover, there are inconsistencies in findings regarding the role of dementia in the pain experience, especially in experimental research [29]. Studies that rely on self-report, and are reporting lower levels of pain in dementia, are confounded by the limitations in ability to provide self-report that can result from the dementing process. Nonetheless, neuroimaging research on central nervous system processing revealed significantly greater pain-related activations in patients with Alzheimer's disease (i.e. dorsolateral prefrontal cortex, mid cingulate cortex and insula; [30]) and some research focusing on nonverbal pain reactions suggested that people with dementia may react with more vigor to painful situations [31]. It is, nonetheless, difficult to reconcile the disparate findings. Pain perception with the progression of dementia remains unclear and further research is needed in order to answer this important question. At the present time, there is no convincing evidence that dementia results in clinically significant reductions in pain-related suffering.

The Clinical Pain Assessment of the Cognitively Intact Older Adult

The successful treatment of pain always relies on appropriate assessment. Regardless of whether pain is acute or persistent, it is important to assess all factors that may contribute to the pain as well as the prospect of remedial or curative actions. With persistent pain, a more comprehensive approach is required, including the evaluation of physical functioning (disability, interference with daily activities), psychosocial function (mood, interpersonal relationships, sleep, cognitive function), beliefs and attitudes to pain (fear of harm, ability to cope, meaning of symptoms) and general quality of life. Each of these aspects of a comprehensive assessment provides information that is essential to development of a tailored pain management program consistent with the specific needs of the older individual [22, 23]. Importantly, understanding the multiple potential contributors and often multifactorial pathway that results in persistent pain is critical in older adults [32].

The first vital step in pain assessment should be by patient self-report whenever possible and may include a structured history that ascertains onset, location, intensity, periodicity, quality, aggravating and relieving factors, and impact of pain [23]. The older adults should be given every opportunity to provide this history and the person taking the history should be a skilled communication partner. Sufficient time, adequate proximity, lighting and sensory assistive devices (i.e. glasses, hearing aid) should be utilized when required. The medical components of an assessment should include making a diagnostic formulation for the cause of pain and this can be more difficult in an older person as they often have pathology in several bodily systems (e.g. musculoskeletal, vascular, neurological) that may contribute to the pain through a variety of different mechanisms. In addition, it is important to evaluate all medications that the patient is already taking, especially in the context of renal or hepatic disease, alertness, cognitive impairment, issues with balance and general frailty, since these problems may restrict the available pharmacological pain treatment options.

The use of psychometric tools can help to provide a standardized assessment of pain and related suffering. Numerous unidimensional and multidimensional self-report measures of pain have been developed and, in general, tools with demonstrated merit in younger adult populations are also thought to be useful with older adults. Several different types of self-report scales exist, including verbal descriptors (i.e. none, mild, moderate, severe), numeric ratings (i.e. 0–10), visual analogue scales, complex qualitative word lists (i.e. McGill Pain Questionnaire; [33]), and more graphic representations, such as the pain thermometer, colored analogue scales or pain faces scales. Several studies directly compare different self-report pain measurement tools and suggest that the verbal descriptor scales are most preferred by older persons and have the strongest evidence of utility, reliability and validity (e.g. [34]). Other acceptable measures include numeric rating scales, the multidimensional McGill Pain Questionnaire [33] and Brief Pain Inventory [35, 36]. There is less uniform support for visual analogue scales and several authors raise concerns when using this measure with older adults ([36] for a discussion of this issue). That said, some research has shown good success with horizontally-presented visual analogues scales that can include changes in color and shape to indicate increasing amounts of pain (e.g. [37]). However, it is important to note that there is no one best measure of pain and a failure to complete one type of scale does not preclude success with other pain assessment tools. In clinical practice it may be best to select tools that are consistent with the personal preference of the individual when it is known, or to try several different types of scales before giving up on the use of self-report tools.

The longer that bothersome pain persists, the greater the probability that the older adult will become depressed, socially withdrawn, and somatically preoccupied. Anger, frustration, loss of ability to cope and increased anxiety also occur as the person tries and fails with a variety of medical and non-medical therapies. As a result, the measurement of mood disturbance and social impacts are now considered as an integral component of any comprehensive clinical evaluation and should be incorporated as a routine part of the assessment plan.

There are a number of standardized tools that have demonstrated reliability and validity for use in older adults (i.e. Geriatric Depression Scale [38,39], Spielberger State-Trait Anxiety Inventory [40,41]). The initial assessment can also include evaluation of other common psychological associations and mediators of pain, including anger, cognitive and behavioral coping strategy use, beliefs and attitudes, psychological strengths (e.g. resilience), stoicism, sleep, spousal bereavement and suicide risk. Developing a better understanding of the persons' social situation, beliefs, attitudes and current coping strategies in relation to their pain, provides an important starting point toward individualizing the eventual management plan and should be considered as a routine part of the clinical assessment.

Chronic pain has a major impact on function and is likely to interfere with many of the activities of daily life. A number of options exist for the measurement of activity levels or disability, ranging from objective measures of uptime/movement and direct observation of activity task performance, through to self-report psychometric questionnaires and activity dairies. The psychometric scales typically used to measure function in geriatric populations such as the Barthel Index and the, Katz ADL scale [42, 43] may be useful to monitor the basic and instrumental activities of daily living in the older adult with chronic pain, although they tend to lack sensitivity and fail to measure the more discretionary activities that are mostly affected by chronic pain (i.e. leisure and pastimes, home maintenance and social interactions). One must also exercise some care with the interpretation of activity measures because activity restriction can also occur as a consequence of a change in social circumstances, medical factors or other concurrent disease states rather than as a consequence of pain. Moreover, regardless of whether measures are via self-report or objective markers, activity performance is highly dependent upon motivational factors and the context in which measurement is undertaken. As a result, studies of chronic pain populations have tended to focus on measures of perceived pain-related interference in activity or self-rated measures of perceived disability (i.e. SF-36, Pain Disability Index [44], Oswestry Disability Questionnaire [45], the Sickness Impact Profile [46]) rather than documenting the actual levels of activity performance. Older adults with chronic pain often respond more dramatically with respect to improvements in function than in pain intensity following an efficacious treatment plan and functional outcomes are often considered as the most important outcome by the older person. For this reason, the measurement of disability and perceived interference should become an essential component of any routine comprehensive assessment.

A Clinical Approach to Pain Assessment in Adults with Dementia

In recent years, we have seen a proliferation of research focusing on the development and validation of observational tools designed to assess pain in persons with cognitive impairments. A detailed review of these is beyond the scope of this chapter but some of the most researched and recommended ones include the Pain Assessment Checklist for Seniors with Limited Ability to Communicate scales (PACSLAC and PACSLAC-II [47, 48]; the DOLOPLUS-II [49] and the Pain in advanced Dementia Scale (PAINAD; [50]). The DOLOPLUS-II has the disadvantage that a considerable portion of its items require knowledge of the patient which may make it more difficult to use in acute situations. The PACSLAC, which is a check list of 60 behaviors, takes less than five minutes to complete and, unlike most other tools of its kind, covers all of the assessment domains that have been recommended by the American Geriatrics Society as being useful in the assessment of older persons. The PACSLAC-II (31 items) is a shorter version of the PACSLAC with psychometric properties that appear to be stronger than the original PACSLAC [47]. With this in mind, we recommend several practical steps in the assessment of older adults with dementia. These steps are adaptations of earlier recommendations by a variety of groups (e.g. [23, 51]).

General guidelines:

In addition to taking into account patient history and physical examination results, we recommend the determination as to whether Mini Mental Status Examination scores [52] are available or can be obtained. This would facilitate determination of patients' ability to provide valid self-report since research suggests that patients with scores of 13 or lower are unlikely to be able to provide valid self-report whereas patients with scores of 18 or higher can typically respond to basic self-report scales such as verbal rating scales [53,54]. Despite this rule of thumb, it is always prudent to attempt self-report with all patients as there are some individuals with low MMSE scores who can reliably self-report pain. The pain assessment can also be supplemented with information from knowledgeable informants who could report on changes on activity patterns and routines as well as other relevant information (typical pain behaviors for the individual). Moreover, as with the assessment of any patient, clinicians should consider all aspects of the pain experience including the psychological consequences of pain and the social environment.

Under ideal circumstances, the clinician would collect baseline observational pain assessment scores on each patient on a regular basis. This would allow for the examination of unusual changes from a patient's usual pattern of scores. However, if assessments are to be repeated over time, it would be important to keep assessment conditions constant. That is, the assessment should be conducted under similar circumstances (e.g. during a routine program of physiotherapy or during a discomforting but necessary transfer), using the same assessment tool.

Self-Report Scales:

There are several self-report tools that have been shown to be valid among seniors with mild to moderate cognitive impairment. These tools include the Coloured Analogue Scale [31, 55], Numeric Rating Scales [53, 54], Verbal Rating Scales (e.g. [32, 53]) and the 21-point Box Scale [53, 56]. Clinicians may choose to check the ability of the patient to understand the scale prior to the assessment (e.g., by asking the patient to point to the parts of the scale that represent the lowest or the highest level of pain [37]. Given that some investigators have reported unusually high numbers of unscorable responses when horizontal visual analogue scales are used among older adults, we would recommend against the use of this tool (see [36] for a discussion of this issue). As others have suggested [51], certain adaptations (e.g. using larger print) may be needed with older adults who present with sensory deficits and the use of synonyms such as "aching" and "hurt" could facilitate self-report among some patients with limited ability to communicate verbally.

Observational Scales:

Reliable and valid tools for use with people who have severe dementia have been reviewed extensively [21–23]. When assessing pain in acute-care settings, tools that primarily focus on evaluation of change over time (i.e. the items have the format of "changes in behavior" or "changes in sleep pattern") should be avoided. Observational assessments during movement-based tasks would be more likely to lead to the identification of underlying pain problems than assessments during rest [22].

Clinicians frequently ask about cut-off scores to determine pain. Some pain assessment tools, such as the PACSLAC-II, do not have specific cut off scores because of recognition of tremendous individual differences among people with severe dementia. Moreover, the typical scores on an assessment tool will vary depending on factors such as the situation during which patients are assessed (e.g. during movement vs. during rest) and the duration of observation. Instead, for patients who are in long-term care or are cared for a chronic problem, it is recommended that pain be assessed on a regular basis (establishing baseline scores for each patient) with the clinician observing score changes over time. Moreover, clinicians can determine whether assessment scores change following the administration of clinically appropriate interventions.

Some of the symptoms of delirium (which is seen frequently in long-term care) overlap with certain behavioral manifestations of uncontrolled pain (e.g. behavioral disturbance) [57]. Clinicians assessing patients with delirium should be aware of this. On the positive side, delirium tends to be a transient state and pain assessment, which can be repeated or conducted when the patient is not delirious, is more likely to lead to valid results. It is important to note also that pain can cause delirium and clinicians should be astute in order to avoid missing pain problems among patients with delirium. Nonetheless, certain tools such as the PACSLAC-II were developed to minimize the extent to which its items overlap with delirium [47]. As a word of caution, clinicians are advised that observational pain assessment tools are only screening instruments and should never be considered to represent definitive indicators for the presence or absence of pain.

Psychological comorbidities of pain in moderate to severe dementia (e.g. depression, agitation) can be evaluated using instruments that rely on caregiver input. These instruments include the Cornell Depression in Dementia Scale [58], the Cohen Mansfield Agitation Inventory [59] and the Alzheimer Disease-Related Quality of Life-Revised (ADRQL-R) measure [60]. Given that agitation can be a consequence of pain, its assessment is especially important both as an index of treatment outcome but also as an indicator of the pain experience.

Psychosocial Interventions

Psychosocial interventions are normally offered either within the context of interdisciplinary treatment or in combination with other treatment modalities such as physiotherapy or pharmacological treatment. Several psychosocial pain management interventions have shown considerable initial promise with older adults although more research needed in this area. With some inconsistencies across studies, cognitive behavior therapy with older adults, who suffer from pain, seems to lead to positive outcomes (e.g. [61, 62]) although sometimes the benefits of the interventions seem to be linked to specific areas of functioning (e.g. pain beliefs, physical role functioning, pain intensity [63]). Acceptance and mindfulness based approaches, that encourage a present moment focus, acceptance of pain and a commitment to live a fulfilling life despite the pain are also showing initial support with older individuals [64–66]. Self-management books (e.g. [67]), specifically tailored to older adults with pain, are also available but require empirical evaluation.

Research with seniors with dementia, who reside in long-term care facilities, has supported the view that the use of regular and routine pain assessment leads to improved pain management practices [68]. Moreover, the success of behavioral mood management interventions, focusing on pleasant activity scheduling, environmental manipulation and other behavioral procedures, in improving patient mood [69, 70] suggests that these types of interventions have the potential of improving the quality of life in pain patients with dementia. Kovach et al. [71] showed that educating caregivers on ways of systematically monitoring pain behaviors and engaging patients in pleasant activities, in conjunction with involving caregivers in efforts to facilitate physical therapy, occupational therapy and other modalities, can facilitate pain management.

Other Non-Pharmacological Approaches to Pain Management

Whenever possible, pain management should be mechanism-based, choosing the most cost-effective and safest approach to the problem in order to optimize health-related outcomes and minimize treatment-related morbidity (Table 40.1). Non-pharmacological approaches may suffice for mild or mild-to-moderate pain (Table 40.2). The care setting may dictate which modalities may be available (e.g. massage by nurse assistants in a long-term care facility), but every effort should be made to integrate these approaches into the chronic pain management care plan, since they may offer appreciable benefits with negligible potential harms.

Pharmacological Therapies

Pharmacological therapies for pain management are used, often in conjunction with non-pharmacologic modalities, when pain and functional limitations persist despite trials of other modalities [72]. A collaborative approach, that includes multiple modalities, and understanding expectations and goals of care are especially critical in older adults with complex medical conditions. First line agents typically include thermal modalities (i.e. hot or cold), especially for management of osteoarthritis (OA) of the hand, knee, or hip OA [73]. Topical agents, including menthol, capsaicin, lidocaine, and diclofenac are particularly appealing in older adults due to improved safety profile from limited systemic absorption.

Acetaminophen (APAP) has been used as a first-line option for mild to moderate pain. While potentially less effective than some non-steroidal anti-inflammatory drugs (NSAIDs), APAP has a more favorable side effect profile as compared to oral non-selective NSAIDs [74]. Long-term use of oral NSAIDs is discouraged in older adults, due to known cardiovascular, gastrointestinal (GI) and renal toxicity [75]. As with all pain medications, the interdisciplinary care team should weigh risks and benefits of NSAID use and aim for the lowest effective dose for brief duration. Opioids are not considered first line management as they have not shown sustained efficacy in symptom or functional improvement. Further, opioids have well characterized adverse effects including falls, mental status changes, constipation, respiratory depression and sometimes death. This class of medications, especially for older adults with dementia, increase the risk of sedation, falls, nausea, and potential for increased agitation [76]. Adjuvant therapies, including antidepressants, antiepileptics or muscle relaxants may be considered on an individual level after the care team carefully weighs the risks and benefits in a given patient [75].

Table 40.1 Pain mechanisms and approaches to therapy.

Pain Type	Underlying Pain Mechanism	Examples	Treatment Approach
Nociceptive	Activation of pain receptors resulting from tissue inflammation (endogenous/ exogenous mediators), mechanical deformation, ongoing injury, tissue destruction, ischemia, visceral obstruction or dilatation.	• Arthritis • Ischemic disorders • Low back pain • Major surgery • Myofascial pain syndromes • Procedural pain	Responds well to traditional analgesic and nonpharmacologic interventions (e.g. heat, ice, acetaminophen, NSAIDs, opioids). Caution with chronic NSAID use in older adults (75)
Neuropathic	Pathology involving peripheral or central nervous system.	• Diabetic neuropathy • Neuropathic back pain • Post-herpetic neuralgia • Post-stroke central or thalamic pain • Postamputation phantom limb pain • Procedural pain • Trigeminal neuralgia	Does not predictably or fully respond to pain management with traditional analgesics; interpatient variability of response to adjunctive agents (e.g. anticonvulsants, antidepressants, local anesthetics), opioids, and a variety of other agents in select cases (calcitonin, snail venom toxin, clonidine, ketamine); often contributes to polypharmacy with traditional and nontraditional analgesic approaches.
Mixed or idiopathic	Mixed or unknown cause and/or mechanism	• Low back pain • Recurrent headache • Vasculitis	Often requires traditional analgesic and nonpharmacologic approaches.
Comorbid Psychological Conditions	Psychiatric conditions/ personality disorders that exacerbate pain behaviors and create a refractory milieu for traditional pain therapy	• Anxiety disorders • Bipolar disorders • Borderline personality disorder • Depression • Dementing illnesses • Schizo-affective disorders	Often requires concurrent psychiatric/psychological management and modification of treatment plan to address concurrent psychological condition.

Table 40.2 Non-pharmacological management of pain in older adults.

Category	Examples
Patient/caregiver education	• Nature and clinical course of pain • Use of pain assessment instruments • Product and dosing information
Cognitive behavioral therapy	• Cognitive restructuring • Relaxation or mindfulness methods • Activity pacing • Involvement in pleasurable activities
Supervised physical therapy	• Flexibility • Strength • Endurance • Range of motion • Enhance postural and gait stability
Assistive devices	• Canes/walkers • Raised chairs/toilet seats • Braces or splints
Adjunctive therapies	• Heat • Cold • Massage • Chiropractic • Acupuncture/acupressure • Transcutaneous electrical nerve stimulation

References

1 Stompor M, Grodzicki T, Stompor T, Wordliczek J, Dubiel M, Kurowska I. (2019) Prevalence of chronic pain, particularly with neuropathic component, and its effect on overall functioning of elderly patients. *Med Sci Monit* **25**:2695–701.

2 Kozak-Szkopek E, Broczek K, Slusarczyk P *et al.* (2017) Prevalence of chronic pain in the elderly Polish population - results of the PolSenior study. *Arch Med Sci* **13**(5):1197–206.

3 Patel KV, Guralnik JM, Dansie EJ, Turk DC. (2013) Prevalence and impact of pain among older adults in the United States: findings from the 2011 National Health and Aging Trends Study. *Pain* **154**(12):2649–57.

4 Larsson C, Hansson E, Sundquist K, Jakobsson U. (2017) Chronic pain in older adults: prevalence, incidence, and risk factors. *Scand J Rheumatol* **46**(4):317–25.

5 Fox PL, Raina P, Jadad AR. (1999) Prevalence and treatment of pain in older adults in nursing homes and other long-term care institutions: a systematic review. *CMAJ* **160**(3):329–33.

6 Takai Y, Yamamoto-Mitani N, Okamoto Y, Koyama K, Honda A. (2010) Literature review of pain prevalence among older residents of nursing homes. *Pain ManagNursing* **11**(4):209–23.

7 Ferrell BR, Novy D, Sullivan MD *et al.* (2001) Ethical dilemmas in pain management. *J Pain* **2**(3):171–180.

8 Li J, Snow AL, Wilson N *et al.* (2015) The quality of pain treatment in community-dwelling persons with dementia. Dement Geriatr Cogn Dis Extra **5**(3):470–81.

9 Nawai A, Leveille SG, Shmerling RH, van der Leeuw G, Bean JF. (2017) Pain severity and pharmacologic pain management among community-living older adults: the MOBILIZE Boston study. *Aging Clin Exper Res* **29**(6):1139–1147.

10 Bullock L, Bedson J, Jordan JL, Bartlam B, Chew-Graham CA, Campbell P. (2019) Pain assessment and pain treatment for community-dwelling people with dementia: A systematic review and narrative synthesis. *Int J Geriatr Psychiatry* **34**(6):807–21.

11 Hemmingsson E, Gustafsson M, Isaksson U *et al.* (2018) Prevalence of pain and pharmacological

pain treatment among old people in nursing homes in 2007 and 2013. *Eur J Clin Pharmacol* **74**(4):483–88.

12 Morrison RS, Siu AL. (2000) A comparison of pain and its treatment in advanced dementia and cognitively intact patients with hip fracture. *J Pain Symptom Manage* **19**(4):240–8.

13 Proctor WR, Hirdes JP. (2001) Pain and cognitive status among nursing home residents in Canada. *Pain Res Manag* **6**(3):119–25.

14 Balfour JE, O'Rourke N. (2003) Older adults with Alzheimer's disease, comorbid arthritis and prescription of psychotropic medications. *Pain Res Manag* **8**(4):198–204.

15 Sandvik R, Selbaek G, Kirkevold O, Husebo BS, Aarsland D. (2016) Analgesic prescribing patterns in Norwegian nursing homes from 2000 to 2011: trend analyses of four data samples. *Age Ageing* **45**(1):54–60.

16 Jensen-Dahm C, Gasse C, Astrup A, Mortensen PB, Waldemar G. (2015) Frequent use of opioids in patients with dementia and nursing home residents: a study of the entire elderly population of Denmark. *Alzheimer Dement* **11**(6):691–9.

17 Makris UE, Higashi RT, Marks EG *et al.* (2015) Ageism, negative attitudes, and competing co-morbidities–why older adults may not seek care for restricting back pain: a qualitative study. *BMC Geriatrics* **15**(1):39.

18 Martin R, Williams J, Hadjistavropoulos T, Hadjistavropoulos HD, MacLean M. (2005) A qualitative investigation of seniors' and caregivers' views on pain assessment and management. Can J Nurs Res **37**(2):142–64.

19 Gibson SG, Chambers CT. (2004) Pain over the life span: A developmental perspective. In: Hadjistavropoulos T, Craig KD, eds. *Pain: Psychological Perspectives*. Lawrence Erlbaum Associate, Mahweh. pp. 113–154.

20 Kaasalainen S, Coker E, Dolovich L *et al.* (2007) Pain management decision making among long-term care physicians and nurses. West J Nurs Res **29**(5):561–80.

21 Hadjistavropoulos T, Herr K, Prkachin KM *et al.* (2014) Pain assessment in elderly adults with dementia. *Lancet Neurol* **13**(12):1216–27.

22 Herr K, Coyne PJ, Ely E, Gélinas C, Manworren RC. (2019) Pain assessment in the patient unable to self-report: clinical practice recommendations in support of the ASPMN 2019 position statement. *Pain Manag Nurs* **20**(5):404–17.

23 Hadjistavropoulos T, Herr K, Turk DC *et al.* (2007) An interdisciplinary expert consensus statement on assessment of pain in older persons. *Clin J Pain* **23**(Suppl 1):S1–43.

24 Kaasalainen S, Coker E, Dolovich L *et al.* (2007) Pain management decision making among long-term care physicians and nurses. *West J Nurs Res* 29(5):561–80.

25 Lautenbacher S, Kunz M, Strate P, Nielsen J, Arendt-Nielsen L. (2005) Age effects on pain thresholds, temporal summation and spatial summation of heat and pressure pain. *Pain* **115**(3):410–8.

26 Lautenbacher S. (2012) Experimental approaches in the study of pain in the elderly. *Pain Med* **13**(suppl 2):S44–50.

27 Lautenbacher S, Peters JH, Heesen M, Scheel J, Kunz M. (2018) Age changes in pain perception: a systematic-review and meta-analysis of age effects on pain and tolerance thresholds. Neurosci Biobehav Rev **75**:104–13.

28 El Tumi H, Johnson M, Dantas P, Maynard M, Tashani O. (2017) Age-related changes in pain sensitivity in healthy humans: a systematic review with meta-analysis. *Eur J Pain* **21**(6):955–64.

29 T Binnekade T, Van Kooten J, Lobbezoo F *et al.* (2017) Pain experience in dementia subtypes: a systematic review. *Curr Alzheimer Res* **14**(5):471–85.

30 Cole LJ, Farrell MJ, Duff EP, Barber JB, Egan GF, Gibson SJ. (2006) Pain sensitivity and fMRI pain-related brain activity in Alzheimer's disease. *Brain* **129**(11):2957–65.

31 Hadjistavropoulos T, LaChapelle DL, MacLeod FK, Snider B, Craig KD. (2000) Measuring movement-exacerbated pain in cognitively impaired frail elders. *Clin J Pain* **16**(1):54–63.

32 Weiner DK, Marcum Z, Rodriguez E. (2016) Deconstructing chronic low back pain in older adults: summary recommendations. *Pain Med* **17**(12):2238–46.

33 Melzack R. (1975) The McGill Pain Questionnaire: major properties and scoring methods. *Pain* **1**(3):277–299.

34 Herr KA, Spratt K, Mobily PR, Richardson G. (2004) Pain intensity assessment in older adults: use of experimental pain to compare psychomet-

ric properties and usability of selected pain scales with younger adults. *Clin J Pain* **20**(4):207–19.

35 Cleeland CS. (1991) *The Brief Pain Inventory*. University of Texas MD Anderson Cancer Center, Houston.

36 Gauthier L, Gagliese L. (2011) Assessment of pain in older persons. In: Turk D, Melzack R, eds. *Handbook of Pain Assessment*. The Guilford Press: New York. pp. 242–59.

37 Scherder EJ, Bouma A. (2000) Visual analogue scales for pain assessment in Alzheimer's disease. *Gerontology* **46**(1):47–53.

38 Yesavage JA, Brink TL, Rose TL *et al*. (1982) Development and validation of a geriatric depression screening scale: a preliminary report. *J Psychiatr Res* **17**(1):37–49.

39 Parmelee PA, Lawton MP, Katz IR. (1989) Psychometric properties of the Geriatric Depression Scale among the institutionalized aged. *Psychological Assessment: A Journal of Consulting and Clinical Psychology* **1**(4):331.

40 Spielberger CD, Gorsuch RL, Lushene R, Vagg PR, Jacobs GA. (1983) Manual for the State-Trait Anxiety Inventory. Consulting Psychologists Press, Palo Alto.

41 Nesselroade JR, Mitteness LS, Thompson LK. (1984) Older adulthood: Short-term changes in anxiety, fatigue, and other psychological states. *Res Aging* **6**(1):3–23.

42 Collin C, Wade D, Davies S, Horne V. (1988) The Barthel ADL Index: a reliability study. *Int Disabil Stud* **10**(2):61–3.

43 Katz S, Ford AB, Moskowitz RW, Jackson BA, Jaffe MW. (1963) Studies of illness in the aged: the index of ADL: a standardized measure of biological and psychosocial function. *JAMA* **185**(12):914–19.

44 Tait RC, Chibnall JT, Krause S. (1990) The Pain Disability Index: psychometric properties. *Pain* **40**(2):171–82.

45 Fairbank JC, Couper J, Davies JB, O'Brien JP. (1980) The Oswestry Low Back Pain Disability Auestionnaire. *Physiotherapy* **66**(8):271–3.

46 Gilson BS, Gilson JS, Bergner M et al. (1975) The sickness impact profile. Development of an outcome measure of health care. *Am J Public Health* **65**(12):1304–10.

47 Chan S, Hadjistavropoulos T, Williams J, Lints-Martindale A. (2014) Evidence-based development and initial validation of the pain assessment checklist for seniors with limited ability to communicate-II (PACSLAC-II). *Clin J Pain* **30**(9):816–24.

48 Fuchs-Lacelle S, Hadjistavropoulos T. (2004) Development and preliminary validation of the pain assessment checklist for seniors with limited ability to communicate (PACSLAC). *Pain Manag Nurs* **5**(1):37–49.

49 Wary B, Doloplus C. (1999) Doloplus-2, une échelle pour évaluer la douleur. *Soins gérontologie* (19):25–7.

50 Warden V, Hurley AC, Volicer L. (2003) Development and psychometric evaluation of the Pain Assessment in Advanced Dementia (PAINAD) scale. *J Am Med Dir Assoc* **4**(1):9–15.

51 Herr K, Coyne PJ, Key T et al. (2006) Pain assessment in the nonverbal patient: position statement with clinical practice recommendations. *Pain Manag Nurs* 7(2):44–52.

52 Folstein MF, Folstein SE, McHugh PR. (1975) "Mini-mental state". A practical method for grading the cognitive state of patients for the clinician. *J Psychiatr Res* **12**(3):189–98.

53 Chibnall JT, Tait RC. (2001) Pain assessment in cognitively impaired and unimpaired older adults: a comparison of four scales. *Pain* **92**(1-2):173–86.

54 Weiner D, Peterson B, Logue P, Keefe F. (1998) Predictors of pain self-report in nursing home residents. *Aging (Milano)* **10**(5):411–20.

55 McGrath PA, Seifert CE, Speechley KN, Booth JC, Stitt L, Gibson MC. (1996) A new analogue scale for assessing children's pain: an initial validation study. *Pain* **64**(3):435–43.

56 Jensen MP, Miller L, Fisher LD. (1998) Assessment of pain during medical procedures: a comparison of three scales. *Clin J Pain* **14**(4):343–9.

57 Hadjistavropoulos T, Voyer P, Sharpe D, Verreault R, Aubin M. (2008) Assessing pain in dementia patients with comorbid delirium and/or depression. *Pain Manag Nurs* **9**(2):48–54.

58 Alexopoulos GS. (2002, 2005) *The Cornell Scale for Depression in Dementia: administration and Scoring Guidelines*. Cornell Institute of Geriatric Psychiatry, White Plains.

59 Cohen-Mansfield J. (1991) *Instruction Manual for the Cohen-Mansfield agitation inventory (CMAI)*. Research Institute of the Hebrew Home of Greater Washington, Rockville.

60 Kasper JD, Black BS, Shore AD, Rabins PV. (2009) Evaluation of the validity and reliability of the

Alzheimer Disease-related Quality of Life Assessment Instrument. *Alzheimer Dis Assoc Disord* **23**(3):275–84.

61 Lunde L, Nordhus IH, Pallesen S. (2009) The effectiveness of cognitive and behavioural treatment of chronic pain in the elderly: a quantitative review. *J Clin Psychol Med Settings*. **6**(3):254–62.

62 Nicholas MK, Asghari A, Blyth FM et al. (2013) Self-management intervention for chronic pain in older adults: a randomised controlled trial. *Pain* **154**(6):824–35.

63 Waters S, Woodward J, Keefe F. (2005) Cognitive-behavioral therapy for pain in older adults. In: Gibson S, Weiner D, eds. *Pain in Older Persons*. IASP Press, Seattle. pp. 239–69.

64 Morone NE, Lynch CS, Greco CM, Tindle HA, Weiner DK. (2008) "I felt like a new person." The effects of mindfulness meditation on older adults with chronic pain: qualitative narrative analysis of diary entries. *J Pain* 9(9):841–8.

65 Morone NE, Greco CM, Weiner DK. (2008) Mindfulness meditation for the treatment of chronic low back pain in older adults: a randomized controlled pilot study. *Pain* **134**(3): 310–9.

66 McCracken LM, Jones R. (2012) Treatment for chronic pain for adults in the seventh and eighth decades of life: a preliminary study of acceptance and commitment therapy (ACT). *Pain Medicine* **13**(7):861–7.

67 Hadjistavropoulos T, Hadjistavropoulos HD. (2019) *Pain Management for Older Adults: A Self-Help Guide*, 2nd edn. Wolters Kluwer, Philadelphia

68 Fuchs-Lacelle S, Hadjistavropoulos T, Lix L. (2008) Pain assessment as intervention: a study of older adults with severe dementia. *Clin J Pain* **24**(8):697–707.

69 Teri L, McKenzie G, LaFazia D. (2005) Psychosocial treatment of depression in older adults with dementia. *Clinical Psychology: Science and Practice* **12**(3):303–16.

70 Teri L, Logsdon RG, Uomoto J, McCurry SM. (1997) Behavioral treatment of depression in dementia patients: a controlled clinical trial. *The Journals of Gerontology Series B: Psychological Sciences and Social Sciences* **52**(4):P159–66.

71 Kovach CR, Logan BR, Noonan PE et al. (2006) Effects of the Serial Trial Intervention on discomfort and behavior of nursing home residents with dementia. *Am J Alzheimers Dis Other Demen* **21**(3):147–55.

72 Qaseem A, Wilt TJ, McLean RM, Forciea MA, Clinical Guidelines Committee of the American College of Physicians. (2017) Noninvasive treatments for acute, subacute, and chronic low back pain: a clinical practice guideline From the American College of Physicians. *Ann Intern Med* **166**(7):514–30.

73 Kolasinski SL, Neogi T, Hochberg MC *et al.* (2020) 2019 American College of Rheumatology/Arthritis Foundation guideline for the management of osteoarthritis of the hand, hip, and knee. *Arthritis Rheumatol* **72**(2):220–33.

74 Bannuru RR, Schmid CH, Kent DM, Vaysbrot EE, Wong JB, McAlindon TE. (2015) Comparative effectiveness of pharmacologic interventions for knee osteoarthritis: a systematic review and network meta-analysis. *Ann Intern Med* **162**(1):46–54.

75 2019 American Geriatrics Society Beers Criteria® Update Expert Panel, Fick DM, Semla TP, Steinman M, Beizer J, Brandt N, *et al.* (2019) American Geriatrics Society 2019 updated AGS Beers Criteria® for potentially inappropriate medication use in older adults. *J Am Geriatr Soc* **67**(4):674–94.

76 Erdal A, Ballard C, Vahia IV, Husebo BS. (2019) Analgesic treatments in people with dementia-how safe are they? A systematic review. *Expert Opin Drug Saf* **18**(6):511–22.

Chapter 41

Pain in children

See Wan Tham[1], Jeffrey L. Koh[2], & Tonya M. Palermo[3]

[1] *Department of Anesthesiology and Pain Medicine, University of Washington School of Medicine, Seattle Children's Hospital and Research Institute, Seattle, Washington, USA*

[2] *Department of Anesthesiology and Peri-Operative Medicine, Oregon Health and Science University, Portland, Oregon, USA*

[3] *Department of Anesthesiology and Pain Medicine, Pediatrics and Psychiatry, University of Washington School of Medicine, Seattle Children's Hospital and Research Institute, Seattle, Washington, USA*

Introduction

Children and adolescents have unique needs that should be considered in the assessment and management of pain. Across childhood, there is tremendous variability in neurocognitive development, physiology, and behavioral and emotional maturation that contribute to differences in presentations of pain. Moreover, the child's determinants of health are nested within their hereditary genetics, family function and the social-ecological system. These variabilities and vulnerabilities can define the pain experience and its trajectory as a chronic condition. Irrespective of whether pain is a symptom of a medical condition or a primary diagnosis, the evaluation and management can be challenging for the treating clinician. In this chapter, we review the considerations in managing pediatric chronic pain, including a discussion of its impact; a description of clinical evaluation and evidence-based management approaches.

Etiology and significance of recurrent and chronic pain in children

Chronic or recurrent pain in children may be associated with underlying medical conditions, such as arthritis or inflammatory bowel disease. Pain may also be associated with life-limiting and/or life-threatening medical conditions, which may include cancer, end-stage and palliative conditions. However, the most frequent form of chronic pain in children is when pain is the primary condition, not accounted for by another disease process. Examples are chronic headaches, musculoskeletal pain, functional abdominal pain or complex regional pain syndrome (CRPS). All forms of chronic pain irrespective of etiology can result in physical and psychosocial impairment and negatively impact children's quality of life, such that pain itself becomes a primary or additional chronic problem.

Epidemiological studies provide prevalence estimates of recurring or persisting pain in 15–30% of children and adolescents [1, 2]. The most common locations involve the head, limbs, abdomen and back. Recurrent and chronic pain can lead to significant daily interference and pain-related disability for an estimated 5–8% of children and adolescents [3]. Of concern are decrements in their ability to function in important life roles, including high rates of school absenteeism, poor academic achievement, as well as reduced participation in physical, social, recreational and peer activities [4]. Parents and family members

Clinical Pain Management: A Practical Guide, Second Edition. Edited by Mary E. Lynch, Kenneth D. Craig, and Philip W. Peng.

may also be impacted such as through increased distress in caring for the child and financial hardship.

Conceptual models of chronic pain

Central to contemporary models of chronic pain are the interrelationships amongst physical, cognitive, affective and social factors that influence pain and disability – commonly referred to as biopsychosocial model of pain [5]. Current conceptualizations recognize the importance of each domain to understand pain in a comprehensive manner. The basis of assessment stems from elucidating the etiology of chronic and recurrent pain, of which central and peripheral nervous system mechanisms are implicated [6]. Processes of central sensitization and deficiencies in endogenous pain modulation are proposed to underlie persistent pain. More recently, neuroimmune and neuroendocrine interactions have been investigated to extend our understanding of chronic pain conditions. For example, the involvement of the brain-gut axis in functional abdominal pain syndromes, and structural and functional brain changes in complex regional pain syndrome [7, 8]. Ongoing research highlights the complexity of pain mechanisms and the extensive systemic physiological involvement within each individual.

Using the framework of the biopsychosocial model, assessment of factors from each domain may organize a comprehensive approach to understanding the pain experience. From the biological and physiological standpoint, influences of age, sex, and aggregated family history of chronic pain have been highlighted. For example, females generally report higher pain intensity, longer lasting and more frequent pain than males [9]. With respect to psychological factors, children's anxiety, depressive and catastrophizing symptoms have been found to have strong associations with pain intensity and pain-related disability [10]. Social and environmental factors such as the role of parental influences have also been recognized as important in explaining the interindividual variability in children's response to pain [11].

More recently, the World Health Organization's International Classification of Functioning, Disability and Health (ICF) has been used to provide a framework for understanding the context and treating the impact of disease. In the evaluation of a health condition such as chronic pain, the environmental and personal factors of the child are incorporated, and overall activity and participation levels are assessed. This provides an understanding of the two primary concepts: "functioning" and "disability". Functioning refers to physiological and anatomical integrity, which supports the ability to participate in activities and life roles. In contrast, disability highlights impairment in body function and structures, limiting activities and restricting participation [12]. With this approach, interventions can be systematically tailored to optimize the child's health related quality of life as the primary target for treatment.

One of the challenges in treating pediatric chronic pain is the limited data on the natural history of pain. Available research suggests that up to half of children with chronic pain continue to have severe symptoms in adulthood [13, 14]. However, this also reflects that a large proportion of children and adolescents experience resolution and reduction in pain symptoms. This perspective allows for a more optimistic view in the treatment of pediatric chronic pain. The neuroplasticity of the pediatric nervous system has been proposed to contribute to the higher rates of resolution of pediatric pain compared to adult chronic pain conditions, although there is a paucity of data. Therefore, further research is critical to identify the risk factors across the biopsychosocial model that predict childhood pain, and to evaluate for vulnerabilities that maintain pain and disability during childhood through to adulthood. This will then give rise to the development of effective preventative and intervention strategies that may negate a lifelong trajectory of pain and disability [15].

Clinical practice: evaluation and treatment

Evaluation

The goals of the evaluation are to identify the etiology of pain, medical/psychological comorbidities, understand the context and impact of pain across all domains of functioning, and establish a therapeutic relationship. A productive way to initiate the history is to elicit the patient's and parents' narratives about the pain, rather than beginning with targeted questions. Further prompts about the pain history can then be provided. Throughout the evaluation, providing reassurance, rapport and validation of the pain problem will enhance receptivity of parents and child to the treatment approach. Details on the medical and psychological assessment are covered extensively in other texts [16].

In addition to the primary pain symptoms, children with chronic pain commonly suffer from comorbidities such as insomnia, anxiety or depression. Given the bidirectional relationships between sleep, pain and mood, it is important to identify potential concerns in these areas, as these comorbidities may interfere with rehabilitation. Standardized measures may be helpful to assess each domain of functioning (pain experience, psychological/physical functioning, disability) [17]. This can allow for objective monitoring of pain and function over time.

Treatment approach

The interdisciplinary model is the recommended treatment approach for pediatric chronic pain. An integrated rehabilitation strategy across disciplines has been shown to be more successful, in contrast to single target treatment that emphasizes complete symptom resolution or cure [18]. The team may consist of a pediatrician, anesthesiologist, nurse practitioner, pediatric psychologist, pediatric psychiatrist and physical or occupational therapist. To enhance team performance, key features include using a consistent treatment approach, providing clear and cohesive messaging to families, and maintaining regular communication.

It is recognized that education on the etiology of recurrent and chronic pain may be a driver of change in behaviors. When the pain experience is not validated or the diagnosis of chronic pain not understood, there is a risk that families may continue to seek further investigations and consultations, rather than engage in appropriate self-management for pain. The International Association for the Study of Pain recognized that contemporary pain education is a central component of treatment (www.iasp-pain.org). Providing information on scientific concepts to explain pain, its function, and biological processes has been found to be associated with reduced pain and disability, reduced catastrophizing, increased self-efficacy, and increased participation in rehabilitation [19].

Unfortunately, dedicated pediatric pain treatment facilities remain limited, with most centers located in major urban cities. Even when pediatric trained clinicians and resources are available, effective treatment may be limited by time, expense, insurance or system barriers. Hence, primary care physicians (PCPs) should be kept informed of management plans so they can provide continuity support and care coordination for families. If experts in chronic pain cannot be located, the PCP can assemble a team of knowledgeable professionals. The PCP can educate the team on chronic pain and establish a treatment plan with the psychologists and therapists. Under the guiding principle of rehabilitation, providers can often participate in treatment even when they do not have expertise in pediatric chronic pain.

We broadly review the evidence base for chronic pain treatment in children. The primary goals are to reduce pain-related disability and improve children's pain experience. Interventions may include psychological treatments, physical therapy, pharmacological strategies, complementary and alternative treatments, and other emerging therapies.

Psychological treatments

Psychological treatments play important roles in modifying pain experiences, emotional, behavioral, social and familial factors that contribute to pain-related disability. Several meta-analytic reviews have documented the efficacy of psychological therapies, showing benefits for reducing pain and disability [20]. A number of treatments are classified under the umbrella of psychological therapies. This includes cognitive behavioral therapy (CBT), behavioral strategies (e.g. biofeedback, relaxation training), cognitive strategies (e.g. hypnosis, guided imagery), acceptance and commitment therapy (ACT) and mindfulness approaches. The most commonly researched psychological therapy is CBT. CBT programs incorporate elements of behavioral and cognitive strategies. The goals are to enhance children's coping skills by instructing them in behavioral and cognitive skills to promote different thoughts and behaviors; which in turn, enhance coping abilities and self-efficacy and reduce the negative effects of having chronic pain. CBT also involves considerable work with parents to teach them ways to support their children and modify social contingencies such as implementing behavioral plans, rewarding the child for participation in therapies or attendance at school. Emerging research has identified reduction in functional a connectivity between brain regions in individuals after CBT treatment as a potential mechanism underlying improved pain symptoms [21].

Given the importance of parents in facilitating treatment, parents may also be targets for interventions. Parents can experience high levels of stress, pain catastrophizing and family conflict whilst caring for a child with pain. Moreover, parents may promote maladaptive behaviors in children through misguided protective strategies, e.g. excessive attention to pain complaints [22]. In providing parents with strategies to reduce distress and skills to help children cope, they may alter the trajectory of pain and disability for a child [23].

Further data are needed to understand to understand the efficacy of other interventions such as biofeedback and ACT [24]. Specifically, biofeedback has undergone empirical evaluation in children with migraine and tension headaches; ACT has received promising support for youth with chronic pain; and more recently mindfulness-based approaches have received increasing attention.

Physical therapy (PT) and occupational therapy (OT) interventions

PT and OT programs are important aspects of pain treatment. Most commonly, these interventions target musculoskeletal deconditioning, gait abnormalities, restricted physical range of motion and sensitization of painful body parts. Strategies to support child participation in physical activities include goal setting, activity pacing and graded exposure to pain-related activities. The majority of studies describing PT-based interventions in children with chronic pain have focused on exercise programs in youth with widespread musculoskeletal pain and localized musculoskeletal pain (e.g. CRPS). These studies have demonstrated increased function and significantly reduced pain. For pain related to CRPS, intensive in-patient rehabilitation as well as outpatient PT has been effective [25]. However, the frequency and intensity of exercise necessary to accomplish symptom reduction remains unclear at this time for other types of pain conditions [26].

Pharmacological treatments

There is limited evidence on pharmacologic treatment for children with chronic non-malignant pain. To date, treatment is largely based on anecdotal evidence or derived from adult literature rather than controlled clinical studies in children [27]. The most commonly prescribed agents are anticonvulsants (e.g. gabapentin, pregabalin), antidepressants (e.g., amitriptyline, duloxetine), and non-steroidal anti-inflammatory agents [28]. In the adolescent population, extrapolation of adult data may be reasonable considering that presumed mechanisms of pain may be similar to adults and that neuro-physiological development more closely resembles adults. In contrast, for younger children, medications may be associated with adverse effects not commonly observed in adults. For example, gabapentin has been associated with higher rates of neuropsychiatric effects in children under 12 years of age, that is not commonly reported in adults [29]. This highlights the importance for safety and efficacy studies in pediatrics and clinical decision making based on the risk and benefits of pharmacologic treatment.

There is a limited role for opioid therapy for children with chronic non-malignant pain [30]. For acute pain management, pain related to cancer and in life-limiting conditions, opioids have been extensively studied. For these populations, education regarding the risk and benefit ratio, including physiological and psychological dependence, safe and responsible handling of opioids are important discussion points. Federal and statewide legislation have been implemented for opioid prescribing and should be referred to in the prescribing process. Finally, opioid therapy should be considered as part of an interdisciplinary treatment plan.

Due to the lack of evidence-based pediatric research for most medications used in chronic pain, dosing is usually based on clinical experience or derived from dosing guidelines for the approved use of the medication (e.g. gabapentin for epilepsy). Dosing range guidelines are beyond the scope of this chapter but can be found in several published textbooks [31]. The guiding principles should include appropriate low dose at initiation, monitor for adverse effects, and discontinuation in the absence of efficacy as part of the interdisciplinary approach.

Complementary and alternative medicine (CAM) therapies

Many parents seek out CAM such as acupuncture, yoga and herbal remedies. There has been some efficacy found for the use of acupuncture in postoperative period and for chemotherapy-induced nausea and vomiting; however, this remains limited for the treatment of pain. From a safety standpoint, the risk of adverse events has been demonstrated to be low in pediatric populations, providing a low risk profile in the treatment regimen [32]. In addition to acupuncture, these alternative therapies require further study to support their use in children.

Other treatment modalities

Remote or digital health interventions: Barriers such as geographic distance from treatment centers, long wait lists in interdisciplinary pain clinics and lack of availability of pain providers are major issues limiting accessibility of children to evidence-based pain care. Remote delivery of treatments has become increasingly utilized to address these issues with access, most commonly delivered as digital health interventions through Internet-based programs or smartphone applications [33]. At this time, the majority of evidence for remote interventions is psychological treatments in pediatric chronic pain [20]. Following the World Health Organization declaration of the COVID-19 pandemic, there has been a tremendous increase in telehealth services. Patient satisfaction with treatment is high; although further data are needed to understand the efficacy of remote delivery of interventions. This is an area of important development as there is high potential for wider availability of evidence-based pain treatment for children.

Intensive interdisciplinary pain treatment programs: A small number of intensive interdisciplinary pain treatment programs have been developed around the world to address more complex chronic pain in youth who have not made adequate progress with traditional outpatient therapies. This includes a range of programs that provide intensive treatment either through outpatient or inpatient services. Therapies encompass physical, occupational and psychological therapy in a highly supportive and structured environment. Programs have demonstrated effectiveness, with improvements in children's physical functioning and disability after treatment, and that are maintained at follow up [34]. Unfortunately, the availability of these programs remained limited due to high cost, available expertise and limited resources.

Summary: a treatment algorithm

As shown in Figure 41.1, a treatment algorithm for pediatric chronic pain management begins with assembling a treatment team. The team lays the groundwork by providing education to the child and family, to engage their participation in the evaluation and treatment. The team partners with the family to formulate the plan and collaboratively set goals. This will include improving the child's functioning (physical, school, social) through enhancing the child's participation in physical activities, coping skills and addressing comorbidities such as poor sleep, anxiety or depression. Throughout treatment, the team supports the child and parents by providing developmentally specific information to champion the child's management plan and addressing the needs of parents. Specific therapies will generally involve a multimodal approach with psychological interventions, physical and rehabilitation therapies and/or complementary and alternative therapies. Pharmacologic therapies may be incorporated to enhance the implementation of these therapies. Routine follow-up is useful to encourage the child's participation in therapies and provide feedback on progress toward interim goals.

The evaluation and treatment of pediatric chronic pain can indeed present unique challenges. However, using the biopsychosocial model to guide the evaluation process, identify and treat the risk factors across different domains of functioning, can thereby reduce disability and improve the lifelong quality of life for the child with recurrent or chronic pain.

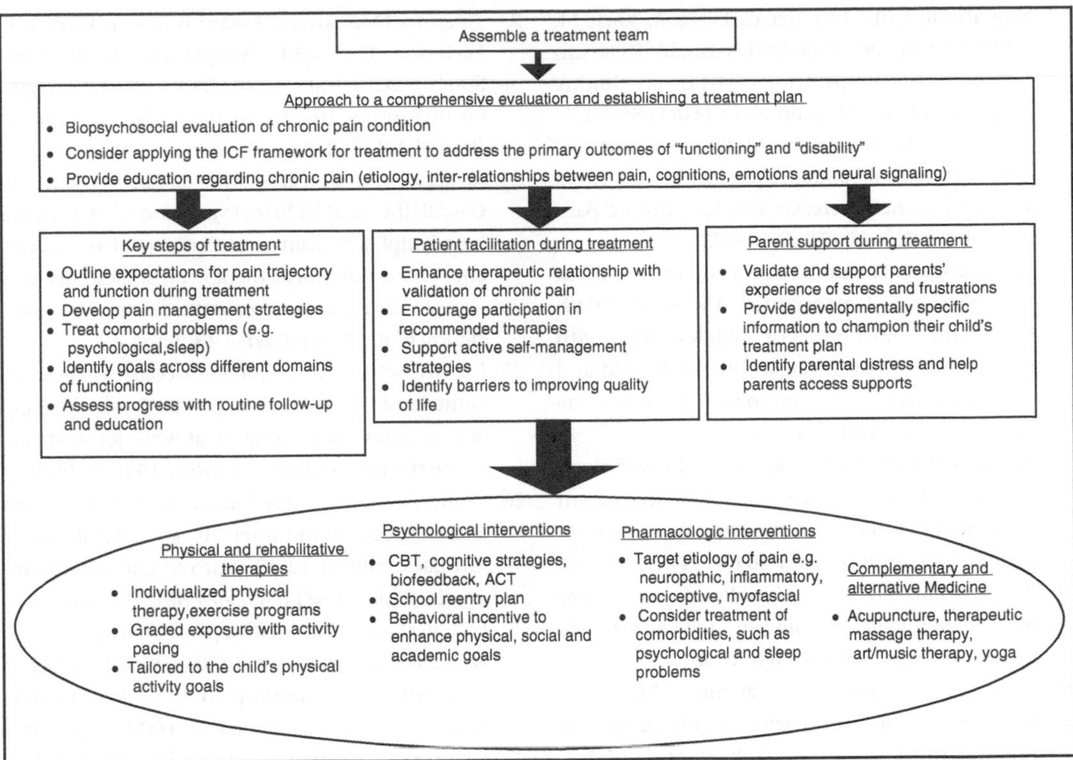

Figure 41.1 A treatment algorithm for pediatric recurrent and chronic pain.

References

1 Stanford EA, Chambers CT, Biesanz JC, Chen E. (2008) The frequency, trajectories and predictors of adolescent recurrent pain: a population-based approach. *Pain* **138**(1):11–21.

2 King S, Chambers CT, Huguet A, MacNevin RC, McGrath PJ, Parker L *et al.* (2011) The epidemiology of chronic pain in children and adolescents revisited: a systematic review. *Pain* **152**(12):2729–38.

3 Huguet A, Miro J. (2008) The severity of chronic pediatric pain: an epidemiological study. *Pain* **9**(3):226–36.

4 Groenewald CB, Tham SW, Palermo TM. (2020) Impaired school functioning in children with chronic pain: a national perspective. *Clin J Pain* **36**(9):693–9.

5 Liossi C, Howard RF. (2016) Pediatric chronic pain: biopsychosocial assessment and formulation. *Pediatrics* **138**(5):e20160331.

6 Ji RR, Nackley A, Huh Y, Terrando N, Maixner W. (2018) Neuroinflammation and central sensitization in chronic and widespread pain. *Anesthesiology* **129**(2):343–66.

7 Powell N, Walker MM, Talley NJ. (2017) The mucosal immune system: master regulator of bidirectional gut-brain communications. *Nat Rev Gastroenterol Hepatol* **14**(3):143–59.

8 Shokouhi M, Clarke C, Morley-Forster P, Moulin DE, Davis KD, St Lawrence K. (2018) Structural and functional brain changes at early and late stages of complex regional pain syndrome. *J Pain* **19**(2):146–57.

9 LeResche L, Mancl LA, Drangsholt MT, Saunders K, Von Korff M. (2005) Relationship of pain and symptoms to pubertal development in adolescents. *Pain* **118**(1–2):201–9.

10 Fisher E, Heathcote LC, Eccleston C, Simons LE, Palermo TM. (2018) Assessment of pain anxiety, pain catastrophizing, and fear of pain in children and adolescents with chronic pain: a systematic review and meta-analysis. *J Pediatr Psychol* **43**(3):314–25.

11 Palermo TM, Chambers CT. (2005) Parent and family factors in pediatric chronic pain and disability: an integrative approach. *Pain* **119**(1–3):1–4.

12 Nugraha B, Gutenbrunner C, Barke A, Karst M, Schiller J, Schafer P *et al.* (2019) The IASP classification of chronic pain for ICD-11: functioning properties of chronic pain. *Pain* **160**(1):88–94.

13 Walker LS, Dengler-Crish CM, Rippel S, Bruehl S. (2010) Functional abdominal pain in childhood and adolescence increases risk for chronic pain in adulthood. *Pain* **150**(3):568–72.

14 Kashikar-Zuck S, Cunningham N, Peugh J, Black WR, Nelson S, Lynch-Jordan AM *et al.* (2019) Long-term outcomes of adolescents with juvenile-onset fibromyalgia into adulthood and impact of depressive symptoms on functioning over time. *Pain* **160**(2):433–41.

15 Palermo TM. (2020) Paie key role of psychological interventionsn presvention and management must bein in childhood: the key role of psychological interventions. *Pain* **161**:S114–21.

16 Palermo TM. (2012) *Cognitive-Behavioral Therapy for Chronic Pain in Children and Adolescents*. Oxford University Press, New York.

17 Tham SW, Wilson, A.C., Palermo T.M. (2014) Measurement of heath-related quality of life and physical function. In: *McGrath PJ*, Stevens, B.J., Walker, S.M., Zempsky, W.T., eds. *Oxford Textbook of Paediatric Pain*. Oxford University Press, Oxford.

18 Simons LE, Sieberg CB, Pielech M, Conroy C, Logan DE. (2013) What does it take? Comparing intensive rehabilitation to outpatient treatment for children with significant pain-related disability. *J Pediatr Psychol* **38**(2):213–23.

19 Louw A, Zimney K, Puentedura EJ, Diener I. (2016) The efficacy of pain neuroscience education on musculoskeletal pain: A systematic review of the literature. *Physiother Theory Pract* **32**(5):332–55.

20 Fisher E, Law E, Dudeney J, Eccleston C, Palermo TM. (2019) Psychological therapies (remotely delivered) for the management of chronic and recurrent pain in children and adolescents. Cochrane Database Syst Rev **4**:CD011118.

21 Lazaridou A, Edwards RR. (2016) Getting personal: the role of individual patient preferences and characteristics in shaping pain treatment outcomes. *Pain* **157**(1):1–2.

22 Wilson AC, Moss A, Palermo TM, Fales JL. (2014) Parent pain and catastrophizing are associated with pain, somatic symptoms, and pain-related disability among early adolescents. *J Pediatr Psychol* **39**(4):418–26.

23 Palermo TM, Law EF, Essner B, Jessen-Fiddick T, Eccleston C. (2014) Adaptation of Problem-Solving Skills Training (PSST) for parent caregivers of Youth with chronic Pain. *Clin Pract Pediatr Psychol* **2**(3):212–23.

24 Kemani MK, Kanstrup M, Jordan A, Caes L, Gauntlett-Gilbert J. (2018) Evaluation of an intensive interdisciplinary pain treatment based on acceptance and commitment therapy for adolescents with chronic pain and their parents: a nonrandomized clinical trial. *J Pediatr Psychol* **43**(9):981–94.

25 Lee BH, Scharff L, Sethna NF, McCarthy CF, Scott-Sutherland J, Shea AM *et al.* (2002) Physical therapy and cognitive-behavioral treatment for complex regional pain syndromes. *J Pediatr* **141**(1):135–40.

26 Fanucchi GL, Stewart A, Jordaan R, Becker P. (2009) Exercise reduces the intensity and prevalence of low back pain in 12–13 year old children: a randomised trial. *Aust J Physiother* **55**(2):97–104.

27 Eccleston C, Fisher E, Cooper TE, Gregoire MC, Heathcote LC, Krane E, *et al.* (2019) Pharmacological interventions for chronic pain in children: an overview of systematic reviews. *Pain* **160**(8):1698–707.

28 Egunsola O, Wylie CE, Chitty KM, Buckley NA. (2019) Systematic review of the efficacy and safety of gabapentin and pregabalin for pain in children and adolescents. Anesth Analg **128**(4):811–9.

29 Lee DO, Steingard RJ, Cesena M, Helmers SL, Riviello JJ, Mikati MA. (1996) Behavioral side effects of gabapentin in children. *Epilepsia* **37**(1):87–90.

30 Busse JW, Wang L, Kamaleldin M, Craigie S, Riva JJ, Montoya L *et al.* (201) Opioids for chronic noncancer pain: a systematic review and meta-analysis. *JAMA* **320**(23):2448–60.

31 Rastogi SC, F. (2014) Drugs for neuropathic pain. In: McGrath PJ, Stevens B.J.,Walker S.M., Zempsky W.T., eds. (2014) *Oxford Textbook of Paediatric Pain*. Oxford University Press, Oxford. pp. 495.

32 Jindal V, Ge A, Mansky PJ. (2008) Safety and efficacy of acupuncture in children: a review of the evidence. *J Pediatr Hematol Oncol*. **30**(6):431–42.

33 Keogh E, Rosser BA, Eccleston C. (2010) e-Health and chronic pain management: current status and developments. *Pain* **151**(1):18–21.

34 Simons LE, Sieberg CB, Conroy C, Randall ET, Shulman J, Borsook D *et al.* (2018) Children with chronic pain: response trajectories after intensive pain rehabilitation treatment. *J Pain* **19**(2):207–18.

Chapter 42

Pain in individuals with intellectual disabilities

Abagail Raiter[1], Alyssa Merbler[2], Chantel C. Burkitt[1,3], Frank J. Symons[3], & Tim F. Oberlander[4,5]

[1] *Gillette Children's Specialty Healthcare, St. Paul, Minnesota, USA*
[2] *Department of Educational Psychology, University of Minnesota, Minneapolis, Minnesota, USA*
[3] *Special Education Program, Department of Educational Psychology, University of Minnesota, Minneapolis, Minnesota, USA*
[4] *Department of Pediatrics, School of Population and Public Health, Faculty of Medicine, University of British Columbia, University of British Columbia, Vancouver, British Columbia, Canada*
[5] *Complex Pain Service, British Columbia Children's Hospital, Vancouver, British Columbia, Canada*

Introduction & Overview

Expression of pain by individuals with intellectual and related developmental disabilities (e.g. cerebral palsy) and disorders (e.g. autism) is frequently ambiguous and its recognition by caregivers and health care providers can be highly subjective. The potential for ambiguity and subjectivity presents a tremendous challenge for clinicians, researchers, individuals with disabilities and their families. Even when pain-specific behaviors are present, such behaviors may be regarded as altered, blunted or confused with other sources of generalized stress, arousal or, in the extreme, misinterpreted as a manifestation of a behavior disorder of psychological origin. There is no reason, however, to believe that pain is any less frequent in the lives of someone with an intellectual or related developmental disability that alters the way they communicate or that such an individual would be insensitive or indifferent to pain.

Until the early 2000s, pain in people with intellectual disability (ID) received little scientific attention and as study participants, individuals with ID have been historically and systematically excluded from pain and related research. This is starting to change [1]. The International Association for the Study of Pain (IASP) updated their definition of pain in 2020 to *"an unpleasant sensory and emotional experience associated with, or resembling that associated with, actual or potential tissue damage"* [2]. The IASP definition is accompanied by a critical note stating that *"verbal description is only one of several behaviors to express pain; inability to communicate does not negate the possibility that a human or a nonhuman animal experiences pain"* [2]. In this sense, our task is to recognize that all features of an individual's behavioral and physiologic repertoire may function as legitimate indices of pain expression and experience and develop strategies to manage this universal, but highly individual, human condition.

The purpose of this chapter is to provide an overview of several issues inherent to assessing and managing pain among children and adults with intellectual and

Clinical Pain Management: A Practical Guide, Second Edition. Edited by Mary E. Lynch, Kenneth D. Craig, and Philip W. Peng.

developmental disabilities (IDD). Wherever possible, our focus is specific to intellectual disability as distinct from but related to the concept of developmental disability (e.g. cerebral palsy is a developmental disability in which some children also have intellectual disability, but some do not). It is beyond the scope of the chapter to provide an exhaustive review, for more information, readers are directed to Oberlander and Symons [3], Siden and Oberlander [4], Doody and Baily [5] or Barney et al. [1]. The chapter begins by defining intellectual disability to clarify the clinical population and then briefly reviews the scope of the problem of pain among individuals with ID. Recent developments in assessment approaches are discussed and specific tools are described. Issues and approaches to pain management are then presented. Readers will note that the chapter and its citation pattern reflect the current reality of our knowledge in this area – much of the research addressing issues in pain and ID has focused on the scope of the problem and assessment in pediatric populations with very little work specific to management [1].

Defining ID and Conceptual Issues

The American Association on Intellectual and Developmental Disabilities (AAIDD) currently defines ID as a disability with onset by 18 years of age characterized by significant limitations in both intellectual functioning and in adaptive behavior, which may cover many everyday social and practical skills [6]. Adaptive behavior can include tasks such as literacy, social problem solving, safety or occupational skills. Evidence of these limitations must be evident before adulthood. AAIDD emphasizes the assessment of ID must include all available information, including considering the cultural, linguistic and community contexts of the individual [6].

Regardless of the degree of ID and the underlying neurological condition, functional limitations frequently confound the presentation of pain in individuals with intellectual and developmental disabilities [7]. Given that the most common approach to pain assessment is based on self-report, how can pain be assessed and managed when the typical means of verbal or nonverbal communication or cognition is altered or absent? In the absence of easily recognized verbal or motor-dependent forms of communication, it remains uncertain if the pain experience itself is different or whether only the expressive manifestations are altered. Indeed, without easily recognizable means of communication or functional motor skills, pain may remain under recognized and under treated. Despite the potential for altered nociception and pain expression, there is no evidence that cognitively or motor impaired individuals are spared any of the miseries of a noxious experience [8].

[1] Note on terminology: there are many terms in use professionally and scientifically with respect to individuals with significant intellectual impairments including mental retardation, intellectual disability, severe neurological impairment and cognitive impairment. For the purposes of this chapter, the term 'intellectual disability' will be used.

Scope of the Problem of Pain in Individuals with ID

Epidemiology

There is a limited but emerging database regarding the epidemiology of pain among children and adults with ID, with varying levels of pain reported across studies [9]. Hauer et al. [10] reported pain occurring weekly in 44% of children with moderate to profound cognitive impairment and almost daily in 41-42% of children with severe cognitive impairment. Breau et al. [11] documented 78% of children with moderate to profound ID (N=94) experienced some type of pain over a four-week period, with 62% experiencing nonaccidental pain, as reported by caregivers. Each week, 35-52% of participants had pain. The mean duration was more than nine hours per week and nonaccidental pain had a mean rating of six out of ten. Those with more severe limitations reported more nonaccidental pain. Similarly, Stallard and colleagues [12], reported 74% of their sample of children with ID (N=34) experienced some form of pain over a two-week period, with 68% having pain rated as moderate to severe. Most troubling was that none of the children were reported to be receiving any type of pain management.

Some studies of adults with ID have produced similar prevalence estimates. An early investigation of chronic pain in adults with ID and cerebral palsy found 67% of their sample reported pain lasting more than 3 months. Many of the pain types listed had a mean duration of greater than 10 years, with a report of up to 20 years in one case, and 56% of individuals reported they had daily pain [13]. More recently, a secondary analysis of health interviews of individuals with ID found that 67% of participants reported living with pain [14]. Other studies have reported lower chronic pain prevalence estimates including 13% and 15% of adults with ID [15, 16]. Overall, there is a wide range of pain prevalence estimates with the upper bound tending to be in the 60-70% range suggesting the need for more routine and systematic assessment and treatment considerations.

Pain Sources and Risk Factors

Whether from a single or multifactorial cause (e.g. genetic/metabolic disorders, multi-organ syndromes, traumatic brain injury or disorders of unknown origin), ID can be associated with multiple sources of acute and chronic pain. It can present as acute or chronic and be from internal or external sources. Adults with ID often have multiple medical conditions [17], many of which can result in pain or are associated with chronic pain (e.g. fractures, dental problems, arthritis). Activities of daily living may involve the use of assistive devices for positioning and mobility (e.g. walkers, seating systems, manual and power wheelchairs), which can cause discomfort and/or pain [18]. Dislocated hips, pressure sores from skin breakdown and repetitive use injuries occur and must be considered. Splinting and casting may be required for the prevention and treatment of contractures and can be associated with pain. For some, eating and swallowing are difficult and special feeding techniques or enterostomy feeds are required. Feeding tubes can result in gastric distention, tugging or pulling of the tube or skin breakdown at the tube site are a potential cause of pain on an everyday basis. Constipation should also be considered a common source of discomfort.

Motor impairments, such as those in cerebral palsy, may be characterized by increased tone, spasms, increased deep tendon reflexes and clonus, coupled with weakness and loss of dexterity. Spasticity and spasms can cause significant discomfort through waking and sleeping hours [19]. Treatment of spasticity frequently involves invasive procedures. High tone/spasticity may be treated through surgical intervention (selective dorsal rhizotomy) or by surgical implantation of an intrathecal baclofen pump, while pharmacologic management of tone may include intramuscular injection of botulinum toxin A [19.20]. Non-invasive therapies can also contribute heavily to frequent pain; adult patients with cerebral palsy report that their memories of pain in childhood center around regular physical therapy sessions and stretching [21].

Although the nociceptive pain of surgery may seem obvious, there are times when repeated surgery or direct trauma to a nerve results in long lasting neuropathic pain [22]. Neuropathic pain can be difficult to identify and treat but should be considered in individuals with severe neurological impairments (SNI) associated with ID with prolonged pain after an intervention. Another potential source of pain is central in origin (i.e., thalamic injury), where the pain afferents appear to be activated without an ongoing input either from tissue damage or peripheral nerve injury [22, 23]. The major evidence for central pain comes from the observation of pain behavior in children with advancing neurodegenerative diseases such as Krabbe disease, children with severe neurological impairments, adults with thalamic strokes and Alzheimer's disease, but the pain mechanisms associated with severe degenerative or severe neurological impairment and associated conditions remain to be fully explained [24.25]. Even with a determined search for an underlying cause, one is frequently faced with the likelihood that the final diagnosis becomes a "medically unexplainable pain" [26], leading to a therapeutic dead-end whereby without a diagnosis, treatment is often delayed or may not begin at all. In such cases, even with a potentially identified source, limited and effective communication only compounds the complexity of effective pain treatment.

Pain Assessment Tools

While individuals with ID are at increased risk for experiencing pain, often compounded by co-occurring conditions, specific assessment tools designed for individuals with ID remain limited and have only emerged within the last two decades. In this section, we briefly outline a number of pain assessment scales (see Table 42.1) designed to evaluate pain specifically among children and adults with ID (for more detailed reviews specific to scale development, see Belew et al. [27]; Breau, McGrath, & Zabalia [3]). The scales reviewed in Table 42.1 were designed and developed specifically for individuals with ID, however scales from other vulnerable populations

Table 42.1 Pain assessment tools for children and adults with intellectual disabilities (ID)

Pain Scale	Brief Description	Items	Psychometric Properties	Recommendations
Child Pain Scales				
Pain Indicator for Communicatively Impaired Children (PICIC) Stallard et al.[12]	-200 pain cues derived from caregiver interview narrowed to 6 main cues	6	-Showed accuracy -Not retested for validity or reliability	-Short and simple -Possible preliminary measure of pain
Pediatric Pain Profile (PPP) Hunt et al.[31]	-Semi-individualized measure providing predetermined categories of behaviors which can be added to by the parent/ caregiver	20	-Valid, reliable and sensitive measure for each individual child -When specific behaviors are added, the measure does not generalize across children	-May distinguish individual child's good days from bad days -May be well suited for monitoring pain for an individual over time
Non-Communicative Children's Pain Checklist-Revised (NCCPC-R) Breau et al.[29]	-Observational assessment tool quantifies pain responses observed by parents and caregivers -Post-operative version available	30	-Reliable and valid in detecting pain	-Useful across populations and settings -Consistently accurate with short observation times and by those unfamiliar with the child
The Chronic Pain Assessment Toolbox for Children with Disabilities Kingsnorths et al.[36]	-Culmination of pediatric assessment tools created to implement standardized pain assessment practices in clinical settings	15	-All assessment tools selected for use in the Toolbox are reliable and valid in screening and detecting pain	-Useful when making real time clinical decisions for patients
Adult Pain Scales				
The Pain and Discomfort Scale (PADS) Bodfish et al.[42] Phan et al.[53]	-Measures pain and discomfort during a standardized physical examination (PEP: pain examination procedure)	18	-High inter-rater reliability -Sensitivity to pain	-Useful in isolating the location/ source of pain
Non-Communicating Adult Pain Checklist (NCAPC) Lotan et al.[35]	-Adapted the NCCPC-R to assess acute pain in adults with ID	21	-High internal consistency -Sensitive to pain	-The NCAPC is recommended currently for assessing acute or procedural pain in adults with ID.

(neonates, elderly) have been adapted for use with children with ID (e.g. the revised FLACC) [28].

The scales developed for individuals with ID to date focus on identifying a variety of possible pain signs in children and adults [29-31]. These include vocalizations (e.g. cry, scream, moan), facial expressions, movement (both increased and decreased), change in muscle tone (increased and decreased), guarding/protection and changes in everyday activity (social interaction, eating and sleeping) [29, 32]. It is important to consider that children with more significant ID may show different behavioral signs than those with mild ID. For example, scores of adaptive function domains (social and communication) were significantly related to the types of pain behaviors observed in children with ID post-operatively using the Non-Communicating Child's Pain Checklist-Postoperative Version (NCCPC-PV) [33].

As there is great variation in pain related behaviors, no measure covers all settings. Scales vary in administration time and have been designed for initial assessment or repeated evaluation for acute, post-operative and/or chronic pain. They are often completed by caregivers, as self-report can be difficult or absent [32, 34]. Some measures offer a wide range of possible behaviors that might reflect pain across a population of children/youth with SNI, while others are highly specific and sensitive to a particular child (e.g. Paediatric Pain Profile [PPP]) and are not completely generalizable. Other measures fall somewhere in between (e.g. r-FLACC).

While the use of pain assessments has been limited in clinical settings, developments have transpired within the last decade to advance evidence-based pain assessments. The Holland Bloorview's Chronic Pain Assessment Toolbox for Children with Disabilities (hereafter "toolbox" Table 42.1) was created with the objective of standardizing assessment approaches among clinicians to promote earlier identification and management of chronic pain. Items in the toolbox include 7 assessment tools appropriate for assessing chronic pain interference and 8 tools to assess chronic pain coping [35]. The toolbox includes two of the pain assessments tools for children found in Table 42.1 (Non-Communicative Children's Pain Checklist-Revised [NCCPC-R]; PPP), as well as additional assessment tools to assist clinicians in their efforts to accurately assess chronic pain in children with disabilities [32, 34, 35].

Other measurement approaches focus on establishing sensitive and specific measures of nonverbal facial pain displays (e.g. facial action unit activity) [36] and biobehavioral reactivity (e.g. heart rate variability [HRV], respiration rate) [37]. Not all studies have found relations between self-reported pain intensity and physiological variables, however, and the clinical utility of these approaches remains to be established [38].

Pain Management

Where to begin? Attempting to identify the source and origin of pain in individuals with ID is challenging yet essential. Reviews published in 2017 [5] and 2020 [1] outlined the challenges of pain management in ID, including a continued lack of quality evidence of the effectiveness of treatment approaches, including some gold-standard approaches. Despite a lack of evidence for specific treatments, the use of a standardized approach, when possible, can lead to significant improvements for individuals with severe disabilities [39].

A clinician taking a pain history can be guided by using an established, symptom cluster assessment tool, such as those offered by Lotan [34], Breau [40] and Hunt [31]. A symptom cluster assessment approach can provide a profile of typical everyday behaviors, how they have changed during a defined period of pain," and other associated changes in everyday function/activities. An alternative but complementary approach was developed by Bodfish et al. [41] based on pairing assessment with an examination. A thorough, systematic interview can also provide clinicians with information about pain or potentially painful health conditions. Turk et al. [14] used the *OK Health Checklist* during a health interview with adults with ID capable of self-report in which an informant can indicate whether they have pain in up to 12 specific body areas (e.g. head, legs), with pictures of each part and clear straightforward non-jargon words to guide the interview. The use of the visual and verbal aids helped the participants better describe their health experiences compared to initially being asked open-ended questions. The responses using the *OK Health Checklist* closely aligned with their caregivers' report, whereas health experiences were under-reported compared to caregiver response when only asking open-ended questions.

Even when using these structured approaches key questions should still be considered (Table 42.2). For those who cannot self-report, appreciating changes from a baseline set of behaviors observed by experienced caregivers compiled to reflect a longitudinal perspective may be the most reliable measure of pain/distress available. A detailed history should include an account of known baseline behaviors or physical conditions, temporal sequences, known stressors, and an understanding of the typical repertoire of verbal and nonverbal cues used to communicate pain and a variety of affective states. The context of the pain behavior itself and the individual and his/her family broadly is crucial and should be considered during assessment and management. For example, caregiver report of a child displaying pain when changing a diaper may indicate possible hip subluxation or sacral decubitus ulcers; whereas pain reported repeatedly after eating or upon laying down suggests gastroesophageal reflux. It may be helpful for caregivers to keep notes of their child's activities and behaviors to identify any changes. Additionally, aspects of co-occurring health conditions (e.g. scoliosis) may create additional risks [45-47].

Beyond a pain history, a detailed review of all systems (gastrointestinal, etc.), medications, allergies, diet, and recent procedures remains essential. A helpful mnemonic, "The PQRST," is listed in Table 42.3 to identify pain qualities and guide assessment (e.g. the Region of pain). Another helpful technique is to ask the family to make a brief home video recording of the behavior they suspect may be a pain sign or that seems idiosyncratic and possibly indicative of a suspected painful experience. Watching the video with the parents develops understanding and agreement about the exact nature of the complaint. The influence of the caregiver's perceptions and social setting and individual factors of the patient are also key to understanding the child's pain experience [42]. This includes the individual's previous painful experiences and treatments (if any), their relationships with the individuals involved in their care (caregivers, health professionals), how pain expression has been modeled in their family, community and/or culture, and the caregiver's beliefs. These factors may influence the behaviors of the participant or the caregiver's interpretation of their child's behavior.

Finally, during the physical examination, careful observation, with guidance by experienced caregivers examining for specific areas of discomfort or injury is essential. Throughout the exam, one should observe the individual's facial and vocal reactions to manipulations [the logic underlying Bodfish et al.'s [41] pain examination procedure (PEP) combined with the Pain and Discomfort Scale [PAD]), as well as the reaction of the parent or caregiver (as a proxy for self-report; a "gut-reaction" or intuition) can sometimes help more than asking them for a more complex evaluation of pain behaviors]. In the search for the source of "irritability of unknown origin" (IUO) one should consider a broad differential diagnosis as illustrated in Figure 42.1. Again, considerations of pain expression within the context of the individual's experiences and abilities, social interactions and culture should be considered.

Table 42.2 What to ask when taking a pain history

Key questions to consider in assessing pain in an individual with ID

- What is the underlying neurological condition/process?
- What is the developmental level?
- How might these factors influence pain system function and the expression of distress associated with the pain experience?
- What is the usual behavioral and health condition: baseline condition and nature of everyday function?
- Usual means of communication
- Caregivers' views and understanding of what is happening
- Role of intercurrent illness
- Differential diagnosis: what else is going on?

Table 42.3 A structured approach to exploring the nature of pain symptoms

The P-Q-R-S-T--exploring the nature of pain symptoms (adapted from [4])

P–palliative or provocative factors for the pain, role of parents, professionals etc.

Q–quality of pain (burning, stabbing, aching, etc.), quantity of pain (impact of pain on daily life – magnitude of pain problem)

R–region of body affected

S–severity of pain (usually 1-10 scale)

T–temporal character (how long has it existed, when does it appear e.g. after meals, in the morning, etc.)

Pain prevention and education are broad strategies to reduce overall pain experiences for individuals with ID. Prevention strategies can include individualized

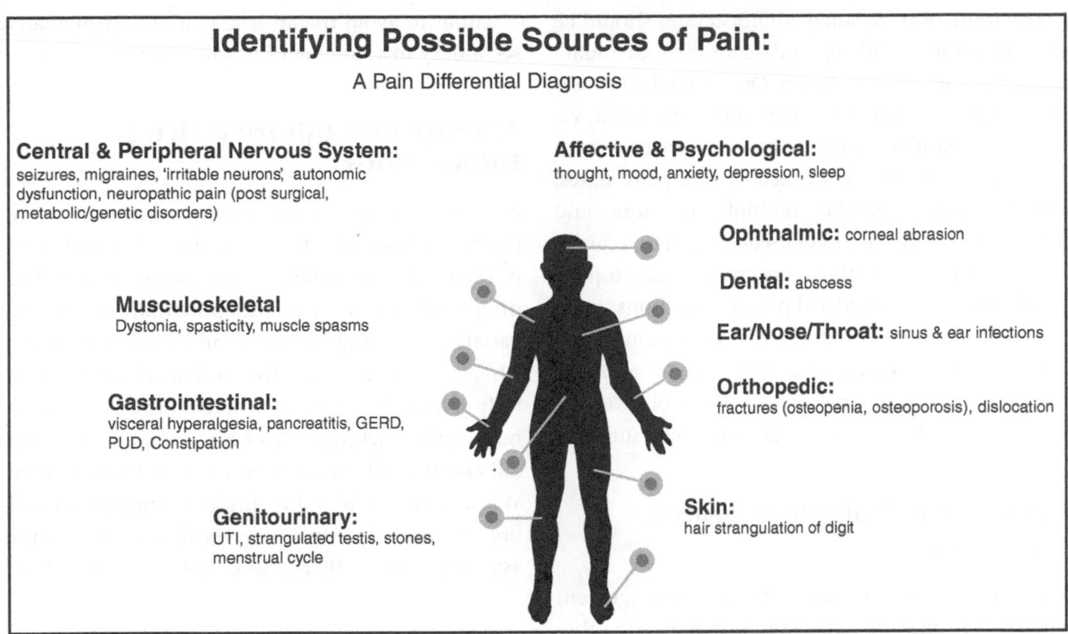

Figure 42.1 Developing a differential diagnosis for irritability of unknown origin (IUO) (Oberlander TF, personal communication, 2021) (Abbreviations: GERD: gastroesophageal reflux disease; PUD: peptic ulcer disease; UTI: urinary tract infection)

adaptions of daily activities to prevent pain or large-scale strategies like surveillance programs for known painful conditions associated with ID and related developmental disabilities, such as dislocations [43]. Caregiver education can include both primary and secondary caregivers, such as staff who work with the individual in school or day programs, and can provide information (e.g. signs of pain) or tools to facilitate communication between caregivers and health professionals [44]. Finally, as described above, education and specific interview strategies taught to healthcare professionals during a healthcare assessment (e.g. visual aids and simple language) can help an individual with ID better report their health [14].

Moving forward

Optimal pain management focuses on identifying the underlying pathology leading to a diagnosis and treatment plan, reducing distress and facilitating a return to baseline function. However, even with a careful history and thoughtful approaches investigating irritability, sources of pain frequently remain uncertain. A diagnosis in this setting may not always be possible, however, and even after a careful empiric evaluation, identification of exacerbating and mediating factors, an empiric medication trial and careful ongoing evaluation may be the only available management options. The success of pain management in this setting requires three key elements: 1) a clearly identified plan including pharmacologic and non-pharmacologic options, 2) coordinated communication and decision making among the individual (to the greatest extent possible), caregivers and clinicians alike and 3) a process for ongoing evaluation to keep this management plan on track especially when the pain has not resolved.

Analgesics

In general, one follows the same principles for pharmacotherapy in the cognitively impaired that are used in other populations with chronic pain, but several unique factors should be considered for individuals with ID (see Chapters 14 and 18-24). In this population, route of administration may be more complex, and there is evidence that individuals with ID may experience more drug-related side effects. Additionally, aspects of co-occurring health conditions (e.g. scoliosis) may create additional risks [45-47].

The route of medication administration should be the least invasive and appropriate for the individual's condition and sources of pain. Oral or g-tube route is preferable. Subcutaneous medications delivered via indwelling catheters may be an appropriate way to administer opioids for selected, severe pain states, with the added pain of multiple injections and reduced muscle mass, intramuscular injections can be avoided. Topical anesthetic creams or other topical agents should be considered prior to injections, venipuncture, refills of intrathecal baclofen pumps and other cutaneous procedures. Silver nitrate and sulcrate in zinc oxide can be very effective topical agents for controlling local irritation at gastric tube sites.

Non-Pharmacological Management Approaches

Acute procedural or postoperative pain management requires the same imaginative approach used in other health care settings. Simple nonpharmacological approaches may be helpful, as well as preventative pain strategies. Educating primary caregivers may help in pain assessment and allow differentiation of non-specific arousal behavior from pain behavior. Similarly, maintaining communication with the inpatient treatment team will provide access to the accumulated knowledge of how the individual reacts to pain and prior treatments and improve the management of ongoing or pre-existing problems.

Depending on the individual's ability to communicate or responsiveness to external stimulation behavioral interventions such as distraction, guided imagery and hypnosis, psychotherapy and virtual reality can be used for individuals with ID. Virtual reality (VR) is an emerging distraction technique that may be effective for managing pain in clinic (procedural or post-operative). The use of VR is drastically increasing in typically developing populations with evidence of pain reduction [48]. As described in Barney et al. [1] VR is currently being introduced in clinical procedure settings (e.g. during botulinum toxin injects, casting) for individuals with developmental disabilities. Clinical trials are ongoing. Physical measures such as massage, touch, heat or cold therapy also may be helpful [49, 50]. Effective coordinated teamwork, including an overall case manager and a map of where the pain fits into the individual's life (i.e., drawing a "pain map"), is essential to avoid therapeutic failure that may arise secondary to a number of possible factors.

Therapeutic failure & drug interactions

Among individuals where multiple medications are needed to manage a diverse number of conditions it is especially important to be aware of potential drug interactions and the potential for genetic variation in drug response and metabolism (see Chapters 18-24). Even the best medications carefully selected to meet specific conditions related to nociceptive, neuropathic or inflammatory pain still fail and the critical question we need to ask is why? While many factors may underlie therapeutic failure, we need to consider critical potential factors associated with therapeutic failure (Table 42.4).

Table 42.4 Why even after you have done everything, treatment still fails.

Factors that might explain therapeutic failure:

1. Limited knowledge & bias about pain in individuals with intellectual disabilities
2. Impact of an altered neurological system:
   a. What do we know about the underlying neurological disorder that influences function of the pain system?
3. Limited access to pain experience:
   a. Is an assessment of pain possible using a standard tool?
   b. Have we targeted the right symptom endpoint?
4. Diagnosis in doubt:
   a. Have we searched for "irritability of unknown origin"?
   b. Multiple comorbid conditions (i.e. sleep disturbances, nutrition, intercurrent infection)?
5. Using the right drugs, but they are still not effective
   a. Pharmacokinetic, pharmacodynamic and pharmacogenetic factors
   b. Drug – drug interactions
   c. Drug – environmental interactions (i.e. interactions with tobacco smoke, grapefruit juice)
6. Contextual Factors
   a. Lack of a "Pain Map" highlighting key sources of pain (nociceptive, inflammatory or neuropathic sources)
   b. Diagnostic uncertainty among clinicians and family members
   c. Multiple caregivers but poorly coordinated health care
   d. Lack of a case manager

Recognizing that pain, at its core, is a self-appraisal condition and pain assessment and management requires a caregiver's or clinician's belief about the presence of the pain experience in individuals with ID or other disabilities is essential. Historically, individuals with disabilities were thought to be insensitive to pain [51]. This belief contrasts emerging evidence that some individuals with ID may be more sensitive to pain and may be more likely to develop chronic pain [8]. Therefore, being mindful of society and individual beliefs and biases of pain in individuals with disabilities may result in better pain assessment and management. Further, Barney et al. [1] and Doody et al. [5] both highlight the problem of observers underestimating or misinterpreting pain, including the patient's parents. Caregiver beliefs about their child's disability and pain provide another potential source of bias in pain assessment and management.

Summary

In the past decade tremendous strides have been taken in recognizing the problem of pain among individuals with ID, although many of the same challenges remain [1, 5]. Problems with the definition of pain are readily recognized, as is the fact that conventional approaches to assessment are limited. A great deal of effort has improved assessment techniques that include a broader range of possible pain indicators beyond verbal self-report. Despite this, caution should be exercised when using any of the tools described in this chapter, as their development and use has been under very specific circumstances in most cases. Regardless of the instruments used, it is clear that systematic pain assessments should be routinely undertaken, regardless of the disability, particularly when extraordinary behavior or context dictates the possibility that pain is present. The development of pain assessment tools for adults with ID is in its infancy, thus, a multifaceted approach to pain assessment and its management is necessary. Although efforts to understand the nature of pain in the context of a neurological injury leading to an ID are underway, we need to focus on the individual, his/her typical behavior and their own experience as an individual living with pain.

Acknowledgements

T. F. O. is the R. Howard Webster Professorship in Brain Imaging and Child Development (UBC). FS & CB were supported, in part, from NIH/NICHD Grant No. 73126 & 94581 and additional support from the Mayday Fund; as well as the University of Minnesota (Distinguished McKnight Professorship [FS]) and the College of Education + Human Development (Birkmaier Chair [FS]). We are very grateful to Ursula Brain for her thoughtful editorial contribution preparing this chapter.

References

1 Barney CC, Andersen RD, Defrin R, Genik LM, McGuire BE, Symons FJ. (2020) Challenges in pain assessment and management among individuals with intellectual and developmental disabilities. *Pain Rep* **5(4)**:e21.

2 Raja SN, Carr DB, Cohen M *et al.* (2020) The revised International Association for the Study of Pain definition of pain: concepts, challenges, and compromises. *Pain* **161(9)**:1976–82.

3 Oberlander TF, Symons FJ. (2006) *Pain in children and adults with developmental disabilities*. Paul H. Brookes, Towson.

4 Siden H, Oberlander TF. (2008) Pain management for children with a developmental disability in a primary care setting. In: Walco GA, Goldschneider KR, eds. *Pain in Children: A Practical Guide for Primary Care*. Humana Press, New York.pp. 29–37.

5 Doody O, Bailey ME. (2017) Pain and pain assessment in people with intellectual disability: issues and challenges in practice. *Br J Learn Disabil* **45(3)**:157–165.

6 Schalock RL, Borthwick-Duffy SA, Bradley VJ *et al.* (2009) *Intellectual Disability: Definition, Classification, and Systems of Supports*. 11th Edn.American Association on Intellectual and Developmental Disabilities, Silver Spring.

7 Abu-Saad HH. (2000) Challenge of pain in the cognitively impaired. *Lancet* **356(9245)**:1867–8.

8 Sobsey, D. (2006). Pain and disability in an ethical and social context. In: T. F. Oberlander & F. J. Symons, *Pain in children & adults with developmental disabilities* (pp. 19–39). Paul H Brookes Publishing Co.

9 Bottos, S., & Chambers, C. T. (2006). The epidemiology of pain in developmental disabilities. In: T. F. Oberlander & F. J. Symons (eds), *Pain in children & adults with developmental disabilities* (pp. 67–87). Paul H Brookes Publishing Co.

10 Hauer J, Houtrow AJ. (2017) Pain assessment and treatment in children with significant impairment of the central nervous system. *Pediatrics* **139**(6):e20171002.

11 Breau LM, Camfield CS, McGrath PJ, Finley GA. (2003) The incidence of pain in children with severe cognitive impairments. *Arch Pediatr Adolesc Med* **157(**12**)**:1219–26.

12 Stallard P, Williams L, Lenton S, Velleman R. (2001) Pain in cognitively impaired, non-communicating children. *Arch Dis Child* **85(**6**)**:460–2.

13 Schwartz L, Engel JM, Jensen MP. (1999) Pain in persons with cerebral palsy. *Arch Phys Med Rehabil* **80(**10**)**:1243–6.

14 Turk V, Khattran S, Kerry S, Corney R, Painter K. (2012) Reporting of health problems and pain by adults with an intellectual disability and by their carers. *J Appl Res Intellect Disabil.***25**(2):155–65.

15 McGuire BE, Daly P, Smyth F. (2010) Chronic pain in people with an intellectual disability: under-recognised and under-treated? *J Intellect Disabil Res* **54(**3**)**:240–245.

16 Walsh M, Morrison TG, McGuire BE. (2011) Chronic pain in adults with an intellectual disability: Prevalence, impact, and health service use based on caregiver report. *Pain* **152(**9**)**:1951–7.

17 Beange H, McElduff A, Baker W. (1995) Medical disorders of adults with mental retardation: a population study. *Am J Ment Retard* **99(**6**)**:595–604.

18 Ehde DM, Jensen MP, Engel JM, Turner JA, Hoffman AJ, Cardenas DD. (2003) Chronic pain secondary to disability: a review. *Clin J Pain* **19(**1**)**:3–17.

19 Chang E, Ghosh N, Yanni D, Lee S, Alexandru D, Mozaffar T. (2013) A review of spasticity treatments: Pharmacological and interventional approaches. *Crit Rev Phys Rehabil Med* **25(**1-2**)**:11–22.

20 Shamsoddini A, Amirsalari S, Hollisaz MT, Rahimniya A, Khatibi-Aghda A. (2014) Management of spasticity in children with cerebral palsy. *Iran J Pediatr* **24(**4**)**:354–351.

21 Kibele A. (1989) Occupational therapy's role in improving the quality of life for persons with cerebral palsy. *Am J Occup Ther Off Publ Am Occup Ther Assoc* 43(6):371–7.

22 Costigan M, Scholz J, Woolf CJ. (2009) Neuropathic pain: A maladaptive response of the nervous system to damage. *Annu Rev Neurosci* **32**:1–32.

23 Colloca L, Ludman T, Bouhassira D *et al.* (2017) Neuropathic pain. *Nat Rev Dis Prim* **3**:17002.

24 Appelros P. (2006) Prevalence and predictors of pain and fatigue after stroke: a population-based study. *Int J Rehabil Res* **29(**4**)**:329–33.

25 Cole LJ, Farrell MJ, Duff EP, Barber JB, Egan GF, Gibson SJ. (2006) Pain sensitivity and fMRI pain-related brain activity in Alzheimer's disease. *Brain* **129(**Pt 11**)**:2957–67.

26 Mayer EA, Bushnell MC. In: EA Mayer, MC Bushnell (eds), *Functional Pain Syndromes: Presentation and Pathophysiology*. IASP Press; Seattle: 2009. pp. 531–565.

27 Belew JL, Barney CC, Schwantes SA, Tibboel D, Valkenburg AJ, Symons FJ. (2013) Pain in children with intellectual or developmental disabilities. In: McGrath PJ, Stevens BJ, Walker SM, Zemsky WT, eds. *Oxford Textbook of Paediatric Pain*, 1st edn. Oxford University Press, Oxford.

28 Malviya S, Voepel-Lewis T, Burke C, Merkel S, Tait AR. (2006) The revised FLACC observational pain tool: Improved reliability and validity for pain assessment in children with cognitive impairment. *Paediatr Anaesth* **16(3)**:258–65.

29 Breau LM, McGrath PJ, Camfield CS, Finley GA. (2002) Psychometric properties of the non-communicating children's pain checklist-revised. *Pain* **99(**1-2**)**:359–57.

30 Collignon P, Giusiano B. (2001) Validation of a pain evaluation scale for patients with severe cerebral palsy. *Eur J Pain* **5(**4**)**:433–42.

31 Hunt A, Goldman A, Seers K *et al.* (2004) Clinical validation of the paediatric pain profile. *Dev Med Child Neurol* **46(**1**)**: 9–18.

32 Breau LM, McGrath PJ, Camfield C, Rosmus C, Allen Finley G. (2000) Preliminary validation of an observational pain checklist for persons with cognitive impairments and inability to communicate verbally. *Dev Med Child Neurol* **42(**9**)**:609–16. doi:10.1017/S0012162200001146

33 Dubois A, Capdevila X, Bringuier S, Pry R. (2010) Pain expression in children with an intellectual disability. *Eur J Pain* **14(**6**)**:654–60.

34 Lotan M, Moe-Nilssen R, Ljunggren AE, Strand LI. (2009) Reliability of the Non-Communicating

Adult Pain Checklist (NCAPC), assessed by different groups of health workers. *Res Dev Disabil* **30(4)**:735–45.

35 Kingsnorth S, Townley A, Provvidenza C *et al.* (2014) Chronic pain assessment toolbox for children with disabilities: Section 3.0: Chronic pain assessment tools. Holland Bloorview Kids Rehabilitation Hospital. Available at: https://hollandbloorview.ca/research-education/knowledge-translation-products/chronic-pain-assessment-toolbox-children. Accessed October 23 2021.

36 Nader R, Oberlander TF, Chambers CT, Craig KD. (2004) Expression of pain in children with autism. *Clin J Pain* **20(2)**:88–97.

37 Oberlander TF, O'Donnell ME, Montgomery CJ. (1999) Pain in children with significant neurological impairment. *J Dev Behav Pediatr* **20(4)**:235–43.

38 Benromano T, Pick CG, Merick J, Defrin R. (2017) Physiological and behavioral responses to calibrated noxious stimuli among individuals with cerebral palsy and intellectual disability. *Pain Med (United States)* **18(3)**:441–453.

39 Siden HB, Carleton BC, Oberlander TF. (2013) Physician variability in treating pain and irritability of unknown origin in children with severe neurological Impairment. *Pain Res Manag* **18(5)**:254–8.

40 Breau LM, Camfield CS, McGrath PJ, Finley GA. (2004) Risk factors for pain in children with severe cognitive impairments. *Dev Med Child Neurol* **46**(6):364–71.

41 Bodfish J, Harper V, Deacon J, Symons FJ. (2001) *Identifying and Measuring Pain in Persons with Developmental Disabilities: A Manual for the Pain and Discomfort Scale (PADS).* Western Carolina Center Research Reports, Asheville.

42 Craig KD. (2015) Social communication model of pain. *Pain* **156(7)**:1198–9. doi: 10.1097/j.pain.0000000000000185. PMID: 26086113.

43 Hägglund G, Andersson S, Düppe H, Lauge-Pedersen H, Nordmark E, Westbom L. (2005). Prevention of dislocation of the hip in children with cerebral palsy. The first ten years of a population-based prevention programme. *J Bone Jt Surg - Ser B* **87(1)**:95–101.

44 Genik LM, Millett GE, McMurtry CM. (2019) Facilitating respite, communication, and care for children with intellectual and developmental disabilities: preliminary evaluation of the caregiver pain information guide. *Clin Pract Pediatr Psychol* **84(4)**:359–68.

45 Arnold LE. (1993) Clinical pharmacological issues in treating psychiatric disorders of patients with mental retardation. *Ann Clin Psychiatry* **5(3)**:189–97.

46 Ramstad K, Jahnsen R, Skjeldal OH, Diseth TH. (2011) Characteristics of recurrent musculoskeletal pain in children with cerebral palsy aged 8 to 18 years. *Dev Med Child Neurol* **53(11)**:1013–8.

47 Rabach I, Peri F, Minute M *et al.* (2019) Sedation and analgesia in children with cerebral palsy: a narrative review. *World J Pediatr* **15(5)**:523–40.

48 Wittkopf PG, Lloyd DM, Coe O, Yacoobali S, Billington J. (2020) The effect of interactive virtual reality on pain perception: a systematic review of clinical studies. *Disabil Rehabil* **42(26)**:3722–33.

49 Chan JSL, Tse SHM. (2011) Massage as therapy for persons with intellectual disabilities: a review of the literature. *J Intellect Disabil* **15(1)**:47–62.

50 Doody O, Bailey ME. (2019) Interventions in pain management for persons with an intellectual disability. *J Intellect Disabil* **23(1)**:132–144.

51 Allely CS. (2013) Pain sensitivity and observer perception of pain in individuals with autistic spectrum disorder. *Sci World J* **2013**:916178.

52 Phan A, Edwards CL, Robinson EL. (2005) The assessment of pain and discomfort in individuals with mental retardation. *Res Dev Disabil* **26(5)**:433–9.

Chapter 43

Pain and psychiatric illness

Michael Butterfield

Department of Psychiatry, Faculty of Medicine, University of British Columbia, Vancouver, British Columbia, Canada

In the not-so-distant past, individuals who experienced chronic pain without an identifiable "organic" cause of their pain were often characterized as being psychopathological [1]. Historically it was thought that the mental illness was the underlying etiology for the pain that these individuals were experiencing. We now know that there are many underlying neurobiological aetiologies that lead to the development and maintenance of chronic pain and that chronic pain can exist in the presence or absence of a psychiatric disorder [2, 3]. Of note, pain is rarely the primary symptom of any psychiatric disorder [4]. That being said, individuals can experience physical manifestations of underlying emotional distress and occasionally this sensation can be pain. This has been termed "somatization" [5]. However, pain is rarely the dominant symptom and is usually accompanied by a number of other physical sensations. In the past, somatization was a term that was often used in a pejorative manner. However, more recently the term somatization has been reclaimed to more effectively and positively describe these physical sensations while facilitating the conceptualization of a mind-body connection [6]. With this in mind, we can begin to see how psychiatric symptoms overlap with symptoms associated with chronic pain such as fatigue, sleep disturbance and cognitive disruption with the hope that concurrent treatment of these symptoms in a holistic, patient-centered approach will improve patient outcomes.

In this chapter, high rates of comorbidity, overlapping symptom profiles and neurobiological aetiologies will be discussed to highlight the importance of detection and treatment of psychiatric disorders in individuals with pain since comorbidity of psychiatric illness and chronic pain negatively affects prognosis and treatment success [7].

Mood Disorders

Depressive disorders are one of the most common psychiatric disorders in individuals that suffer from chronic pain. Chronic pain is most commonly comorbid with major depressive disorder (MDD), with prevalence rates of comorbidity being 27% in primary care clinics [7]. Interestingly, studies have shown that in general pain clinics the prevalence of MDD is approximately 52% and in some subspecialty pain clinics such as dental pain clinics, prevalence rates can be as high as 85%[7]; highlighting the profound association between chronic pain and mood disorders. Persistent depressive disorder on the other hand is not as strongly associated with chronic pain with a prevalence of between 1 to 9% [8]. The combined prevalence of bipolar I and bipolar II disorder with chronic pain ranges between 1 to 21%[8]. Of note, in patients with bipolar I or bipolar II disorder, the prevalence of migraine is almost twice the prevalence rate of the general population with some studies showing a prevalence rate of 24% [9, 10]. The focus of the rest of this section will primarily be on the comorbidity between MDD and chronic pain.

Clinical Pain Management: A Practical Guide, Second Edition. Edited by Mary E. Lynch, Kenneth D. Craig, and Philip W. Peng.

Not only is MDD a common comorbidity of chronic pain but it also increases the risk of the development of chronic pain. It has been shown that there is a positive correlation between MDD symptom severity and pain severity over time [11]. Further, some clinical features of pain disorders including severity of pain, duration of pain and pain location may be indicative of the presence of a depressive disorder. Individuals with pain lasting greater than 6 months are at four-fold increased the risk of developing MDD and individuals with three or more sites of pain are at an eight-fold increased risk [7, 12]. Finally, individuals with back pain, fibromyalgia, temporomandibular joint disorder and chronic abdominal pain have the highest probability of developing a depressive disorder [13-16].

The importance of identifying MDD in individuals with chronic pain cannot be emphasized enough. The presence of a MDD is a better predictor of disability than pain severity or duration and leads to higher treatment resistance for both pain and depression [7]. One of the most important reasons for identifying individuals with comorbid MDD and chronic pain is that this population is more likely to have thoughts of suicide than individuals with MDD alone and the risk of completing suicide is two to three times higher [17]. Therefore, it is of utmost importance for any health care professional treating individuals with pain to be able to properly identify the presence of a depressive disorder in their patient population.

Given the consistent findings of highly prevalent comorbidity and synchronicity between depressive symptoms and pain, there has been a significant amount of research focused on identifying shared pathways and common mechanisms between pain and depression. We know that the pathophysiology of both chronic pain and depression can involve dysfunctional serotonergic and noradrenergic signaling [8, 18]. The abnormal ascending serotonergic and noradrenergic signalling to the brain leads to the signs we see and symptoms of depression whereas the abnormal descending signalling can impact pain perception [19]. Additionally, there are a number of different brain regions that are known to function abnormally in both depressive and pain disorders including the anterior cingulate cortex, dorsolateral prefrontal cortex and insula [8, 18].

With this shared mechanism of overlapping neurotransmitter systems in mind, it is not surprising that serotonin-norepinephrine reuptake inhibitors (SNRIs) have been shown to effectively treat both depressive symptoms and pain. Duloxetine has been the most studied medication for the treatment of concurrent MDD and chronic pain with significant positive response rates for both pain and depression, though in some studies the improvements in pain are independent of changes in depressive symptom severity [11]. Interestingly, ketamine (NMDA receptor antagonist) has been shown to be an effective treatment for treatment-resistant depression and is used for management of treatment-resistant neuropathic pain, again suggesting shared mechanistic pathways [20, 21].

In addition to pharmacological interventions, psychotherapeutic treatments such as cognitive behavioral therapy and mindfulness-based therapies have been demonstrated to lead to sustained improvements in a number of functional domains in both depressive and pain disorders with very few side effects. Therefore, these treatments should be considered first line treatments in individuals with this comorbidity [8, 11].

Anxiety Disorders

Anxiety disorders are also some of the most common comorbid psychiatric disorders in individuals living with chronic pain [22]. Anxiety disorders are defined as disorders of excessive fear and anxiety and related behavioral disturbances. Individuals with anxiety disorders often overestimate the danger in the situations they fear or avoid. This is of particular importance in individuals with chronic pain who can experience pain-related fear and subsequent avoidance of physical activity. This avoidance can further perpetuate pain-related disability and the maintenance of the pain symptoms [23].

Epidemiological studies show an increased prevalence of anxiety disorders in various pain disorders including osteoarthritis, chronic back pain and migraine. Individuals with back pain are two to three times more likely to have a panic disorder, agoraphobia or social anxiety disorder; and three times more likely to have a diagnosis of generalized anxiety disorder or post-traumatic stress disorder [22, 24].

A direct correlation has been shown between the severity of the anxiety symptoms and the severity of pain and pain-associated disability [25, 26]. Interestingly, having a past history of an anxiety disorder without any active symptoms also increases the odds ratio of having a more severe pain with a high level of disability [25]. Conversely, a high level of pain that interferes with daily activities is associated with more severe anxiety symptoms and a decreased chance of responding to treatment for certain anxiety disorders [27].

Like in depressive disorders, there are common neurobiological circuits and altered areas of activity in certain brain regions in anxiety and chronic pain disorders. Dysfunction of the regulation of the noradrenergic system is commonly seen in both chronic pain and anxiety disorders leading to impaired descending pain inhibition and increased arousal and sympathetic overdrive, respectively [19, 28]. Anxiety disorders are thought to result in part from disruption of balance of neural activity between higher cognitive regions and emotional regions in the brain. One of the regions that is commonly observed to have altered activity in anxiety disorders is the limbic cortex, which includes the insular cortex and cingulate cortex. These regions integrate the sensory, affective and cognitive components of pain and functional abnormally in individuals with chronic pain [29].

Treatment options for anxiety disorders and pain disorders are often overlapping and complementary. Some of the most effective treatments for anxiety disorders and chronic pain disorders are psychotherapeutic treatments such as cognitive behavioral therapy [30, 31]. The focus of cognitive behavioral therapy in individuals with anxiety disorders and chronic pain is to interrupt the fear avoidance cycle by developing alternative thinking patterns in relation to their pain and encouraging and supporting positive behavioral change. From a pharmacological standpoint, there are also a number of medications that are used for treatment of anxiety disorders and pain disorders such as SNRIs, pregabalin and gabapentin [31, 32].

Trauma and Stressor Related Disorders

Trauma and stressor-related disorders are very common in individuals suffering from chronic pain. This group of disorders is characterized by exposure to a traumatic or stressful event and in some cases of people living with chronic pain, can be well understood within an anxiety- or fear-based context. The most common of these disorders seen in chronic pain populations include adjustment disorder and post-traumatic stress disorder (PTSD) [26, 33].

The DSM-5 criteria for an adjustment disorder primarily includes the development of emotional or behavioral symptoms in response to a stressor, which could include the development of chronic pain. These symptoms must also cause significant impairment and/or marked distress that is out of proportion to the severity or intensity of the stressor [33]. Most individuals with chronic pain will develop some emotional or behavioral response to their pain. However, to meet criteria for an adjustment disorder, this response must be out of proportion to what others in their situation would be experiencing. Furthermore, adjustment disorders can present with depressed mood, anxiety symptoms or a combination thereof.

The connection between chronic pain and PTSD has been receiving increased attention and research focus. The primary clinical features of PTSD include exposure to a traumatic event, recurrent and intrusive trauma-related thoughts, persistent avoidance of stimuli associated with the traumatic event, negative alterations in thoughts and mood and marked alterations in arousal and reactivity [34]. The prevalence of post-traumatic stress disorder in people with chronic musculoskeletal pain or low back pain is approximately 10% [26]. When individuals develop chronic musculoskeletal pain as a consequence of a motor vehicle accident, the prevalence of PTSD increases to between 30 to 50% [35]. Conversely, in people with PTSD, approximately 30% of them will describe some type of chronic pain disorder such as back pain or migraines. The prevalence of chronic pain in military veterans and with PTSD increases to 66% [36]. Individuals with chronic pain and PTSD report higher pain severity, increased pain chronicity, more emotional distress, greater pain interference and greater disability than those without a PTSD diagnosis [24, 26, 37].

Similar to both depressive and anxiety disorders, PTSD has a number of shared symptoms with different chronic pain disorders. Individuals with both PTSD and chronic pain have increased somatic hyper-vigilance, lowered pain thresholds and avoidance behaviours as prominent symptom clusters [24]. The combination of these symptom clusters can lead to increased risk of depression and inactivity, reinforcing the pain fear-avoidance cycle. In both disorders, avoidance may be adopted as a means to minimize pain and disturbing thoughts.

The neurobiological underpinnings of PTSD involve abnormal modulation in a number of areas of the brain which are also important in the processing of painful stimuli including the amygdala, insula and prefrontal cortex [38]. Like in certain chronic pain disorders, the noradrenergic system, with its cell bodies in the locus coeruleus, can be dysfunctional in PTSD. This system is often hyperactive, leading to common symptoms of increased autonomic arousal and hypervigilance [39]. This overlap in neurobiological substrates may be one of the reasons why there is more treatment resistance when both PTSD and chronic pain are present.

Treatment for individuals with PTSD and chronic pain should be multi-modal with a trauma-informed care approach [24, 26, 31]. Similar to anxiety and depressive disorders, there is a significant overlap in the types of treatment that are used for management of PTSD and chronic pain. From a psychotherapeutic approach, this includes cognitive behavioral therapy and mindfulness-based therapies. One study that examined the effect of an integrated CBT treatment for pain and PTSD showed significant improvements at 6-month follow-up in all domains, which included PTSD symptoms, depressive symptoms and anxiety symptoms [40]. PTSD symptoms unrelated to pain may be specifically targeted using trauma-focused cognitive therapy or eye movement desensitization and reprocessing (EMDR[1]) [31, 41]. From a pharmacological perspective, the use of medications such as SNRIs or TCAs is encouraged to target both PTSD symptoms and pain, though multimodal analgesia may provide more symptom benefit depending on the patient's individual symptom profile. Other pharmacological treatments that are showing some promising results include the use of cannabinoids and ketamine [42]. However, at this point in time, there is not enough evidence to support the regular use of these medications in this patient population [1].

[1] EMDR is a type of psychotherapy that incorporates having the individual perform specific eye movements or rhythmic stimulation while recalling traumatic experiences. This treatment is associated with desensitization of negative responses to traumatic memories and reduction of PTSD symptoms.

Adjustment Disorders, Somatic Symptom and Related Disorders

With the release of the DSM-5 in 2013, the diagnosis of "pain disorder" was removed and the diagnosis of "somatic symptom disorder (SSD), with predominant pain" was added [34]. This was a major change in how pain as a symptom was viewed as a diagnostic entity from a psychiatric perspective. In SDD, the two main criteria include (1) an individual must have at least one physical symptom that is distressing or results in disruption of daily life (which could include pain) and (2) must exhibit excessive thoughts, feelings and behaviours related to those symptoms [34].

There has been much debate as to the appropriateness of this change in the DSM-5. Overall, this change has been welcomed as it has been a positive step forward with removing the diagnoses of "pain disorder", "somatization disorder" and "undifferentiated somatoform disorder". The criteria for those disorders were thought to be either much too over-inclusive or much too stringent, making the utility of these diagnostic entities quite challenging. Thus, most psychiatrists tended to avoid making these diagnoses and these disorders were often under diagnosed [1].

Studies investigating the utility of the new SSD diagnostic category have shown that the criteria may lead to diagnostic overinflation, with up to 25% of people living with chronic widespread pain meeting criteria for SDD [43]. A high false positive rate of diagnosing of SSD can also lead to underlying medical causes of their symptoms being missed. It has been suggested that somatic symptom disorder has not been adequately field tested in individuals with chronic pain conditions and this in combination with diagnostic inflation lead to a high probability of diagnosing a medical illness, including chronic pain, as a mental illness [33]. In response to these concerns, it has been suggested that individuals who exhibit psychiatric symptoms in response to pain that are thought to be out of proportion should be given a diagnosis of an adjustment disorder [33]. By using the diagnosis of adjustment disorder, in place of SSD, it may decrease stigmatization of the psychiatric symptoms that are often seen in people living with chronic pain. It is important to note that if an individual does meet criteria for another psychiatric disorder, such as MDD or PTSD, then that diagnosis should be made [44].

In summary, as presented in several other chapters in this book, significant progress has been made in our understanding of the pathophysiology of chronic pain, yet unfortunately a quarter of a century has led to no real progress in how pain is treated in the DSM [44]. We are left with diagnostic criteria that have high false positive rates that increase stigmatization and can lead to missed diagnoses and inappropriate treatment [33, 44–46]. Moving forward, it will be important not to over-pathologize psychological distress associated with painful conditions but at the same time identify and treat psychiatric diagnoses when they are present.

Conclusions

Depressive disorders, anxiety disorders, adjustment disorders and PTSD are common comorbidities in individuals with chronic pain. Rarely are these disorders the cause of the pain, but they can exacerbate overall suffering. They often have common symptom profiles and shared pathophysiology. The presence of these psychiatric disorders can have negative effects on treatment outcomes which highlights the importance of early recognition and concurrent treatment of psychiatric disorders in individuals with chronic pain.

References

1 Scamvougeras A, Howard A. (2020) Somatic symptom disorder, medically unexplained symptoms, somatoform disorders, functional neurological disorder: how DSM-5 got it wrong. *Can J Psychiatry* **65**(5):301–5.

2 Okifuji A, Turk DC. (2014) Assessment of Patients with Chronic Pain with or Without Comorbid Mental Health Problems. In: Marchand S., Saravane D., Gaumond I. (eds.) *Mental Health and Pain*. Springer, Paris.

3 Apkarian AV, Bushnell CA, Schweinhardt P. (2013) Representation of Pain in the Brain. In: Mcmahon S, Koltzenburg M, Tracey I, Turk D. (eds.) *Wall & Melzack's Textbook of Pain*, 6th edn. Elsevier, Philadelphia.

4 Gagliese L, Katz J. (2000) Medically unexplained pain is not caused by psychopathology. *Pain Res Manag* **5**(4):251–7.

5 Lipowski ZJ. (1988) Somatization: the concept and its clinical application. *Am J Psychiatry*. **145**(11):1358–68.

6 Boerner KE, Green K, Chapman A *et al.* (2020) Making sense of "somatization": a systematic review of its relationship to pediatric pain. *J Pediatr Psychol* **45**(2):156–69.

7 Bair MJ, Wu J, Damush TM, Sutherland JM, Kroenke K. (2008) Association of depression and anxiety alone and in combination with chronic musculoskeletal pain in primary care patients. *Psychosom Med* **70**(8):890–7.

8 Hooten WM. (2016) Chronic pain and mental health disorders: shared neural mechanisms, epidemiology, and treatment. *Mayo Clin Proc* **91**(7):955–70.

9 Ortiz A, Cervantes P, Zlotnik G *et al.* (2010) Cross-prevalence of migraine and bipolar disorder. *Bipolar Disord* **12**(4):397–403.

10 Stovner LJ, Hagen K, Jensen R *et al.* (2007) The global burden of headache: a documentation of headache prevalence and disability worldwide. *Cephalalgia* **27**(3):193–210.

11 IsHak WW, Wen RY, Naghdechi L *et al.* (2018) Pain and depression: a systematic review. *Harv Rev Psychiatry* **26**(6):352–63.

12 Currie SR, Wang JL. (2004) Chronic back pain and major depression in the general Canadian population. *Pain* **107**(1-2):54–60.

13 Balliet WE, Edwards-Hampton S, Borckardt JJ *et al.* Depressive symptoms, pain, and quality of life among patients with nonalcohol-related chronic pancreatitis. *Pain Res Treat* 2012:978646.

14 Dersh J, Gatchel RJ, Mayer T, Polatin P, Temple OR. (2006) Prevalence of psychiatric disorders in patients with chronic disabling occupational spinal disorders. *Spine (Phila Pa 1976)* **31**(10):1156–62

15 Giannakopoulos NN, Keller L, Rammelsberg P, Kronmüller KT, Schmitter M. (2010) Anxiety and depression in patients with chronic temporomandibular pain and in controls. *J Dent* **38**(5): 369–76.

16 Uguz F, Çiçek E, Salli A *et al.* (2010) Axis I and Axis II psychiatric disorders in patients with fibromyalgia. *Gen Hosp Psychiatry* **32**(1):105–7.

17 Tang NKY, Crane C. (2006) Suicidality in chronic pain: A review of the prevalence, risk factors and psychological links. *Psychol Med* **36**(5):575–86.

18 Sheng J, Liu S, Wang Y, Cui R, Zhang X. (2017) The link between depression and chronic pain: neural mechanisms in the brain. *Neural Plast* **2017**:9724581.

19 Stahl S, Briley M. (2004) Understanding pain in depression. *Hum Psychopharmacol* **19**(Suppl.1): 9–13.

20 Cohen SP, Bhatia A, Buvanendran A *et al.* (2018) Consensus guidelines on the use of intravenous ketamine infusions for chronic pain from the American Society of Regional Anesthesia and Pain Medicine, the American Academy of Pain Medicine, and the American Society of Anesthesiologists. *Reg Anesth Pain Med* **43**(5):521–46.

21 Phillips JL, Norris S, Talbot J *et al.* (2019) Single, repeated, and maintenance ketamine infusions for treatment-resistant depression: a randomized controlled trial. *Am J Psychiatry* 176(5):401–9.

22 Velly AM, Mohit S. (2018) Epidemiology of pain and relation to psychiatric disorders. *Prog Neuro-Psychopharmacology Biol Psychiatry* **87**(Pt B):159–67.

23 Lucchetti G, Oliveira AB, Mercante JPP, Peres MFP. (2012) Anxiety and fear-avoidance in musculoskeletal pain. *Curr Pain Headache Rep* **16**(5):399–406.

24 Asmundson GJG, Coons MJ, Taylor S, Katz J. (2002) PTSD and the experience of pain: research and clinical implications of shared vulnerability and mutual maintenance models. *Can J Psychiatry* **47**(10):930–937.

25 De Heer EW, Gerrits MMJG, Beekman ATF *et al.* (2014) The association of depression and anxiety with pain: a study from NESDA. *PLoS One* **9**(10):1–11.

26 Asmundson GJG, Katz J. (2009) Understanding the co-occurrence of anxiety disorders and chronic pain: state-of-the-art. *Depress Anxiety* **26**(10):888–901.

27 Teh CF, Morone NE, Karp JF *et al.* (2009) Pain interference impacts response to treatment for anxiety disorder. *Depress Anxiety* **26**(3):222–8.

28 Morris LS, McCall JG, Charney DS, Murrough JW. (2020) The role of the locus coeruleus in the generation of pathological anxiety. *Brain Neurosci Adv* **4**:239821282093032.

29 Martin EI, Ressler KJ, Binder E, Nemeroff CB. (2009) The neurobiology of anxiety disorders: brain imaging, genetics, and psychoneuroendocrinology. *Psychiatr Clin North Am* **32**(3): 549–75.

30 Eccleston C, Morley SJ, Williams AC. (2013) Psychological approaches to chronic pain management: evidence and challenges. *Br J Anaesth* **111(1)**:59–63.

31 Katzman MA, Bleau P, Blier P *et al.* (2014) Canadian clinical practice guidelines for the management of anxiety, posttraumatic stress and obsessive-compulsive disorders. *BMC Psychiatry* **14**(Suppl.1):S1.

32 Mu A, Weinberg E, Moulin DE, Clarke H. (2017) Pharmacologic management of chronic neuropathic pain. *Can Fam Physician* **63:(**11):844–52.

33 Katz J, Rosenbloom BN, Fashler S. (2015) Chronic pain, psychopathology, and DSM-5 somatic symptom disorder. *Can J Psychiatry* **60**(4):160–7.

34 American Psychiatric Association. DSM-5. In: *Diagnostic and Statistical Manual of Mental Disorders*, 5th Edn.

35 Beck JG, Coffey SF. (2007) Assessment and treatment of posttraumatic stress disorder after a motor vehicle collision: empirical findings and clinical observations. *Prof Psychol Res Pract* **38**(6):629–39.

36 Otis JD, Keane TM, Kerns RD. (2003) An examination of the relationship between chronic pain and post-traumatic stress disorder. *J Rehabil Res Dev* **40**(5):397–406.

37 Benedict TM, Keenan PG, Nitz AJ, Moeller-Bertram T. (2020) Post-traumatic stress disorder symptoms contribute to worse pain and health outcomes in veterans with PTSD compared to those without: a systematic review with meta-analysis. *Mil Med* **185**(9-10):E1481–91.

38 Moeller-Bertram T, Keltner J, Strigo IA. (2012) Pain and post traumatic stress disorder - review of clinical and experimental evidence. *Neuropharmacology* **62**(2):586–97.

39 Naegeli C, Zeffiro T, Piccirelli M *et al.* (2018) Locus coeruleus activity mediates hyperresponsiveness in posttraumatic stress disorder. *Biol Psychiatry* **83**(3):254–62.

40 Otis JD, Keane TM, Kerns RD, Monson C, Scioli E. (2009) The development of an integrated treatment for veterans with comorbid chronic pain and posttraumatic stress disorder. *Pain Med* **10**(7):1300–11.

41 Chen Y, Hung K, Tsai J, Chu H, Chung M, Chen S. (2014) Efficacy of eye-movement desensitization and reprocessing for patients with posttraumatic-stress disorder: a meta-analysis of randomized controlled trials PLoS One **9** (8):e103676.

42 Yehuda R, Hoge CW, McFarlane AC *et al.* (2015) Post-traumatic stress disorder. *Nat Rev Dis Prim* **1**:15057.

43 Frances A. (2013) The new somatic symptom disorder in DSM-5 risks mislabeling many people as mentally ill. *BMJ* **346**:f1580.

44 Lynch ME. (2015) What is the latest in pain mechanisms and management? *Can J Psychiatry* **60**(4):157–9.

45 Frances A. (2013) DSM-5 somatic symptom disorder. *J Nerv Ment Dis* **201**(6):530–1.

46 Dimsdale JE. (2011) Medically unexplained symptoms : a treacherous foundation for somatoform disorders? *PSC* **34**(3):511–513.

Chapter 44

Basic principles in acute and perioperative pain management in patients with opioid tolerance

Benjamin Matson[1,2], James Chue[1], & Oscar A. de Leon-Casasola[1,2]

[1] *Department of Anesthesiology, The Jacobs School of Medicine at the University of Buffalo, Buffalo, New York, USA*
[2] *Division of Pain Medicine, Roswell Park Comprehensive Cancer Institute, Buffalo, New York, USA*

Background

Pain in the perioperative setting is unique in some ways. The most relevant is that the pain is the result of intentional trauma. This uniqueness allows us to study and understand in a 'before and after' comparison. We can then apply this understanding to predict and anticipate pain and then be prepared to treat it. To accomplish this goal of pain control in the perioperative setting we rely on our understanding not just of anatomy and physiology, but also on surgical principles such as the gentle handling of tissues [1]. The therapeutic targets are chosen along criteria of safety, efficacy and ease of access.

Neurophysiology of Pain

Sensing pain begins with converting the biophysical activity into a transmittible message in the process known as transduction. Transduction happens via the activation of specific neuron types with specific features. One of these features is a projection of their dendrites into fibers which penetrate connective tissues such as the skin [2]. Though slightly thickened at the terminal end, these fibers lack a complex sensory structure, do not formally engage another cell and thus are known as free nerve endings (FNE). Some FNE will be activated by moderate heat or cold (thermoception), some by light touch (mechanoreception) and others by painful (nociception) amounts of temperature, touch and chemicals [2, 3].

The cell membranes of neurons regulate the electric charge between the cell's interior and exterior through ion channels. A class of ion channels particularly relevant to nociceptor neurons is Transient Receptor Potential (TRP) channels [3]. They allow the passage of positively charged ions like calcium and sodium in a proportion of 8:1 when open. Upon activation, the channel opens and the ions rush in depolarizing the cell. This initiates an action potential which is then transmitted across the cell. There are several classes of TRP channel and it is the specific TRP channels in the cell membrane which determine whether the nociceptor is activated by chemicals, by temperature or by mechanical stress. This model of FNE and TRP channels alone does not account for episodes of increased pain (hyperalgesia) or increased sensitivity to noxious stimulation (allodynia) that are seen after injury. In their baseline state some nociceptors are effectively silent. The routine stimulus is not enough to activate the TRP channel and transduce a message of pain. However, after tissue injury the release of chemical

Clinical Pain Management: A Practical Guide, Second Edition. Edited by Mary E. Lynch, Kenneth D. Craig, and Philip W. Peng.

mediators such as serotonin, bradykinin and histamine as well as the decreased pH of the environment change the behavior of the nociceptive neuron [4]. The altered responses to noxious stimuli following tissue injury are collectively described peripheral sensitization. These may directly activate the channel or raise the resting membrane potential making the neuron more easily activated [4, 5, 6]. In addition, the local effects of swelling and increased blood flow of these chemical mediators lead to increased activation of thermal and mechanical nociceptors.

Knowledge of these ion channels allows us to identify some therapeutic targets. Topical capsaicin works by opening the TRPV1 channel long enough to defunctionalize the neuron, preventing it from transducing painful stimuli. However, capsaicin can induce an unpleasant sense of warmth when first applied which makes it unsuitable for perioperative pain management. Similarly, topical camphor exerts its effect through TRPM8. Less specific to nociception, voltage sensitive sodium channels in the neuron are susceptible to local anesthetics (LAs). The local anesthetic prevents the channel from permitting sodium to flow into the cell, thus preventing the action potential. Applying surgical principles of gentle tissue handling and preservation of blood supply reduce tissue damage. This decreases the release of inflammatory chemical mediators thus diminishing peripheral sensitization. Nonsteroidal anti-inflammatory drugs (NSAIDs) and intravenous local anesthetic also exert an effect against peripheral sensitization by interrupting the inflammatory chemical mediator signaling.

The first order nociceptive neuron's cell body resides near the spinal cord in a dorsal root ganglion. It is these neuron's dendritic fibers that extend to the FNE throughout the body. Two subtypes of primary neurons exist, Aδ (A delta) and C. These primary neurons pass their action potential messages via synapse to spinal cord neurons. This process is known as transmission.

Both Aδ (A delta) and C fibers are small and slow in comparison to other nerve fiber types. C fibers are smaller, slower than Aδ and have no myelin while Aδ are thinly myelinated. C fibers also branch closer to the cell body and will innervate a larger distribution of tissue than Aδ fibers. Consequently, sensations from Aδ fibers are more discrete and localized than the diffuse sensations carried on C fibers. Both Aδ and C fibers synapse with second order neurons in Rexed laminae II and V of the dorsal horn of the spinal cord.

When an action potential travelling on a neuron reaches the end of the cell involved in synapse it triggers the release of neurotransmitters into the synaptic cleft. The neuron produces these neurotransmitters and packages them into closed synaptic vesicles. The release of synaptic vesical contents into the cleft is mediated through the activation of voltage gates calcium channels (VGCCs). The excitatory neurotransmitters released by pain neurons include substance P, calcitonin related gene peptide (CGRP), brain derived neurotrophic factor (BDNF) and glutamate [7, 8]. In opposition, when presynaptic opioid receptors are activated, this hyperpolarizes the resting membrane potential of the neuron decreasing the release of these excitatory neurotransmitters [9]. A particular type of glutamate receptor, *N*-methyl-d-aspartate (NMDA), in the post-synaptic neuron in the spinal cord induces hyperexcitability when activated. NMDA receptor (NMDAR) activation in glial cells around the primary neuron contribute to central sensitization.

The anatomy and physiology of transmission present several potential therapeutic targets. Identification of the nerve through which the C and/or Aδ fibers are traveling and then bathing it in local anesthetic will stop pain transmission; and there are many well described peripheral nerve blocks. Gabapentin and pregabalin bind to the α2δ subunit of VGCCs modulating signal transmission at the synapse. Both have been shown to reduce pain and opioid requirements in the perioperative setting. Local anesthetic and opioid can be delivered via an epidural catheter. The local anesthetic will cover a broader area of the body than a peripheral nerve block. The opioid will decrease pain transmission by reducing release of excitatory neurotransmitters at the synapse. Ketamine antagonizes the NMDAR, reducing peripheral sensitization and interrupting pain transmission, and can be given as a continuous infusion.

Transmission continues from the dorsal horn of the spinal cord through the spinothalamic and spinoreticulothalamic tracts. These tracts communicate with the ventral posterolateral (VPL), ventral posterior inferior (VPI) and other nuclei in the thalamus, the mesencephalic reticular formation, the periaqueductal gray (PAG) and tectum of the brain stem. Perception of pain occurs as these structures communicate via the third order neurons with the cerebral cortical structures such as the primary somatosensory cortex.

Pain signals are modulated significantly in the brainstem and midbrain. There are projections into the limbic structures and hypothalamus which mediate the emotional and visceral responses to pain. Opioid receptors in the PAG, rostral ventral medulla (RVM), caudate nucleus, nucleus raphe magnus and others perform a similar function as in the spinal cord by hyperpolarizing their target neurons. This decreases the pain signal transmission when activated by endogenous ligands and pharmaceuticals.

The PAG, nucleus raphe magnus, locus coerulus and others comprise a circuit that when activated suppresses painful signals. This is the descending inhibitory pathway. The opioid receptor plays a different role here. Neurons in the RVM which can suppress ascending painful signals are at baseline kept inactive by neurons in the PAG. When opioid receptors in these PAG neurons are activated, this "off switch" is disengaged activating the RVM neurons to suppress these ascending signals [10]. Thus, opioids play two distinct roles in pain attenuation depending on the where the opioid receptors are located.

Cannabinoid receptors (CBR) have been found to play a role pain perception as well. When opioid receptors are repeatedly activated it is found that increasing doses of opioids are required to achieve the same level of analgesia. This physiological tolerance can develop rapidly. By antagonizing the CBR2, tolerance is mitigated [11]. This restores the efficacy of opioid receptor activation to provide analgesia. Acetaminophen metabolites antagonize the CBR2.

In synthesis, the full armamentarium of perioperative analgesia is extensive. The choice of pre-, intra- and post-operative analgesia should be tailored to the patient and the surgery. The intravenous formulation of pregabalin is in limited use and no intravenous gabapentin is available, thus oral gabapentinoids can be given pre-operatively for the decreased pain transmission benefit. Both acetaminophen and Cox-2 inhibitors can be given at the same time as the gabapentinoid [12]. Respectively these promote opioid receptor sensitivity and diminish peripheral sensitization. The preoperative period is also the window to initiate regional anesthesia in the form of a peripheral nerve block or epidural catheter delivering local anesthetic and an opioid [13]. The factors influencing the choice of peripheral nerve block versus epidural, and the spinal level of the epidural, are numerous. However, these effectively stop transmission and should be discussed with the anesthesiologists in advance. After the initiation of sedation or anesthesia, local anesthetic infiltration prior to incision blocks transduction but requires waiting the full time for onset. During the intraoperative phase both the surgeon and anesthesiologist play a role. Good surgical technique including gentle tissue handling and preservation of blood supply curb peripheral sensitization. Lidocaine infusions have been shown to decrease post-operative pain[12] via their anti-inflammatory effect [14]. A ketamine infusion, which can also be continued post-operatively, diminishes central sensitization and transmission at the level of the spinal cord [15]. In the postoperative window, acetaminophen, NSAIDs/COX-2 inhibitors, peripheral nerve blocks (via catheter placement), epidural infusions, lidocaine and ketamine infusions, can be continued. The most widely recognized form of perioperative analgesia, oral and intravenous opioids to enhance the descending inhibitory pathway, is ultimately the last.

Practical Management

In clinical practice it is evident that every patient for every surgery does not require every intervention. However, clinicians may encounter patients who do require such intensive management. The Division of Pain Medicine at Roswell Park Comprehensive Cancer Center has found the population of patients who do require the highest level of coordination between the surgeon, the operative anesthesiologist and the post-operative pain medicine consultant are those who present to the surgical suite with tolerance to opioids. There is not sufficient evidence in the literature to support formal guidelines such as Procedure Specific Postoperative Pain Management (PROSPECT) in this specific population. This is our approach to multi-modal analgesia [16] in these patients based on the joint American Pain Society, American Society of Regional Anesthesia and American Society of Anesthesiology Guidelines on the Management of Postoperative Pain [16]. We define an opioid tolerant patient as one who shows clinical signs of tolerance and has tolerated for more than one week a total daily oral dose of at least 60 mg of morphine or its equivalent. We use this conversion of equivalent doses: transdermal fentanyl 25 mcg/hr, oxycodone 30 mg, oxymorphone 25 mg, hydromorphone 8 mg, hydrocodone 60 mg [17].

In the preoperative holding area, 30-60 minutes prior to the start of surgery, the patient is given an oral dose of gabapentin, celecoxib and acetaminophen unless contraindicated. A gabapentin dose of 300 mg followed by a tapering dose has been shown to reduce the incidence of neuropathic pain and decrease post-operative opioid use [18]. Our typical gabapentin dose is 600 mg for patients <60 years of age, 300 mg for patients 60-69 years and no typical dose (avoidance) in patients 70 years and above. This guideline-based gradation is influenced by empirical post-anesthesia care unit holding times due to excessive sedation. We dose celecoxib at 400 mg for patients <65 years of age with normal renal function, 200 mg for those 65 and above or with creatinine clearance of 30-50 mL.min-1 and held for those with more significant renal impairment. Celecoxib is contraindicated in patients who undergo coronary artery bypass grafting. A celecoxib dose of 400 mg given this way was shown to reduce post-operative pain scores and opioid consumption [19]. The need of an opioid rescue dose is reduced from 91% to 63% [20] and the time of the first post-operative rescue dose of opioids is increased from 2.3 hours to 6.6 hours [20]. Acetaminophen has been shown to reduce opioid consumption post-operatively by 33% [21]. If the patient cannot tolerate oral feedings post-operatively then we convert to IV acetaminophen until such time as they can.

Intraoperatively, the surgical site is infiltrated with long-acting local anesthetic as appropriate for the specific surgical procedure [16]. When significant pain is expected beyond the duration of the local anesthetic, continuous infusion of local anesthetic peripheral regional anesthesia is used. Such catheters are placed via standardized regional techniques when appropriate or surgically when necessary. Ketamine and lidocaine infusions are also started intraoperatively. Ketamine infusion is started with a 0.5 mcg.kg-1 bolus and continued at 10 mcg.kg-1.min-1. In overweight patients we use a dosing weight formula: dosing weight = ideal weight + (actual weight – ideal weight)/3. The infusion is continued until hospital discharge without a weaning period or until pain is satisfactorily controlled. Lidocaine infusion is started with a 1.5 mg.kg-1 bolus and continued at 2 mg.kg-1.hr-1 into the post-operative period.

It is preferred that these patients receive appropriate regional anesthesia. This is particularly important in patients who are having major thoracic or abdominal surgery and are at risk for cardiac or pulmonary complications or post-operative ileus [16]. In the setting of an epidural placed pre-operatively, a 5-10 mL dose of ropivacaine 0.5% is given 10-15 minutes prior to the incision. Then a continuous infusion of ropivacaine 0.2% and morphine 0.010%, or 5 mg morphine in 50 mL, is given at a rate of 4-6 mL.hr-1. This infusion is continued postoperatively via patient controlled epidural analgesia (PCEA) with an initial basal rate of 3 mL.hr-1 for those <55 years and 2mL.hr-1 for those older. Bolus doses of 2 mL with a lock-out of 10 minutes are ordered. If sufficient analgesia cannot be obtained even by increasing the basal rate to 5 mL.hr-1, then the solution is changed to ropivacaine 0.2% and hydromorphone 0.004%, or 2 mg hydromorphone in 50 mL. We retain the capacity to compound custom concentrations of ropivacaine, bupivacaine, morphine, hydromorphone and fentanyl as necessary. Providing the PCEA in this way has given excellent pain control and prevented physiologic signs of opioid withdrawal [22-24].

For patients whose regional anesthesia is not an epidural or for whom there is no appropriate regional technique, we provide patient controlled analgesia (PCA) starting in the post-anesthesia care unit (PACU). In these opioid tolerant patients, our preferred opioids are hydromorphone or sufentanil because of their greater intrinsic efficacy. Opioid tolerance in the spinal cord has been demonstrated to have both time dependent [25] and dose dependent [26] components. We then expect these patients have superior analgesia with small but frequent changes to a continuous infusion. However, continuous infusions, i.e. the basal rate, have not been shown to improve analgesia quality or reduce opioid consumption and carry significant risks of morbidity [27]. Still, in the cases where the patient takes long acting or time release opioids which cannot be continued post-operatively, we calculate a basal rate based on their long acting opioid requirements. For this purpose we consider a daily dose of 100 mg of oral morphine, 10-60 mg of oral methadone, 50 mg of oral oxycodone, 12 mg of oral hydromorphone, or 25 ug.hr^{-1} of transdermal fentanyl is equivalent to

2-3 mg of IV hydromorphone or 2-4 ug.hr-[1] of IV sufentanil [28]. Initially the bolus dose is set at 20% of the basal hourly dose. The patient is then evaluated every six hours and bolus doses adjusted until 2-3 boluses per hour provide satisfactory analgesia. Whether given as a PCA or a PCEA we proceed with the expectation that the opioid tolerant patient will require more days of therapy than the opioid naïve patient [29. 30]. In the setting where ketamine or lidocaine was not initiated intraoperatively or was discontinued before recovery, these infusions can still be initiated post-operatively. Ketamine may be started in the post-operative period at 5 mcg.kg-1.min-1 and titrated every 6 hours to analgesia or a maximum of 10 mcg.kg-1.min-1. The limiting factor in the dose can be side effects of diplopia, sedation, dysphoria and dizziness. We have not found a need for routine benzodiazepines. Instead we favor a temporary reduction in the dose until the cognitive side effects have resolved. The lidocaine infusion can be started 2 mg.kg-1.hr-1 without a loading bolus. The patient should be monitored regularly for signs of local anesthetic toxicity. These signs include ringing in the ears (tinnitus), numbness of the lips or tongue, new metallic taste and cardiac dysrhythmias.

Summary

The ideal pain management in the perioperative setting improves the patient experience and enhances their recovery from surgery. Harms are reduced by tailoring the management strategy to include only the necessary and effective treatment modalities. To achieve both simultaneously requires understanding of the anatomy and biochemical basis of pain. Historic practice patterns of opioid monotherapy have given way to protocolized multimodal regimen. Future work is to be done to refine these protocols to the patient and surgery specific level.

References

1 Blalock A. (1952) William Stewart Halsted and His Influence on Surgery. *Proc R Soc Med* **45**(8):555–561.

2 Dominy N. (2009) Evolution of sensory receptor specializations in the glabrous skin. In: Squire L., ed. *Encyclopedia of Neuroscience*, Vol 4. Academic Press, Waltham. pp. 39–42.

3 Christensen AP, Corey DP. (2007) TRP channels in mechanosensation: direct or indirect activation? *Nat Rev Neurosci* **8**(7):510–21.

4 Amaya F, Izumi Y, Matsuda M, Sasaki S. (2013) Tissue injury and related mediators of pain exacerbation. *Curr Neuropharmacol* 11(6):592–7.

5 Bolay H, Moskowitz M. (2002) Mechanisms of pain modulation in chronic syndromes. *Neurology* **59**(5 Suppl 2):S2–7.

6 Graven-Nielsen T, Arendt-Nielsen L. (2002) Peripheral and central sensitization in musculoskeletal pain disorders: an experimental approach. *Curr Rheumatol Rep* **3**(4):313–21.

7 Alvarez, F, Kavookjian AM, Light AR. (1993) Ultrastructural morphology, synaptic relationships, and CGRP immunoreactivity of physiologically identified c-fiber terminals in the monkey spinal cord. *J. Comp. Neurol* **329**(4):472–90.

8 Lever IJ, Bradbury EJ, Cunningham JR *et al.* (2001) Brain-derived neurotrophic factor is released in the dorsal horn by distinctive patterns of afferent fiber stimulation. *J Neurosci* **21**(12):4469–77.

9 Heinke, B, Gingl E, Sandkühler J. (2011) Multiple targets of μ-opioid receptor-mediated presynaptic inhibition at primary afferent Aδ- and C-Fibers. *J Neurosci* **31**(4):1313–22.

10 Lueptow, LM, Fakira AK, Bobeck EN. (2018) The contribution of the descending pain modulatory pathway in opioid tolerance. *Front Neurosci* **12**:886.

11 Lin X, Dhopeshwarkar AS, Huibregtse M, Mackie K, Hohmann AG. (2018) Slowly signaling G protein-based CB2 cannabinoid receptor agonist LY28288360 suppresses neuropathic pain with sustained efficacy and attenuates morphine tolerance and dependence. *Mol Pharmacol* **93**(2):49–62.

12 Joshi GP, Bonnet F, Kehlet H, PROSPECT collaboration. (2013) Evidence-based postoperative pain management after laparoscopic colorectal surgery. *Colorectal Dis* **15**:146–155.

13 Fischer HBJ, Simanski CJP, Sharp C *et al.* (2008) A procedure-specific systematic review and consensus recommendations for postoperative analgesia following total knee arthroplasty. *Anaesthesia* **63**(10):1105–23.

14 Cassuto J, Sinclair R, Bonderovic M. (2006) Anti-inflammatory properties of local anesthetics and their present and potential clinical implications. *Acta Anaesthesiol Scand* **50**(3):265–82.

15 Himmelseher S, Durieux ME. (2005). Ketamine for perioperative pain management. *Anesthesiology* **102**(1):211–20.

16 Chou R, Gordon DB, de Leon-Casasola OA *et al.* (2016) Management of postoperative pain: a clinical practice guideline from the American Pain Society, the American Society of Regional Anesthesia and Pain Medicine, and the American Society of Anesthesiologists' Committee on Regional Anesthesia, Executive Committee, and Administrative Council. [published correction appears in *J Pain* (2016) 17(4):508-10. Dosage error in article text]. *J Pain* **17**(2):131–57.

17 FDA. Extended-release (ER) and long-acting (LA) opioid analgesics Risk Evaluation and Mitigation Strategy (REMS). Updated 06/2015. Available at: www.fda.gov/downloads/drugs/drugsafety/postmarketdrugsafetyinformationforpatientsandproviders/ucm311290.pdf. Accessed April 21, 2021.

18 Hurley RW, Cohen SP, Williams KA, Rowlingson AJ, Wu CL *et al.* (2006) The analgesic effects of perioperative gabapentin on postoperative pain: a meta-analysis. *Reg Anesth Pain Med* **31**(3):237–47.

19 Buvanendran A, Kroin JS, Della Valle CJ, Kari M, Moric M, Tuman KJ. (2010) Perioperative oral pregabalin reduces chronic pain after total knee arthroplasty: a prospective, randomized, controlled trial. *Anesth Analg.* **110**(1):199–207.

20 Derry S, Moore, RA. (2013) Single dose oral celecoxib for acute postoperative pain in adults. *Cochrane Database Syst Rev* **10**:Cd004233.

21 Sinatra RS, Jahr JS, Reynolds LW, Viscusi ER, Groudine SB, Payen-Champenois C. (2005) Efficacy and safety of single and repeated administration of 1 gram intravenous acetaminophen injection (paracetamol) for pain management after major orthopedic surgery. *Anesthesiology* **102**(4):822–31.

22 de Leon-Casasola OA, Lema MJ. (1992) Epidural sufentanil for acute pain control in a patient with extreme opioid dependency. *Anesthesiology* **76**(5):853–6.

23 de Leon-Casasola OA, Lema MJ. (1994) Epidural bupivacaine/sufentanil therapy for postoperative pain control in patients tolerant to opioid and unresponsive to epidural bupivacaine/morphine. *Anesthesiology* **80**(2):303–9.

24 de Leon-Casasola OA, Myers DP, Donaparthi S, Bacon DR, Peppriel J, Rempel J, Lema MJ. (1993) *A comparison of postoperative epidural analgesia between patients with chronic cancer taking high doses of oral opioids versus opioid-naive patients. Anesth Analg* **76**(2):302–7.

25 Wiesenfeld Z, Gustafsson LL. (1982) Continuous intrathecal administration of morphine via an osmotic minipump in the rat. *Brain Res* **247**(1):195–7.

26 Stevens CW, Monashy MS, Yaksh TL. (1988) Spinal infusion of opiate and alpha-2 agonists in rats: tolerance and cross-tolerance studies. J Pharmacol Exp Ther**244(1)**: 63-70.

27 *Principles of Analgesic Use in the Treatment of Acute Pain and Cancer Pain*, 6th edn. American Pain Society, Glenview.

28 de Leon-Casasola O. (2008) Implementing therapy with opioids in patients with cancer. *Oncol Nurs Forum* **35** Suppl:7–12.

29 Kossmann B, Dick W, Bowdler I. (1984) Modern aspects of morphine therapy. In Wilkes E and Napp Laboratories, eds. *Advances in Morphine Therapy: International Congress and Symposium Series/Royal Society of Medicine*, London.

30 Pfeifer B.L, Sernacker HL, Ter Horst U M, Porges SW. (1989) Cross-tolerance between systemic and epidural morphine in cancer patients. *Pain* **39**(2):181–7.

Index

Note: *Italic page numbers* indicate figures, **bold page numbers** indicate tables

Clinical Pain Management: A Practical Guide, Second Edition. Edited by Mary E. Lynch, Kenneth D. Craig, and Philip W. Peng.

D

E

F

Q

R

T